Female Urology

Female Urology

EDITED BY

Elroy D. Kursh, MD

Professor of Urology
Case Western Reserve University School of Medicine
Cleveland, Ohio

Edward J. McGuire, MD

Professor of Urology
University of Texas School of Medicine
Director, Division of Urology
Hermann Hospital
Houston, Texas

WITH 35 CONTRIBUTORS

J. B. LIPPINCOTT COMPANY
Philadelphia

Acquisitions Editor: Mary K. Smith
Assistant Editor: Anne Geyer
Indexer: Lillian R. Rodberg
Cover Designer: Tom Jackson
Production Manager: Janet Greenwood
Production Service: Editorial Services of New England, Inc.
Compositor: Circle Graphics
Printer/Binder: Arcata Graphics-Kingsport

6 5 4 3 2 1

Library of Congress Cataloging-in-Publication Data

Female urology / edited by Elroy D. Kursh and Edward J. McGuire; with 35 contributors.
        p.   cm.
    Includes bibliographical references and index.
    ISBN 0-397-51154-X
    1. Urogynecology. I. Kursh, Elroy D.   II. McGuire, Edward J.
    [DNLM: 1. Genital Diseases, Female.   2. Urologic Diseases.
3. Urinary Incontinence.   WJ 190 F3299 1994]
RG484.F463 1994
616.6--dc20
DNLM/DLC
for Library of Congress   93-5545
                                                                                     CIP

The authors and publisher have exerted every effort to ensure that drug selection and dosage set forth in this text are in accord with current recommendations and practice at the time of publication. However, in view of ongoing research, changes in government regulations, and the constant flow of information relating to drug therapy and drug reactions, the reader is urged to check the package insert for each drug for any change in indications and dosage and for added warnings and precautions. This is particularly important when the recommended agent is a new or infrequently employed drug.

To Dee, Matt, Franci, and Herman,
and in memory of Sara

and

To Paula, Megan, Colleen, and Briget McGuire
and Allison

Contributors

RODNEY A. APPELL, MD

Head, Female Urodynamics Section
Department of Urology
The Cleveland Clinic Foundation
Cleveland, Ohio

JERRY G. BLAIVAS, MD

Clinical Professor
Department of Urology
New York Hospital–Cornell
  Medical Center
New York, New York

MICHAEL B. CHANCELLOR, MD

Assistant Professor
Department of Urology
Jefferson Medical College
  of Thomas Jefferson University
Thomas Jefferson University Hospital
Philadelphia, Pennsylvania

JOHN O. L. DeLANCEY, MD

Associate Professor
Department of Obstetrics and Gynecology
University of Michigan Medical School
Ann Arbor, Michigan

JACK S. ELDER, MD

Professor of Surgery–Urology
Case Western Reserve University School of
  Medicine;
Director, Pediatric Urology
University Hospitals of Cleveland
Cleveland, Ohio

THOMAS E. ELKINS, MD

Professor and Chairman
Department of Obstetrics and Gynecology
Louisiana State University
Baton Rouge, Louisiana

DEBORAH R. ERICKSON, MD

Assistant Professor
Department of Surgery, Division of Urology
Pennsylvania State University School
  of Medicine;
Attending Physician, Division of Urology
Milton S. Hershey Medical Center
Hershey, Pennsylvania

GARY J. FAERBER, MD

Instructor, Section of Urology
Department of Surgery
University of Michigan
Ann Arbor, Michigan

CHRISTOPHER C. FITZPATRICK, MD

Senior Registrar/Assistant Master
Department of Obstetrics and Gynecology
Coombe Lying-in Hospital
Dublin, Ireland

JENELLE FOOTE, MD

Midtown Urology
Atlanta, Georgia

GAMAL M. GHONIEM, MD

Associate Professor of Urology
Tulane University
New Orleans, Louisiana

W. TERRY JONES, MD

Community Hospitals of Indianapolis
Indianapolis, Indiana

ELROY D. KURSH, MD

Professor of Urology
Case Western Reserve University School
  of Medicine
University Hospitals of Cleveland
Cleveland, Ohio

GARY E. LEACH, MD

Associate Clinical Professor of Urology
University of California, Los Angeles School
  of Medicine;
Chairman of Urology
Southern California Permanente Medical
  Group
Los Angeles, Calfornia

NANCY A. LITTLE, MD

Assistant Professor of Urology
University of Texas Health Science Center
San Antonio, Texas

EDWARD J. MCGUIRE, MD

Professor and Director
Division of Urology
University of Texas Medical School
  at Houston;
Director, Division of Urology
Hermann Hospital
Houston, Texas

FRIEDHELM NOLL, MD

Department of Urology
University of Witten-Herdecke
Schwelm, Germany

PAT D. O'DONNELL, MD

Professor of Surgery and Urology
University of Cincinnati School of Medicine
University of Cincinnati Medical Center
Cincinnati, Ohio

C. LOWELL PARSONS, MD

Professor of Urology
University of California, San Diego Medical
  Center
San Diego, California

JOHN F. RANDOLPH, JR., MD

Assistant Professor and Chief
Division of Reproductive Endoscopy
University of Michigan Medical School
Ann Arbor, Michigan

SHLOMO RAZ, MD

Professor of Surgery–Urology
University of California, Los Angeles School
  of Medicine
UCLA Center for Health Sciences
Los Angeles, California

MARTIN I. RESNICK, MD

Lester Perskey Professor and Chairman
Department of Urology
Case Western Reserve University School
    of Medicine
University Hospitals of Cleveland
Cleveland, Ohio

NEIL M. RESNICK, MD

Assistant Professor of Medicine
Harvard Medical School;
Chief of Gerontology
Director of Continence Center
Brigham & Women's Hospital
Boston, Massachusetts

MICHAEL L. RITCHEY, MD

Section of Urology
University of Michigan Medical School
Ann Arbor, Michigan

RICHARD A. SCHMIDT, MD

Professor of Urology
University of Colorado Health Sciences Center
Denver, Colorado

FRIEDHELM SCHREITER

Head, Department of Urology
University of Witten-Herdecke
Schwelm, Germany

STEVEN W. SIEGEL, MD

St. Paul Urologic Surgeons
St. Paul, Minnesota

J. PATRICK SPIRNAK, MD

Associate Professor of Urology
Case Western Reserve University;
Director of Urology
MetroHealth Medical Center
Cleveland, Ohio

ERNEST M. SUSSMAN, MD

Clinical Fellow, Division of Urology
UCLA Center for Health Sciences
Los Angeles, California

PATRICK J. SWEENEY, MD

Department of Urology
Case Western Reserve University School
    of Medicine
Cleveland, Ohio

MARK D. WALTERS, MD

Head of the Section of General Gynecology
Director, Urologic Gynecology
The Cleveland Clinic Foundation
Cleveland, Ohio

JULIAN H. WAN, MD

Section of Urology
University of Michigan Medical School
Ann Arbor, Michigan

ALAN J. WEIN, MD

Professor and Chairman
Division of Urology
University of Pennsylvania School
    of Medicine;
Chief of Urology
Hospital of the University of Pennsylvania
Philadelphia, Pennsylvania

BRIAN H. WINDLE, MD

Assistant Professor of Surgery
Case Western Reserve University School
    of Medicine;
Acting Chief, Division of Plastic and
    Reconstructive Surgery
University Hospitals of Cleveland
Cleveland, Ohio

PHILIPPE E. ZIMMERN, MD

Assistant Associate Clinical Professor
  of Urology
University of California, Los Angeles School
  of Medicine;
Co-Director, Urodynamic Laboratory
Kaiser Sunset Medical Center
Los Angeles, California

Women account for approximately 25 percent of all visits to urologists and, obviously, 100 percent of visits to gynecologists. Urologists entering practice are often surprised by the numbers of women expecting them to provide special care for a variety of nonsurgical and surgical problems. Unfortunately, their residency training often leaves them ill prepared to deal with the types of problems facing them in a routine urological practice. Likewise, gynecologists are often frustrated by their own lack of knowledge regarding a variety of urogynecological problems. It is apparent that in order to better serve female patients, research and education in the field of urogynecology is sorely needed.

Fortunately, the expanding need for development in this field is being addressed by some physicians, and urogynecology is being recognized as an important area of health care delivery. Many of the problems treated in this specialty are unique to women. A successful outcome requires a clear understanding of anatomy, pathology, and physiology of the various diseases and the use of sound medical and surgical principles and judgment.

This new textbook presents a comprehensive, current review of female urology designed to enhance the education of urologists, gynecologists, or any other physicians caring for women. The book is organized differently from similar textbooks in that it presents the material in what we believe is a more logical approach based on our current understanding of the pathophysiology of the various diseases and problems in women. The book is subdivided into eight major areas of female urology; a number of chapters review separate problems under these major headings. The major areas covered are (1) anatomy and physiology, (2) detrusor incontinence, (3) urethral incontinence, (4) management of genital and pelvic prolapse, (5) injuries to the urogenital organs, (6) vesicovaginal fistula, (7) urgency frequency syndromes, and (8) other conditions. An eminent team of contributors has been assembled. The book is well illustrated, particularly the various surgical procedures utilized in this special area of urogynecology. We believe that this textbook will be a valuable addition to your professional library and one that you will refer to often.

E. D. K.
E. J. McG.

Contents

IV. Management of Genital and Pelvic Prolapse

V. Injuries to the Urogenital Organs

VI. Vesicovaginal Fistula

VII. Urgency Frequency Syndromes

VIII. Other Conditions

Female Urology

I

Anatomy
and Physiology

1

Functional Anatomy of the Female Pelvis

John O. L. DeLancey

The pelvic floor is a collection of tissues that span the opening within the bony pelvis. It lies at the bottom of the abdominopelvic cavity and forms a supporting layer for the abdominal and pelvic viscera (Fig. 1-1). The best way to appreciate its structural role is by placing a hand on the pelvic contents through an abdominal incision and pressing in a caudal direction. The muscles, ligaments, viscera, and fasciae that resist this downward force are the pelvic floor. They include all of the structures that lie between the pelvic peritoneum and the vulvar skin. Together they form a multifaceted structural unit. In addition to supporting the abdominal and pelvic organs and maintaining continence of urine and feces, the pelvic floor must also allow for intercourse and parturition as well as for evacuation of excretory products.

There are three supportive layers to the pelvic floor: the endopelvic fascia, levator ani muscles, and the perineal membrane/external anal sphincter. A fourth layer consists of the external genital muscles, but these small muscles are more directly related to sexual function than to support.

The first layer of the pelvic floor is formed by the pelvic viscera and their connections to the pelvic walls by the endopelvic fascia (Fig. 1-2). Neither the fascia alone nor the organs themselves are responsible for the strength of this layer. It is the combination of these two structures that provides support. The next layer is a sheetlike muscular diaphragm (the pelvic diaphragm) that is formed by the levator ani muscles and its superior and inferior fasciae (Fig. 1-3). This layer of muscle spans the opening in the bony pelvis in much the same way that the respiratory diaphragm spans the opening formed by the bottom of the rib cage. Although anatomy textbooks usually show this muscle shaped as a deep bowl, it is a horizontal sheet in the living individual that has an anteriorly placed midline cleft (the urogenital hiatus) through which the urethra, vagina, and rectum pass.

The third layer in the pelvic floor, the perineal membrane (urogenital diaphragm), lies immediately below the levator ani muscles at the level of the hymenal ring (Fig. 1-4). In the male it forms an uninterrupted sheet that spans the anterior triangle of the pelvic outlet in front of the bituberous diameter. In the female, however, it is incomplete, with a large opening provided for the vagina to pass through. Therefore, rather than forming a supportive sheet as it does in the male, the perineal membrane in the female attaches the edges of the vagina to the ischiopubic ramus. It also provides lateral attachments for the perineal body as well as support for the urethra.

In addition to these major supportive layers,

3

Female Urology, edited by Elroy D. Kursh and Edward McGuire. J. B. Lippincott, Philadelphia, © 1994.

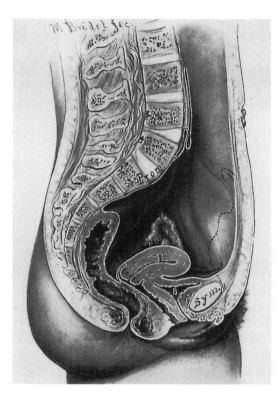

Figure 1-1. The relationship between the pelvic floor and the abdominal cavity. (From Kelly HA. Gynecology. Used with permission of the Department of Art as Applied to Medicine. Johns Hopkins Medical School.)

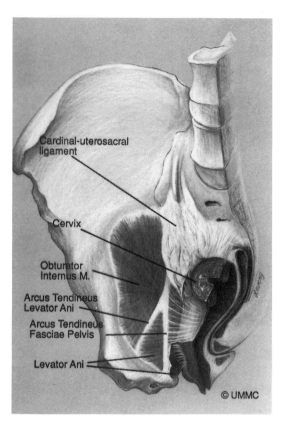

Figure 1-2. Sagittal section of the pelvis showing the connections of the cervix and vagina to the pelvic walls. Fibers going from the vagina to the arcus tendineus fasciae pelvis represent the pubocervical fascia. The corpus of the uterus has been removed, as have the bladder and urethra.

a fourth layer lies below the perineal membrane and consists of the ischiocavernous, bulbocavernosus, and superficial transverse perineal muscles. Although these muscles are frequently mentioned as being important to closure of the introitus, they are too small and weak to provide any substantial support. As previously mentioned, they relate primarily to the vestibular bulb and clitoris and probably have their major function in the sexual response.

Before considering the details of pelvic floor structure, a brief discussion of its function may prove helpful in understanding the more detailed anatomy that follows. The primary support for the pelvic organs comes from the levator ani muscles, which close off the pelvic floor so that

structures lying above them rest on their upper surface. The effectiveness of this closure can be appreciated by recognizing that a small, frictionless, spherical object placed in the upper vagina would remain in place without falling out of the vagina despite a complete lack of attachment to any surrounding structures. In a similar way, the uterus is held in the pelvis by the activity of these muscles, which close the pelvis below this level. The layer of endopelvic fascia and ligaments that attach the uterus and other pelvic organs to the pelvic side walls is important during relaxation of the levator ani muscles but is not under tension

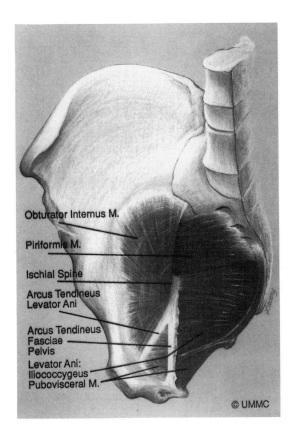

Obturator Internus M.

Piriformis M.

Ischial Spine

Arcus Tendineus
Levator Ani

Arcus Tendineus
Fasciae
Pelvis

Levator Ani:
Iliococcygeus
Pubovisceral M.

© UMMC

Figure 1-3. *Muscles of the levator ani are shown after removal of the pelvic organs. Note the relatively horizontal shelf that they form.*

as long as the muscles function normally and keep the pelvic floor closed.

The ligaments and fasciae are also called on to support the pelvic organs when the levator ani muscles have been damaged. In this situation, the muscles no longer close the pelvic floor, and the organs must depend on their fascial attachments to prevent them from prolapsing. The perineal membrane lies below the levator ani muscles and attaches the lateral vaginal wall to the bony pelvis and also assists in supporting the perineal body. This support is probably not important in the resting state because the perineal body can descend an inch during relaxation of the levator ani muscles. This suggests that the perineal membrane becomes active in sup-

port during relaxation of the levator ani but not when the levators are in their normal state of contraction.

What Is the Pelvic Floor Attached To?

The supportive layers described above fill the cylindrical space that lies within the pelvic bones. They attach to the pelvic side walls and span the intervening area. The term *pelvic side wall* is used to refer to the vertical walls of the pelvis to which the pelvic floor attaches (Fig. 1-5). The structures that form these walls can best be understood by considering the circular space of the pelvis as the face of the clock with 12 o'clock being at the pubic symphysis. The region from 11 o'clock to 1 o'clock is formed by the pubic bones and pubic symphysis. The region from 1 o'clock to 3 o'clock represents the region where the arcus tendineus stretches over the obturator internus muscle, suspended between the pubic bone and the ischial spine. At 3 o'clock, the bony pelvis is exposed in the region of the ischial spine, and from this point to 5 o'clock the piriformis muscle, coccygeus muscle, and sacrospinous ligament occupy the greater sciatic foramen and delimit its lower border. The posterior aspect of the pelvis from 5 o'clock to 7 o'clock is where the sacrum lies. The remainder of the circle is completed symmetrically with its opposite side.

These walls form the point of origin for the pelvic floor, and it is the connection between the pelvic floor and the pelvic walls that provides for the structural support of the abdominopelvic cavity.

What Role Does the Endopelvic Fascia Play in Supporting the Pelvic Viscera?

As previously mentioned, the first layer of the pelvic floor is formed by the endopelvic fascia and the pelvic organs it connects to the pelvic walls. The endopelvic fascia is a fibromuscular tissue that consists of collagen, elastin, and

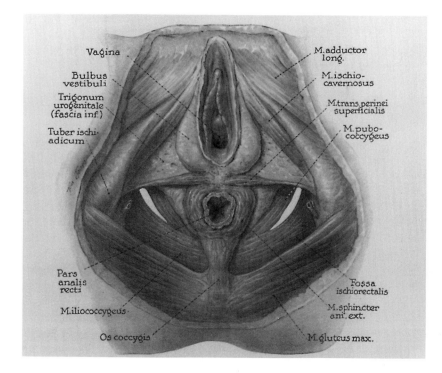

Figure 1-4. *Urogenital diaphragm (trigonum urogenitale) as seen from below. (From Anson BJ. Human Anatomy. Philadelphia, WB Saunders, 1950:361.)*

smooth muscle. Its structure varies considerably in different areas of the pelvis. The cardinal ligaments, for example, are primarily perivascular connective tissue, whereas the rectal pillars have fewer blood vessels and more fibrous tissue. These visceral ligaments and fasciae serve to attach the pelvic organs laterally to the pelvic side walls, and the combination of viscera and their connections forms a supportive layer (Fig. 1-6). As previously mentioned, this can be appreciated by pushing downward on the pelvic contents through an abdominal incision and feeling the ligaments and fascia come tight as downward force is applied.

The upper vagina, cervix, and uterus are attached by a broad sheet of endopelvic fascia to the pelvic side walls. This sheet is usually referred to as the cardinal uterosacral ligament complex. It originates over the region of the greater sciatic foramen and lateral sacrum to insert into the side of the cervix as well as the upper one third of the vagina. Although the cardinal and uterosacral ligaments are given separate names, they are a single unit, with the uterosacral ligaments being the visible medial margin of this continuous body of tissue. In this region, the endopelvic fascia consists of perivascular collagen and elastin but also contains a considerable amount of nonvascular smooth muscle as well as autonomic nerves to the uterus and bladder.[1,2] These ligaments are usually thought of as running transversely from the pelvic wall to the vagina and cervix. Actually they are vertical in orientation, so they suspend the organs from above. To appreciate their functional characteristics, it is necessary to think about their orientation in the standing individual rather than in the supine woman usually observed

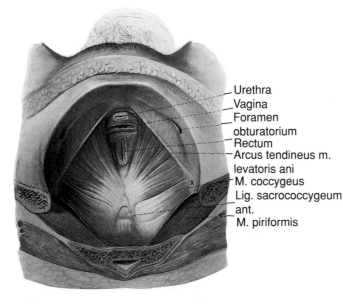

Urethra
Vagina
Foramen
obturatorium
Rectum
Arcus tendineus m.
levatoris ani
M. coccygeus
Lig. sacrococcygeum
ant.
M. piriformis

Figure 1-5. *Pelvic walls and levator ani muscles (shown but not labeled). Ischial spine (X). (From H. Peham and J Amreich. Operative Gynecology. Vol. 1. Philadelphia, J.B. Lippincott, 1934:178.)*

in the operating or examining room. Their vertical orientation is obviously better suited to suspending these organs than a transverse orientation, as has sometimes been suggested.

Below the level of the uterus, the endopelvic fascia continues to attach the upper one third of vagina to the pelvic walls in the same way that the cardinal and uterosacral ligaments provide attachment for the uterine cervix[3] (Fig. 1-7). The middle one third of the vagina is attached laterally to the pelvic walls more directly by the pubocervical and rectovaginal fasciae. These are downward continuations of the cardinal and uterosacral ligaments. They attach the lateral margin of the vagina on each side to the pelvic side wall. These lateral attachments of the vagina stretch it from one side of the pelvis to the other so that its anterior wall forms a horizontal sheet on which the bladder can rest. Posteriorly the attachment of the vagina to the pelvic side wall forms a similar sheet that prevents the rectum from prolapsing forward and represents the rec-

tovaginal fascia. Although these fasciae (pubocervical and rectovaginal) are sometimes considered to be separate sheets in themselves, they are only a combination of the vaginal wall and its attachment to the pelvic side wall.

In the past, these ligaments and fasciae have been considered to be the most important elements of pelvic support. Biomechanical considerations, however, would suggest that fibrous tissue is poorly suited to maintain the kind of constant load that intra-abdominal pressure and gravity place on them. The persistent misconception that fibrous ligaments are the primary supports of the pelvis comes from the fact that these are the tissues used in operations that repair defective support. Because these procedures are generally successful, this type of empiric surgery is effective, yet this should not create the impression that these tissues are normally the ones that hold the uterus, cervix, and vagina in place. The muscular tissues of the levator ani are much better suited to supporting this constant load. They

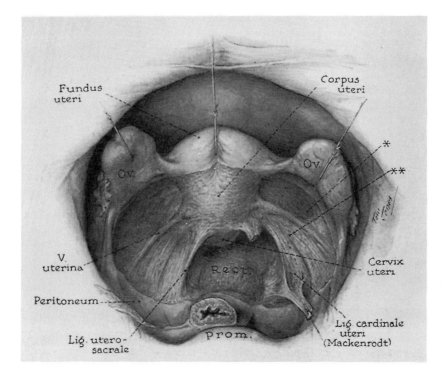

Figure 1-6. *Uterus and supportive ligaments. *Clear space in broad ligament; **cardinal-uterosacral ligament complex. (From Anson BJ. Human Anatomy. Philadelphia, WB Saunders, 1950:371.)*

can constantly renew themselves and do not have the kind of elongation and breakage that connective tissue has under tension.

Levator Ani Muscles

Few clinicians have seen the levator ani muscles in their entirety, and most find them difficult to comprehend. The problem involved in understanding their form and function has been recognized and is aptly stated by Dickinson, who observed that: "There is no muscle in the body whose form and function is more difficult to understand than the levator ani."[4] Many of these misconceptions about these muscles come from the fact that their shape is greatly distorted by the embalming process. As a result, most of the illustrations in anatomic textbooks bear little

resemblance to what clinicians encounter in the examining room.[5]

The levator ani muscle has two different parts (Fig. 1-8). The first is a thick, U-shaped band of muscle that arises from the pubic bones. It attaches to the lateral walls of the vagina and rectum as well as sending fibers behind the rectum as a sling that pulls the rectum toward the pubic bones. This part of the muscle is often called the pubococcygeus but is referred to herein as the pubovisceral muscle, as is described later.[6,7] The second component is the iliococcygeus, which is a thin sheet of muscle that arises from the pelvic side wall on either side and inserts into a midline raphe behind the rectum.

There are several aspects of the pubovisceral muscle's structure that are important to pelvic floor function. Although this is a single continuous body of muscle, it has several portions.

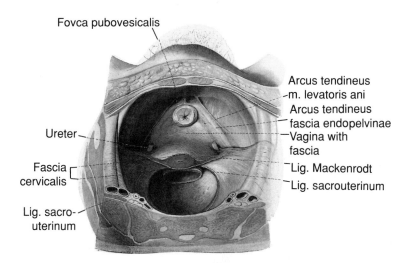

Fovca pubovesicalis

Arcus tendineus
m. levatoris ani
Arcus tendineus
fascia endopelvinae
Vagina with
fascia
Lig. Mackenrodt
Lig. sacrouterinum

Ureter

Fascia cervicalis

Lig. sacro-
uterinum

Figure 1-7. Upper layer of support showing the cervix after the uterine corpus has been removed as well as the vagina and their lateral attachments to the pelvic walls.

There are fibers that originate in the pubic bone and attach to the vagina. These are called the pubovaginalis. Other fibers go to the anus and rectum and are called the puboanalis and puborectalis. Some of these latter fibers also form the thick band that passes behind the rectum and forms a sling that pulls the rectum forward toward the pubic bone. There are a few fibers in this area that also go back to attach to the coccyx, and this portion has been called the pubococcygeus. The overall term *pubovisceral muscle* more correctly represents the multifaceted nature of this sling of tissue than the term *pubococcygeus*, which implausibly calls attention to the unimportant attachment of two relatively immovable structures, the pubes and coccyx. The pubovisceral muscle has considerable bulk and can be palpated during pelvic examination as a distinct ridge just above the hymenal ring along each lateral wall of the pelvis. The function of this muscle is to pull the rectum, vagina, and urethra anteriorly toward the pubic bones and to compress their lumens closed.

The iliococcygeus muscle arises from the arcus tendineus levator ani, which is a fibrous band that is suspended between the pubic bone and the ischial spine. It is a thin, membranous sheet whose muscle fibers join in the midline as a median raphe behind the rectum. It forms a horizontal sheet that helps to support the pelvic viscera and also has some function in pulling these organs anteriorly toward the pubic bones. The posterior margin of the muscle lies at the sacrospinous ligament, where it fuses with the fibers of the coccygeal muscle. This latter muscle goes from the sacrum to the ischial spine and represents a developmental vestige of the tail-wagging muscle of lower quadrupeds. It is undergoing degeneration, and because it attaches to immovable structures, it has no function. It is sometimes considered part of the pelvic diaphragm. It is not a part of the levator ani muscles because it cannot elevate the anus.

As is true of the striated muscle of the external anal sphincter, the levator ani muscles exhibit constant activity.[8] In addition, they may be contracted to increase the closure of the pelvic floor during increases in abdominal pressure. The constant activity of this muscle is poorly understood but is critical to pelvic support. It is a separate phenomenon from voluntary contraction because many individuals in whom these

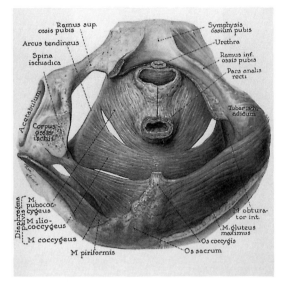

Figure 1-8. Levator ani muscles as seen from below. (From Anson BJ: Human Anatomy. Philadelphia, WB Saunders, 1950:366.)

muscles are flaccid at rest can still forcefully contract them voluntarily. Because the levator ani muscles maintain closure of the pelvic floor, the viscera that lie above them can rest on this muscular shelf. The constant modulation of muscular activity maintains closure under many different circumstances and keeps the ligaments from becoming stretched. This muscular support is a critical factor in pelvic support because fibrous tissues, when subjected to constant tension, elongate.

Perineal Membrane

The perineal membrane (urogenital diaphragm) is a fibrous layer that spans the anterior triangle of the pelvic outlet (see Fig. 1-4). It attaches laterally to the ischiopubic ramus approximately 1 to 2 cm above its lower (caudal) margin. Medially it fuses with the side walls of the vagina and perineal body. Previous descriptions have often shown two layers of fascia with a layer of muscle in between (the deep transverse perineal muscle).

This erroneous concept of the urogenital diaphragm has been corrected by Oelrich, whose description of the striated urogenital sphincter muscle and the perineal membrane is discussed later in this chapter.[9] The perineal membrane has some smooth muscle and a few striated muscle fibers associated with it that do fit the term *deep transverse perineal muscle*, but there is no superior fascia of the diaphragm as had previously been supposed.

The anterior portion of the perineal membrane is intimately connected with the distal portion of the urethra and with the urethral musculature. The structural features of this region are described later in a consideration of the anatomy of urinary continence.

Perineal Body

The mass of fibrous tissue that lies between the vagina and the anus is called the perineal body. It is an ill-defined mass of dense connective tissue that does not have distinct borders. Its connective tissue is fused anteriorly with the vaginal wall. Laterally it receives fibers from the bulbocavernosus and superficial transverse perineal muscles as well as the perineal membrane. A significant portion of what is clinically identified as the perineal body is occupied by the external anal sphincter, and it is the anococcygeal raphe that connects the external anal sphincter to the coccyx, which forms the dorsal attachment of the perineal membrane. Downward descent of the perineal body is limited by these connections, especially the connections to the ischiopubic rami.

When the perineal body is incised or torn apart during the process of vaginal birth and not reapproximated, the supportive effect of the posterior portions of the perineal membranes is weakened. It is through the interconnections of these two sides in the perineal body that support of the perineal body is maintained. This is not the only support of the pelvic outlet because the levator ani muscle provides a strong upward traction on this area, but normal continuity of the perineal membrane through the perineal body also assists in supporting the outlet. The attachments of the bulbocavernosus and superficial transverse perineal muscles into the perineal body are probably less important than the levator ani muscle because of the relatively small bulk of muscle that the former muscles represent.

Continence Anatomy

The portion of the pelvic floor that influences the bladder and urethra has special importance to urinary incontinence and receives separate consideration here.

URINARY BLADDER

The urinary bladder has sometimes been described as having several distinct layers to its muscular wall. In the dome of the bladder, this is not the case. Here there is a generally amorphous and interlacing network of muscle fibers. There are occasional areas where these muscle fibers are parallel to one another, but there is no particular layered arrangement that has any functional importance.

In contrast, the base of the bladder contains a much thicker and more organized musculature than does the dome. There is a distinct loop of fibers that passes from the dorsal lateral aspect of the bladder in front of the vesical neck to return to the posterior aspect of the bladder on the contralateral side. This U-shaped band of muscle fibers is referred to as the detrusor loop, and its functional significance is not entirely known. Between the detrusor loop and the lumen of the lower urinary tract, there is a specialized area of smooth muscle known as the urinary trigone that extends posteriorly from the internal urinary meatus to end at the ureteral orifices. The smooth muscle in this area is continuous with the musculature of the ureters, and some fibers pass into the urethra. The trigonal musculature has a circular extension that surrounds the internal urinary meatus for the first

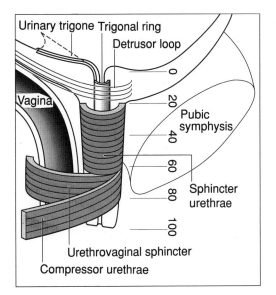

Figure 1-9. *Location of various structures along the urethra. (Copyright University of Michigan, 1989.)*

0.5 to 1 cm of the urethral lumen's length (Fig. 1-9). This circular group of fibers has been referred to as the trigonal ring.[10]

From the internal to the external urinary meatus, the structures that surround the urethral lumen vary[11] (see Fig. 1-9). The region where the bladder and urethra join is known as the vesical neck. This is the part of the lower urinary tract where the urethral lumen is surrounded by detrusor and trigonal musculature. The striated muscle of the urethra has not yet begun in this area, and so it is entirely influenced by the autonomic nervous system. Alpha-adenergic blockade causes this area of the urethra to dilate, and when this occurs, stress urinary incontinence can be present despite normal urethral support. Whether the alpha-adenergic innervation goes to the detrusor loop or the trigonal musculature is not completely established. The bladder neck smooth muscle has special functional significance because it is the area surrounded by this tissue that is open in patients who have type III urinary incontinence.

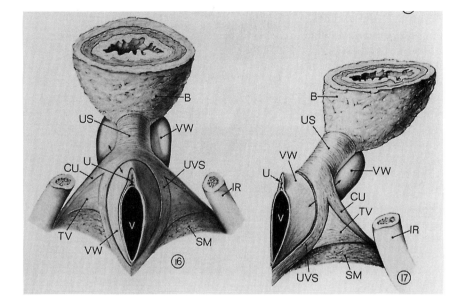

Figure 1-10. *Striated urogenital sphincter muscle seen from below after removal of the perineal membrane and pubic bones. US, Urethral sphincter; UVS, urethrovaginal sphincter; CU, compressor urethrae; B, bladder; IR, ischiopubic ramus; TV, transverse vaginae muscle; SM, smooth muscle; U, urethra; V, vagina; VW, vaginal wall. (From Oelrich TM: Anat Rec 1983;205:223, with permission of Alan R. Liss.)*

URETHRA

The urethra extends from the outer surface of the bladder to the external urinary meatus. There is a considerable quantity of longitudinally oriented smooth muscle that lies immediately below the mucosa in this area from the level of the bladder down to the external urinary meatus. This layer becomes less and less prominent as one approaches the external meatus.

Outside of the longitudinal smooth muscle is a layer of circular smooth muscle. This layer is extremely thin and poorly developed in the woman and often difficult to identify, even under histologic examination. Outside the circular smooth muscle layer is the prominent striated urogenital sphincter muscle or rhabdosphincter[9] (Fig. 1-10). This muscle is a single body of striated muscle that has two different portions that are continuous with one another. It is made up primarily of muscle fibers suited to maintaining constant tone.[12] The upper portion is circularly oriented and forms the sphincter urethrae. This is what has been traditionally referred to as the rhabdosphincter. The second portion lies at the distal end of the striated urogenital sphincter muscle and is not circular in orientation but consists of two bands of fibers that arch over the ventral surface of the urethra with the concave portion of the arch pointing dorsally. One band of these fibers originates in the perineal membrane and is called the compressor urethra, whereas the other encircles the wall of the vagina and is referred to as the urethrovaginal sphincter muscle. These are the muscles that were previously referred to by the somewhat confusing term deep transverse perineal muscle. The urethral sphincter extends from approximately 20% to 60% of total urethral length, where 0 is the internal meatus and 100 is the external meatus. The compressor urethrae and urethral vaginal sphincter are found in the distal-most portion of the urethra from 60% to 80% of total urethra length.[11]

This striated urogenital sphincter is not capable of keeping an individual continent during times of increases in intraabdominal pressure. In individuals with myelodysplasia, in whom this sphincter is intact, stress urinary incontinence occurs if the internal sphincter is not normally innervated and the vesical neck is open. The striated urogenital sphincter is probably a backup mechanism that comes into play when the detrusor muscle contracts inappropriately or when there is sufficient increase in abdominal pressure to force urine past the internal urinary meatus. When excised during radical vulvectomy, it may convert someone who has marginal continence to total incontinence by removing this backup sphincteric mechanism.[13]

The support and position of the urethra are critically important to stress urinary incontinence. Although there have been many different theories that have attempted to explain stress urinary incontinence based on angles, ligaments, or sphincters, none of these theories provides a satisfactory explanation for all observations concerning stress urinary incontinence. Despite this imperfect understanding, few would argue with the observation that poor urethral support is somehow associated with this condition. It seems to be the support of the proximal urethra that is specifically the factor associated with loss of continence during increases in intraabdominal pressure.

Previous studies have suggested that the proximal urethra is attached to the pubic bone by ligamentous structures called the posterior pubourethral ligaments. This arrangement, whereby the urethra is attached to the pubic bones by ligamentous bands, is not plausible because fluoroscopic examination shows that an individual can move the proximal urethra backward and forward by contraction and relaxation of the levator ani muscle.[14] Also, the position of the proximal urethra is above the insertion of the

supposed *pubourethral ligaments* into the pubic bones so that the structural arrangement would not allow the ligaments to elevate the vesical neck.[15]

The support of the proximal urethra is perhaps best described by Bonney in 1922 and illustrated in his paper on urinary incontinence in which he demonstrated the way in which the pubocervical fascia lies underneath the proximal area of the vesical neck and is attached to the pubic bones anteriorly through the arcus tendinous fascia pelvis. To understand the anatomy of urethral support, a brief review of the space of Retzius anatomy is appropriate.

When the bladder is pulled backward away from the inner surface of the pubic bones to expose the vesical neck, a white band of tissue is visible on either side that goes from the inner surface of the lower portions of the pubic bones back to the ischial spine (Fig. 1-11). This is the arcus tendineus fasciae pelvis. It lies on the medial surface of the levator ani muscles near the pubic bones. A second tendinous arch (the arcus tendineus levator ani), which serves as the origin of the iliococcygeus muscle, begins near the top of the pubic rami and passes diagonally down toward the ischial spine to fuse with the arcus tendineus fascia pelvis approximately 3 to 4 cm anterior to the ischial spine. Therefore, these two tendinous arches are fused in their more dorsal portions. In this region near the ischial spine, these two tendinous arches lie on the inner surface of the obturator internus muscle. Spanning the space between the fascial arch on the left and right is a sheet of fibromuscular tissue on which the base of the bladder rests. This is the pubocervical fascia, and its attachments laterally are to the arcus tendineus fasciae pelvis. The upper portion of this area is continuous with the suspensory ligaments of the uterus (the cardinal and uterosacral ligaments).

The tissues that provide urethral support have two lateral attachments: a fascial attachment and a muscular attachment[16] (Fig. 1-12). The fascial attachment of the urethral supports connects the periurethral tissues and anterior vaginal wall to the arcus tendineus fasciae pelvis

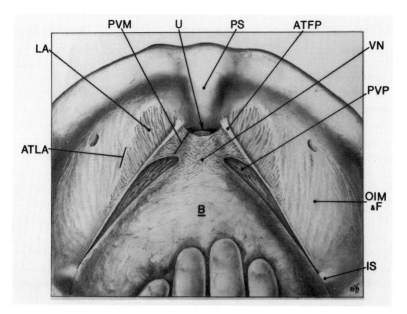

Figure 1-11. *Space of Retzius (drawn from cadaver dissection).*
Pubovesical muscle (PVM) *can be seen going from vesical neck* (VN) *to*
arcus tendineus fasciae pelvis (ATFP) *and running over the paraurethral*
vascular plexus (PVP). ATLA, *Arcus tendineus levator ani;* B, *bladder;*
IS, *ischial spine;* LA, *levator ani muscles;* OIM&F, *obturator internus*
muscle and fascia; PS, *pubic symphysis;* U, *urethra. (From DeLancey*
JOL: Neurol Urodyn 1989;8:53, with permission of Alan R. Liss.)

and are called the paravaginal fascial attachments.[17] The muscular attachment connects
these same periurethral tissues to the medial
border of the levator ani muscle.[18] These attachments allow the continuous activity of the levator ani muscle, along with the fascial attachments, to maintain the position of the vesical
neck. Separation of the endopelvic fascia from
the arcus tendineus fasciae pelvis is an anatomic
factor responsible for stress incontinence in
many (but not all) women[17] and has been demonstrated using magnetic resonance imaging.

The way in which these structures influence
urinary continence is poorly understood. The
current concept of pressure transmission is based
on the observations that intraurethral pressure
rises simultaneously with intraabdominal pressure during a cough.[19] The supposition that this
occurs because a portion of the urethra lies

within the abdomen is not based on any direct
anatomic observation and is anatomically im-
plausible. The urethra lies immediately adjacent
to and fuses with the vagina throughout its
course, and there is no specific layer that the
urethra perforates that would separate the intra-
abdominal urethra from an extraabdominal region. The interplay between the endopelvic
fascia and the urethra is almost certainly responsible for these increases in intraurethral pressure
that have been observed, but further study is
necessary to illuminate the anatomic factors responsible for this phenomenon. The height of the
urethra relative to some reference plane that supposedly divides the intraabdominal space and
the extraabdominal space can be discarded as an
explanation because many patients who have a
significant cystourethrocele have a urethra that
lies entirely outside the body and yet have per-

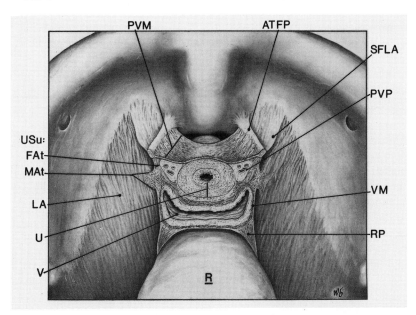

Figure 1-12. *Cross section of the urethra (U), vagina (V), arcus tendineus fasciae pelvis (ATFP), and superior fascia of levator ani (SFLA) just below the vesical neck (drawn from cadaver dissection). Pubovesical muscles (PVM) lie anterior to urethra and anterior and superior to paraurethral vascular plexus (PVP). The urethral supports (USu) (the pubourethral ligaments) attach the vagina and vaginal surface of the urethra to the levator ani muscles (MAt, muscular attachment) and to the superior fascia of the levator ani (FAt, fascial attachment). R, Rectum; RP, rectal pillar; VM, vaginal wall muscularis. (From DeLancey JOL: Neurol Urodyn 1989;8:53, with permission of Alan R. Liss.)*

fectly good stress continence. In contrast, there are a number of individuals whose urethra has been returned to a normal position and who persist in having stress incontinence despite this normal support.

Summary

There are a series of factors that are important to support of the female pelvic organs. The levator ani muscles in the normal individual close the pelvic floor and are responsible for the primary support in the nulliparous individual. Damage to these muscles or deterioration with aging allows the pelvic floor to open somewhat. In this instance, the fibrous tissues of the pelvis (endopelvic fascia) must suspend the vagina and uterus and provide support for the urinary tract and rectum. Secondary failure of these ligaments gives rise to the various types of genital prolapse. Failure of the cardinal uterosacral ligament complex is manifested as uterine prolapse when the uterus is present or vaginal prolapse after the uterus has been removed. Failure of the pubocervical fascia is associated with a cystourethrocele, and failure of the rectovaginal fascia is associated with a rectocele. Isolated damage to the perineal body and external genital muscle can give rise to some gaping of the introitus but is not specifically associated with genital prolapse unless other damage is also present.

The specific nature of urethrovesical support depends on the attachment of the pubocervical fascia to the arcus tendineus on either side. This support is intimately intertwined with the connection of the endopelvic fascia in this area to the levator ani muscles, which allows the position of the urethra to be influenced by contraction and relaxation of these muscles.

Our current treatments of genital prolapse and urinary incontinence are primarily empiric. Although we are currently quite successful in alleviating stress urinary incontinence and most obvious genital prolapse, we frequently fail to restore normal urinary function or coital function. As we begin to understand the physiology of the pelvic floor better, we will be able to target our therapy more specifically to the individual defects that are present.

References

1. Range RL, Woodburne RT. The gross and microscopic anatomy of the transverse cervical ligaments. Am J Obstet Gynecol 1964;90:460.
2. Campbell RM. The anatomy and histology of the sacrouterine ligaments. Am J Obstet Gynecol 1950;59:1.
3. DeLancey JOL. Anatomic causes of vaginal prolapse after hysterectomy. Am J Obstet Gynecol 1992;166:1717.
4. Dickinson RL. Studies of the levator ani muscle. Am J Dis Wom 1889;22:897.
5. Richter K. Lebendige anatomie der vagina. Geburtshilfe Frauenheilkd 1966;26:1213.
6. Lawson JO. Pelvic anatomy. I. Pelvic floor muscles. Ann R Coll Surg Engl 1974;54:244.
7. Lawson JO. Pelvic anatomy. II. Anal canal and associated sphincters. Ann R Coll Surg Engl 1974;54:288.
8. Parks AG, Porter NH, Melzak J. Experimental study of the reflex mechanism controlling muscles of the pelvic floor. Dis Colon Rectum 1962;5:407.
9. Oelrich TM. The striated urogenital sphincter muscle in the female. Anat Rec 1983;205:223.
10. Huisman AB. Aspects on the anatomy of the female urethra with special relation to urinary continence. Contrib Gynecol Obstet 1983;10:1.
11. DeLancey JOL. Correlative study of paraurethral anatomy. Obstet Gynecol 1986;68:91.
12. Gosling JA, Dixon JS, Critchley HOD, Thompson SA. A comparative study of the human external sphincter and periurethral levator ani muscles. Br J Urol 1981;53:35.
13. Reid GC, DeLancey JOL, Hopkins MP, Roberts JA, Morley GW. Urinary incontinence following radical vulvectomy. Obstet Gynecol 1990;75:852.
14. Muellner SR. Physiology of micturition. J Urol 1951;65:805.
15. Noll LE, Hutch JA. The SCIPP line—an aid in interpreting the voiding lateral cystourethrogram. Obstet Gynecol 1969;33:680.
16. DeLancey JOL. The pubovesical ligament, a separate structure from the urethral supports ("pubourethral ligaments"). Neurol Urodynam. 1989;8:53.
17. Richardson AC, Edmonds PB, Williams NL. Treatment of stress urinary incontinence due to paravaginal fascial defect. Obstet Gynecol 1981;57:357.
18. DeLancey JOL. Structural aspects of the extrinsic continence mechanism. Obstet Gynecol 1988;72:296.
19. Enhorning G. Simultaneous recording of the intravesical and intra-urethral pressures. Acta Obstet Gynecol Obstet (Suppl) 1961;276:1.

2

Congenital Abnormalities

Patrick J. Sweeney

Jack S. Elder

The urinary and genital systems in the female are closely interrelated not only in regard to their anatomic location, but also their embryologic origin. Each system may be adversely affected by common misadventures in its development, and genitourinary anomalies are one of the most common congenital defects in the human. This chapter reviews normal and abnormal development of the urogenital system in the female.

Normal Development of the Urogenital Tract

The urinary and genital systems develop from the intermediate mesoderm, located along the length of the developing embryo in humans. The intermediate mesoderm migrates ventrally to form paired urogenital ridges. Each urogenital ridge subsequently differentiates into two distinct regions: the nephrogenic cord and the gonadal ridge, which develop into the urinary and genital systems.[1,2]

DEVELOPMENT OF THE FETAL KIDNEY

Each nephrogenic cord gives rise to three successive excretory units: the pronephros, the mesonephros, and the metanephros or definitive kidney[3] (Fig. 2-1). The pronephros forms as a transitory nonfunctional structure in the cephalic region of the nephrogenic cord during the fourth week of development. The pronephric duct develops in a craniocaudal direction, reaching the dorsolateral portion of the cloaca by the fifth week of development. By this time, the pronephros has degenerated and been replaced by the mesonephros, which forms in the thoracolumbar portion of the nephrogenic ridge. S-shaped tubules of the mesonephros communicate and empty into the degenerating cranial portion of the pronephric duct, which is now termed the mesonephric duct. The prominent tissue of the mesonephros and the medially developing gonads form the paired urogenital ridges. The mesonephros forms progressively in a cranial to caudal direction during the second month, with the cranial portion regressing before completion of the caudal mesonephros. The mesonephric tubules subsequently empty into the mesonephric duct and continue to regress until the end of the second month. A few of these caudalmost tubules remain as vestigial structures, the epoophoron and the paraoophoron.[4]

The mesonephric, or wolffian duct, reaches the cloaca by the fifth week of development, and the ureteral bud develops as a diverticulum near the caudal end of the mesonephric duct. The

Female Urology, edited by Elroy D. Kursh and Edward McGuire. J. B. Lippincott, Philadelphia, © 1994.

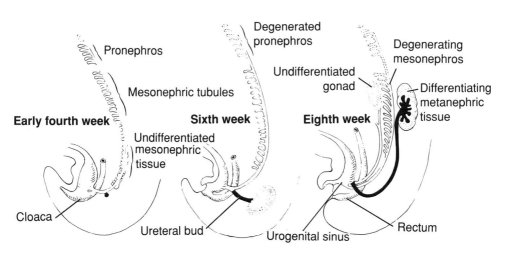

Figure 2-1. *Schematic representation of the development of the nephric system. Only a few of the tubules of the pronephros are present early in the fourth week, while the meso-nephric tissue differentiates into mesonephric tubules that progressively join the meso-nephric duct. The first sign of the ureteral bud from the mesonephric duct is seen at this time. At 6 weeks, the pronephros has completely degenerated. The ureteral bud grows dorsocranially and meets the metanephric blastema. At 8 weeks, there is cranial migration of the differentiating metanephros. (From Tanagho EA, McAninch JW (eds): Smith's General Urology, 13th ed. Norwalk, Appleton & Lange, 1992.)*

ureteral bud grows in a dorsocranial direction to reach the metanephric blastema, the most caudal region of the nephrogenic ridge. The ureteral bud undergoes a series of branchings and becomes the collecting system, including the ureter, renal pelvis, calyces, and collecting tubules, and the metanephric blastema becomes the renal parenchyma.

DEVELOPMENT OF THE CLOACA AND UROGENITAL SINUS

The terminal portion of the hindgut forms the cloaca (Fig. 2-2). Its termination at the ventral caudal portion of the embryo, the cloacal membrane, is a region where ectoderm and endoderm lie in apposition without intervening mesoderm. Subsequent growth of mesenchyme lateral to the cloacal membrane results in tissue elevations known as the labioscrotal swellings. Similar growth of mesodermal tissue cranial to the cloa-

cal membrane results in formation of the genital tubercle, or the precursor of the phallus.[5] The cloaca receives the allantois cranioventrally and the mesonephric ducts laterally. It gradually undergoes division by the urorectal septum, which forms as a coronal wedge of tissue growing caudad between the allantois and the hindgut. The urorectal septum then fuses with the cloaca during the sixth week, forming a ventral urogenital membrane and a dorsal anal membrane. During the sixth week the urogenital membrane disintegrates, opening the urogenital sinus into the amniotic cavity. The region of the urogenital sinus cranial to the entrance of the mesonephric ducts is referred to as the vesicourethral canal, and caudal to their insertion is the definitive urogenital sinus.[3] The allantoic portion of the vesicourethral canal subsequently becomes obliterated, forming a connective tissue band referred to as the urachus or the medial umbilical ligament. The bladder forms as the cranial portion

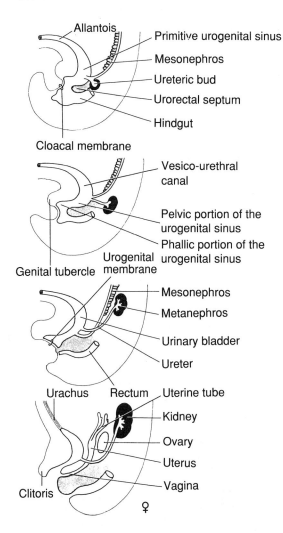

Figure 2-2. *Diagrams showing division of the cloaca into the urogenital sinus and the rectum; absorption of the mesonephric ducts; development of the urinary bladder, urethra, and urachus; and changes in the location of the ureter. (From Moore KL: The Developing Human. Philadelphia, WB Saunders, 1973.)*

of the remaining vesicourethral canal, with the terminal region of the mesonephric duct becoming absorbed into the dorsal caudal wall as the ureteral orifice and trigone. The remainder of the mesonephric duct migrates caudally and medially, joining the urogenital sinus with the fused paramesonephric (or müllerian) ducts to form

the müllerian (Müller's) tubercle (Fig. 2-3). The caudalmost region of the vesicourethral canal forms the female urethra. Outbuddings of the most cranial portion of the urethra form the paraurethral (or Skene's) glands in females, whereas homologous buds in the male lead to formation of the prostate.[4] The urethral orifice opens caudal to the genital tubercle in the vestibule, as does the caudal true urogenital sinus, which forms the distal fifth of the vagina. The labial swellings grow posterior and lateral to the vestibule to form the posterior commissure and the labia majora. Urethral folds develop into the labia minora. Bartholin's glands (homologous to Cowper's glands in the male) grow into the labia majora as invaginations of the vestibular endoderm.

DEVELOPMENT OF THE GENITAL SYSTEM

Although genetic sex is determined at fertilization, early development of the genital system proceeds identically in both sexes until the seventh or eighth week. The paramesonephric, or müllerian duct, develops as an evagination of the coelomic epithelium just lateral to the mesonephros at the sixth week. Caudal to the mesonephros, the bilateral müllerian ducts grow caudomedially to pass ventral to their closely associated mesonephric duct and fuse. The fused terminal portion meets the urogenital sinus as a swelling between the entrance of the mesonephric ducts known as the müllerian tubercle.[3] The association between the paramesonephric and the mesonephric duct is so close that müllerian duct development cannot proceed in the absence of the mesonephric (wolffian) duct.[7]

Meanwhile at about the fourth week, the multipotential primordial germ cells migrate from the yolk sac to the gonadal ridges medial to the nephrogenic ridge. These cells enter the mesenchyme of the gonadal ridge and are incorporated into the primary sex cords by the sixth week.[1] The indifferent stage of the developing genital system is thus completed.

Phenotypic differentiation proceeds according to a series of complex steps dependent on the

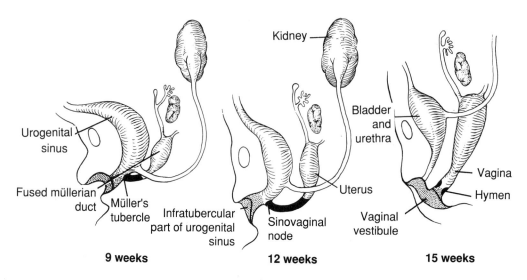

Figure 2-3. *Differentiation of the urogenital sinus and the müllerian ducts. At 9 weeks, the urogenital sinus receives the fused müllerian ducts at Müller's tubercle (sinovaginal node), which is solidly packed with cells. As the urogenital sinus distal to Müller's tubercle becomes wider and more shallow (15 weeks), the urethra and fused müllerian ducts develop separate openings. The distal part of the urogenital sinus forms the vaginal vestibule and the lower third of the vagina (shaded area), and the portion above Müller's tubercle forms the urinary bladder and entire female urethra. The hymen is formed at the junction of the sinovaginal node in the urogenital sinus. (From Tanagho EA, McAninch JW (eds): Smith's General Urology, 13th ed. Norwalk, Appleton & Lange, 1992.)*

presence or absence of the testis-organizing factor, the H-Y antigen.[1] During the seventh week, in the presence of the H-Y antigen, local secretion of testosterone leads to differentiation of the testis, penis, and scrotum, whereas local secretion of müllerian-inhibiting factor leads to regression of the müllerian ducts and persistence of the male ductal system. Ovarian development begins between the 8th and 10th weeks, and the primordial germ cells undergo repeated mitotic divisions from the 8th through the 20th week of gestation. In the absence of testosterone, the mesonephric ducts regress, and the müllerian ducts develop into the fallopian tubes, uterus, and upper two thirds of the vagina (Table 2-1).

The sinovaginal bulb forms as a solid mass of cells between the caudal aspect of the fused müllerian ducts and the dorsal wall of the urogenital sinus. These cells proliferate to produce a vaginal plate, which elongates to increase the distance between the uterus and the urogenital sinus (Fig. 2-4). At 11 weeks, the inner cells of the vaginal plate begin to degenerate caudally, forming the vaginal lumen.[1] A thin membrane, the hymen, remains fused until late in fetal life, separating the vaginal plate from the urogenital sinus.[8] The upper two thirds of the vagina is of müllerian duct origin, and the lower one third is derived from the urogenital sinus.

From the 9th through the 12th weeks of gestation, differentiation of the external genitalia in the female and male diverges. In the female, the genital tubercle bends ventrally, the lateral portions of the genital swellings enlarge to form the labia majora, the urethral folds persist as the labia minora, and the posterior aspect of the genital swellings fuse in the midline to form the posterior fourchette (Fig. 2-5).

Table 2-1. *Female and Male Homologous Structures*

EMBRYONIC STRUCTURE	FEMALE	MALE
Mesonephric duct	Duct of epoophoron	Epididymis
	Gartner's duct	Vas deferens and seminal vesicles
		Ejaculatory ducts
	Vesicular appendage	Appendix epididymidis
	Ureter, renal pelvis	Ureter, renal pelvis
	Trigonal structure	Trigonal structure
Müllerian duct	Uterine tubes	Appendix testis
	Uterus	Prostatic utricle
	Vagina (upper ⁴/₅)	
Müller's tubercle	Site of hymen	Verumontanum
Sinovaginal bulb from urogenital sinus	Lower ¹/₃ of vagina	Part of prostatic utricle
Junction of sinovaginal bulb and urogenital sinus	Hymen	Disappears normally (remnants probably from posterior urethral valves)
Urogenital sinus		
Ventral and pelvic part	Urinary bladder (except the trigone)	Urinary bladder (except the trigone)
	Entire urethra	Supramontanal part of prostatic urethra
Phallic or urethral portion	Vaginal vestibule	Inframontanal part of prostatic urethra
		Membranous urethra
Genital tubercle	Clitoris	Penis
Urethral folds	Labia minora	Penile urethra
Genital swelling	Labia majora	Scrotum
Gubernaculum	Ligament of ovary	Gubernaculum
	Round ligament of uterus	
Genital glands	Ovary	Testis

Cloacal and Urogenital Sinus Abnormalities

Defects in partitioning of the cloaca result not only in visceral malformations, but also in defects of the perineal musculature and genitalia. The defects may include cloacal malformations or urogenital sinus abnormalities, which occur only in boys, or exstrophic abnormalities (cloacal exstrophy, bladder exstrophy, epispadias).[9] These disorders often require a multidisciplinary approach with various pediatric surgical subspecialists to minimize mortality, preserve renal function, provide urinary and fecal continence, and maximize quality of life.

Failure of the urorectal septum to divide the cloaca in the sixth week of gestation leads to a *cloacal malformation*, in which there is a common canal into which the bladder, uterus, and rectum empty. The Latin word *cloaca* means sewer. The variety of configurations or varying depths of cloaca and urethrovaginal canal probably reflect variations in arrest of development of the urorectal septum.[10] The cloacal malformation is associated with a high incidence of urologic defects, including vesicoureteral reflux, ureterocele, ectopic ureter, renal agenesis, and urethralization of the female phallus (Fig. 2-6A), as well as vaginal and uterine septation with hydrocolpos.[11-13] Similarly, there may be associated anomalies of the upper gastrointestinal tract, the cardiovascular system, and the spinal cord or spine.[9] The diagnosis is generally confirmed shortly after birth, although extensive diagnostic evaluation may be necessary to delineate the true extent of the malformation, which may be initially misdiagnosed in 50% of patients.[14] Physical examination reveals absence of

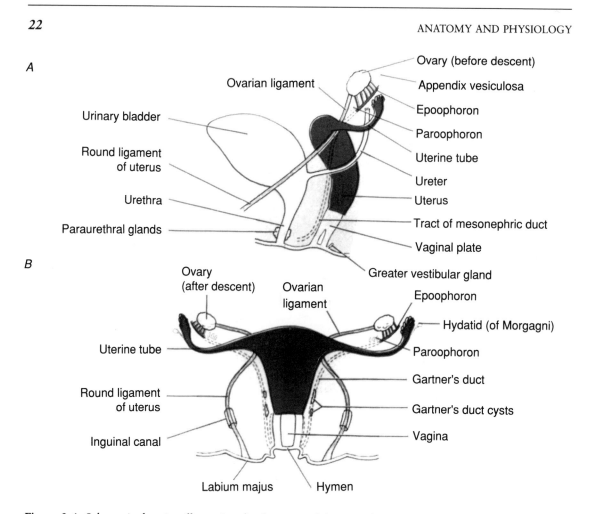

Figure 2-4. *Schematic drawing illustrating development of the reproductive system in 12-week fetus (A) and a female newborn (B). (From Moore KL: The Developing Human. Philadelphia, WB Saunders, 1973.)*

the rectum with a common cloacal opening. Anatomic variability is delineated by a series of tests, which may include a cloacagram (contrast radiograph of the cloacal sinus), voiding cystourethrogram, intravenous pyelogram, abdominal ultrasound or computed tomography (CT) scan, and endoscopy of the cloacal tract. The gastrointestinal tract usually is diverted surgically with a colostomy early in life, whereas definitive repair of the defect is undertaken when the patient is several years old. In some cases, the bladder empties into the vagina, which fills with urine and causes extrinsic compression of the lower urinary tract. Management in such newborns includes intermittent catheterization of the vagina. The posterior sagittal approach to these malformations has resulted in improved continence without permanent intestinal and urinary diversion.[11,15]

If the urorectal septum forms normally but there is abnormal differentiation of the vesicourethral canal from the true urogenital sinus (which normally constitutes the distalmost portion of the vagina), a common drainage outlet of the uterovaginal secretions and urine is formed, termed a *urogenital sinus abnormality*. This con-

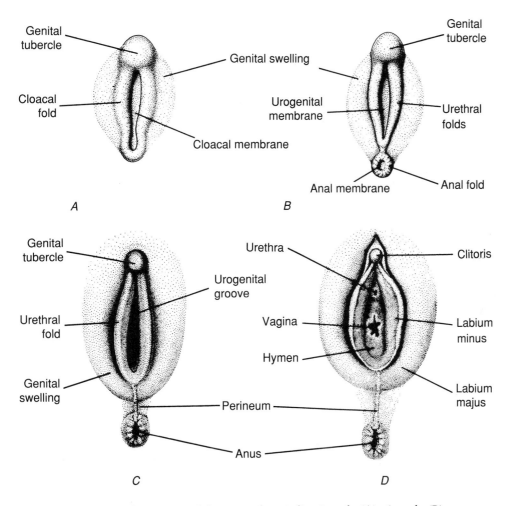

Figure 2-5. *The indifferent state of the external genitalia: 4 weeks (A), 6 weeks (B). Development of the external genitalia in the female: 5 months (C), newborn (D). (From Langman J: Medical Embryology, 3rd ed. Baltimore, Williams & Wilkins, 1975.)*

dition may be associated with other abnormalities of the urinary tract, such as absence or duplication of the ureters, renal agenesis, or renal ectopia. It may also be the result of female pseudohermaphroditism due to congenital adrenal hyperplasia.[9]

Exstrophy, as proposed by Marshall and Muecke, is a condition that results from an abnormally enlarged or persistent cloacal membrane with associated defects in the lower abdominal wall and genitalia.[16] It can be classified as either cloacal or bladder exstrophy, the latter occurring when the urorectal septum has fully formed before rupture of the cloacal membrane. An epispadias defect with bifid clitoris is almost always associated with exstrophy but may occur alone if the perforation occurs later (and therefore distally) in vesicourethral development (Fig. 2-6B). The upper urinary and genital tracts are usually normal, with anomalies such as phallic, urethral, and müllerian duplication most commonly occurring with cloacal exstrophy.[17] There-

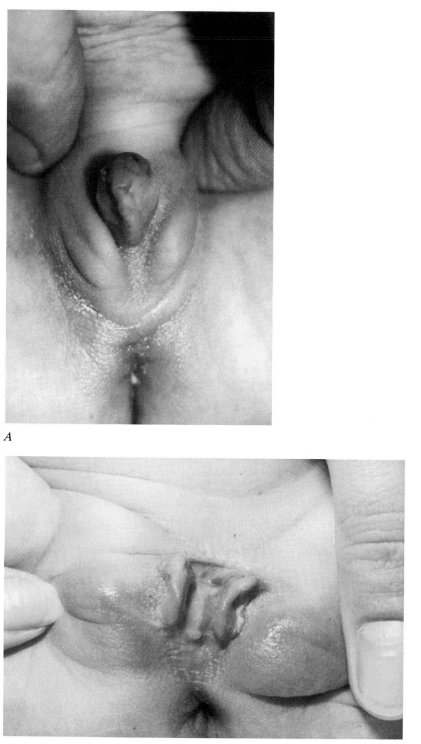

A

B

Figure 2-6. (A) *Female with prune belly syndrome and phallic urethra.* (B) *Female with epispadias without exstrophy.*

fore, these patients may have a normal reproductive potential, although their offspring have a 1 in 70 chance of sharing their condition.[18] The exstrophy complex is generally repaired by multiple staged procedures, including primary vesical and lower abdominal wall closure (preferably within the first 72 hours after birth) with delayed reconstruction of the bladder neck, urethra, and bifid clitoris. Epispadias in the female may go unrecognized until a lack of continence is noted and the bifid clitoris is verified; definitive repair may then be undertaken.[9]

Urethral Anomalies

Congenital anomalies of the urethra are rare in females. Hypospadias may occur but is generally asymptomatic, with only occasional note of a double voiding pattern. The urethra is a common site of ectopic ureteral orifices, which generally occur in the posterior midline (Fig. 2-7).

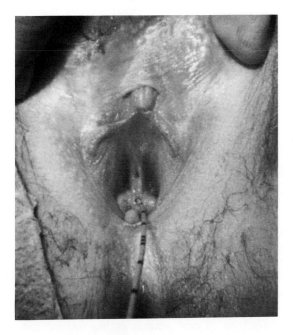

Figure 2-7. Female with ectopic ureter draining into urethrovaginal septum.

Urethral diverticula are usually an acquired phenomenon, occurring most commonly with local abscess formation in Skene's glands. They may also occur congenitally in association with blind-ending ureters.[19] Urethral valves, more common in males, occur rarely in females as well.[20]

Much has been written about congenital distal urethral stenosis, and the subject remains controversial. This term is used to define a fibrous ring causing narrowing of the distal urethra, possibly leading to recurrent urinary tract infections or a dysfunctional interrupted voiding pattern in young girls.[21] The ring is not present at birth but generally appears in all girls in the first few months of life. It later disappears at puberty.[22] Many have bladder instability documented by cystometrogram, and a *spinning-top urethra* with dilation from the bladder neck to the ring may be demonstrable by voiding cystourethrography[23] (Fig. 2-8). Urethral calibration may be similar to normal controls.[24] Treatment in the past has consisted of urethral dilation with sounds, although more conservative treatment with anticholinergics and suppressive antibiotics is generally favored at this time.

Uterovaginal (Müllerian) Abnormalities

Uterovaginal anomalies result from alterations in the formation and fusion of the ductal septum between the fused müllerian ducts and have an incidence of 1 : 250 to 1 : 1000. These abnormalities may be classified into disorders of medial fusion, vertical fusion, or in failure of development, also known as aplasia.[10] Uterovaginal anomalies frequently are present in girls with anorectal or cloacal anomalies. For example, in girls with imperforate anus, 35% have an internal genital abnormality, most commonly bicornuate uterus or uterus didelphys, whereas 70% of girls with a uterovaginal malformation are reported to have a cloacal or anorectal anomaly.[26, 27] In addition, as many as 55% to 70% of females with unilateral renal agenesis have associated internal genital

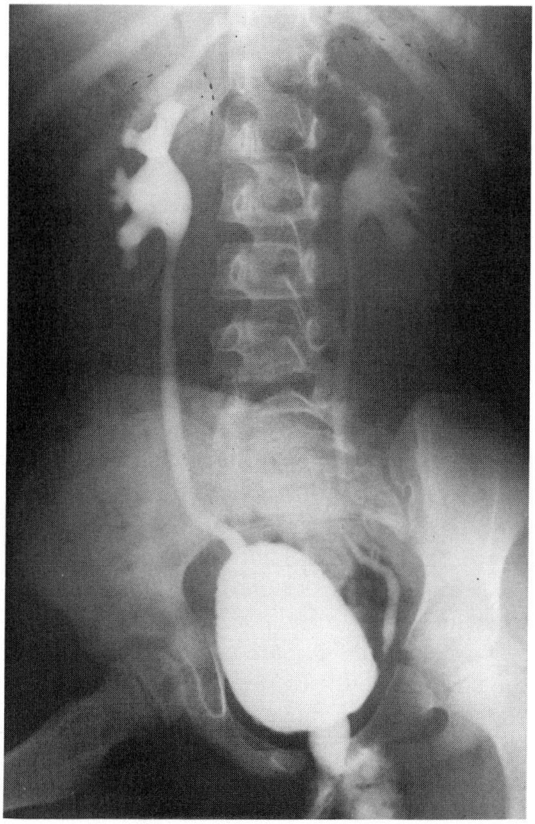

Figure 2-8. Voiding cystourethrogram demonstrating spinning-top urethra and bilateral vesicoureteral reflux.

anomalies.[28] Incomplete müllerian fusion occurs in association with multisystem anomalies in numerous genetic disorders, including the autosomal dominant hand-foot-genital syndrome, the autosomal recessive McKusick-Kaufman (hydrometrocolpos-polydactyly) syndrome, the MURCS association (müllerian duct aplasia, renal aplasia, and cervicothoracic somite dysplasia), the Mayer-Rokitansky-Küster-Hauser syndrome (vaginal agenesis), and the Beckwith-Wiedemann syndrome (macroglossia, omphalocele, macrostomia, and bicornuate uterus).[29–31]

DISORDERS OF MEDIAL FUSION

Complete or partial failure of the müllerian ducts to fuse medially results in a variety of duplication anomalies of the uterovaginal tract (Fig. 2-9). Complete failure of medial fusion results in uterus didelphys with vaginal duplication. More commonly, partial fusion of müllerian structures occurs, resulting in complete or partial bicornuate uterus, complete or partial septate uterus, or an arcuate uterus. These conditions usually are associated with persistence of the longitudinal septum through the vagina to a varying degree. If no obstructive component exists, these malformations often are not diagnosed until later in life, when the woman is evaluated for infertility or dyspareunia. These patients generally are able to become pregnant but may have repeated spontaneous miscarriages or obstetric malpresentation at the time of delivery.[32] Treatment consists of partial or total resection of the vaginal septum and wedge metroplasty of the uterine septum, if indicated.[33]

Obstruction of a uterine-hemivagina complex may occur in cases of uterine didelphys with double vagina (Fig. 2-10). Although rare, this condition is almost always associated with ipsilateral renal agenesis.[34–36] The condition results from incomplete ipsilateral mesonephric duct formation, resulting in abnormal müllerian duct development with resultant noncommunion of the vagina with the urogenital sinus.[37] This condition may present as an abdominal mass secondary to hydrocolpos in the newborn[35,38] but more commonly presents at menarche with the development of hydrohematocolpos and an "extrinsic" vaginal mass associated with cyclic abdominal pain. Careful physical and radiologic evaluation of the genitourinary tract is necessary and may include vaginoscopy, intravenous pyelography, abdominopelvic ultrasound, and CT scan.[27] Treatment may vary from vaginal excision of the septum to removal of the uterovaginal segment if it is only rudimentary or infected.[39] Pregnancy in noncommunicating rudimentary bicornuate uterine horns has been reported and may result in sudden life-threatening hemor-

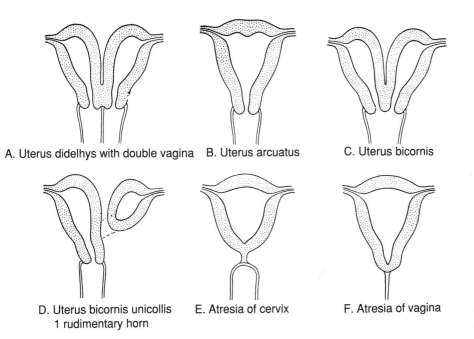

A. Uterus didelhys with double vagina   B. Uterus arcuatus   C. Uterus bicornis

D. Uterus bicornis unicollis
1 rudimentary horn   E. Atresia of cervix   F. Atresia of vagina

Figure 2-9. (A–F) *Schematic representation of the main abnormalities of the uterus and vagina caused by persistence of the uterine septum or obliteration of the lumen of the uterine canal. (From Langman J: Medical Embryology, 3rd ed. Baltimore, Williams & Wilkins, 1975.)*

rhage.[25] Cerclage may be indicated in women with a patent hemiuterus who are diagnosed as having this disorder at the time of pregnancy because there is a high rate of spontaneous abortion.[39]

DISORDERS OF VERTICAL FUSION

Abnormal caudal development of the müllerian duct or abnormal canalization of the vaginal plate results in vertical fusion anomalies, characterized by a blind-ending vagina with varying degrees of septation. In the most severe cases, there is nearly complete absence of the vagina with a thick plate of mesodermal-based tissue separating the vaginal space (derived from the distal urogenital sinus) from a normal uterus. In less severe cases, there is a thin partial or complete transverse vaginal septum. Overall these abnormalities occur in approximately 1 in 80,000

females. The position of the septum is variable and is generally classified as being high, mid, or low vaginal, with estimated incidences of 46%, 35%, and 19%.[40] Upper transverse vaginal septae are often incomplete, whereas they are usually obstructive in the lower third of the vagina.[41]

The diagnosis of complete transverse vaginal septum often is made in childhood following the development of hydrocolpos, which presents as a midline abdominal mass on physical examination (Fig. 2-11). Ultrasound demonstrates a large midline sonolucent mass with debris and may show hydronephrosis if there is extrinsic ureteral compression. Further enlargement of the mass can result in lower extremity lymphedema owing to compromised venous return.[34] If the diagnosis is delayed until puberty, cyclic abdominal pain with lack of menstrual flow and an enlarging lower abdominal mass secondary to hydrometrocolpos result.

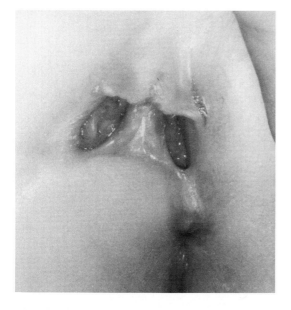

Figure 2-10. Infant with vaginal duplication.

The surgical treatment of this condition depends on patient age as well as the position and thickness of the intervening septum and varies from simple excision of the septum to a pull-through vaginoplasty[41,42] (Fig. 2-12).

Hydrocolpos may also be diagnosed in the neonate with imperforate hymen. These patients usually present with a bulging cystic interlabial mass or may have a palpable abdominal mass. An ultrasound should be performed to verify the diagnosis as well as to rule out the presence of hydronephrosis due to mass effect, although usually these patients have no other associated congenital defects. These patients may also present at puberty, with an estimated incidence of 1 in 2000 women.[43] Definitive treatment is generally achieved by the creation of a cruciate hymenotomy, with oversewing of the wound edges with absorbable sutures and placement of a small drain to prevent wound adhesion. Fertility is usually identical to that of the normal population once the defect is repaired.[44]

DISORDERS OF DEVELOPMENT (APLASIA)

Vaginal agenesis is the second most common cause of primary infertility in women (after gonadal dysgenesis), occurring in 1 in 4000 to 5000 females.[41] Although this condition usually results from aplasia of the müllerian ducts, it may also result from vaginal atresia or failure of canalization of the vaginal plate.[29] Typically the ovaries and fallopian tubes are normal, but the uterus is rudimentary. When there is bilateral uterine obstruction owing to müllerian aplasia, the incidence of urinary tract anomalies is low. The Mayer-Rokitansky-Küster-Hauser syndrome usually refers to patients with vaginal agenesis, although it has been proposed that the syndrome refer to the entire spectrum of müllerian anomalies in females with normal endocrine status and without associated anorectal or cloacal malformations.[31] This broad classification results in the inclusion of disorders of both vertical and medial fusion and is therefore associated with up to a 40% incidence of renal anomalies, including renal agenesis, renal ectopy, horseshoe kidney, and duplex ureteral systems.[29,31,45] Skeletal anomalies occur in approximately 10% of these patients as well.[46,47]

Girls with vaginal agenesis are phenotypically normal females at birth, with a blind-ending introitus that may go unnoticed. Diagnosis is confirmed by bimanual physical examination and abdominal ultrasound when the patient presents for evaluation of amenorrhea. Vaginal agenesis may be distinguished from a transverse vaginal septum or an imperforate hymen by the absence of a normal uterus and the presence of a normal hypothalamic-pituitary-ovarian endocrine axis. Treatment consists of creation of a neovagina through the use of skin grafts, soft tissue flaps, or bowel segments and generally is performed late in the teenage years.[33,42,47–52]

Mesonephric (Wolffian) Duct Remnants

The wolffian duct frequently persists to varying degrees in girls. The vestigial remnant of this

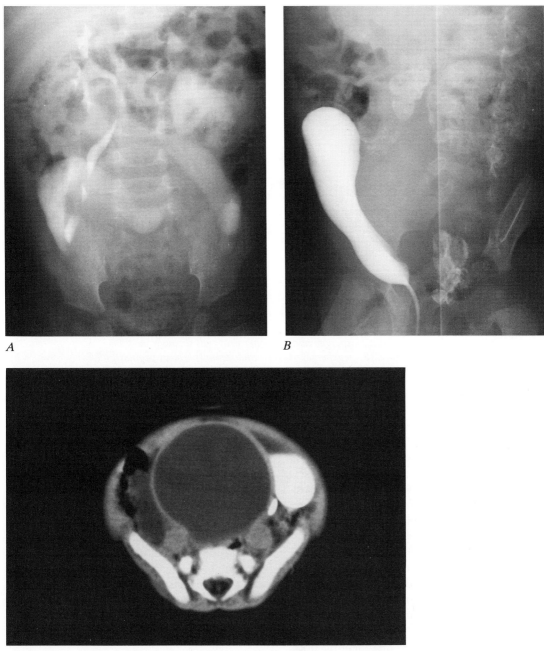

Figure 2-11. (A) *Intravenous pyelogram showing left hydroureteronephrosis and bilateral ureteral deviation. Arrow points to displaced bladder.* (B) *Voiding cystourethrogram in same patient demonstrating displacement of the bladder without reflux.* (C) *CT scan, same infant, with hydrocolpos secondary to transverse vaginal septum.*

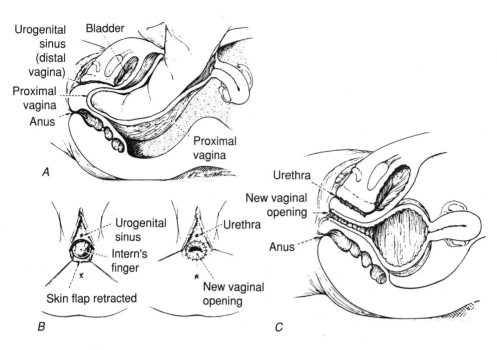

Figure 2-12. (A–C) *Ramenofsky-Raffensperger abdominoperineal pull-through vaginoplasty. (From Ramenofsky ML, Raffensperger JG: An abdominal-perineal-vaginal pull-through: A definitive treatment of hydrometrocolpos. J Pediatr Surg 6:381, 1971.)*

ductal system may occur in infants as a thin cuboidally lined nonsecretory system parallel to the fallopian tube in the broad ligament. Tubules in the lateral portion of the broad ligament are referred to as the epoophoron, and those more medially are known as the paraoophoron. Benign cysts occasionally arise from these structures but usually are of little clinical significance. Cystic structures at the level of the fallopian os, referred to as hydatids of Morgagni, are thought to be terminal remnants of the müllerian duct and on rare occasion become evident by undergoing torsion.[53]

Caudally the regressing mesonephric duct lies within the muscular wall of the cervix and vagina. Cystic lesions of varying size may form in these sites in up to 1% of women and are referred to as Gartner's duct cysts[54] (see Fig. 2-4). These cysts typically are asymptomatic and benign, although they may cause symptoms such as dys-

pareunia or irritative voiding symptoms owing to mass effect. Rarely they have been found to communicate with the ureter and an ipsilateral dysplastic kidney, representing a variant of an ectopic ureter.[55,56] These cysts may be distinguished from other cystic lesions of the pelvis by abdominal or transvaginal ultrasound as well as coronal magnetic resonance imaging.[54] If troublesome, they may be managed by simple incision and drainage, although occasionally marsupialization or complete excision of these lesions is necessary.

Abnormalities of the Introitus

Physical examination of the newborn and young female external genitalia can be difficult but is increasingly important because of the increase in requests for genital examinations in girls who may have been sexually abused.[57–62] Abnormal findings vary from benign congenital or acquired disorders to malignant or traumatic changes.

A normal physical examination of the introitus of a newborn or young girl reveals paired labia majora of variable prominence relating to the stage of maturity. Ventrally a single hooded clitoris is present in the midline. The labia minora, less prominent than the majora, are paired as well and fuse in the dorsal midline to form a thin membranous connection with the vulva known as the posterior fourchette. An avascular flat midline streak between the posterior fourchette and hymen, referred to as the linea vestibularis, is present in 25% to 85% of neonates.[58,59] The urethral meatus lies in the ventral midline midway between the clitoris and hymen. The hymen, which embryologically represents the termination of the müllerian duct, has a variable appearance in normal girls.[59–62] Various morphologic shapes such as annular, fimbriated, punctate, septate, cribriform, dentate, crescentic, and tulip-shaped hymens have been described, with the annular type appearing most commonly.[59] Ventral hymenal clefts are present in 35% of normal neonates.[59]

In a study of sexually abused and nonabused young girls, it appeared that clefts dorsal to the 3 to 9 o'clock position were present only in the abused group. Similarly, a hymenal opening of greater than 5 mm is uncommon in the nonabused population. Overall the hymen seems to be thicker and more elastic than previously regarded and may not show evidence of trauma in young girls with known sexual penetration. Abnormal features noted more frequently, but not exclusive to, the sexually abused group include labial erythema, vascularity or friability, labial adhesions or scars, an attenuated hymen, and intravaginal synechiae.[60,61]

Abnormalities of the Vulva

Clitoromegaly and virilization of the labioscrotal folds are categorized as disorders of intersex. The most common cause of ambiguous genitalia

in the newborn is congenital adrenal hyperplasia (CAH), most commonly secondary to an autosomal recessive 21-hydroxylase deficiency in a 46,XX female (Fig. 2-13). Other common causes include mixed gonadal dysgenesis, male pseudohermaphroditism (46,XY male with incomplete virilization), and true hermaphroditism. Girls with CAH may have a relatively normal appearing male phallus, but because the ovaries remain intra-abdominal, the "scrotum" (fused labioscrotal folds) is empty. In less severe cases, there may be clitoromegaly without fusion of the labioscrotal folds. Prompt recognition and evaluation of genital ambiguity are crucial because many neonates with CAH experience potentially life-threatening salt-wasting during the first few weeks. A complete diagnostic evaluation should include physical examination, serum karyotype, analysis of serum and urinary electrolytes and steroid levels, and genitography performed by the pediatric urologist or pediatric general surgeon. Gender assignment in the neonate with ambiguous genitalia depends on the specific disorder and the potential for phallic growth. Girls with CAH are always reared as females and undergo feminizing genitoplasty when their endocrine status is stable. A discussion of the surgical correction of intersex disorders is beyond the scope of this chapter, although several reviews are available.[63–68]

Fusion of the posterior portion of the labia without clitoral hypertrophy in patients without maternal or congenital androgenic influence is uncommon but may result in some families as an autosomal dominant disorder with incomplete penetrance. Evaluation proceeds identically to that of the intersex disorders, and the condition is corrected surgically by vulvovaginoplasty.[69]

A labial adhesion is an acquired disorder in which the labia minora are exposed to an inflammatory process and become adherent in the midline, resulting in a thin line of adherence from the clitoris to the posterior fourchette (Fig. 2-14). The average age at presentation is 2.5 years; 90% of girls are younger than 6 years of age. Most patients are symptomatic, with a urinary tract infection or incontinence occurring when

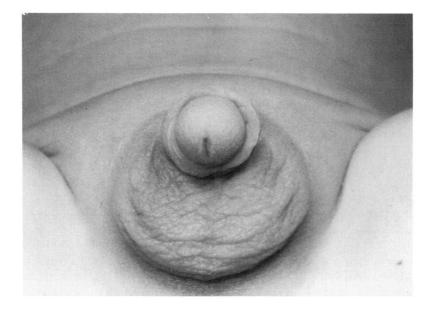

Figure 2-13. Newborn female with adrenogenital syndrome. Labioscrotal folds (scrotum) are empty.

the child stands after voiding, resulting from vaginal voiding.[69,70] Labial adhesions initially may be managed by applying estrogen cream to the vulva three times daily for 10 days but usually is ineffective. Most girls undergo formal lysis of the adhesion as an office procedure. Application of estrogen cream for 1 week following lysis of the adhesion allows recornification of the raw labial surface and prevents recurrent adhesions from forming.

Labial ectopy is a rare condition analogous to the ectopic scrotum and has been associated with ipsilateral renal agenesis.[71]

A strawberry hemangioma is an uncommon lesion in infancy that has a strong predilection for the anogenital region in females. This lesion represents a proliferation of immature capillary vessels. A hemangioma typically is obvious at birth and may undergo rapid growth in the first 6 months of life. These lesions usually are self-limited, however, often undergoing spontaneous involution by 7 years of age.[72] Ulceration and bleeding often can be controlled by conservative

measures, although argon-laser treatment under local anesthesia is helpful for problematic lesions.[73]

Although clitoral hypertrophy in the newborn can result from excessive androgen exposure in the prenatal or postnatal period, it must be distinguished clinically from a normal but prominent clitoris. Clitoral size usually stabilizes at 27 weeks' gestation, remaining essentially unchanged until the first birthday. At times, however, the clitoris may appear abnormally enlarged in the premature child[74] (Fig. 2-15). Infants with a clitoral breadth less than 6 mm or a clitoral index less than 10 mm are normal, whereas those with higher values should undergo evaluation for intersex disorders.[75] Clitoral enlargement also may occur in girls with severe chronic vulvovaginitis[76] or neurofibromatosis.[77]

Duplication of the clitoris occurs primarily in girls with an exstrophic anomaly, as previously discussed. In a girl with a normal abdominal wall, it may be the only visible feature on physical examination indicative of complete epi-

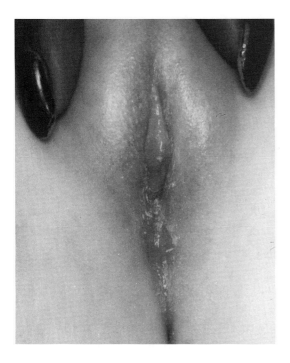

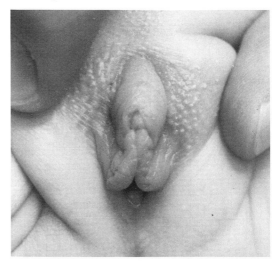

Figure 2-15. Clitoral hypertrophy in premature infant with gonad in left labium majorum, karyotype 46,XX. Labial mass was normal ovary with inguinal hernia.

Figure 2-14. Labial adhesion.

spadias. These girls have total urinary incontinence. Surgical correction consists of clitoroplasty in conjunction with bladder neck reconstruction.

The detection of an interlabial mass in an infant often is of tremendous concern to the child's family and referring physician. Careful evaluation and knowledge of the causes of interlabial masses, however, generally allow one to make the diagnosis promptly.[78]

In the newborn, a paraurethral cyst results from retained secretions in Skene's glands, secondary to ductal obstruction (Fig. 2-16A). The cyst displaces the meatus in an eccentric manner. Urethral obstruction and infection of the cyst, however, are rare. Most of these cysts regress in size during the first 4 to 8 weeks of life, although occasionally it is necessary to incise them.

Urethral prolapse has an appearance of erythematous, inflamed protruding mucosa surrounding the urethral meatus (Fig. 2-16B). It occurs almost exclusively in black girls between 1 and 9 years of age with an average age of 4

years. The most common signs are bloody spotting on the underwear or diaper, although dysuria or perineal discomfort also may occur. For obvious reasons, sexual abuse is suspected in many of these cases until the diagnosis of urethral prolapse is made. There is no known relationship between external genital trauma and urethral prolapse. Initial treatment is the application of estrogen cream three times daily to the prolapsed urethra for 2 to 3 weeks and Sitz baths. If these measures do not cause resolution of the inflammatory process, typically the child continues to exhibit bloody spotting, and formal excision is recommended.[79,80]

A prolapsed ureterocele may present as a cystic mass protruding from the urethral meatus and occurs in approximately 10% of young girls with a ureterocele (see Fig. 2-16C). When the ureterocele is prolapsed, the child typically is extremely irritable. Although the urethra is difficult to identify, the hymen and vagina generally can be determined to be in a normal position. Nearly all of these are associated with a nonfunctioning upper pole segment. Evaluation includes

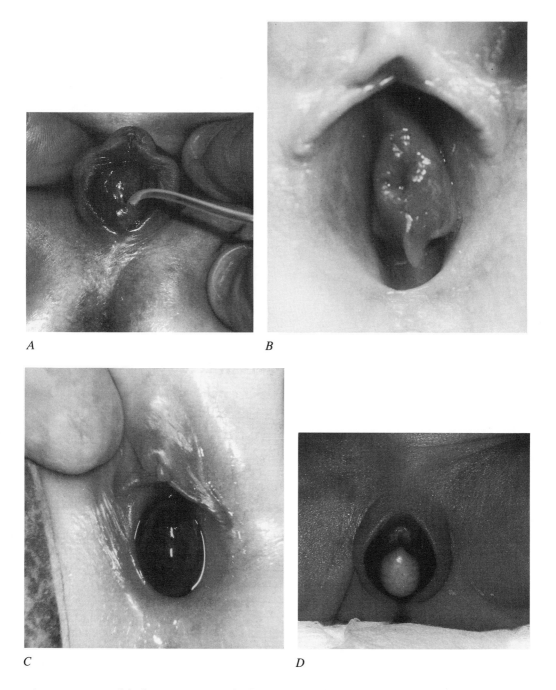

Figure 2-16. *Interlabial masses: Paraurethral cyst (A), urethral prolapse (B), prolapsed ectopic ureterocele (C). Intravenous pyelogram demonstrated obstructed upper pole of right kidney. (D) Imperforate hymen with hydrocolpos.*

renal ultrasound to identify a dilated upper pole segment as well as the ureterocele in the base of the bladder. These children should also undergo a voiding cystourethrogram and a renal functional study such as an intravenous pyelogram or renal scan. Upper pole heminephrectomy and removal of as much ureter as possible through a flank incision or dorsal lumbotomy allow decompression of the ureterocele.[81]

Sarcoma botyroides (rhabdomyosarcoma) is another cause of interlabial mass. The lesion may be visible as a firm grapelike mass protruding from the vagina and may be detected by palpating a vaginal mass on bimanual examination. The diagnosis and histologic type (usually embryonal) are established by biopsy.

An imperforate hymen appears as a bulging interlabial mass in the newborn with retained vaginal secretions that result from stimulation by maternal estrogens (see Fig. 2-16A). Because of its elasticity, the vagina may contain as much as 1 liter of mucus.[41] Usually a simple incision (hymenotomy) allows satisfactory drainage of the imperforate hymen. Signs of upper tract obstruction, which result from extrinsic compression from the mass, generally resolve following decompression of the hydrocolpos.

Uterovaginal prolapse usually occurs in the newborn with meningomyelocele, possibly owing to altered innervation of the pelvic musculature.[41] Often temporary support with a rubber nipple or pessary restores the uterus to its normal position.

References

1. Moore KL. The developing human. 4th ed. Philadelphia: WB Saunders, 1988:246.
2. Tanagho EA. Embryology of the genitourinary system. In: Tanagho EA, McAninch JW, eds. Smith's general urology. 13th ed. Norwalk, CT: Appleton & Lange, 1992:18.
3. Aydelotte MB. Developmental anatomy. In: Buchsbaum HJ, Schmidt JD, eds. Gynecologic and obstetric urology. Philadelphia: WB Saunders, 1982:3.
4. Langman J. Medical embryology. 4th ed. Baltimore: Williams & Wilkins, 1981:234.
5. Maizels M. Normal development of the urinary tract. In: Walsh PC, Retik AB, Stamey TA, Vaughan ED Jr, eds., Campbell's urology. 6th ed. Philadelphia: WB Saunders, 1992: 1301.
6. Tanagho EA. Developmental anatomy and urogenital abnormalities. In: Raz S, ed. Female urology. Philadelphia: WB Saunders, 1983:3.
7. Gruenwald P. The relation of the growing mullerian duct and its importance for the genesis of malformations. Anat Rec 1941;81:1.
8. George FW, Wilson JD. Embryology of the genital tract. In: Walsh PC, Retik AB, Stamey TA, Vaughan ED Jr, eds. Campbell's urology. 6th ed. Philadelphia: WB Saunders, 1992:1496.
9. Jeffs RD. Exstrophy, epispadias and cloacal and urogenital sinus abnormalities. Pediatr Clin North Amer 1987;34:1253.
10. Bast JD. Embryology of the urogenital system and congenital anomalies of the female genital tract. In: Pernoll ML, ed. Current obstetric and gynecologic diagnosis and treatment. 7th ed. Norwalk: Appleton & Lange, 1991:56.
11. Hendren WH. Cloacal malformations. In: Walsh PC, Retik AB, Stamey TA, Vaughan ED Jr, eds. Campbell's urology. 6th ed. Philadelphia: WB Saunders, 1992:1822.
12. Sotolongo JR, Gribetz ME, Saphir RL, et al. Female phallic urethra and persistent cloaca. J Urol 1983;130:1186.
13. Tam PKH, Parikh DH, Rickwood AMK. Urethralization of the female phallus with absent urogenital sinus. Br J Urol 1990;66:551.
14. Allen TD, Husmann DH. Cloacal anomalies and other urorectal septal defects in female patients: A spectrum of anatomical abnormalities. J Urol 1991;145:1034.
15. Ricketts RR, Woodard JR, Zwiren GT, et al. Modern treatment of cloacal exstrophy. J Pediatr Surg 1991;26:444.
16. Marshall VM, Muecke EC. Variations in exstrophy of the bladder. J Urol 1962;88:766.
17. Flanigan RC, Casale AJ, McRoberts JW. Cloacal exstrophy. Urology 1984;23:227.
18. Shapiro E, Lepor H, Jeffs RD. The inheritance of the exstrophy-epispadias complex. J Urol 1984;132:308.
19. Orikasa S, Metoki R, Ishikawa H, et al. Congenital urethral and vesical diverticula allied to blind-ending ureters. Urology 1990;35:137.
20. Cherrie RJ, Leach GE, Raz S. Obstructing urethral valve in a woman: A case report. J Urol 1983;129:1051.
21. Lyon RP, Smith DR. Distal urethral stenosis. J Urol 1963;89:414.
22. Fisher RE, Tanagho EA, Lyon RP, et al. Urethral calibration in newborn girls. J Urol 1969;102:67.

23. Saxton HM, Borzyskowski M, Mundy AR, et al. Spinning top urethra: Not a normal variant. Radiology 1988;168:147.
24. Immergut M, Culp D, Flocks RH. The urethral caliber in normal female children. J Urol 1967; 97:693.
25. Sharp HC. Reproductive tract disorders. In: Danforth DN, Scott JR, eds. Obstetrics and gynecology. 5th ed. Philadelphia: JB Lippincott, 1986: 561.
26. Fleming SE, Hall R, Gysler M, et al. Imperforate anus in females: Frequency of genital tract involvement, incidence of associated anomalies, and functional outcome. J Pediatr Surg 1986; 21:146.
27. Tolete-Velcek F, Hansbrough F, Kugaczewski J, et al. Uterovaginal malformations: A trap for the unsuspecting surgeon. J Pediatr Surg 1989;24:736.
28. Anderson KA, McAninch JW. Uterus didelphys with left hematocolpos and ipsilateral renal agenesis. J Urol 1982;127:550.
29. Simpson JL, Carson SA. Etiology of mullerian duct anomalies. In: Sciarra JJ, ed. Gynecology and obstetrics. Vol 5. Philadelphia: JB Lippincott, 1990:90.
30. Chitayat D, Hahm SYE, Marion RW, et al. Further delineation of the McKusick-Kaufman hydrometrocolpos-polydactyly syndrome. Am J Dis Child 1987;141:1133.
31. Tarry WF, Duckett JW, Stephens FD. The Mayer-Rokitansky syndrome: Pathogenesis, classification and management. J Urol 1986;136:648.
32. Carzy MP, Steinberg LH. Vaginal dystocia in a patient with a double uterus and a longitudinal vaginal septum. Aust NZ J Obstet Gynecol 1989; 29:74.
33. Rock JA. Surgical correction of uterovaginal anomalies. In: Sciarra JJ, ed. Gynecology and obstetrics. Vol 1. Philadelphia: JB Lippincott, 1990:70.
34. Sayer T, O'Reilly PH: Bicornuate and unicornuate uterus associated with unilateral renal aplasia and abnormal solitary kidney: Report of 3 cases. J Urol 1986;135:110.
35. Burbige KA, Hensle TW. Uterus didelphys and vaginal duplication with unilateral obstruction presenting as a newborn abdominal mass. J Urol 1984;132:1995.
36. Gilsanz V, Cleveland RH. Duplication of the mullerian ducts and genitourinary malformations (part I). Radiology 1982;144:793.
37. Gilsanz V, Cleveland RH, Reid BS. Duplication of the mullerian ducts and genitourinary malformations (part II). Radiology 1982;144:797.
38. Tran ATB, Arensman RM, Falterman KW. Diagnosis and management of hydrohematometrocolpos syndrome. Am J Dis Child 1987;141:632.
39. Golan A, Langer R, Bukovsky I, et al. Congenital anomalies of the mullerian system. Fertil Steril 1989;51:747.
40. Rock JA, Zacur HA, Dlugi AM, et al. Pregnancy success following surgical correction of imperforate hymen and complete transverse vaginal septum. Obstet Gynecol 1982;59:448.
41. Rock JA, Azziz R. Genital anomalies in childhood. Clin Obstet Gynecol 1987;30:682.
42. Ramenofsky ML, Raffensperger JG. An abdomino-perineal pull through for definitive treatment of hydrometrocolpos. J Pediatr Surg 1971; 6:381.
43. Parazzini F, Cechetti G. The frequency of imperforate hymen in northern Italy. Int J Epidemiol 1990;19:763.
44. Rock JA, Schlaff WD. The obstetric consequences of uterovaginal anomalies. Fertil Steril 1985; 43:681.
45. Griffin JE, Edwards C, Madden JD, et al. Congenital absence of the vagina: The Mayer-Rokitansky-Kuster-Hauser syndrome. Ann Intern Med 1976;85:224.
46. Stephens FD. The Mayer-Rokitansky syndrome. J Urol 1986;135:109.
47. Bernhisel MA, London SN, Haney AF. Unusual mullerian anomalies associated with distal extremity abnormalities. Obstet Gynecol 1985; 65:291.
48. Rock JA, Reeves LA, Retto H, et al. Success following vaginal creation for mullerian agenesis. Fertil Steril 1983;39:809.
49. Johnson N, Lilford RJ, Batchelor A. The free-flap vaginoplasty: A new surgical procedure for the treatment of vaginal agenesis. Br J Obstet Gynaecol 1991;98:184.
50. Lilford RJ, Johnson N, Batchelor A. A new operation for vaginal agenesis: Construction of a neovagina from a rectus abdominus musculocutaneous flap. Br J Obstet Gynaecol 1989;96: 1089.
51. Farber MA, Mitchell GW. Surgery for congenital absence of the vagina. Obstet Gynecol 1978; 51:364.
52. Tolhurst DE, vanderHelen TWTS. The treatment of vaginal atresia. Surg Gynecol Obstet 1991; 172:407.
53. Muckle CW. Developmental abnormalities of the female reproductive organs. In: Sciarra JJ, ed. Gynecology and obstetrics. Philadelphia: JB Lippincott, 1990:4:121.
54. Lee MJ, Yoder IC, Papanicolaou N, et al. Large gartner duct cyst associated with solitary crossed

ectopic kidney: Imaging features. J Comput Assist Tomogr 1991;15:149.

55. Watanabe K, Ogawa A, Inoue Y, et al. Single vaginal ectopic ureter via gartner's duct cyst spontaneously perforating into bladder. J Urol 1989;142:1044.

56. Sheih CP, Hung CS, Wei CF, et al. Cystic dilatations within the pelvis in patients with ipsilateral renal agenesis or dysplasia. J Urol 1990;144:324.

57. Adams JA, Horton M. Is it sexual abuse? Clin Pediatr 1989;28:146.

58. Kellogg ND, Parra JM. Linea vestibularis: A previously undescribed normal genital structure in female neonates. Pediatrics 1991;87:926.

59. Berenson A, Heger A, Andrews S. Appearance of the hymen in newborns. Pediatrics 1991;87:458.

60. Emans SJ, Woods ER, Flagg NT, et al. Genital findings in sexually abused, symptomatic, and asymptomatic girls. Pediatrics 1987;79:778.

61. Herman-Giddens ME, Frothingham TE. Prepubertal female genitalia: Examination for evidence of sexual abuse. Pediatrics 1987;80:203.

62. Jenny C, Kuhns MLD, Arakawa F. Hymens in newborn female infants. Pediatrics 1987;80:399.

63. Perlmutter AD, Reitelman C. Surgical management of intersexuality. In: Walsh PC, Retik AB, Stamey TA, Vaughan ED Jr, eds. Campbell's urology. 6th ed. Philadelphia: WB Saunders, 1992:1951.

64. Donahoe PK, Powell DM, Lee MM. Clinical management of intersex abnormalities. Curr Prob Surg 1991;28:516.

65. Coran AG, Polley TC. Surgical management of ambiguous genitalia in the infant and child. J Pediatr Surg 1991;26:812.

66. Gonzalez R, Fernandez ET. Single-stage feminization genitoplasty. J Urol 1990;143:776.

67. Karlin G, Brock W, Rich M, Pena A. Persistent cloaca and phallic urethra. J Urol 1989;142:1056.

68. Greenfield SP, Rutigliano E, Steinhardt G, Elder JS. Genitourinary tract malformations and maternal cocaine abuse. Urology 1991;37:455.

69. Klein VR, Willman SP, Carr BR. Familial posterior labial fusion. Obstet Gynecol 1989;73:500.

70. Capraro V, Greenberg H. Adhesions of the labia minora. Obstet Gynecol 1972;39:65.

71. So EP, Brock W, Kaplan GW. Ectopic labium and VATER association in a newborn. J Urol 1980;124:156.

72. Sasaki GH, Pang CY, Whittliff JL. Pathogenesis and treatment of infant skin strawberry hemangiomas: Clinical and in vitro studies of hormonal effects. Plast Reconstr Surg 1984;73:359.

73. Achauer BM, VanderKam VM. Ulcerated anogenital hemangioma of infancy. Plast Reconstr Surg 1991;87:861.

74. Huffman JW. Some facts about the clitoris. Postgrad Med 1976;60:245.

75. Riley WJ, Rosenbloom AL. Clitoral size in infancy. J Pediatr 1980;96:918.

76. Dershwitz RA, Levitsky LL, Feingold M. Vulvovaginitis: A cause of clitoromegaly. Am J Dis Child 1984;138:887.

77. Griebel ML, Redman JF, Kemp SF, et al. Hypertrophy of the clitoral hood: Presenting sign of neurofibromatosis in female child. Urology 1991;37:337.

78. Elder JS. Congenital anomalies of the genitalia. In: Walsh PC, Retik AB, Stamey TA, Vaughan ED, eds. Campbell's urology. 6th ed. Philadelphia: WB Saunders, 1992:1920.

79. Lowe FC, Hill GS, Jeffs RD, et al. Urethral prolapse in children: Insights into etiology and management. J Urol 1986;135:100.

80. Johnson CF. Prolapse of the urethra: Confusion of clinical and anatomic characteristics with sexual abuse. Pediatrics 1991;87:722.

81. Caldamone AA, Snyder HM, Duckett JW. Ureteroceles in children: Follow-up of management with upper tract approach. J Urol 1984;131:1130.

3

Physiology of the Lower Urinary Tract

Michael B. Chancellor

Jerry Blaivas

The urinary bladder is optimally suited for the storage and expulsion of urine. The normal bladder unconsciously stores a large volume of urine with little or no change in intravesical pressure. Continence is maintained by the sphincteric action of the vesical neck and urethra, which maintains a watertight seal despite wide fluctuations in intravesical and intra-abdominal pressures. Timely expulsion of urine is volitionally controlled. It is a coordinated event characterized by opening of the urethra, detrusor contraction, and unobstructed voiding. During storage and expulsion of urine, the ureterovesical junctions remain competent, thereby preventing ureteral reflux. Neurologic integration and coordination of these events occur in the rostral pons in the area known as the pontine micturition center.[1–6]

Because of the complex neurologic regulation of the bladder and urethra, virtually every neuropathic disease process can and often does cause bladder dysfunction. Common neurologic disorders associated with lower urinary tract dysfunction include multiple sclerosis, cerebrovascular accidents, myelodysplasia, Parkinson's disease, spinal cord injury, herniated discs, and diabetes mellitus. Abdominal and pelvic surgery and pelvic trauma can also cause neuropathic bladder. Examples include radical hysterectomy and abdominal-perineal resection.[7–9]

Anatomy

The lower urinary tract may be conceptualized as being composed of a reservoir and a sphincter. They are functionally distinct but anatomically indistinct. On gross inspection, the muscle fibers and mucosa of the bladder blend with those of the vesical neck and urethra. No sphincter or valve mechanism can be seen with the naked eye. Rather the sphincter comprises a unique arrangement of smooth and striated muscle of the vesical neck and proximal urethra interlaced with collagenous and elastic tissue. In addition, the mucosal lining of the urethra keeps its walls coapted and forms a watertight seal.[10]

DETRUSOR

The bladder comprises the detrusor proper and the trigone.[11–15, 89] The detrusor consists of interlacing bundles of smooth muscle fibers that are not arranged in distinct layers. Rather the individual bundles freely criss-cross with one another and do not seem to follow any particular pattern.[15, 16] There is a tendency for the outer and inner layers to form a longitudinal orientation, particularly as they approach the vesical neck. The trigone is a triangular area bounded superolaterally by the ureteral orifices and inferiorly by the bladder neck.

Female Urology, edited by Elroy D. Kursh and Edward McGuire. J. B. Lippincott, Philadelphia, © 1994.

The normal bladder has high compliance as demonstrated by its ability to hold increasing amounts of urine without a corresponding rise in intravesical pressure by virtue of elastic and vesicoelastic properties of the bladder wall.[17] Elasticity allows the bladder wall to stretch to a certain degree without any increase rise in tension. The ratio of the change in intravesical volume to the change in intravesical pressure is termed *compliance*.

URINARY SPHINCTER

The urinary sphincter can be divided into the internal sphincter and the external sphincter. The internal sphincter (bladder neck and proximal urethra, including the prostatic urethra in men) is composed mainly of smooth muscles. The external sphincter is composed mainly of skeletal muscles.

Internal Sphincter

The smooth muscle urethral sphincter consists of the bladder base with its investment of the distal end of the ureters and the extensions into the urethra.[14, 18] Bands of smooth muscle loop around the posterior aspect of the bladder base in two distinct groups. A superficial group, known as Heiss's loop, lies cranial to the precervical arc, and a deeper group lies caudal to the precervical arc. According to Woodburne, these loops of smooth muscle do not encircle the vesical neck and, further, do not provide the anatomic configuration to account for sphincteric function.[15] Rather he described dense elastic tissue in the vesical neck region and theorized that the vesical neck was maintained in a closed position by the passive properties of this tissue.

The muscles of the internal sphincter are arranged in both longitudinal and circular orientations. From a functional and teleologic standpoint, the presence of both longitudinal and circular fibers in the vesical neck and urethra provides the substrate for understanding both the mechanism of micturition and the means for providing urinary continence. In this schema, contraction of the longitudinal fibers would serve to shorten and widen the urethra during micturition, thus opening the urethra for unobstructed voiding. Contraction of the circular fibers would aid in maintaining continence; relaxation, either actively or passively, would open the urethra for micturition. The proportion and functional significance of longitudinal and circular fibers remain a subject of controversy. Moreover, there are major differences between the two sexes. Most authors agree that in both sexes there are longitudinal or helical bundles of smooth muscle that extend from the detrusor base into the prostatic urethra in the male and for almost the whole urethra in females.

In the male, there is an additional rather well-defined, circularly oriented smooth muscle group just below the vesical neck.[13, 19] According to Gil-Vernet, these fibers are located in an intermediate position between an inner longitudinal and an outer transverse layer.[19] Hutch believed that this proximal urethral circular smooth muscle is identical to the prostatic capsule and that this structure is the primary involuntary *internal sphincter*.[13] Gosling, however, denies that this is a urinary sphincter; rather he believes it to be a genital sphincter that prevents the retrograde ejaculation of semen during sexual intercourse.[16] Elbadawi believes that the urethral smooth musculature is both anatomically and functionally contiguous with the deep trigone, whereas Gosling and Dixon stated that there is a functional and anatomic division between these two structures at the vesical neck.[20–22] According to the latter proposal, the smooth muscle of the urethra consists of fibers of much smaller diameter than those of the deep trigone. Moreover, according to Gosling, the orientation of the smooth muscle in the urethra is predominantly longitudinal and helical, not circular.[16]

External Sphincter

The external urinary sphincter is composed of both urethral and periurethral muscles. Striated muscle fibers are of two varieties. Fibers within the wall of the urethra are smaller than those located periurethrally and are generally slow twitch in character. The periurethral muscle is a mix of slow-twitch and fast-twitch fibers. Slow-twitch muscle has a rich mitochondrial population and is resistant to fatigue. It is believed to be important in maintaining continence at rest. Fast-twitch fibers are characterized by a high glycogen content and easy fatigue. They maintain continence during acute stress, such as coughing and laughing.[21,23–26]

The intraurethral portion surrounds the middle third of the female urethra and is composed mostly of slow-twitch muscle fibers.[22] In the male, the muscle is even more prominent and often extends to the vesical neck.[25,27,28] Gosling believes that this represents the primary urethral sphincter in women.[16]

The external sphincter muscle, composed of striated muscle fibers and under voluntary control, lies between the fascial layers of the urogenital diaphragm. In females, it is condensed around the middle third of the urethra. In the male, these muscle fibers start at the apex of the prostate and surround the membranous urethra. The striated muscles of the pelvic floor (levator ani) act as an indirect sphincter and contribute to sphincteric function.

Urethral Closure and Urinary Continence

The muscle of the urethra compresses the connective and vascular tissues that form the inner part of the urethral wall and molds these soft pliable tissues to form a watertight seal. The elastic tension and urethral connective tissues and the compression by the urethral smooth muscle are fairly uniformly distributed along the functional length of the urethra, but the effect of the striated muscle is more localized. As a result, there is a zone of maximal urethral compression in the region of the striated sphincter. Experimental studies suggest that the smooth and striated muscle components of the distal sphincter mechanism each contribute about 50% of the tension exerted by the sphincter.[29] The urethral sphincter is supported by the muscles, ligaments, and fascial attachments of the pelvic floor.

The neural regulation of the internal and external sphincter is complex and not completely understood. We know that detrusor contraction is preceded by relaxation of the urethra. Detrusor stretch (bladder filling) reflexly produces an increase in urethral tone. The influence of detrusor stretch is probably a sacral reflex, but modulation by suprasacral neural pathways is likely.

Neurophysiology

Early students of neurophysiology believed that micturition was a simple spinal reflex the afferent and efferent pathways of which resided in the second through fourth segments of the sacral spinal cord and that this reflex was supplemented by a number of *cephalospinal reflexes.*[30–34]

Afferent pathways innervating the lower urinary tract are those passing in the pelvic nerve to the sacral spinal cord (S2-4). These afferents are small-diameter fibers that are linked with tension receptors in the bladder wall. Afferent pathways from striated muscle sphincters and from the urethra, which transmit sensations of warm, cold, pain, and passage of urine, travel in the pudendal nerve to the sacral cord (S2-4). Studies in animals have revealed that bladder afferent neurons contain a number of peptides.[35] These neurons were identified in sacral dorsal root ganglia by retrograde dye-labeling techniques. A large percentage of bladder afferents contained vasoactive intestinal polypeptide (VIP), substance P, cholecystokinin, leucine enkephalin, bombesin, and somatostatin. Coexistence of neurotransmitters in the same cells has been shown. The physiologic significance of peptide coexistence in afferents is uncertain. It has been speculated, however, that substance P and VIP may be excitatory transmitters in afferents and that enkephalin may be an inhibitory modulator, which functions to block the release of excitatory transmitter.[35]

CEREBRAL CORTEX

Many studies have demonstrated that different parts of the brain are involved in inhibition and facilitation of the micturition reflex. In general terms, the tonic activity of the cerebral cortex and midbrain is inhibitory.[36-39] The superior medial portion of the frontal lobes and the corpus callosum have been identified as the area of major detrusor innervation. This is deducted from careful correlation of bladder function and clinical neurologic lesions of the cerebral cortex. It is interesting that the cerebrocortical areas for innervation of the bladder and periurethral striated muscle are geographically distinct. Because the bladder and the sphincter are midline structures, they receive bilateral innervation from all levels of the central nervous system. Clinical studies of patients with frontal lobe lesions have confirmed the release of reflex detrusor activity with cerebral diseases.[38,40-42]

The micturition reflex can be voluntarily inhibited by contraction of the urethral and periurethral striated musculature, which is dependent on neural connections between the frontal cortex and Onuf's nucleus.[1] Contraction of these muscles during micturition interrupts the urinary stream and, probably through a reflex mechanism, inhibits the micturition reflex.

PONTINE MICTURITION CENTER

The micturition reflex is coordinated, not in the sacral spinal cord as was formerly believed, but rather in the rostral brain stem in a region known as the pontine mesencephalic reticular formation.[1,30,31,43,44] This region of the brain stem has been designated the pontine micturition center; the sacral reflex arc is called the sacral micturition center. When the neural pathways between the pontine and sacral micturition center are intact, micturition is achieved by activation of the micturition reflex, which results in a coordinated series of events consisting of relaxation of the striated urethral musculature, detrusor contraction, and opening of the bladder neck and urethra. Neurologic lesions that interrupt these pontine-sacral pathways usually result in uncoordinated micturition in the form of detrusor-external sphincter dyssynergia.[1,45]

SPINAL CORD

The innervation of the lower urinary tract is derived from three sets of peripheral nerves: sacral parasympathetic (pelvic nerve), thoracolumbar sympathetic (hypogastric nerve and sympathetic chain), and sacral somatic nerve (pudendal nerve).[38,46,47]

Vertebral levels T11-L1 (nerve levels S2-4) is the center for micturition control. Trauma to this level of the cord results in detrusor areflexia. Lesions above the sacral micturition center generally result in a bladder with reflex activity but lacking volitional control (detrusor hyperreflexia). It is important to remember that trauma and spinal cord disease are often incomplete, and mixed patterns of bladder dysfunction often result[48] (Fig. 3-1).

PELVIC PLEXUS, GANGLION, AND MOTOR END PLATES

Efferent parasympathetic fibers are carried in the ventral roots of the second to fourth sacral segments. These roots merge to form the pelvic nerve (nervi erigentes), the anatomy of which varies considerably among different species.[49,50] Fibers of the pelvic nerve meet those of the hypogastric nerve to form the pelvic plexus. The pelvic plexus is a fine, multibranched group of nerve fibers that sends twigs of fibers to the bladder and urethra without ever forming an identifiable nerve trunk. Most of the efferent fibers synapse again in pelvic ganglia in or near the walls of the bladder and urethra. Because of their close proximity to the end organ, these peripheral ganglia have been designated the urogenital short neuron system by Elbadawi and Schenk.[51] This short neuronal system has extensive interconnections with sympathetics throughout the wall of the bladder and urethra.

Histochemical studies have shown that the ganglia of the short neuron system is composed predominantly of three types of cells: cholinergic, adrenergic, and small, intensely fluorescent neurons.[20,52] The presence of this short neuron

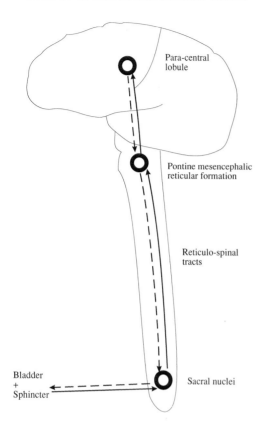

Figure 3-1. Major neurologic pathways involved in micturition. The micturition reflex is integrated in the pontine micturition center. Suprapontine influences may be either facilitatory or inhibitory. Neural connections between the pontine and sacral micturition centers traverse the lateral columns of the spinal cord. These pathways are necessary for coordination of the micturition reflex. Connections between the frontal cortex and pudendal nucleus control voluntary contraction and relaxation of the rhabdosphincter and pelvic floor muscles.

system ensures that the bladder and urethra cannot become completely denervated by neurologic lesions. Even radical surgery, such as abdominoperineal resection of the rectum, does not ablate the short neuronal system. Thus the proper term for neurologic lesions of the preganglionic neuron or for more central lesions is *decentralization* rather than *denervation*.[53]

Bladder filling causes a gradual increase in the discharge of pelvic nerve afferents. After synapse in the sacral spinal cord, probably by way of an interneuron, there is increased efferent pudendal nerve activity, which results in increasing electromyographic activity of the striated urethral and periurethral musculature.[38,44] This has been termed the *guarding reflex*.[23]

SACRAL PARASYMPATHETIC NERVES

The pelvic nerve is the primary parasympathetic nerve involved in micturition. Acetylcholine is the primary neurotransmitter at both the preganglionic and postganglionic synapse. Administration of acetylcholine or electrical stimulation of the pelvic nerve results in detrusor contraction.[11,38,54–57] The detrusor contraction that results from electrical stimulation is partially resistant to blockade by atropine.[58,59] The effect of pelvic nerve stimulation and administration of acetylcholine on the urethral musculature is not well understood. Various studies have shown an increase in urethral resistance,[56,60] a decrease,[61–63] or no change.[11] The nucleus of the pelvic nerve is located in the interomedial lateral cell column of the second to fourth segments of the sacral spinal cord.[38,64] Afferent fibers are axonal projections from the dorsal spinal root ganglia, although there is evidence that in some species a proportion of the afferent fibers are located in the ventral root as well.[65]

THORACOLUMBAR SYMPATHETIC NERVES

The role of the sympathetic nervous system in micturition has been controversial. Studies in the cat have provided information that seems to be applicable to humans.[46,66–70] The sympathetics promote the storage of urine by two mechanisms, both of which are mediated by alpha adrenoceptors.[35] The first action is closure of the vesical neck and proximal urethra; the second is inhibition of neural transmission from the preganglionic to the postganglionic parasympathetic nerve. In addition, relaxation of the body of the detrusor is accomplished by way of a beta adrenoceptor.[71-75] The sympathetics appear to play little or no role in sensory function. According to Learmonth, presacral neurectomy had no effect on either bladder or urethral function in humans.[76]

The cell bodies of the sympathetic nerves are located in the intermedial lateral cell column of the tenth thoracic to the second lumbar segments of the spinal cord. Efferent fibers traverse the ventral roots and synapse in the prevertebral ganglia of the lumbar sympathetic chain. From here they branch out to form the presacral plexus, which bifurcates to form the right and left hypogastric nerves. The hypogastric nerve consists of multiple tiny strands, not a single nerve trunk. The hypogastric nerve joins the pelvic nerves to form the pelvic plexus. Within the pelvic plexus and the walls of the bladder and urethra, there are sympathetic ganglia, which are part of the urogenital short neuron system. This intramural neuronal network is thought to be an important modulator of reflex activity that affects micturition.

During filling, there is direct sympathetic stimulation of alpha adrenoceptors, which maintains closure of the vesical neck and proximal urethra.[35,37,39] Relaxation of the body of the detrusor is accomplished by way of a sympathetic beta adrenoceptor.[37,44,71] The role and significance of this mechanism in human physiology, however, has not been well defined.

After pelvic injury, neural recovery may involve neural modulation or reorganization. de Groat and associates showed that removal of the pelvic nerve caused reorganization such that hypogastric nerve stimulation led to large bladder contraction, suggesting existence of sympathetic pathways for the contractions by way of the pelvic nerve.[77] Injury to the sympathetic innervation can have devastating consequences. Bilateral hypogastric nerve transections after retroperitoneal nerve transection, such as after radical hysterectomy, result in an open bladder neck, which can cause type 3 stress urinary incontinence in both sexes and retrograde ejaculation in men. Animal and clinical experience suggest that the hypogastric nerve is the major pathway of bladder neck contraction at ejaculation.[78,79]

SOMATIC NERVES

The pudendal nerve is the primary innervation of the striated muscles of the pelvic floor and the rhabdosphincter. Horseradish peroxidase studies have clearly demonstrated that the cell bodies of the pudendal nerve originate in Onufrowicz's (Onuf's) nucleus in the anterior horn of the S2-4.[80,81] The cells of Onuf's nucleus are smaller and more spherical than the other cells in the anterior horn, and they are resistant to the degenerative process that destroys other anterior horn cells in amyotrophic lateral sclerosis.[82] This probably accounts for the observation that there may be a disparity in the neurologic involvement of the bladder and striated sphincter in patients with certain neurologic disorders, such as multiple sclerosis and myelodysplasia.[1,83]

MECHANISMS CONTROLLING MICTURITION

During urine storage, a low level of afferent activity in the pelvic nerve and possibly also in the proprioceptive afferents in the pudendal nerve initiates reflex efferent firing in sympathetic and somatic pathways to the bladder base and urethra, whereas the parasympathetic efferent outflow to the bladder body is quiescent. During micturition, a high level of vesical afferent activity reverses the pattern of efferent outflow, producing firing in the parasympathetic pathways and inhibition of the sympathetic and somatic pathways.[38,84] These reflexes occur in their simplest form in infants. With maturation, these reflexes are subject to modulation and voluntary control by supraspinal centers.[38]

The central mechanisms that coordinate the autonomic and somatic component of micturition require the integrative action of neuronal populations at various levels of the central nervous system. Electrical stimulation in the rostral brain stem in the region of the dorsolateral pontine reticular formation elicited detrusor contractions and firing in the parasympathetic efferent pathways to the bladder (Figs. 3-2 through 3-4).

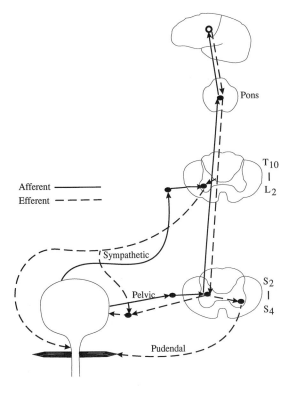

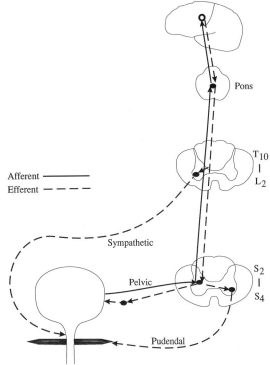

Figure 3-2. *Physiology of micturition, storage phase. During bladder filling, detrusor pressure remains fairly constant. There is a gradual increase in electrical activity of the urethral and periurethral striated muscles, and urethral pressure remains greater than intravesical pressure, thus maintaining continence. The micturition reflex is inhibited by pelvic, pudendal, and sympathetic reflexes, which maintain closure of the vesical neck and inhibition of the micturition reflex (see text for details).*

Figure 3-3. *Physiology of micturition, voiding phase. The first recordable event during the micturition reflex is a sudden and complete relaxation of the striated urethral and periurethral muscles. This is followed almost immediately by a fall in urethral pressure and a rise in detrusor pressure. When the proximal urethra becomes isobaric with the bladder, flow commences. The vesical neck and urethra gradually widen during voiding and achieve their widest caliber at peak flow. The inhibitory reflexes are shut off, and transmission across the pelvic ganglion results in detrusor contraction.*

Storage Phase of Micturition Cycle

During the storage phase, the ureters transport urine to the bladder at physiologic rates ranging from approximately 20 to 100 ml/hour. As the bladder fills with urine, its walls begin to stretch, and it assumes a roughly spherical shape. The thickness of the bladder wall diminishes, and the individual muscle cells increase their length. Because the ureter is fixed by its attachment to the superficial trigone and Waldeyer's sheath, its intramural portion is stretched. Accordingly the

lumen becomes longer and narrower, increasing the resistance to flow. This serves to prevent vesicoureteral reflux.

The behavior of the bladder as it stretches is due to a combination of active and passive forces that arise from its component parts. Elastin, collagen, and smooth muscle (when it is not contracting) are the main tissues responsible for the passive properties of the bladder; the contractile

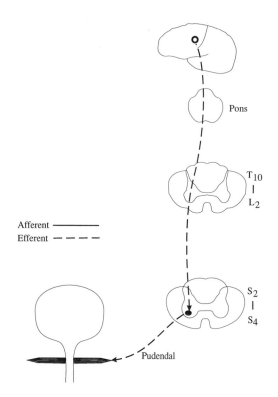

Figure 3-4. *Physiology of micturition, termination of micturition. Interruption of the stream is accomplished by voluntary contraction of the rhabdosphincter and periurethral striated musculature.*

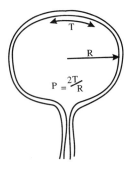

Figure 3-5. *Law of LaPlace for a sphere. Because the radius for different bladders at the similar bladder volume is approximately the same, differences in pressure must be due to differences in bladder wall tension. P, Pressure; R, radius; T, tension.*

elements of smooth muscle account for the active behavior.[85–89]

During physiologic bladder filling, the bladder exhibits a property known as accommodation, in which it accepts large volumes of urine at very low intravesical pressure. The magnitude of the pressure rise is usually in the range of 0 to 20 cm H_2O. The relationship between pressure and volume is determined by the Law of LaPlace, which, for a sphere, states: $P = 2T/R$, where P is detrusor pressure, T is bladder wall tension, and R is the radius of the bladder. Because the radius is approximately the same for any given bladder volume, pressure is dependent on the bladder wall tension (Fig. 3-5). Bladder wall tension is determined by the active and passive properties

of its constituent parts, including smooth muscle fibers, collagen, and elastic tissue.

The relationship between pressure and volume is usually expressed as compliance. Compliance is defined as the change in volume divided by the corresponding change in pressure. Clinical measurement of bladder compliance, however, is difficult for several reasons. First, compliance is strongly influenced by a number of factors, including the rate of bladder filling, the duration of filling, hysteresis, and the activity of the smooth muscle. Second, compliance changes during different parts of the filling curve. Third, the numeric value of compliance varies considerably depending on the volume interval over which it is measured[86] (Fig. 3-6).

CONTINENCE DURING STORAGE

A straightforward view of urinary continence is that during bladder filling urethral pressure remains greater than intravesical pressure. The difference between intravesical and intraurethral pressure is termed the *urethral closure pressure*. The mechanism by which the urethral closure pressure is maintained is only incompletely understood. First, the *resting* urethra has a much

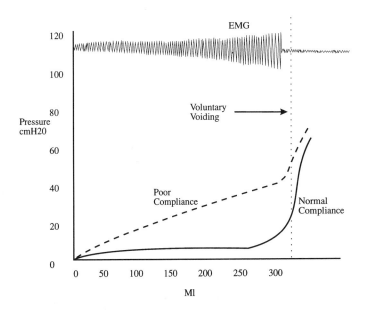

Figure 3-6. *Cystometrogram of two patients, one with normal compliance and another status–post–radical colon surgery, with diminished compliance. Electromyographic activity of the external sphincter demonstrates coordinated sphincter activity with complete relaxation at onset of voluntary voiding in both patients.*

higher pressure than the bladder, usually in the range of 40 to 80 cm H_2O. This relatively high pressure in the urethra is due to a number of factors, some active and some passive. Active forces include the tone of the intraurethral smooth and striated muscle as well as the contribution derived from the periurethral striated musculature of the pelvic diaphragm. Passive forces include the contributions of elastic and collagen fibers and *inner wall softness*.[10]

An acute rise in intra-abdominal pressure, such as occurs during coughing, laughing, and physical activity, is normally transmitted equally to the bladder and proximal urethra, so the net change in closure pressure is zero.[90] In women, it has been documented that the transmission of pressure has both an active and a passive component.[91] The active component appears to be due to a reflex contraction of the striated mus-

culature, but it has not been determined whether this is intraurethral or periurethral muscle. The passive component is dependent on the *intra-abdominal position* of the vesical neck and proximal urethra. When the musculofascial supporting structures weaken, descent of the vesical neck and proximal urethra is accompanied by unequal transmission of pressure. When intravesical pressure exceeds urethral pressure, stress incontinence ensues (Fig. 3-7).

URINARY STORAGE PROBLEMS

The most common cause of "irritative" voiding symptoms is involuntary detrusor contractions. There are numerous causes of involuntary bladder contractions, including neurologic, secondary to long-term bladder outlet obstruction, and idiopathic. The presence of involuntary detrusor

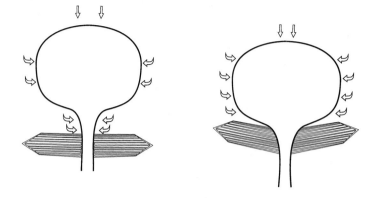

Figure 3-7. *The passive component of urinary continence. The drawing on the left illustrates a normal anatomic relationship with simultaneous transmission of intra-abdominal pressure to both the bladder and the proximal urethra. On the right, the musculo-fascial support is weakened with descent of the bladder neck and proximal urethra. There is unequal transmission of intra-abdominal pressure, and stress incontinence ensues.*

contractions should not by themselves be considered objective evidence of a neurologic lesion. The definition of an involuntary bladder contraction is a sudden rise in bladder pressure that is not volitional. Detrusor hyperreflexia refers to involuntary bladder contractions secondary to neurologic pathology. In contrast, in the absence of a neurologic lesion, the condition is termed *detrusor instability.*

The therapeutic regimen of involuntary detrusor contractions is predicated on its underlying pathophysiology. For example, when involuntary contractions are secondary to bladder outlet obstruction, the relief of the obstruction usually results in abolition of the involuntary detrusor contractions. In other cases, when no obstruction is noted, the treatment of choice has been anticholinergic medication, such as propantheline bromide or oxybutynin chloride. Other therapeutic modalities include behavior modification, functional electrical neural stimulation (transcutaneously, percutaneously, or by direct stimulation of nerve roots), surgical *denervation procedures*, and operations designed to

increase bladder capacity, such as augmentation cystoplasty.

SPHINCTER ABNORMALITIES

Stress incontinence due to hypermobility describes a condition in which there is abnormal descent of the proximal urethra when the patient increases intra-abdominal pressure, that is, during coughing or straining. The proximal urethra herniates through the pelvic floor. Consequently, the increased intra-abdominal pressure is unequally transmitted to the bladder and urethra. Leakage occurs as intravesical pressure exceeds intraurethral pressure. The sphincter itself is relatively normal; it is capable of maintaining a watertight seal, but it cannot withstand the effects of increased pressure. Therefore any operation designed to prevent descent of the proximal urethra (the suspension operations) is generally successful in effecting a cure.

Intrinsic sphincter deficiency describes a second condition in which the urethra no longer functions as a sphincter (type 3 stress incontinence). It cannot maintain a watertight seal, and therefore leakage occurs with the slightest provocation. The cause of sphincteric failure is almost always either neurologic injury or a history of multiple prior surgeries.[92,93] The standard procedures described to alleviate stress incontinence have no role in the management of these patients. The creation of a pubovaginal sling, however, has been the treatment of choice.[92] In men, the insertion of an artificial urinary sphincter has met with reasonable success.

BLADDER INSTABILITY DURING STORAGE PHASE

From a clinical perspective, detrusor overactivity has been attributed to a variety of causes. In certain neurologic disorders, such as multiple sclerosis and stroke, the cause and effect relationship is obvious and well studied. In others, such as inflammation and infection, the relationship is mere conjecture. Other causes for detrusor instability include urethral and bladder trauma, bladder outlet obstruction, aging, and anxiety neurosis.[94–99] Because of a lack of a clear understanding of the pathophysiology of the unstable bladder, attempts to improve the management of this condition have been frustrating.[100]

When muscle strips from normal, idiopathic detrusor instability and detrusor hyperreflexia patients were compared under isometric conditions in an organ bath, spontaneous contractions developed more often in the unstable and hyperreflexic muscles and were of greater amplitude and frequency.[97] This suggests that the pathophysiology of involuntary detrusor contraction is common to both idiopathic detrusor instability and detrusor hyperreflexia.

It has been hypothesized that imbalances of the neurotransmitters that control and modulate the micturition reflex may be responsible for some cases of detrusor overactivity. VIP, which is known to inhibit detrusor contractions, has been found in reduced concentration in the bladder of patients with detrusor instability.[101] The spinal and cerebral enkephalinergic system has also been implicated because of its inhibitory effect on the bladder.[35]

Voiding Phase of the Micturition Cycle

The micturition reflex is initiated by relaxation of the periurethral and intraurethral striated muscles.[1] This is signaled by a fall in urethral pressure and a rise in detrusor pressure as voiding ensues. The vesical neck and urethra gradually open during micturition and assume their widest cross-sectional area during the steady state of peak flow.[102] During voiding, the entire proximal urethra in both sexes is isobaric with the bladder.[103,104] There is a variable fall in pressure at the membranous urethra in the male and the distal urethra in the female. The micturition reflex requires neurologic integration in the pontine micturition center. Neurologic lesions that interrupt the pathways between the pontine micturition center and the sacral micturition center usually result in uncoordinated micturition in the form of detrusor–external sphincter dyssynergia. Neurologic lesions above the pontine micturition center that leave these pathways intact result in involuntary micturition, but the micturition reflex remains intact, and the mechanics of micturition remain normal.[1]

Opening of the bladder neck to initiate voiding probably is achieved by relaxation of the vesical outlet by the same parasympathetic discharge that induces micturition contraction of the detrusor body. Controversy exists as to its exact mechanism, be it active opening or passive pulling open by bladder neck contraction. Bladder neck closure is likely secondary to sympathetic neural discharge. Sympathetic stimulation, whether neurologic or pharmacologic, can interrupt micturition while in progress.[20]

HYDROMECHANICS

In the simplest of terms, voiding is accomplished when the expulsive properties of the bladder overcome the resistance to the flow of urine offered by the urethra. Hydrodynamic principles can be applied to the lower urinary tract. The bladder is conceptualized as a pump and the urethra as a pipe. The bladder, by contracting, provides the energy for propelling urine through the urethra. The resistance offered by the urethra determines what the flow rate is for any given detrusor contraction.

Calculation of the effective cross-sectional area of the urethra at the *flow rate controlling zone* is the most direct measurement of urethral resistance in a collapsible tube.[102] Direct measurement of urethral cross-sectional area, however, is not readily available. A probe using the field-gradient principle was used to measure related values of urethral cross-sectional areas and pressure.[105, 106]

An estimation of the urethral resistance can be made, in the simplest possible way, by plotting detrusor pressure and urine flow simultaneously during micturition. In a pressure/flow plot, the intercept of the tracing with the pressure axis gives the urethral opening pressure, the overall slope of the tracing reflects the general trend in the outlet resistance, and the deflections of the tracings signify dynamic changes in outlet resistance. During flow, synchronous unidirectional changes in pressure and flow are due to changes in detrusor contractility; inverse changes in pressure and flow are due to changes in urethral resistance. For example, a concomitant increase in detrusor pressure and a fall in uroflow can be due only to an increase in urethral resistance to the flow of urine; similarly, a concomitant rise in detrusor pressure and uroflow can be due only to increased detrusor contractility.

NEUROLOGIC CONSIDERATIONS DURING VOIDING

Normally micturition is voluntarily initiated at an appropriate and socially convenient time when afferent impulses from the bladder and urethra signal the need to void. Once the sensation of the need to void is experienced, it is normally possible to suppress both the sensation and the act of micturition for a considerable length of time.

Although there is some disagreement as to the exact neural mechanisms by which the micturition reflex is regulated, it is generally agreed that the pontine micturition center plays a major role.[1, 30, 31, 39, 41, 107] The concept of a micturition reflex and a micturition threshold is important for understanding the neurophysiology of micturition. The specifics, however, are poorly understood. For example, there does not appear to be a single stimulus that initiates the micturition reflex. Rather it is probably regulated by a series of neural events that exert their influence through one or more mechanisms that alter the micturition threshold. It has been demonstrated that the threshold of micturition is raised by descending neural influences from the frontal and cingulate cortex, hypothalamus, and midbrain; by the medial region of the pons and medulla; by raising the threshold for micturition; and by activation of colonic, genital, and perineal afferents. The micturition threshold is lowered by increasing activation of pelvic (vesical) afferents and by activity of the dorsolateral pons and mammilary bodies.[32–34, 36, 38, 39] The inhibitory action of the endorphins has been alluded to earlier, but their clinical relevance remains to be determined.

The first recordable event in the activation of the micturition reflex is cessation of efferent pudendal nerve activity and relaxation of the striated muscles.[1] Concomitantly there is suppression of sympathetic activity; the net result is that the inhibitory effects of sympathetic stimulation are aborted. This permits transmission of neural impulses across the pelvic ganglion, and efferent postganglionic firing results in detrusor contraction. Inhibition of vesical neck stimulation permits opening of the urethra.

A number of different neural reflex mechanisms have been proposed that facilitate, sustain, and terminate the micturition reflex.[34, 39] The role of these reflexes in human physiology, however, is speculative. The interested reader is referred to the original publications for a more complete description.

Neurologic diseases, such as spinal cord injury, transverse myelitis, multiple sclerosis, and myelodysplasia, which can interrupt this *long routed micturition reflex*, usually result in uncoordinated micturition called *detrusor–external sphincter dyssynergia*.[1, 45, 108] Suprapontine neurologic lesions, such as cerebrovascular accident, tumor, Parkinson's disease, and normal pressure hydrocephalus, usually result in loss of control over the micturition reflex without detrusor–external sphincter dyssynergia.[1,109]

BLADDER EMPTYING PROBLEMS

Incomplete bladder emptying is secondary to either bladder outlet obstruction or impaired detrusor contractility. Although impaired detrusor contractions may be attributable to myogenic, neurogenic, or psychological origin, no current diagnostic method distinguishes between these entities. Most neurologic causes of detrusor abnormalities, however, are associated with other neurologic deficits. For example, a neurologic lesion that affects the second through fourth segments of the sacral spinal cord usually results not only in detrusor areflexia, but also perianal anesthesia, poor anal tone, absent voluntary control of the anal sphincter, and absence of the bulbocavernosus reflex.

Noncholinergic, Nonadrenergic Neurotransmitter

It has been known for many years that electrical stimulation of the ventral sacral roots resulted in noncholinergic, nonadrenergic, atropine-resistant contraction of the detrusor.[58] This has given rise to an extensive search for neurotransmitters in addition to norepinephrine and acetylcholine. Among the more prominent candidates for this substance are the "purinergic" amines, particularly adenosine triphosphate (ATP), and the neuropeptides, including VIP, substance P, and the enkephelins.[110–116]

Some purines and neuropeptides appear to modify bladder and urethra activity.[112] Burnstock and colleagues first suggested that ATP might be the neurotransmitter involved in atropine-resistant, electrically induced detrusor contractions.[117] There is sufficient evidence to support the contention that ATP functions as an excitatory transmitter at the postganglionic neu-romuscular junction and an inhibitory transmitter at the ganglion. Many studies have confirmed that ATP is released during transmural electrical stimulation and that administration of ATP causes contraction of detrusor strips in humans, rats, rabbits, and guinea pigs.[117–122]

de Groat and Kawatani have postulated an important role for opioid peptides in the regulation of micturition.[35] Immunohistochemical studies have demonstrated a high concentration of leucine enkephalin in proximity to Onuf's nucleus and the parasympathetic nucleus in the sacral spinal cord and in the pontine mesencephalic reticular formation of the brain stem.[112] It has been further shown that exogenous enkephalins generally have an inhibitory effect on micturition. Three types of opioid receptors have been identified: gamma, mu, and kappa. Gamma enkephalins inhibit transmission from the preganglionic to the postganglionic parasympathetic neuron by blocking the release of acetylcholine. The net effect of this is to inhibit detrusor contractions. Mu and gamma enkephalins inhibit the micturition reflex at the brain stem level. Kappa enkephalins appear to have no effect on the micturition reflexes. The effect of exogenous enkephalins can be blocked by naloxone, an opioid antagonist. Moreover, even in the absence of exogenous enkephalin administration, naloxone has a facilitatory effect on micturition, suggesting that endogenous enkephalins normally play a regulatory role in micturition. It has been postulated that the neuropeptides function primarily as neuromodulators or cotransmitters rather than primary neurotransmitters.[35]

VIP has been demonstrated throughout the bladder, but it is found in highest concentrations in the trigone and bladder base. Coincidentally VIP has been also found in high concentrations in the gastroesophageal junction and the pylorus. Accordingly it has been postulated that VIP is important in smooth muscle with a sphincteric function, possibly mediating noncholinergic, nonadrenergic relaxation of smooth muscle sphincter.[111,113] Studies have shown that approximately 10% to 15% of cholinergic pelvic ganglion cells contain VIP.[35] Administration of VIP has been shown to cause inhibition of detrusor contractions induced by electrical stimulation and by administration of parasympathetic and sympathetic agonists.[35, 123–125] In another study, the concentration of VIP was reduced in patients with detrusor instability, suggesting the possibility that loss of VIP inhibition may be a cause of this disorder.[35, 114] VIP has also been demonstrated in afferent pelvic and hypogastric nerves and in their spinal cord projections.

Substance P may be important in the afferent limb of the micturition reflex. The systemic administration of capsaicin, a substance P antagonist, caused depression of the micturition reflex in rats. Substance P has also been shown to cause contraction of detrusor smooth muscle and to enhance the contractions induced by electrical field stimulation.[126]

A number of studies have implicated prostaglandins in the modulation of vesicourethral function. The actions of prostaglandins, however, are resistant to tetrodotoxin; hence their role relation to autonomic neuroeffector is unlikely.[127] Prostaglandin E_1 and E_2 have been shown to cause relaxation of human detrusor and urethra, whereas prostaglandin $F_{2\alpha}$ caused contraction.[128, 129]

The basic framework of lower urinary tract is established, and most bladder and sphincter functions can be explained. With the rapid rate of scientific advances, more fascinating but more complex data are being published. We are now aware of sympathetic and parasympathetic interaction peripherally at both the ganglionic and the prejunctional levels. Cholinergic, adrenergic, and noncholinergic, nonadrenergic neurotransmitters may be involved in modulating discharges through these axons, functioning probably as cotransmitters.[47, 74, 130]

In various micturition disorders (*i.e.*, recurrent urinary tract infections, aging, neurogenic bladder, sensory urgency, and interstitial cystitis), physiologic, pharmacologic, and structural changes can occur. Further, experimental studies indicate that sex hormones alter the structure and distribution of cholinergic and adrenergic innervation of the bladder.[20, 131] Such influences would not only have an important bearing on our understanding of bladder physiology, but also may offer innovative therapeutic treatments.

Hormonal Effect on Physiology

The urinary bladder is an estrogen-sensitive organ. Estrogen and progesterone receptors are present in the trigone and urethra. The urethral mucosa decreases in thickness and atrophies after menopause.[132–134] Administration of estrogens to postmenopausal women produces increases in urethral pressure and mucosal thickness and blood vessel engorgement.[135] The density of urethral alpha-sympathetic receptors and sensitivity to alpha agonists is also increased when estrogen is administered.[136–138] The concentrations of estradiol receptors in the urethra and bladder were about 10 to 20 times lower than those in the uterus.[136] Although there is no established minimum for the number of receptors required to define a target cell, an almost doubling of urethral tissue weight in rabbits after 4 days of estradiol treatment suggests that the female urethra is an estrogen-responsive tissue.[136] A study by Longhurst and associates showed that, at least in the rat, ovariectomy has a negligible effect on urinary bladder function.[139] In their model, 4 months after ovariectomy, there were no overt effects on micturition characteristics or bladder mass, but significant decreases in contractile responses of bladder strips occurred. Estradiol treatment prevented the ovariectomy-induced decreases in contractile responsiveness but in addition caused increases in water consumption and urine output. The ability to modulate neurotransmitter receptor density by sex steroid hormones may have important clinical implications in the future.

References

1. Blaivas JG. The neurophysiology of micturition: A clinical study of 550 patients. J Urol 1982; 127:958.
2. Dixon J, Gosling J. Structure and innervation in

the human. In: Torrens M, Morrison JFB, eds. The physiology of the lower urinary tract. London: Springer-Verlag, 1987.

3. Fletcher TF, Bradley WE. Neuroanatomy of the bladder-urethra. J Urol 1978;119:153.

4. Uhlenhuth E, Hunter DW Jr, Loechel WF. Problems in the anatomy of the pelvis. Philadelphia: JB Lippincott, 1953.

5. Griffiths DJ. The mechanics of micturition. In: Yalla SV, Elbadawi A, McGuire EM, Blaivas JG, eds. The Principles and practice of neurourology and urodynamics. New York: Macmillan, 1988: 96–105.

6. Tanagho EA. Interpretation of the physiology of micturition. In: Hinman F Jr, ed. Hydrodynamics of micturition. Springfield, IL: Charles C Thomas, 1971: 18–40.

7. Blaivas JG, Barbalias GA. Characteristics of neural injury after abdominal perineal resection of the rectum. J Urol 1983;129:84.

8. McGuire EJ, Urodynamic evaluation after abdominal-perineal resection and lumbar intervertebral disc herniation. Urology 1975;6:63.

9. Yalla SV, Andriole G. Vesicourethral dysfunction following pelvic visceral ablative surgery. J Urol 1984;132:503.

10. Zinner NR, Sterling AM, Ritter RC. Role of inner wall softness in urinary continence. Urology 1980;16:115.

11. Fagge CH. On the innervation of the urinary passages in dogs. J Physiol 1902;28:304.

12. Hutch JA. A new theory of the anatomy of the internal urinary sphincter and the physiology of micturition, Invest Urol 1965;3:36.

13. Hutch JA. Anatomy and physiology of the bladder, trigone and urethra. New York: Appleton-Century-Crofts, 1972.

14. Tanagho EA, Smith DR. The anatomy and function of the bladder neck. Br J Urol 1966;38:54.

15. Woodburne RT. Anatomy of the bladder and bladder outlet. J Urol 1968;100:474.

16. Gosling JA, Dixon JS, Humpherson JA: Functional anatomy of the urinary tract: An integrated text and color atlas. Edinburg: Churchill-Livingstone, 1993.

17. Zinner NR, Ritter RC, Sterling AM. The mechanism of micturition. In: Chrisholm GD, Williams DE, eds. Scientific foundations of urology. London: Heineman, 1976.

18. Hutch JA. A new theory of the anatomy of the internal urinary sphincter and the physiology of micturition. IV. The urinary sphincteric mechanism. J Urol 1967;97:705.

19. Gil-Vernet S. Morphology and function of vesico-prostatourethral musculature. Treviso: Edizioni Canova. 1968.

20. Elbadawi A. Neuromorphologic basis of vesicourethral function. I. Histochemistry, ultrastructure, and function of intrinsic nerves of the bladder and urethra. Neurourol Urodynam 1982;1:3.

21. Gosling JA, Dixon JS, Lendon RG. The autonomic innervation of the human male and female bladder neck and proximal urethra. J Urol 1977;118:302.

22. Gosling JA, Dixon JS, Critchley HOD, Thompson SA. A comparative study of the human external sphincter and periurethral levator ani muscles. Br J Urol 1981;53:35.

23. Garry RC, Roberts TDM, Todd JI. Reflexes involving the external urethral sphincter of the cat. J Physiol 1959;149:653.

24. Bazeed MA, Thuroff JW, Schmidt RA, Tanagho EA. Histochemical study of urethral striated musculature in the dog. J Urol 1982;128: 406.

25. Oerlich TM. The urethral sphincter muscle in the male. Am J Anat 1980;158:229.

26. Oerlich TM. The striated urogenital sphincter muscle in the female. Anat Rec 1982;205:223.

27. Hanes RW. The striped compressor of the prostatic urethra. Br J Urol 1970;41:481.

28. Yalla SV, Blunt KJ, Fam BA, et al. Detrusor-urethral sphincter dyssynergia. J Urol 1977; 118:1026.

29. Tanagho EA. The anatomy and physiology of micturition. Clin Obstet Gynecol 1978;5:3.

30. Barrington FJF. Relation of hind brain to micturition. Brain 1921;44:23.

31. Barrington FJF. The effect of lesions of the hind and mid-brain on micturition of the cat. Q J Exp Physiol 1925;15:181.

32. Barrington FJF. The component reflexes of micturition in the cat. Parts I & II. Brain 1931; 64:239.

33. Barrington FJF. The localization of the paths subserving micturition in the spinal cord of the cat. Brain 1933;56:126.

34. Barrington FJF. The component reflexes of micturition in the cat. Part III. Brain 1941;64:239.

35. de Groat WC, Kawatani M. Neural control of the urinary bladder: Possible relationship between peptidergic inhibitory mechanisms and detrusor instability. Neurourol Urodynam 1985; 4:285.

36. Bors E, Comarr AE. Neurologic urology. Baltimore: University Park Press, 1971.

37. Elbadawi A. Neuromuscular mechanisms of micturition. In: Yalla SV, Elbadawi A, McGuire EM, Blaivas JG, eds. The principles and practice of neurourology and urodynamics. New York: MacMillan, 1988: 3–35.

38. Kuru M. Nervous control of micturition. Physiol Rev 1965;45:425.

39. Morrison JFB. Bladder control: Role of the higher levels of central nervous system. In: Torrens M, Morrison JFB, eds. The physiology of the lower urinary tract. London: Springer-Verlag, 1987: 237–274.

40. Andrew J, Nathan PW. Lesions of the anterior frontal lobes and disturbances of micturition and defecation. Brain 1964;87:233.

41. Barrington FJF: The central nervous control of micturition. Brain 1928;51:209.

42. Bradley WE, Timm GW, Scott FB. Innervation of the detrusor muscle and urethra. Urol Clin North Am 1974;1:3.

43. Bradley WE, Conway CJ. Bladder representation in the pontine-mesencephalic reticular formation. Exp Neurol 1966;16:237.

44. deGroat WC, Booth AM, Krier J, et al. Neural control of the urinary bladder and large intestine. In: McBrooks C, Koizumi K, Sato A, eds. Integrative functions of the autonomic nervous system. Amsterdam: Elsevier Biomedical Press, 1979.

45. Blaivas JG, Sinha HP, Zayed AAH, Labib KB. Detrusor-external sphincter dyssynergia. J Urol 1981;125:541.

46. deGroat WC, Booth AM. Inhibition and facilitation in parasympathetic ganglia of the urinary bladder. Fed Proc 1980;39:2990.

47. de Groat WC, Kawatani M. Enkephalinergic inhibition in parasympathetic ganglia of the urinary bladder of the cat. J Physiol 1989;413:13.

48. Woodside JR, McGuire EM. Urethral hypotonicity after suprasacral spinal cord injury. J Urol 1979;121:783.

49. Gruber CM. The autonomic innervation of the genitourinary system. Physiol Rev 1933;13:497.

50. Langworthy OR. Innervation of the pelvic organs of the rat. Invest Urol 1965;2:491.

51. Elbadawi A, Schenk EA. A new theory of the innervation of urinary bladder musculature. III. Postganglionic synapses in ureterovesiourethral autonomic pathways. J Urol 1981;105:372.

52. Elbadawi A, Schenk EA. Dual innervation of the mammalian urinary bladder. A histochemical study of the distribution of cholinergic and adrenergic nerves. Am J Anat 1966;119:405.

53. Morgan C, Nadelhaft I, de Groat WC. The distribution of visceral primary afferents from the pelvic nerve within Lissauer's tract and the spinal gray matter and its relationship to the sacral parasympathetic nucleus. J Comp Neurol 1981; 201:415.

54. Nergardh A, Boreus LO. The functional role of cholinergic receptors in the outlet region of the urinary bladder: An in vitro study of the cat. Acta Pharmacol Toxicol (Copenh) 1973;32:467.

55. Brindley GS. Control of the bladder and urethral sphincters by the surgically implantable electrical stimulators. In: Chisolm GD, Williams DF, eds. Scientific foundations in urology. Chicago: Year Book, 1982;464–470.

56. Creed KE, Tulloch AGC. The effect of pelvic nerve stimulation and some drugs on the urethra and bladder of the dog. Br J Urol 1978;50:398.

57. Langworthy OR, Kolb LC, Lewis LG. Physiology of micturition. Experimental and clinical studies with suggestions as to diagnosis and treatment. Baltimore: Williams & Wilkins, 1940.

58. Ambache N, Zar MA. Non-cholinergic transmission by postganglionic motor neurons in the mammalian bladder. J Physiol (Lond) 1970; 210:761.

59. Taira N. The autonomic pharmacology of the bladder. Ann Rev Pharmacol 1972;12:197.

60. Graber P, Tanagho EA. Urethral responses to autonomic nerve stimulation. Urology 1975; 6:52.

61. Elliott TR. The innervation of the bladder and urethra. J Physiol 1906–1907;35:367.

62. Girado JM, Campbell JB. The innervation of the urethra of the female cat. Exp Neurol 1959;1:44.

63. McGuire EJ, Wagner FC Jr. The effects of sacral denervation on bladder and urethral function. Surg Gynecol Obstet 1977;144:343.

64. Yamamoto T, Satomi H, Ise H, et al. Sacral spinal innervation of the rectal and vesical smooth muscles and the sphincteric striated muscles demonstrated by the horseradish peroxidase method. Neurosci Lett 1978;7:41.

65. Coggehsal RE. Law of separation of function of the spinal roots. Physiol Rev 1980;60:716.

66. Norlen L. Influence of the sympathetic nervous system on the lower urinary tract and clinical implications. Neurourol Urodynam 1982;1:129.

67. Barbalias GA, Blaivas JG. Neurologic implication of the pathologically open bladder neck. J Urol 1983;129:780.

68. deGroat WC, Saum WR. Sympathetic inhibition of the urinary bladder and of pelvic ganglionic transmission in cats. J Physiol (Lond) 1972; 214:297.

69. Edvardsen P, Setekleiv J. Distribution of the adrenergic receptors in the urinary bladder of cats, rabbits and guinea pigs. Acta Pharmacol Toxicol 1968;26:437.

70. Levin RM, Wein AJ. Distribution and function of adrenergic receptors in the urinary bladder of the rabbit. Mol Pharmacol 1979;16:441.

71. Benson GS, Wein WJ, Raezer DM, Corriere JN Jr. Adrenergic and cholinergic stimulation and

blockade of the human bladder base. J Urol 1976;116:174.

72. Downie JW, Dean DM, Carro-Ciampi G, Awad SA. A difference in sensitivity to alpha-adrenergic agonists exhibited by detrusor and bladder neck of the rabbit. Can J Physiol Pharmacol 1975;53:525.

73. Ek A, Alm P, Andersson KE, Persson CGA. Adrenergic and cholinergic nerves of the human urethra and urinary bladder: A histochemical study. Acta Physiol Scand 1977;99:34.

74. Nergardh A. The interaction between adrenergic and cholinergic receptor functions in the outlet region of the urinary bladder. Scand Urol Nephrol 1974;8:108.

75. Van Buren GA, Anderson GF. Comparison of the urinary bladder base and detrusor to cholinergic and histaminergic receptor activation in the rabbit. Pharmacology 1979;18:136.

76. Learmonth JR. A contribution to the neurophysiology of the urinary bladder in man. Brain 1931;54:147.

77. de Groat WC, Kawatani M. Reorganization of sympathetic preganglionic connections in cat bladder ganglia following parasympathetic denervation. J Physiol 1989;409:431.

78. Edvardsen P. Nervous control of urinary bladder in cats. IV. Effects of autonomic blocking agents on response to peripheral nerve stimulation. Acta Physiol Scand 1968;72:234.

79. Edvardsen P. Nervous control of the urinary bladder in cats. II. The expulsion phase. Acta Physiol Scand 1968;72:172.

80. Oliver JE, Bradley WE, Fletcher TJ. Spinal cord distribution of the somatic innervation of the external urethral sphincter in the cat. J Neurol Sci 1970;10:11.

81. Tanagho EA, Schmidt RA, Araugo CG. Urinary striated sphincter: What is its nerve supply? Urology 1982;24:415.

82. Rockswold GL, Bradley WE, Chou CM. Innervation of the urinary bladder in higher primates. J Comp Neurol 1980;193:509.

83. Blaivas JG, Scott M, Labib KB. Urodynamic evaluation as a test of sacral cord function. Urology 1979;9:692.

84. deGroat WC, Lalley PM. Reflex firing in the lumbar sympathetic outflow to activation of vesical afferent fibers. J Physiol 1972;226:289.

85. Coolsaet BRLA. Stepwise cystometry. A new method to investigate properties of the urinary bladder. Doctoral thesis. Erasmus University, Rotterdam, 1977.

86. Coolsaet BRLA. Bladder compliance and detrusor activity during the collection phase, Neururol Urodynam 1985;4:263.

87. Van Mastrigt R, Coolsaet BLRA, van Duyl WA. The passive properties of the urinary bladder in the collection phase. Med Biol Eng Comput 1978;16:471.

88. Van Duyl WA. A model for both the passive and active properties of urinary bladder tissue related to bladder function. Neurourol Urodynam 1985;4:275.

89. Tanagho, Smith, DR. Mechanism of urinary continence. I. Embryologic, anatomic and pathologic considerations. J Urol 1968;100:640.

90. Rud T. Urethral pressure profile in continent women from childhood to old age. Acta Obstet Gynecol Scand 1980;59:331.

91. Constantino CE, Govan DE. Spatial distribution and timing of transmitted and reflexly generated urethra pressures in healthy women. J Urol 1982;127:964.

92. Blaivas JG, Jacobs BZ. Pubovaginal fascial sling for the treatment of complicated stress urinary incontinence. J Urol 1991;145:1214–1218.

93. McGuire EM. Urodynamic findings in patients after failure of stress incontinence operations. In: Zinner NR, Sterling AM, eds. Female incontinence. New York: Alan R. Liss, 1981: 351–360.

94. Hafner RJ, Stranton SL, Guy J. A psychiatric study of women with urgency and urgency incontinency. Br J Urol 1977;49:211.

95. Rees DLP, Wickjam JEA, Whitfield HN. Bladder instability in women with recurrent cystitis. Br J Urol 1978;50:524.

96. Frewen WK. The management of urgency and frequency of micturition. Br J Urol 1980;52:367.

97. Kinder RB, Mundy AR. Pathophysiology of idiopathic detrusor instability and detrusor hyperreflexia. Br J Urol 1987;60:509.

98. Fihn SD, Stemm WE. The urethral syndrome. Semin Urol 1983;1:121.

99. Moore KH, Sutherst JR. Response to treatment of detrusor instability in relation to psychoneurotic status. Br J Urol 1990;66:486.

100. Mundy AR, Blaivas JG. Non-traumatic neurological disorders. In: Mundy AR, Stephenson JP, Wein AJ, eds. Urodynamics: Principles, practice and applications. New York: Churchill-Livingstone, 1984: 278–287.

101. Gu J, Blamk MA, Huang WM, Islam KN, et al. Vasoactive intestinal peptide in the normal and unstable bladder. Br J Urol 1983;55:645.

102. Griffiths DJ. Urodynamics: The mechanics and hydrodynamics of the lower urinary tract. Medical Physics Handbooks. Bristol: Adam Hilger, Ltd, 1980.

103. Woodside JR. Micturitional static urethral pressure profilometry in women. Neurourol Urodynam 1982;1:149.

104. Yalla SV, Sharma GVRK, Barsamian EM. Micturitional urethral pressure profile during voiding and the implications. J Urol 1980;124:649.
105. Colstrup H, Mortensen SO, Kristensen JK. A probe for measurements of related values of cross-sectional area and pressure in the resting female urethra. Urol Res 1983;11:139.
106. Sorensen S. Urethral pressure variations in heathy and incontinent women. Neurourol Urodynam 1992;11:549.
107. Barrington FJF. The nervous mechanism of micturition. QJ Exp Physiol 1914;8:33.
108. McGuire EJ, Brady S. Detrusor-sphincter dyssynergia. J Urol 1979;121:774.
109. Khan Z, Hertanu J, Yang WC, et al. Predictive correlation of urodynamic dysfunction in brain injury after cerebrovascular accident. J Urol 1981;126:86.
110. Alm P, Alumets J, Hakanson R, Sundler F. Peptidergic nerves in the genitourinary tract. Neuroscience 1977;2:751.
111. Alumets J, Fahrenkrug R, de Muckadell S, et al. A rich VIP nerve supply is characteristic of sphincters. Nature 1980;280:155.
112. deGroat WC, Kawatani M, Hisamitsu T, et al. The role of neuropeptides in the sacral autonomic reflex pathways of the cat. J Auton Nerv Syst 1983;7:339.
113. Goyal RK, Rathan S, Said SI. VIP as a possible neurotransmitter of non-cholinergic non-adrenergic inhibitory neurons. Nature 1980;288:78.
114. Gu J, Blank MA, Huang WM, et al. Peptide-containing nerves in human urinary bladder. Urology 1984;24:353.
115. Maggi CA, Meli A. The role of neuropeptides in the regulation of the micturition reflex. J Auto Pharmacol 1986;6:133.
116. Andersson PO, Andersson KE, Fahrenkrug J, et al. Contents and effects of substance P and vasoactive intestinal polypeptide in the bladder of rats with and without infravesical outlet obstruction. J Urol 1988;140:168.
117. Burnstock G, Dumsday B, Smythe A. Atropine-resistant excitation of the urinary bladder: The possibility of transmission via nerves releasing purine nucleotide. Br J Pharmacol 1972;44:451.
118. Brown C, Burnstock G, Cocks T. Effect of adenosine 5-triphosphate and B-Y-methylene ATP on the rat urinary bladder. Br J Pharmacol 1979; 65:97.
119. Downie JW, Larsson C. Prostaglandin involvement in contractions in rabbit detrusor by field stimulation and by adenosine 5-triphosphate. Can J Physiol Pharmacol 1981;59:253.
120. Longhurst PA, Belis JA, O'Donnell JP, et al. A study of the atropine-resistance component of the neurogenic response of the rabbit urinary bladder. Eur J Pharmacol 1984;99:295.
121. Levin RM, Ruggieri MR, Wein AJ. Functional effects of the purinergic innervation of the rabbit urinary bladder. J Pharmacol Exp Ther 1985; 236:452.
122. Chancellor MB, Kaplan SA, Blaivas JG. The cholinergic and purinergic components of detrusor contractility in rabbit whole bladder model. J Urol 1992;148:906–909.
123. Klarakov P. Lower urinary tract smooth muscle inhibitory nerve responses. Neurourol Urodynam 1988;7:307.
124. Larsen JJ, Ottesen B, Fahrenkrug J, Fahrenkrug L. Vasoactive intestinal polypeptide in the male genitourinary tract. Invest Urol 1981;19:211.
125. Levin RM, Wein AJ. Effect of vasoactive intestinal polypeptide on the contractility of the rabbit urinary bladder. Urol Res 1981;9:217.
126. Husted S, Sjogren C, Andersson KE. Substance P and somatostatin and excitatory neurotransmission in rabbit urinary bladder. Arch Int Pharmacodyn Ther 1981;252:72.
127. Andersson KE, Ek A, Persson CGA. Effect of prostaglandins on the isolated human bladder and urethra. Acta Physiol Scand 1977;100:165.
128. Andersson KE, Forman A. Effects of prostaglandins on the smooth muscle of the urinary tract. Acta Pharmacol Toxicol (Copenh) 1978; 43:90.
129. Bultitude MI, Hills NA, Shuttleworth KED. Clinical and experimental studies on the action of prostaglandins and their synthesis inhibitors on detrusor muscle in vitro and in vivo. Br J Urol 1976;48:631.
130. Kihara K, Sato K, Ando M, et al. A mechanism of retrograde ejaculation after bilateral hypogastric nerve transection s in the dog. J Urol 1992;148:1307.
131. Mattiasson A, Andersson KE, Elbadawi A, Morgan E, Sjogren C. Interaction between adrenergic and cholinergic nerve terminals in the urinary bladder of rabbit, cat and man. J Urol 1987;137:1017–1019.
132. Batra SC, Iosif CS. 1987. Female urethra: A target for estrogen action. J Urol 1983; 129:418.
133. Iosif CS, Batra SC, Ek A, Astedt B. Estrogen receptors in the human female lower urinary tract. Am J Obstet Gynecol 1981;414:817.
134. Saez S, Martin PM. Evidence of estrogen receptors in the trigone area of human urinary bladder. J Steroid Biochem 1981;15:317.
135. Miodrag A, Castleden CM, Vallance TR. Sex hormones and the female urinary tract. Drugs 1988;36:491.

136. Batra SC, Iosif CS. Female urethra: A target for estrogen action. J Urol 1983;129:418.

137. Shapiro E. Effect of estrogens on the weight and muscarinic cholinergic receptor density of the rabbit bladder and urethra. J Urol 1986;135:1084.

138. Hodgson BJ, Dumas S, Bolling DR, Heesch CM. Effect of estrogen on sensitivity of rabbit bladder and urethra to phenylephrine. J Urol 1978;16:67.

139. Longhurst PA, Kauer J, Leggett RE, Levin RM. The influences of ovariectomy and estradiol replacement on urinary bladder function in rats. J Urol 1992;148:915.

4

Physiology of the Female Genital Tract

John F. Randolph, Jr.

The hallmark of female genital tract physiology is programmed change. Predictable long-term and short-term changes occur in the female genital tract with one overriding purpose, that of procreation. An understanding of the expected changes in the female genital tract that have evolved to promote reproduction facilitates a rational approach to female genital tract abnormalities. This chapter summarizes both the long-term and the short-term changes in female genital tract physiology, with a particular emphasis on the origins and effects of gonadal steroids on the genital tract.

Short-Term Changes— the Menstrual Cycle

The most visible sign of change in the genital tract in reproductive-age women is the menstrual cycle. All events of the menstrual cycle are coordinated to promote the establishment and maintenance of pregnancy or to complete the cycle if pregnancy does not occur in preparation for the next cycle. Loss of cyclicity results in loss of reproductive capacity as well as possible genital tract abnormalities.

The menstrual cycle results from a complex interplay of hormonal and neuroendocrine events reflected in a variety of physiologic changes. This section summarizes the events of the menstrual cycle by looking at individual body compartments and by describing the interplay between compartments.

Normal menstrual cycle length varies from 25 to 30 days with a slight decrease in mean length as a woman ages.[1] The menstrual cycle can be divided into two prominent phases straddling ovulation. The first half of the cycle is the follicular phase, dominated by the development of a mature oocyte in an ovarian follicle with an associated increase in estradiol. This phase of the cycle is also known as the proliferative phase for the characteristic proliferation of endometrium in response to estradiol stimulation. The second half of the cycle is the luteal phase in which the dominant feature is the presence of an active corpus luteum derived from the ovulating follicle and producing progesterone. This is also known as the secretory phase for the characteristic endometrial response to progesterone with gland secretions.

Compartments important in the menstrual cycle include the hypothalamus, pituitary, ovaries, uterus and cervix, and vagina and vulva. The response of the lower urinary tract to cyclic events is also relevant (Table 4-1).

Female Urology, edited by Elroy D. Kursh and Edward McGuire. J. B. Lippincott, Philadelphia, © 1994.

Table 4-1. *Summary of Menstrual Cycle Changes*

BODY COMPARTMENT	FOLLICULAR PHASE	OVULATION	LUTEAL PHASE
Hypothalamus	Accelerating GnRH pulses	Massive GnRH release	Slowing GnRH pulses
Pituitary	Increasing LH release, early FSH dominance	LH and FSH surges	Decreasing LH and FSH
Ovaries	Estradiol secretion from a dominant follicle	Oocyte release	Progesterone secretion from the corpus luteum
Endometrium	Proliferation after superficial shedding	—	Secretion, then decidualization
Cervix	Mucous production	—	Mucous regression
Vagina	Increased epithelial maturation	—	Decreased epithelial maturation
Urethra	Increased epithelial maturation	—	Decreased epithelial maturation

HYPOTHALAMUS

The hypothalamus is that portion of the midbrain immediately beneath the thalamus from which extends the pituitary gland into the sella turcica. The hypothalamus is involved in the control of multiple bodily functions, including thermoregulation, food intake and satiety, and hormonal control of pituitary secretions. Releasing factors from the hypothalamus are transported to the pituitary through the hypothalamic-pituitary portal system to stimulate release of pituitary hormones with resultant systemic effects.

Gonadotropin-releasing hormone (GnRH) is the hypothalamic releasing factor controlling the secretion of the pituitary gonadotropins follicle-stimulating hormone (FSH) and luteinizing hormone (LH).[2] As with most hormones, GnRH is secreted in a pulsatile fashion under a variety of as yet incompletely characterized influences (catecholamines, endogenous opioids, and gonadal steroids).[3] A characteristic change in the pattern of GnRH pulses has been identified across the menstrual cycle.[4] Pulse characteristics include pulse frequency and amplitude.

GnRH pulse frequency in the follicular phase of the cycle has been shown to increase from about one pulse every 90 to 100 minutes during menses to one pulse every 50 to 60 minutes just before ovulation. The initial less frequent pulses favor the release of FSH from the

pituitary with more rapid pulses later in the follicular phase favoring LH release and ultimately an LH surge.[5,6] GnRH pulse amplitude increases dramatically with the development of a mature follicle and contributes to the LH surge signalling for ovulation. Following ovulation, the GnRH pulse generator begins to slow throughout the luteal phase, eventually reaching a frequency of one pulse every 4 to 6 hours in the late luteal phase. This slowing is largely influenced by estradiol and progesterone.[7] With the eventual decline of progesterone and estradiol at the end of the luteal phase, the hypothalamus begins to speed up and initiate follicular development for the next cycle.

PITUITARY

The anterior pituitary secretes a number of hormones in addition to gonadotropins and is influenced principally by releasing factors from the hypothalamus, with major influences through feedback loops by a variety of hormones and factors. FSH and LH released from the pituitary are controlled primarily by GnRH pulse frequency and amplitude with secondary control by ovarian estradiol and other factors such as inhibin. Animal studies have demonstrated direct correlation between LH pulse frequency and GnRH frequency.[8] FSH secretion, however, has not completely correlated with GnRH secretion and has led to speculation of separate control of

FSH release. A putative hypothalamic FSH-releasing factor has not been identified, and many investigators have focused on ovarian feedback as a source of differential regulation.

Mean FSH levels corresponding to preferential FSH secretion begin to increase at the end of the menstrual cycle as gonadal steroid levels fall and the GnRH pulse generator begins to speed up. Mean FSH levels continue to rise through the first half of the follicular phase but then begin to fall as the GnRH pulses become even more frequent and preferentially stimulate LH release. This fall in FSH is also due to a negative feedback effect of rising estradiol levels as well as rising levels of inhibin. There is a smaller but definite surge of FSH coincident with the LH surge and then continual decline until the end of the menstrual cycle, when the negative feedback from the ovary is released and levels again begin to rise.

Mean LH levels begin to rise as the GnRH pulse generator begins to speed up at the end of the menstrual cycle. LH pulse frequency increases in response to GnRH with the resultant increase in mean LH through the follicular phase of the cycle culminating in a massive release of LH, the LH surge. The surge occurs in response to a massive GnRH release from the hypothalamus and is primed by high levels of ovarian estradiol. Mean LH levels then rapidly fall and decline from preovulatory values to a lower steady-state level until the end of the luteal phase.

OVARY

The ovary is both a target organ for gonadotropin stimulation and an endocrine organ producing large amounts of gonadal steroids and other factors. Oocytes are stored in the ovaries, induced to develop and mature, and released from the ovaries in a process coordinated to facilitate pregnancy. A group, or cohort, of follicles is recruited before the onset of a menstrual cycle and begins gonadotropin-independent follicular development. Under the influence of increasing FSH levels, this cohort of follicles is induced to develop further with the eventual selection of a dominant follicle in the midfollicular phase. The dominant follicle is destined to ovulate, whereas the remainder of the cohort undergoes atresia. Coincident with oocyte maturation in the dominant follicle, estradiol production by granulosa cells lining the dominant follicle accelerates, resulting in rising levels of estradiol throughout the latter follicular phase. Peak estradiol levels are reached approximately 2 days before ovulation and contribute both negative feedback, suppressing FSH release, and positive feedback, increasing LH release.[9]

The LH surge initiates the final maturational events of the oocyte, changes the estradiol-producing granulosa cells to estradiol and progesterone-producing luteal cells, and triggers ovulation. Ovulation results from proteolytic enzyme digestion of the wall of the follicle with separation of the oocyte in its cumulus mass and extrusion of the oocyte-cumulus complex by myoepithelial contraction of the follicle.

Luteinized cells begin to produce increasing amounts of progesterone in addition to estradiol, reaching peak levels in the midluteal phase, with a steady decline thereafter. The life span of the corpus luteum is consistently about 14 days with uncertain mechanisms dictating the decline or luteolysis. The corpus luteum can be "rescued" if pregnancy occurs by human chorionic gonadotropin (hCG) derived from trophoblast after implantation in the midluteal phase.[10] Human chorionic gonadotrophin can induce corpus luteum function until a fetal placenta has developed sufficiently to allow the corpus luteum to degenerate at 4 to 6 weeks' postconception. If no conception occurs, progesterone and estradiol levels fall throughout the latter luteal phase. Low levels eventually initiate menses and allow escape of the GnRH pulse generator from negative feedback with the initiation of the next cycle.

UTERUS AND CERVIX

The uterus provides the most visible evidence of reproductive cyclicity as the source of menstrual bleeding. It has long been viewed as primarily a target organ for gonadal steroid stimulation, although there is ample evidence that the uterus also secretes a variety of hormones and factors. The uterine corpus is primarily a sac of smooth muscle lined by endometrium. Endometrium must develop appropriately in every cycle to facilitate implantation and nidation of a conceptus should pregnancy occur. In most of the 300 to 400 cycles in a woman's reproductive life span, conception does not occur, and the endometrium must be shed and redevelop to promote conception in the subsequent cycle.

The endometrium undergoes characteristic histologic and biochemical changes throughout the menstrual cycle in response to gonadal steroids and other factors.[11] The first half of the menstrual cycle is characterized by proliferation of endometrium from the relatively stable basalis layer under the influence of rising levels of estradiol. The three main components of endometrium, epithelial glands, stroma, and blood vessels, all proliferate and increase the thickness of the endometrium fivefold to tenfold. Estrogen receptors are always present in the endometrium and increase under the influence of rising estradiol. Estradiol also induces the development of progesterone receptors, which are essential for later endometrial changes. Endometrial proliferation is the source of the term *proliferative* for this phase of the menstrual cycle. Proliferation continues until ovulation, when progesterone secretion inhibits further growth.

The postovulatory endometrial changes are characterized initially by the secretion of glycogen by endometrial glands into gland lumens and the endometrial cavity under the influence of increasing progesterone. These secretions are used to support the unattached blastocyst in the endometrial cavity before implantation which occurs about 1 week after ovulation if a conception has occurred. Endometrial vessels continue to grow and assume an increasingly tortuous architecture owing to the fixed height of the endometrium. In the latter part of the secretory phase, the endometrial stroma undergoes changes termed *pseudodecidualization*, with enlarged cells

abutting each other and forming a sturdier supporting matrix for a developing implantation. All of these changes require the presence of adequate amounts of progesterone and development of adequate progesterone receptors.

If a pregnancy does not occur, estradiol and progesterone secretion from the corpus luteum fall, resulting in a predictable pattern of endometrial responses. The most dramatic effect is a marked vasomotor response of endometrial arteries with rhythmic vasoconstriction eventually leading to ischemia of the upper two thirds of the endometrium. Vascular integrity is lost with extravasation of blood and eventual coordinated shedding of the ischemic layer. The residual stroma becomes very compact, with bleeding limited by vasoconstriction and estrogen-induced thrombosis of disrupted vessels. Endometrial desquamation occurs within the first 24 hours of menses with visible bleeding lasting 3 to 5 days. Prostaglandins play a prominent role in the endometrial vasomotor response.

The cervix also demonstrates characteristic changes throughout the menstrual cycle in response to gonadal steroids. The two most prominent changes in the cervix involve the diameter of the internal os and changes in cervical mucus secretion.[12] The internal cervical os is constricted except under the influence of peak levels of estradiol in the immediate preovulatory period, when the diameter is increased. The diameter is also somewhat increased during menses with the efflux of the menstrual flow. Cervical mucus is produced by endocervical glands and is generally thick, sticky, and resistant to the passage of sperm or microorganisms. Under the influence of estradiol, the protein latticework of cervical mucus opens with an increase in water content. This results in copious, clear, slippery mucus that can be stretched between two surfaces and demonstrates crystallization when dried on a glass slide. Peak mucus production corresponds with peak estradiol production and peak diameter of the internal cervical os, all facilitating the migration of motile sperm through the cervix to allow conception. With ovulation and the influence of progesterone, the estrogen-induced changes are reversed, restoring the protective mucus barrier to the transcervical passage of pathogens.

VAGINA AND VULVA

Cyclic vaginal changes are less obvious than those seen in the endometrium or cervix. The stratified squamous vaginal epithelium, however, demonstrates the characteristic growth pattern of such epithelium with continuous desquamation of surface cells and replenishment from basal cells.[13] The degree of differentiation and level of desquamation in vaginal epithelium are influenced primarily by gonadal steroids and have been characterized in a number of classification systems. Smaller, more elastic cells from the basal epithelial layer become progressively flatter and broader as they migrate to the epithelial surface with eventual reduction in size of the nucleus. Vaginal epithelium does not normally cornify, and therefore desquamated vaginal epithelial cells have normally not lost the nucleus.

Desquamated vaginal cells most commonly are classified into three groups. Parabasal cells are ovoid cells with plump nuclei and thickened cytoplasm. Intermediate cells are flattened with a polygonal shape but still relatively plump nuclei. Superficial cells are large, flattened, and polygonal with pyknotic dark nuclei. The frequency ratio of these cell types in desquamated vaginal samples reflects the hormonal influence and changes throughout the menstrual cycle. Estrogens promote complete maturation of cells before desquamation. The estrogen-dominant follicular phase is characterized by a predominance of superficial cells. Progesterone promotes desquamation of cells at the intermediate stage. The progesterone-dominant luteal phase is characterized by a predominance of intermediate cells. Androgens typically promote desquamation of all three cell types similar to the pattern seen in inflammatory conditions of the vagina.

The vulva demonstrates little obvious cyclic change in response to patterned fluctuations in gonadal steroids. Vulvar responses are more chronic in nature and are covered later in this chapter.

URETHRA AND BLADDER

Less objective documentation of cyclic changes in urethral and bladder epithelium has been noted, but cytologic studies are available demonstrating cyclic change. Studies of urethral smears have demonstrated cyclic changes across the menstrual cycle similar to those seen in vaginal epithelium.[14] Cytologic studies of urethral cells from urinary sediment have confirmed these findings and have been used to detect ovulation. Estrogen receptors have been identified in the urethra and, taken together with clinical data, suggest consistent cyclic changes throughout the menstrual cycle in response to gonadal steroids.

Long-Term Changes— from Conception to Menopause

An understanding of the evolution of genital tract physiology from conception through the reproductive years is often helpful in understanding changes that occur after the reproductive years. This section provides a broad overview of the time period, including gonadal development and competence with particular attention to the availability and influence of gonadal steroids (Table 4-2).

FETAL PERIOD

The development of the reproductive system from conception to birth can be roughly divided into two time periods. The first half of gestation is characterized by development of the gonads, the reproductive duct systems, and basic neuroendocrine secretory capacity. The second half of gestation is characterized by maturation of these systems.

Germ cells migrate from the yolk sac to the

Table 4-2. The Reproductive Life Span

BODY COMPARTMENT	FETUS	INFANT/CHILD	ADOLESCENT	ADULT	MENOPAUSE
Hypothalamus	Developing GnRH competence	High feedback sensitivity	Falling sensitivity, increasing pulsatility	Cyclic pulsatility	High pulsatility
Pituitary	Developing FSH and LH secretion	Low FSH and LH secretion	Increasing FSH and LH secretion	Cyclic FSH and LH secretion	High FSH and LH secretion
Ovaries	Peak oocyte numbers, estrogen production	Low estrogen, continued atresia	Estrogen secretion, onset of cyclicity	Regular cyclic ovulation	Loss of cyclicity, androgen production
Uterus and tubes	Structural development, endometrial proliferation	Quiescent	Endometrial proliferation, structural maturation	Cyclic endometrial proliferation and shedding	Atrophy
Vagina and vulva	Structural development	Atrophic	Epithelial proliferation and secretion	Cyclic epithelial changes	Atrophy
Urethra	Structural development	Normal function	Normal function	Normal function	Distal atrophy

gonadal ridge at 5 weeks' gestation with evidence of ovarian differentiation within 1 to 3 weeks. The germ cells undergo rapid mitotic division and reach a lifetime maximum of 6 to 7 million oogonia by midgestation. Estradiol synthesis and secretion are first noted in concert with ovarian differentiation, although the contribution to circulating estrogen in comparison with placental estrogens is small. From midgestation on, no further mitotic activity occurs in ovarian germ cells, and the process of initial maturation and atresia of cohorts of cells begins. By birth, the total germ cell complement has been reduced to 2 million cells.

Female genital duct development, including development of estrogen receptors, is largely completed by the end of the first trimester. Vaginal development continues until midgestation.

Production of gonadotropins in the pituitary has been documented as early as 8 weeks' gestation, with rising levels of both LH and FSH detected throughout the first half of pregnancy.[15] Peak levels are reached at midgestation with a decline thereafter. There is evidence that influences by gonadal steroids may provide some neuroendocrine differentiation between males and females, and gonadal steroids are postulated to influence later reproductive and behavioral differences. The central nervous system (CNS) becomes sensitive to the negative feedback effects of gonadal steroids at midgestation, with an increase in sensitivity throughout the rest of gestation. The hypothalamic-pituitary-ovarian axis, however, appears to be remarkably intact later in pregnancy, as evidenced by the not infrequent finding of follicular development in newborn girls.

Systemic influences by placental estrogens and progesterones probably predominate during later gestation with endometrial proliferation and development of breast budding.

NEONATAL PERIOD

Exposure of the infant to placental hormones is abruptly terminated at birth with an immediate reflex rise in gonadotropins due to the loss of negative feedback. Vaginal bleeding in infant girls is common within the first week of life owing to the withdrawal of exogenous estrogens. Breast buds gradually disappear for the same reason.

Over the next 1 to 2 years, the CNS becomes increasingly sensitive to negative feedback from the ovaries, resulting in very low levels of gonadotropins by age 2 years. During this time period, ovarian follicle development is relatively common and sometimes confused with a neoplastic process.

The vaginal epithelium at birth is well differentiated under the influence of placental steroids. With the postnatal drop in steroids, there is a mass exfoliation of the more mature intermediate cell layer with a resultant thin and atrophic epithelium.

CHILDHOOD

Early childhood is characterized by low levels of gonadotropins and resultant low levels of gonadal steroids. Ovarian follicular atresia continues throughout childhood, constantly depleting the germ cell complement. The vaginal epithelium remains thin and atrophic with little evidence of maturation. Between 4 and 10 years of age, there is a slight and gradual increase in gonadotropins but no significant change in gonadal steroids.

PUBERTY

The precise signal for the onset of puberty is unknown but normally occurs somewhere between 8 and 10 years of age.[16] The hypothalamus and pituitary begin to lose the exquisite sensitivity to gonadal steroids characteristic of childhood and demonstrate increasing secretory activity. In response to the increase in gonadotropin pulsatility, ovarian follicular development and estradiol production begin. Gonadotropin secretion and ovarian follicular development eventually coordinate and mature, resulting in ovulatory cycles.

Increasing levels of ovarian estradiol induce

breast budding and further development. The uterus grows in response to estrogen stimulation and changes from a childhood corpus to cervix ratio of 1:1 to an adult ratio of 2:1. Urogenital epithelial proliferation begins with an increasing percentage of intermediate and superficial cells.

Early breast development is the first sign of puberty in about two thirds of pubescent girls. Pubic hair development begins first in the other third, reflecting the almost simultaneous maturation of the hypothalamic-pituitary-adrenal axis. Breast development generally precedes menarche by about 2 years, although the time span is quite variable. The first menses usually precede regular ovulatory cycles by about a year, and the full maturation of the urogenital system may not be complete for several years after menarche.

ADULTHOOD

Adulthood may be considered to extend from the onset of normal reproductive capacity until menopause. It is characterized in normally functioning women by regular menstrual cyclicity as elaborated earlier. There are, however, both short-term and long-term changes in cyclicity characteristic of adulthood.

The most dramatic short-term change in regular cyclicity occurs with pregnancy. If timing and conditions are appropriate, the oocyte released from the dominant follicle encounters viable sperm in the distal third of the fallopian tube within 12 hours after ovulation and is penetrated and fertilized. Embryonic development begins in the fallopian tube, where the embryo stays for the first 3 days postfertilization, presumably under the influence of rising levels of progesterone. The embryo is then transported to the endometrial cavity, where it eventually implants a week after ovulation and fertilization. The bulk of the embryo becomes trophoblast, which eventually develops into placenta and membranes and begins to produce increasing amounts of hCG. Circulating levels of hCG can be detected with sensitive assays within 8 to 9 days after ovulation and fertilization and before the first

missed menses. Human chorionic gonadotrophin functions as LH and "rescues" the corpus luteum, inducing it to continue to produce increasing amounts of progesterone. The progesterone in turn maintains the endometrium, now termed *decidua*, to allow support of the developing pregnancy.

At 4 to 6 weeks' postconception, the corpus luteum regresses for unknown reasons.[17] Trophoblast/placental development has progressed to provide increasing amounts of progesterone to continue the support of pregnancy and replace the corpus luteum. Human chorionic gonadotrophin levels continue to rise throughout the first trimester, reaching a peak at about 12 weeks' gestation with a steady decline thereafter.

The human placenta is a rich source of increasing amounts of progesterone and estrogens throughout pregnancy. Quantitatively the most significant hormone produced is the weak estrogen estriol, which is believed to promote uteroplacental blood flow and growth. A large variety of other steroid and peptide hormones are produced by the placenta, membranes, and fetus, all directed at optimizing fetal growth and development and ultimate birth.

In response to this dramatic change in the hormonal milieu, the female genital tract undergoes dramatic changes. The uterus hypertrophies to accommodate the growing fetus and ultimately to expel the infant and other contents. Supporting ligaments relax. The ovaries become relatively quiescent owing to the negative feedback on the pituitary with reduced gonadotropins. Blood flow to the entire pelvis increases as well as vaginal epithelial turnover. The cytologic pattern is consistent with both estrogen and progesterone exposure with an increase in intermediate cells. Vulvar pigmentation may increase as a result of stimulation of melanocytes.

Increased cardiac output and some increase in striated muscle mass are noted, especially in the proximal lower extremities. Breast areolar development occurs with eventual preparation for lactation.

Initiation of labor in humans is incompletely understood but involves prostaglandins and is not under significant neural control. Regular rhythmic contractions ideally lead to the expulsion of the infant through the dilated cervix and vagina. Significant tearing of cervix, vaginal mucosa, introitus, and pelvic floor striated muscle can occur with childbirth and may contribute to later mechanical problems.

Following delivery of the placenta, there is a rapid decline in circulating gonadal steroids and pregnancy-derived peptide hormones. If the woman does not nurse, cyclic ovarian function is resumed when pregnancy-induced hormones have been cleared, generally 4 to 6 weeks' postpartum. If the woman is nursing, an initial hyperprolactinemic state is maintained to facilitate milk production. The hyperprolactinemia is associated with hypogonadotropism, resulting in persistent anovulation and low estrogen levels. The elevated prolactin levels gradually decline over the next several weeks but are transiently elevated during suckling.[18] These episodic periods of hyperprolactinemia maintain the hypoestrogenic anovulatory state until about 6 months' postpartum, when ovulatory cycles generally resume. There is some variability depending on the frequency and duration of breast-feeding.

Lactational amenorrhea is analogous to menopausal amenorrhea with hot flashes and thinning of the vaginal and vulvar epithelium. Vulvovaginal atrophy can lead to significant dyspareunia.

Long-term changes in the menstrual cycle throughout adulthood are characterized by a gradual decrease in menstrual cycle length throughout a woman's reproductive life span.[1] The mean decrease in cycle span is about 2 days. Subtle differences in menstrual cycle characteristics may be noticeable to some women 10 to 15 years before menopause. Premenopausal cycles are characterized by increasingly frequent abnormal or anovulatory cycles eventually culminating in loss of cyclicity and menopause.

The last decade before menopause is remarkable for a dramatic deterioration in fertility, both in terms of conception and in pregnancy loss rates.[19] There is also an increase in the frequency of conceptions with chromosomal trisomies. Some women demonstrate a decline in mean estrogen levels at this time and may be at risk for premenopausal bone loss owing to the relative hypoestrogenemia.

As a result of a decline in negative feedback from the ovary, pituitary gonadotropin levels variably rise before actual menopause.[20] This may be due to a relative decrease in estrogen or may reflect declining levels of follicular inhibin as cohorts of follicles become smaller. Generally vaginal blood flow and resultant epithelial proliferation and lubrication are adequate for comfortable intercourse until menopause.

MENOPAUSE

The mean age of menopause in the United States is 51.4 years and is defined as the last menstrual period.[21] It is important to remember, however, that menopause simply marks the point in the progressive decrease in ovarian estrogen production when the endometrium is insufficiently stimulated to proliferate and ultimately shed. The continuum of changing ovarian function from the early reproductive years through the premenopausal period shifts in the postmenopausal period away from ovarian estrogen production. It is the hypoestrogenemia of the postmenopausal period that is primarily responsible for the majority of the changes of the female genital tract.

Ovaries maintain steroidogenic activity after menopause, although normal cyclic ovulatory activity dominated by estrogen production is lost. Androgens are the principal secretory products of postmenopausal ovaries, initially with significant secretion followed by a gradual decline. Testosterone secretion increases significantly in early postmenopausal women compared with premenopausal secretion.[22] In conjunction with the dramatic decline in estradiol production, the androgen to estrogen ratio from postmenopausal ovaries is dramatically increased. Androstenedione, a quantitatively greater but relatively weaker androgen, is secreted in smaller amounts by the postmenopausal ovary and is primarily derived from the adrenal glands. Significant amounts of estrogen are produced, however, primarily by conversion of circulating androstenedione and testosterone in peripheral tissues such as fat and muscle.[23] The principal postmenopausal circulating estrogen is estrone, a weaker estrogen than estradiol. Obese women may have significant estrone production and have sufficient estrogen effect to avoid the changes of hypoestrogenemia. These women, however, are at risk for the problems of unopposed estrogen exposure, with endometrial proliferation, irregular bleeding, and the risk of endometrial carcinoma. Slender women are less able to convert androgens to estrogens peripherally and are more likely to suffer hypoestrogenic symptoms.

Postmenopausal ovaries gradually shrink and usually are nonpalpable on pelvic examination several years after menopause. A palpable ovary after this time is a sign of possible ovarian pathology and requires further investigation.

The fallopian tubes diminish in size somewhat with hypoestrogenemia, with a gradual loss of ciliated cells on the tubal mucosa. Estrogen replacement therapy restores tubal mucosa to its premenopausal appearance.

The postmenopausal uterus gradually decreases in size from a premenopausal weight of 75 to 100 g to as little as 25 to 30 g in the geriatric population.[24] The corpus to cervix ratio regresses to the preadolescent measurement of 1:1. The endometrium undergoes atrophy, becoming thin with decreased blood vessels and endometrial glands. Endometrium retains estrogen receptors, however, and is able to respond to estrogen and progesterone in a normal premenopausal fashion. It has been documented that the endometrium in women with premature menopause can be receptive to and support pregnancy when stimulated by exogenous gonadal steroids.[25] Inactive postmenopausal endometrium is somewhat more susceptible to infections owing to its decreased vascularity.

The postmenopausal cervix decreases in size in conjunction with the uterus. The ectocervix usually becomes flush with the vaginal mucosa with migration of the squamocolumnar junction into the endocervical canal. The epithelium of the ectocervix thins and becomes fragile, often bleeding at the time of the Papanicolaou smear.

The postmenopausal vagina undergoes progressive epithelial thinning with loss of cytologic maturation and a shift to a predominantly parabasal cell pattern. Grossly the vaginal epithelium demonstrates a loss of rugae and is either pale or erythematous. Vaginal blood flow decreases, and there is a loss of elasticity with a relative increase in vaginal connective tissue. The vaginal dimensions decrease. The pH of the vagina increases owing to a loss of epithelial glycogen and a decrease in lactic acid production. Vaginitis is more common in a less acidic environment and is a common problem after menopause. Owing to thinning of the vaginal epithelium and the decrease in dimensions and distensibility of the vagina, the epithelium is prone to trauma and resultant "atrophic" bleeding. So-called atrophic vaginitis is responsible for 15% of postmenopausal bleeding.[26] Vaginal fluid is also decreased, usually resulting in decreased lubrication with intercourse. Dyspareunia is common, although regular coital activity provides some protection against atrophic changes. Dyspareunia frequently leads to the vicious cycle of decreased coital activity and progressive atrophy, resulting in the eventual abandonment of sexual intercourse.

The postmenopausal vulva undergoes changes both from hypoestrogenemia and from hormone-independent mechanisms. Pubic hair diminishes, and the labia decrease in size with a loss of subcutaneous fat and elastic tissue in the labia majora and progressive atrophy of the labia minora. Vulvar glands secrete less with sexual arousal, adding to the lubrication problem with intercourse. The vulvar epidermis thins and grossly may appear erythematous and smooth. There may be some slight increase in size of the clitoris, perhaps owing to the increase in androgen to estrogen ratio following menopause.

The bulk of these changes are related to hypoestrogenemia. The loss of subcutaneous fat and elastic tissue and thinning of pubic hair may be general changes related to aging and do not respond well to estrogen replacement therapy. Mechanical changes, especially musculoskeletal, as a result of childbirth trauma or chronic diseases also may contribute to vulvovaginal changes and do not respond to estrogen replacement.

Urethral cytologic studies demonstrate good correlation with vaginal smears and demonstrate a shift to a hypoestrogenic parabasal cell–dominant exfoliative picture.[27] Urethral blood flow decreases postmenopausally, particularly the submucosal plexus. This decrease in vasculature may decrease the urethral pressure and contribute to incontinence.[28] Distal urethral atrophy may increase the risk of ascending urinary tract infections, leading to nocturia, urgency, and voiding difficulties. Estrogen treatment of such symptoms of less than a year's duration results in significant improvement, whereas complaints for more than a year are more resistant to replacement therapy. The more prolonged cases may reflect chronic fibrosis and stricture formation in addition to epithelial atrophy.

ESTROGEN REPLACEMENT THERAPY

Estrogen replacement in physiologic doses generally reverses the majority of postmenopausal genital tract atrophic changes. Estrogen replacement therapy is also strongly promoted for the prevention of postmenopausal osteoporosis and beneficial cardiovascular effects with a favorable influence on circulating lipids. Women without absolute contraindications to estrogen replacement therapy can usually be managed effectively and favorably (Table 4-3).

Most of vulvovaginal atrophic changes improve with estrogen replacement, leading to a significant improvement in sexual functioning, a decrease in atrophic vaginitis and bleeding, and improvement in vulvar pruritus. Subcutaneous loss of fat and elastic tissue does not reverse, and estrogen does not completely restore normal vaginal function without some mechanical activity. Estrogen-primed cytologic changes occur as in the premenopausal state. Epithelial changes occur relatively rapidly, usually within several

Table 4-3. Estrogen Replacement Therapy

ADVANTAGES	DISADVANTAGES
Reverses hypoestrogenic atrophic changes	Promotes endometrial neoplasia if unopposed
Retards osteoporosis	May exacerbate other conditions
Reduces cardiovascular risk	Uncertain association with breast disease
Restores vasomotor stability	

weeks to several months. Blood flow changes require a longer period of therapy and may take 6 to 12 months. There may be some improvement in incontinence and voiding symptoms.

Endometrium responds to estrogen replacement therapy with proliferation. It is imperative to counteract the unchecked proliferative effects of estrogen with progesterone to protect against endometrial hyperplasia and neoplasia. If this important point is kept in mind, estrogen replacement therapy can be offered to most postmenopausal women. Women without a uterus can be managed with estrogen alone or in combination with a progestin. There is some theoretical support for the use of progestins to protect against estrogen-associated breast cancer. Studies to date, however, have failed to link either estrogen to increased breast cancer or progestins to decreased breast cancer conclusively, and many practitioners do not add a progestin to estrogen therapy in the absence of a uterus.

There are multiple therapeutic regimens and options for hormone replacement therapy. Conjugated equine estrogens have enjoyed the widest use in the United States with fairly extensive data on the appropriate dosage and associated problems. For most postmenopausal women, 0.625 mg once daily by mouth is recommended to prevent osteoporosis, alleviate vasomotor symptoms, and restore urogenital and epithelial integrity. The most common regimen in the past has been cyclic therapy with 0.625 mg daily for 21 to 25 days each month with the addition of medroxyprogesterone acetate, 10 mg orally daily, for the last 10 days on estrogen. This regimen provides a predictable cyclic withdrawal bleed and is acceptable therapy to many women.

Many women, however, do not relish the idea of continued menses in the postmenopausal period and have requested alternative therapies. Newer regimens include continuous oral estrogen with cyclic progestin and continuous estrogen and progestin. Current clinical trials are assessing the safety and efficacy of both regimens. Transdermal estrogen is also available for women with difficulties tolerating oral estrogen and is an effective alternative in many situations. The cardioprotective effect of estrogen, however, may be diminished with transdermal administration owing to diminished hepatic effects. A subcutaneous progestin has been approved in the United States for long-term contraception. Subcutaneous implants for postmenopausal hormonal replacement therapy may be approved in the future.

References

1. Treolar AE, Boynton RE, Behn BG, Brown BW. Variation of the human menstrual cycle through reproductive life. Int J Fertil 1967;12:77.
2. Schally AV, Arimura A, Kastin AJ, et al. Gonadotropin releasing hormone: One polypeptide regulates secretion of LH and FSH. Science 1971; 173:1036.
3. Knobil E. The neuroendocrine control of the menstrual cycle. Rec Prog Horm Res 1980;36:53.
4. Marshall JC, Kelch RP: Gonadotropin-releasing hormone: Role of pulsatile secretion in the regulation of reproduction. N Engl J Med 1986;315:1459.
5. Haisenleder DJ, Khoury S, Zmeili SM, et al. The frequency of gonadotropin releasing hormone secretion regulates expression of alpha and luteinizing hormone beta subunit messenger ribonucleic acids in male rats. Mol Endocrinol 1987;1:834.
6. Dalkin AC, Haisenleder DJ, Ortolano GA, Ellis T, Marshall JC. The frequency of gonadotropin releasing hormone (GnRH) stimulation differentially regulates gonadotropin subunit mRNA expression. Endocrinology 1989;125:917.
7. Nippoldt TB, Reame N, Kelch RP, Marshall JC. The roles of estradiol and progesterone in decreasing luteinizing hormone pulse frequency in the luteal phase of the menstrual cycle. J Clin Endocrinol Metab 1989;59:67.
8. Clarke IJ, Cummins JT. The temporal relationship between gonadotropin releasing hormone (GnRH) and luteinizing hormone (LH) secretion in ovariectomized ewes. Endocrinology 1982; 1111:1737.
9. Hoff JD, Quigley ME, Yen SSC. Hormonal dynamics at midcycle: A reevaluation. J Clin Endocrinol Metab 1983;57:792.
10. Van deWiele RL, Bogumil J, Dyrenfurth I, et al. Mechanisms regulating the menstrual cycle in women. Rec Prog Horm Res 1970;26:63.
11. Noyes RW, Hertig AW, Rock J. Dating the endometrial biopsy. Fertil Steril 1950;1:3.
12. Gibor Y, Garcia CJ, Cohen MR, Scommegna A. The cyclical changes in the physical properties of the cervical mucus and the results of the postcoital test. Fertil Steril 1970;21:20.
13. Frost JK. Gynecologic and obstetric clinical cytopathology. In: Novak ER, Woodruff JD, eds. Gynecologic and obstetric pathology. 8th ed. Philadelphia: WB Saunders, 1979:689.
14. Krouse TB. Menopausal pathology. In: Eskin BA, ed. The menopause: comprehensive management. New York: Masson Publishing USA, 1980:9.
15. Kaplan SL, Grumbach MM, Aubert ML. The ontogenesis of pituitary hormones and hypothalamic factors in the human fetus. Maturation of central nervous system regulation of anterior pituitary function. Rec Prog Horm Res 1976; 32:161.
16. Reiter EO, Grumbach MM. Neuroendocrine control mechanisms and the onset of puberty. Ann Rev Physiol 1982;44:595.
17. Csapo AL, Pulkkinen MO, Wiest WG. Effects of luteectomy and progesterone replacement in early pregnant patients. Am J Obstet Gynecol 1973;115:759.
18. Short RV. Breast feeding. Sci Am 1984;250:35.
19. Tietze C. Reproductive span and rate of reproduction among Hutterite women. Fertil Steril 1957;8:89.
20. Sherman BW, West JH, Korenman SG. The menopausal transition. Analysis of LH, FSH, estradiol and progesterone concentrations during menstrual cycles of older women. J Clin Endocrinol Metab 1976;42:629.
21. Jaszmann LJB. Epidemiology of the climacteric syndrome. In: Campbell S, ed. The management of the menopause and postmenopausal years. Baltimore: University Park Press, 1976:12.
22. Judd HL, Judd GE, Lucas WE, Yen SSC. Endocrine function of the postmenopausal ovary: Con-

centrations of androgens and estrogens in ovarian peripheral vein blood. J Clin Endocrinol Metab 1974;39:1020.

23. Grodin JM, Siiteri PK, MacDonald PC. Source of estrogen production in postmenopausal women. J Clin Endocrinol Metab 1973;36:207.

24. Utian WH. Problems of the untreated menopause. In: van Herendael H, van Herendael B, eds. The Climacteric: An Update. Hingham, MA: MTP Press, 1983:104.

25. Sauer MV, Paulson RJ, Lobo RA. A preliminary report on oocyte donation extending reproductive potential to women over 40. N Engl J Med 1990;323:1157.

26. Hammond CB, Maxson WS. Current status of estrogen therapy for the menopause. Fertil Steril 1982;37:5.

27. Smith P. Age changes in the female urethra. Br J Urol 1972;44:667.

28. Corlett RC. Urinary tract disorders. In: Buchsbaum HJ, ed. The Menopause. New York: Springer-Verlag, 1983:134.

II

Detrusor Incontinence

5

Disorders of the Control of Bladder Contractility

Edward J. McGuire

There are several specific causes of uncontrolled bladder contractility, but probably the best recognized are those associated with neural disease or injury.

Neural Etiology

Incontinence related to disorders of the control of bladder contractility can be subdivided by the location of the neural lesion resulting in the abnormality. These can be supraspinal, spinal, or peripheral. Because the association between incontinence and supraspinal disease is circumstantial, incontinence does not by itself suggest an intracerebral process or vice versa; evaluation of incontinence as a symptom in patients with known or suspected neural disease or when a neurogenic process is not suspected involves the following steps.

A history of the pattern of the incontinence, including any suggestion of stress incontinence as well as the precise timing of the incontinence, is important. Does leakage occur in specific circumstances, as, for example, when arising in the morning or returning home (which symptoms are consistent with motor contractile incontinence)? If the leakage occurs only when the subject is upright and not when supine, urethral

dysfunction is likely. Physical examination with attention to anal sphincter tone and perineal sensation as well as deep tendon and pathologic reflexes is important, but these findings even if positive are not usually sufficient for a urologic diagnosis to be established. Specific urologic evaluation includes urinalysis, residual urine determination, and as complete a urodynamic evaluation as possible. Videourodynamics is best because this incorporates a study of bladder storage responses, urethral closing function, and bladder and urethral micturition responses. In lieu of videourodynamic testing, a cystometrogram to determine storage responses and a provocative cystometrogram to determine the degree of detrusor irritability, preferably with a good-quality interference pattern electromyogram, are helpful. The examiner first needs to determine whether the lower urinary tract behaves as if it is completely free of cortical and subcortical control. Next the examiner needs to determine whether the neural lesion appears to separate the working neural circuits from the basal ganglia and cerebellar axis and whether the brain stem center appears to function in control of the phasing and sequence of bladder and urethral activity. Supraspinal, intracerebral lesions, as, for example, a cerebrovascular accident, are associated with absence of cortical

Female Urology, edited by Elroy D. Kursh and Edward McGuire. J. B. Lippincott, Philadelphia, © 1994.

override of detrusor reflex events. Patients with Parkinson's disease (or syndrome) show abnormalities of bladder modulating and contractile facilitory activity, and brain stem lesions have features of both supraspinal and spinal cord lesions. The latter separate the sacral spinal cord segments concerned with lower urinary tract function from the brain stem center, which results in discoordinate bladder and external sphincter responses, short-duration detrusor responses, residual urine, and high bladder pressures.

Neural Lesions

Supraspinal diseases, for example, a space occupying lesion or vascular disease (*e.g.*, hemorrhagic or thrombotic stroke), usually induce acute detrusor areflexia, which is followed by the development of virtually automatic reflex bladder and urethral activity. This kind of bladder dysfunction, which is peculiar to intracerebral disease of all types, is due to uninterrupted function of the brain stem center for reflex lower urinary tract activity. Both bladder storage responses to filling and the micturition response occur relatively normally but are not subordinate to volitional control. Bladder contractility occurs suddenly with little subjective warning, although detrusor and external sphincter responses are coordinate, and the bladder usually empties. Cystometric examination of the bladder shows sudden, unanticipated reflex vesical contractility, which is preceded by a fall in urethral external sphincter activity either measured by pressure or EMG responses. Although most patients do contract their external sphincter when they appreciate that an unwanted bladder contraction is in progress, this is not reflexly determined detrusor sphincter dyssynergia but rather a volitional response to an uninhibited, hyperreflexic detrusor contraction. Subjectively patients do not appear to be able to tell precisely how full their bladder is or what it might do until a bladder contraction is actually in progress. The differential diagnosis in men is obstructive uropathy related to benign prostatic hypertrophy. In women, true outlet obstruction is unusual, and a more common association is stress incontinence associated either with urethral hypermobility or poor closing function of the proximal urethra.

Once incontinence is established, the characteristics of that problem have important consequences for treatment. Not all demented patients (who have a kind of intracerebral disease even if that is not well defined) are incontinent, but those who are are extremely difficult to treat because they do not recognize the incontinence as a problem. Patients with parkinsonism and those suffering from the sequelae of a major cerebrovascular accident are usually troubled by incontinence and are often unable to communicate accurately to caregivers what happens to them when they experience wetting. A degree of patience and understanding is helpful to the urologist in delineating the individual circumstances in which the incontinence occurs. Sometimes patients with almost normal bladder function simply cannot act sufficiently quickly to avoid incontinence because of relative loss of mobility, coupled with an inability to warn caregivers or attendants about a bladder contraction. A cystometrogram may show an unsuppressed bladder contraction, which often occurs at a lower volume than normal, but that finding does not represent the entire explanation for the incontinence.

Patients with Parkinson's disease or syndrome are often incontinent and complain of urgency, frequency, and nocturia. These patients demonstrate residual urine volumes in amounts up to 100 to 200 ml. Urodynamic evaluation shows sudden reflex bladder contractility, a slowly relaxing external sphincter, and early cessation of the bladder contraction before complete emptying. When the latter occurs, there are two possible explanations: (1) The detrusor is weakened, and the energy available for a given micturition cycle is depleted by the work the bladder is forced to do. (2) The contraction is not fully facilitated and ceases on that basis before complete emptying has occurred. Although the former clearly occurs in obstructive uropathy, the latter is more typical of neurogenic conditions, most notably spinal cord injury and parkinsonism. In the latter, it appears that facilitation of lower urinary tract reflex responses to filling, both storage and micturition responses, are incomplete. In men, because of the finding of an enlarged prostate, residual urine, urgency, and frequency, this often leads to prostatectomy. In women, this is more often treated by anticholinergic agents, which makes the detrusor inefficiency worse, as does treatment of the primary disease with drugs with anticholinergic side effects. In contrast, diabetic patients suffering from bladder-related incontinence may require large bladder volumes to generate a reflex detrusor response, and lesser volumes than those required to excite a reflex response are not associated with subjective appreciation of the degree of bladder filling. We have considered the diabetic bladder to be an expression of an afferent denervation process similar to that associated with tabes dorsalis, but there is no concrete proof that this is the case. We do not know if the lesion is central or peripheral nor where in those two broad areas the lesion is. Resnick and Yalla have described in elderly women a syndrome of incontinence and bladder instability with incomplete emptying, which they found particularly difficult to treat.[1] The incidence of this syndrome increases with age. Although the presumptive cause is a poor-quality detrusor contraction, that is not proved, and it is not clear whether the abnormality of bladder emptying is related to a lack of neural facilitation or replacement of bladder muscle with fibrous tissue, which process seems to occur with aging. There may be alternatively some subtle change in the elasticity of the urethra with respect to its urinary conduit function. Some early studies by Sussett and Plante on the vesicoelastic properties of the female urethra have been reopened by Lose and associates in Denmark, and this may help to explain some of the vagaries of detrusor instability in women, particularly elderly women, in whom residual urine is an additional problem.[2,3]

Treatment

Hyperreflexic detrusor contractile responses associated with cerebral disease are distinguished by a lack of early subjective recognition of a detrusor contraction. Occasionally total failure of automatic modulating activity leads to small volume, repetitive contractility and residual urine. Treatment depends on whether the detrusor response is frequent and easily provoked, in which case drug therapy with oxybutynin chloride, 2.5 to 5 mg three times a day, or imipramine 10 to 25 mg three to four times daily, is likely to improve bladder capacity and detrusor control, even if this is not associated with perfect continence. Because warning times for detrusor contractility are short, it is worthwhile to combine drug therapy with a timed, anticipatory voiding schedule, for example, voiding on a 2- to 3-hour basis. Even if the bladder responds to the medication, if urinary sensation does not improve, symptomatic cure may not occur.

If residual urine is present (and even if that does occur, the amount may vary considerably), poor bladder function must be included in the differential diagnosis, along with incomplete neural facilitation and obstructive uropathy. Poor bladder function related, for example, to radiation-induced fibrosis combined with bladder motor instability might best be treated by anticholinergic agents and intermittent catheterization if that can be accomplished. This method of treatment is effective for incontinence associated with poor emptying for other reasons, including parkinsonism and diabetes, but it is difficult to implement in the elderly. If intermittent catheterization can be used, direct instillation of lidocaine (Xylocaine) solution (90 ml of 1% solution in 1000 ml saline), 30 ml, after catheterization or other intravesical anticholinergic agents can be used to circumvent the troublesome side effects associated with oral anticholinergic drugs. If these conservative measures fail, some surgical option must be considered.

Spinal Cord Injury or Disease

Complete or incomplete spinal cord injuries have a profound effect on function of the lower urinary tract. In this regard, "incomplete" lesions refer to spinal cord injuries or diseases characterized by variable sparing of neural function below the level of the lesion. The degree of incompleteness has some relationship to the severity of the lower urinary tract dysfunction, but the relationship is not constant. Patients with some patchy sensory or motor sparing insufficient for useful lower extremely function manifest on occasion nearly normal reflex bladder contractility, whereas others who have regained the ability to walk may never recover useful reflex vesical function.

Traditionally transverse *upper motor neuron* lesions, or those between C1-2 and T11-12 (lesions superior to the sacral cord segments but inferior to the brain stem micturition center), have been associated with reflex vesical contractility, which is both difficult to control and inefficient because of the concomitant development of dyssynergic external sphincter responses. This constellation of lower urinary tract dysfunction, if untreated, induces with time severe uncontrollable reflex bladder contractility, intractable incontinence, residual urine, urinary tract infection, and a risk to upper urinary tract function. Until relatively recently, the precise mechanism whereby this kind of lower urinary tract dysfunction influenced ureteral and renal function was not known. It was difficult to separate problems encountered in women with spinal cord lesions that were the results of urologic management from those that resulted from dysfunction induced by the neural lesion. In the past, women with severe incontinence associated with spinal disease or injury were almost always treated by catheter drainage of one kind or another, and when that failed, supravesical urinary diversion was done. It is now clear that at least some of the upper and lower urinary tract problems encountered in patients with spinal cord lesions, including renal infection, upper tract and bladder stone formation, loss of the bladder as a reservoir, vesicoureteral reflux, and urethral erosion, can be related directly to catheter drainage. A study of equal numbers of women treated by intermittent catheterization or by urethral catheter drainage showed a high degree of association between serious complications and use of an indwelling catheter.[4,5] *Incontinence*, despite chronic catheterization, which was initiated to treat that specific condition, was more of a problem in the catheterized group than the intermittent catheterization group.

A study of patients with neurogenic vesical dysfunction treated at the University of Michigan for upper tract stone disease indicates the superiority of management of the lower urinary tract by methods other than supravesical diversion or chronic catheter drainage.[6] It could be argued that it is the severity of the condition that prompts treatment with catheters or suprapubic tubes and that the outcome is determined by the urologic problem that demands treatment and not the treatment. Men with identical lesions and identical urodynamically identified bladder and urethral dysfunction, however, clearly do better if treated without catheters. Those treated by sphincter ablative procedures and condom catheter drainage do much better in terms of overall outcome with respect to renal function, stone formation, urethral integrity, autonomic dysreflexia, hypertension, and bladder cancer than those treated with catheters or supravesical diversion. Obviously women cannot be treated effectively by sphincterotomy and condom catheter drainage, but a study of both male and female spinal cord–injured patients (128), with a mean follow-up of 5 years, indicates that early use of intermittent catheterization with suppression of reflex bladder activity as soon as that occurs is associated with a 96% rate of perfect continence on an every 4 hour intermittent catheterization program.[7] This in turn is associated with preservation of a flat bladder pressure volume curve and the total lack of development of high pressure repetitive detrusor sphincter dyssynergia. Preservation of low bladder storage pressures is associated with maintenance of perfectly normal upper urinary tracts. This kind of excellent outcome has also been recorded after sphincterotomy in men, presumably as a result of the effects of that procedure on bladder pressures. Urinary leakage occurs at a pressure determined by the sphincterotomy. If that pressure is low, for example, less than 20 cm H_2O, this appears to prevent the repetitive interaction of a contracting bladder and a high pressure external sphincter, which leads to progressive loss of bladder compliance and a consequent risk to the upper urinary tract.

Once detrusor sphincter dyssynergia has been well established for some time, restoration of normal bladder storage activity becomes more difficult. For example, 25% of patients with upper motor neuron lesions treated by intermittent catheterization in the University of Michigan series never required any drug therapy to maintain low pressure areflexic vesical activity. Patients treated by methods designed to encourage reflex voiding or by catheter drainage for periods longer than 3 to 4 months after injury become much more difficult to treat effectively by intermittent catheterization and drugs alone, as are those patients who present at 5 to 6 years after injury with a major complication related to upper urinary tract function. In these patients, continued management by the method associated with the development of upper tract disease is not a reasonable option, but conversion to a tubeless low pressure reservoir system is much more difficult at this stage than if that kind of treatment is begun early.

Multiple Sclerosis

Multiple sclerosis is a progressive, but incomplete, multifocal neural process with devastating effects on lower urinary tract function and control. There are three basic patterns of lower urinary tract dysfunction in multiple sclerosis. All are associated with the same symptoms, which thus have no differential value. The symptoms include urgency, frequency, a feeling of inability to urinate, and incontinence with little warning.

On evaluation, 10% of these patients show a large residual urine and an areflexic bladder on cystometry. Treatment by intermittent catheterization often (60%) leads to recovery of totally uninhibited reflex vesical contractility associated with a dyssynergic sphincter within 1 to 2 months. For that reason, if intermittent catheterization is feasible in such patients, we usually begin anticholinergic agents at the same time, hoping to prevent the recovery of basically useless reflex contractility and detrusor sphincter dyssynergia. About 25% of multiple sclerosis patients show minimal residual urine volumes and by cystometry uninhibited bladder contractility without detrusor sphincter dyssynergia. Such patients can be treated either by timed voiding or by small doses of anticholinergic agents and timed voiding. Once established, this pattern tends to be stable for long periods of time. It is almost invariably encountered in patients with stable multiple sclerosis who progress slowly (if at all) over a 4- to 5-year period of observation.

The most common problem encountered in multiple sclerosis patients occurs in 66% of those who present to urologists. The findings are a moderate (100 to 200 ml) residual urine volume and overt detrusor sphincter dyssynergia on cystometry with an EMG or by a videourodynamic study. Most patients can be treated successfully by anticholinergic agents and intermittent catheterization. Although intermittent catheterization is the best alternative for treatment, there are rare circumstances in which it cannot be used. In these cases, catheters should be a treatment of absolute last resort. One of two extremely bad outcomes occurs in more than 60% of patients so treated in a 5-year period. These include serious, irreversible, upper tract damage leading to urosepsis and death (50%, 5-year mortality in the University of Michigan series of patients who refused management other than catheter drainage) and erosion of the urethra with consequent constant incontinence. The latter, a kind of catheter-induced sphincterotomy, may spare the upper urinary tract but often leads to larger and larger catheters and balloons in an effort to obviate the severe incontinence until diversion is the treatment of last resort.

Urodynamic Monitoring

In any patient with spinal neural disease or injury, low pressure bladder storage of urine to those volumes associated either with reflex contractile bladder activity or with intermittent catheterization should be monitored periodically urodynamically. Most women are not managed by reflex voiding, so practically speaking cystometry to those volumes obtained by intermittent catheterization should be done on a regular basis. The chief expression of deterioration in bladder function or control in women is incontinence, which usually prompts an immediate visit to the urologist. It should be kept in mind that approximately two-thirds of patients treated by intermittent catheterization are bacteriuric at any given time, and thus a positive culture result is not usually related to the incontinence except indirectly. Therefore treatment with an antibiotic for a presumed infection that is thought to cause the sudden incontinence is usually futile. Indeed, the escape of the bladder from control with elevated pressures and incontinence is usually responsible for the symptomatic (febrile) infection rather than the other way around. With that in mind, the bacteriuria and the unstable bladder responses should be treated simultaneously.

Peripheral Lesions

There are some poorly defined peripheral, or apparently peripheral, lesions, which can be associated with uninhibited bladder contractility and incontinence. The best defined condition, and that is not very well defined, occurs after an episode of prolonged bladder distention, often related to trauma; surgery, particularly surgery for stress incontinence; childbirth; and occasionally in cases of an undiagnosed central herniated intervertebral disc. These patients present initially with detrusor areflexia with large resid-

ual urine volumes and often a history of unsuccessful attempts to induce voiding by urethral dilation, urethrotomy, placement of suprapubic tubes, and administration of bethanechol chloride or alpha-blocking agents. The cause is usually undeterminable, and a cystometrogram and EMG or a videourodynamic study shows no subjective appreciation of bladder filling and no increase in EMG activity despite bladder overfilling. The bladder is found to be large and low pressure; therefore intermittent catheterization is almost always used for management. For most patients, this method works well, and although they are often disappointed with a lack of recovery of reflex bladder activity, management by intermittent catheterization is safe and well tolerated.

A small group of patients, however, do recover reflex vesical contractility, which is quite normal, coordinate, and effective with regard to bladder emptying, but it occurs totally automatically with no warning, and the subject simply cannot control it. Neither can she initiate volitional micturition, apparently as a result of loss of all bladder sensation. Where a neural lesion that would produce this kind of bladder dysfunction would be located is difficult to imagine, but for various reasons, it almost has to involve the sensory neural apparatus within the bladder itself. That would be the neural apparatus that is activated during filling and provides information necessary for the cortical appreciation of lower urinary tract events. If this is the case, the afferent pathway that generates reflex storage and micturition responses cannot be identical to that which subserves cortical appreciation of bladder and urethral events because the storage and micturition responses in this circumstance work perfectly normally in the total absence of any cortical ability to control reflex lower urinary tract function. That in fact fits with some other disparate clinical detail, such as the complex of symptoms and findings in *interstitial cystitis*, in which intense urinary urgency is associated with normal bladder behavior under anesthesia, suggesting that the disease involves an abnormal bladder sensory mechanism related to cortical appreciation of bladder events but one that does not affect the sensory apparatus subserving reflex storage and micturition responses. In any event, treatment of totally acerebral but normal reflex micturition is not possible with drugs and intermittent catheterization and almost always requires reservoir replacement or subtotal cystectomy and augmentation of the bladder with bowel and then intermittent catheterization. In this respect, the bladder dysfunction is identical to that seen in patients with high spinal cord injury who survive the acute injury and become totally respirator dependent. Some of these patients show perfectly normal automatic reflex contractility, which is totally avolitional and acerebral and impossible to treat once established except (in men) by condom catheter drainage.

References

1. Resnick NM, Yalla SV. Detrusor hyperactivity with impaired contractile function: An unrecognized but common cause of incontinence in elderly patients. JAMA 1987;257:3076.
2. Sussett JG, Plante P. Studies of urethral pressure profile. Part II: Urethral pressure profile in female incontinence. J Urol 1980;123:70.
3. Lose G, Colstrup H, Thind P. Urethral elastance in healthy and stress incontinence women. Neurourol Urodynam 1989;8:371.
4. McGuire EJ, Savastano JA. Long term follow up of spinal cord injury patients managed by intermittent catheterization. J Urol 1983;129:775.
5. McGuire EJ, Savastano JA. Comparative urologic outcome in females with spinal cord injury. J Urol 1986;135:730.
6. Wan J, Fleenor S, Kielczewski P, et al. Upper tract status of patients with neurogenic dysfunction presenting with upper tract stone disease. J Urol 1992;148:1126.
7. McGuire EJ, Noll F, Maynard JF. A pressure management system for the neurogenic bladder after spinal cord injury. Neurourol Urodynam 1991; 10:223.

6

Disorders of Bladder Compliance

Gamal M. Ghoniem

Compliance, in physical terms, is the inverse of stiffness. Bladder compliance usually is described in clinical practice as being good (high) or poor (low). More specific description is generally avoided because of the lack of standard values for normal and abnormal compliances. A highly compliant bladder permits storage of a large volume of urine under low pressure and is considered a safe system. Low bladder compliance, in which storage of urine is under high pressure, predisposes the patient to infection, impairment of urinary tract anatomy, and deterioration in renal function.

The passive properties of the bladder wall are responsible for the degree of compliance noticed during the early stages of bladder filling. The physiologic response of a normal bladder to filling is an almost imperceptible change in intravesical pressure. In addition to the passive component, an active, neurogenic component is responsible for the changes of the pressure curve toward the end of filling (Fig. 6-1).

Two components make up the detrusor response to volume increments: an active component that is due to smooth muscle activity and a passive component that is related to the viscoelastic properties of the bladder wall.[1] The passive component was initially suggested by Nesbit and Lapides and by Ruch and Tang.[2,3]

The bladder wall is composed of smooth muscle, mucosa, submucosa, and connective tissue that contains elastin and collagen. The interaction of these components causes definite viscoelastic behavior of the bladder tested. The active component is produced by the bladder smooth muscle cells, which are not in a silent state but have properties of a pacemaker; the smooth muscles are stimulated by stretch to produce tone.[4] This tone of the bladder is a continued state of stress that is controlled by central and peripheral nervous reflexes.[5]

Compliance Measurement

The degree of bladder compliance is determined from a cystometrogram and is calculated by dividing the volume change (Δ V) by the change in detrusor pressure (Δ Pdet) during the change in bladder volume (Δ V/Δ Pdet) and is expressed as milliliters per centimeters of water.[6]

Compliance can be calculated simply from intervesical pressure change, and it is not necessary to determine detrusor pressure. Because it calculates the changes of pressure, rather than absolute values, it is unnecessary to measure rectal (abdominal) pressure simultaneously. This is a clinical advantage that saves time, decreases patient discomfort, and gives reliable results.

Female Urology, edited by Elroy D. Kursh and Edward McGuire. J. B. Lippincott, Philadelphia, © 1994.

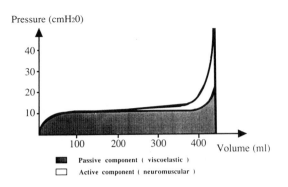

Figure 6-1. *Components of bladder compliance. The active components become more prominent toward full bladder capacity.*

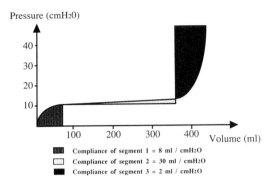

Figure 6-2. *Pressure changes during filling. In segments I and III, the calculated compliance is low compared with segment II (defined as initial compliance).*

In a typical cystometrogram, there are generally three segments of pressure change in response to the volume infused (Fig. 6-2). Because each segment may indicate different values of compliance, every effort should be made to identify in which segment the compliance is measured.

The first segment to be noted is brief, and calculations of compliance show a high value. This initial rise of pressure (resting bladder pressure) is of no clinical significance but is relative to the abdominal pressure (weight of viscera) and the status of the deformed bladder cavity. In the latter, if the measuring urodynamic catheter enters a smaller compartment of the folding cavity, a higher pressure is recorded. This is more pronounced when using carbon dioxide for gas cystometry. Therefore, for all practical reasons, this short segment should be omitted from calculations. In our practice, the *resting bladder pressure* is "zeroed" before filling.

The degree of compliance in segment II, where most of the filling occurs, is more important. Defined as *initial compliance* previously, it is calculated from the segment of cystometry between segment I and a steep rise of pressure.[7]

Terminal compliance (segment III) may also be calculated. A correlation between initial and terminal compliance has been reported previously.[7] It may be inaccurate, however, to attribute all the pressure rise in segment III to bladder

wall properties (active and passive) when there is a phasic (long and sustained) bladder contraction. One way to overcome this inaccuracy is to stop the infusion intermittently and observe the pressure behavior. If a continuous rise of pressure is noted, a contraction is in progress, and the pressure values are therefore invalid for terminal compliance calculation.

In the case of detrusor hyperreflexia, it is reasonable to calculate compliance from the pressure value between contractions and the corresponding volume. Bladder hyperreflexia may occur with or without low compliance (Figs. 6-3 and 6-4).

At present, the active and passive components of compliance cannot be distinguished or segregated numerically. Terms such as *tone, hypertonic, hypotonic, spastic,* and *tonus limb* should be avoided until the different components of compliance can be accurately measured. Because complete blocking of the smooth muscle cannot be achieved in the awake state, it is impossible to perform a cystometrogram with the bladder wall in a purely passive state, to differentiate between the neurogenic and viscoelastic components of compliance. Moreover, in a neurogenic bladder, there is evidence of an atropine-resistant component that is not fully understood.[8]

For an easy clinical determination of compli-

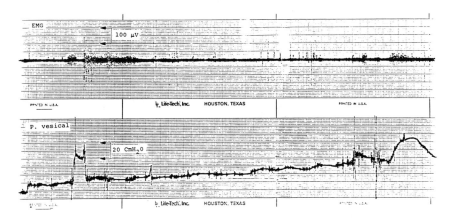

Figure 6-3. *A 17-year-old meningomyelocele patient with sphincter dyssynergia and low bladder compliance (3.3 ml/cm H_2O). The patient has grade 2 right vesicoureteral reflux and recurrent urinary tract infections.*

ance, we have found that *initial compliance* can be calculated reliably by simple cystometry without monitoring abdominal pressure. Moreover, it characterizes that segment of the cystometrogram where most of the filling occurs. The term *compliance* is used because it describes the slope of the pressure curve without the necessity of defining the mechanism that produces that curve.

The factors affecting compliance measurement are infusion rate and the condition of the bladder before testing. The speed of stretching the bladder wall (strain) directly affects the resultant pressure (force). Very slow elongation of the smooth muscles in the bladder wall produces a smaller pressure. Moreover, fast infusion rates decrease membrane rest potentials and increase the frequency of active potentials. This stimulates more of the active component of compliance, obscuring the actual passive (vesicoelastic) element. Klevmark showed that physiologic filling values produce essentially no pressure rise.[9]

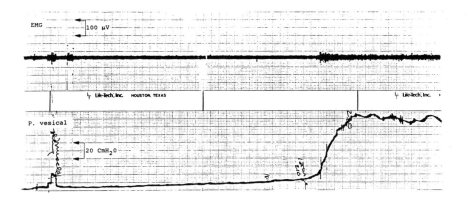

Figure 6-4. *A 15-year-old meningomyelocele patient with sphincter dyssynergia and reasonable bladder compliance (17.5 ml/cm H_2O). The patient has normal upper tracts, no vesicoureteral reflux, and no urinary tract infections.*

In contrast, sudden increase of the volume causes the bladder wall to respond with an increase in intravesical pressure. For calculation of bladder compliance, a slow filling rate is preferred, to avoid activation of the smooth muscles.

If the bladder has been overstretched or insufficient time has been allowed before repeating a cystometrogram, lower pressure values and subsequently higher compliance may be anticipated.[10] In contrast, having an indwelling catheter for even a few days decreases compliance.

Compliance and Outlet Resistance

There is a direct relationship between bladder compliance and outlet resistance. Theoretically if the most rigid system studied has a hole big enough to permit fluid leakage during filling, the pressure rise, if any, is minimal. The presence of a patulous outlet, vesicoureteral reflux, or bladder diverticuli leads to a measurement of compliance lower than its actual value. Occlusion of refluxing ureteral orifices by a Fogarty balloon catheter gives more realistic values of bladder compliance. Likewise, in a case of patulous urethra, the bladder neck should be occluded by a Foley's balloon.[11, 12]

The relationship between outlet resistance and compliance goes beyond mechanical concepts. Wang and colleagues showed that repeated urethral dilatation in patients with meningomyelocele gradually improves both bladder compliance and continence.[13] One possible explanation for this intriguing phenomenon may be the aborting of excitatory reflexes originating from the urethra to the bladder. McGuire suggested a direct inhibition of the detrusor motor neurons in the sacral spinal cord because of increased afferent pudendal nerve activity generated by receptors in the striated sphincter.[14–16] Such a reflex was first described in humans by Kock and Pompeius, who noted an inhibition of bladder contractile activity as initiated by anal distention.[17] Sundin and colleagues have proposed a similar pudendal nerve–mediated inhibition of bladder activity during nerve stimulation but mediated through hypogastric nerve activity.[18] That could be also true in female patients who have irritative symptoms (so-called urethral syndrome) but experience relief after urethral dilatation. Moreover, in some patients who demonstrate no significant changes of detrusor pressure drop during voiding, after transurethral balloon dilatation of the prostate, their irritative symptoms, especially nocturia, improved.[19]

Compliance and Upper Tracts

Under normal circumstances, bladder filling occurs with minimal pressure rise, a property called *accommodation*. Accommodation of urine is due to normal vesicoelastic properties and the influence of sympathetic, and possibly parasympathetic, systems on bladder filling. In pathologic conditions resulting in low compliance, this property is lost totally or in part. The resultant filling under increasing intravesical pressures is limited only by the outlet resistance. The best example of the latter condition is found in patients with meningomyelocele.

Smith showed that in untreated meningomyelocele patients there is gradual deterioration of the upper and lower urinary tracts.[20] These changes were profound in patients with evidence of obstruction in the posterior urethra, noted by Smith as a neurogenic spasm. In 58% of the untreated patients studied, structural changes in the urinary tract developed by the time the patient was 3 years old. Upper urinary tract deterioration in these children was related closely to elevated intravesical pressure.[21–25]

In a study of 61 patients with myelodysplasia, Ghoniem and associates found that 31 had upper tract deterioration as detected by excretory urography, ultrasound, and renal scan studies.[26] The urodynamic findings in those patients were characterized by a significant higher leak pressure and lower bladder compliance than the other group with normal upper tracts. Improving bladder compliance either by pharmacologic therapy or surgery results in stabilization or improvement of the upper tracts in most of those patients.[27,28]

Compliance and Continence

The relationship between bladder compliance and continence is a direct one, with the outlet resistance as a determining factor. When the intravesical pressure exceeds outlet resistance, incontinence occurs. The major difference between central (sacral or sacral root lesion) and peripheral (pelvic plexus) injury is in their effects on this sphincteric mechanism. Central injuries may interfere with the external sphincteric mechanism but do not influence the internal sphincteric function. On the contrary, peripheral lesions, including those due to sympathetic injury, may interfere with the internal sphincteric function, leading to varying degrees of open bladder neck, but they do not influence the external sphincteric mechanism. In management of voiding dysfunction in patients with sacral lesions, the internal sphincteric mechanism is usually intact, and continence is possible. In the case of peripheral denervation with sympathetic injury, causing lower urethral resistance, continence may be difficult to achieve.

Disorders Producing Low Compliance

A standard cut-off value for low compliance has not been established, but a value of 10 ml/cm H_2O is a strong prognosticator for upper tracts at risk. A value of 10 to 20 ml/cm H_2O is considered abnormally low compliance. A value above 20 ml/cm H_2O is considered normal compliance. A definition of abnormally high compliance would be difficult and probably not of clinical importance, but bladder volume would be a factor. Volumes above 750 ml with a compliance of above 100 ml/cm H_2O are considered abnormally high compliance, but one should realize that an occasional perfectly normal subject will void to completion with values above 750 ml.

NEUROGENIC BLADDER

A suprasacral spinal cord lesion results in bladder hyperreflexia and low compliance, which is mainly neurogenic. Early treatment with anticholinergics usually controls both. Structural changes, however, eventually occur in the muscle, nerve, and interstitium.[29] Eventually some bladders become refractory to treatment and require augmentation cystoplasty.

Sacral lesions affect compliance in different ways. Complete intradural sacral rhizotomy in dogs resulted in a significant increase in passive properties and low compliant bladders.[30] Histologic studies showed increased collagen content, smooth muscle hypertrophy, and hyperplasia. Division of the posterior sacral roots produces arreflexia and increased capacity. In contrast, long-term results of selective anterior sacral root division include a decrease in both capacity and compliance.[31,32]

Low compliance as a result of bladder decentralization is due to both morphologic and innervation changes. Sundin and others noted the appearance of normally undetected detrusor adrenergic nerve terminals after decentralization in humans and cats.[33,34] Hanno and associates observed in cats that after decentralization synapses reorganize in the vesical wall ganglia with new cholinergic excitatory inputs from the hypogastric nerve.[35] In primates, compliance and capacity losses after decentralization can be partially restored by phenoxybenzamine, supporting the concept that detrusor adrenergic terminals are hyperactive after decentralization.[36]

Low compliance impairs bladder function and causes filling under high pressure. Even in the absence of reflux, upper urinary tract deterioration can be anticipated, as in meningomyelocele patients.[7,22,26,28]

Complete sacral denervation to treat hyperactive neurogenic bladder has been advocated for some time. This usually abolishes detrusor reflex activity, which is at least temporary. It also impairs the function of the external sphincteric mechanism and in men may result in impotence. McGuire and Wagner showed that complete sacral denervation resulted in loss of anal sphincter and detrusor and urethral skeletal muscular activity, but resting urethral smooth muscular sphincter tone was unaffected.[37] So in a lower motor neuron lesion without perineal floor electromyography activity, transurethral resection of the bladder neck, especially in women, is not acceptable because of the expected high risk of incontinence.

It is suggested that the denervation supersensitivity tests may not accurately determine the nature and degree of bladder and urethral denervation, and they are known to produce false-positive and false-negative results.[38]

PELVIC SURGERY

Clinical studies of bladder function after a radical pelvic operation are conflicting. At least a portion of the confusion involves the timing of evaluation postoperatively. Radical pelvic surgery may alter bladder function through many processes because the sympathetic pathways are highly susceptible to injury. Hanno and co-workers found that parasympathetic decentralization results in adrenergic hyperinnervation of the detrusor.[35] Some clinical studies suggest that compliance changes may be seen frequently but only temporarily after a radical pelvic operation and that detrusor motor denervation occurs in only a small number of patients.

During rectal surgery, nerve injury can occur from direct injury of the parasympathetic nerves and the posterior part of the pelvic plexus, especially in men.[39] In addition, traction injury (neuropraxia) may occur during rectal mobilization. Bladder dysfunction due to the latter is usually temporary.

Gerstenberg and colleagues reported on 26 consecutive patients who had undergone abdominal perineal resection.[40] This is probably the only series with consecutive patients; other studies are highly selective and have not included consecutive patients. They reported that bladder arreflexia occurred postoperatively in 7.7%. These were 6-month and 12-month evaluations, excluding the early postoperative evaluations,

which probably had a high percentage of temporary bladder dysfunction. Blaivas and Barbalias reported on 13 male patients with voiding dysfunction after an abdominal perineal resection.[41] Three of these patients showed a bladder capacity of less than 250 ml with an open bladder neck and involuntary contractions. In addition, four patients had problems with storage and emptying. Pudendal nerve injury usually occurs during the perineal portion of the dissection. According to Blaivas, he found 38% had parasympathetic denervation, 54% had pudendal denervation, and 100% had sympathetic denervation.

Low and associates noted a uniform decrease in compliance without arreflexia in 20 women immediately after radical abdominal hysterectomy.[42] In a selected group of patients referred for voiding dysfunction after radical pelvic surgery, Sislow and Mayo evaluated and identified a higher proportion with abnormal compliance (18 out of 31) compared with patients with conal cauda equina injury (4 out of 33).[43] Roman-Lopez and Barclay found abnormal compliance in 95% of 31 radical vaginal hysterectomy patients studied serially 21 to 169 days postoperatively.[44] Only 2 of their 31 patients had arreflexic bladders. In a 5- to 15-year study by Fraser, abnormal cystometrograms were found in 20 out of 45 women after abdominal hysterectomy.[45] Woodside and McGuire reported on three patients who within 13 months of radical hysterectomy had decreased compliance associated with upper tract dilatation.[46]

During hysterectomy, the risk of damage to the pelvic plexus is only slight because the bulk of the pelvic plexus lies below the cardinal ligament. Sympathetic in addition to parasympathetic nerve injury may occur in patients with higher stage disease after dissection in the vicinity of the cardinal ligaments and in those who require extensive vaginal cuff removal. Forney found 50% occurrence of bladder hypertonia (low compliance) and incompetent bladder neck after radical hysterectomy.[47] Yalla and Andriole suggested that a finding of a decreased bladder capacity (low compliance) and incompetent bladder neck is consistent with sympathetic denervation, whereas decreased activity or bladder arreflexia with decreased proprioception sensation and increased bladder capacity is consistent with parasympathetic denervation.[48] In such radical pelvic surgery, however, usually a combination of the two could be expected.

Case History

A 45-year-old black woman underwent a radical abdominal hysterectomy for cervical carcinoma. Seven months postoperative, she was admitted to the hospital with fever, chills, bilateral flank pain, and incontinence. The patient also complained of difficulty in voiding and progressive incontinence. Urodynamic evaluation revealed a postvoid residual urine of 500 ml and arreflexic low bladder compliance. Intravenous urography showed bilateral hydronephrosis (Fig. 6-5), which was relieved immediately after drainage by a Foley catheter (Fig. 6-6). The patient did not have vesicoureteral reflux and had low closing pressures at the level of the proximal urethra as demonstrated by videofluorourodynamics. The patient was treated with intravenous antibiotics according to the urine culture sensitivity results, and the bladder was drained by an indwelling catheter. All of her general symptoms resolved within 3 days, and the patient was instructed in clean intermittent catheterization technique. This patient was started on anticholinergic medications (oxybutynin, 5 mg three times a day) and intermittent catheterization after treatment of pyelonephritis. The patient continued to do well on that regimen with no evidence of return of bladder function up to 1 year of followup.

Causes of bladder dysfunction after radical pelvic surgery include nerve injury either direct or by traction, direct vesical trauma, traumatic aseptic pericystitis, loss of bladder base support, tumor invasion of nerves, and prostatic obstruction in males.[49-54] Other factors contributing to dysfunction postoperatively are stretch injuries (urinary retention), radiation, and infection.

Urodynamic evaluation in patients undergoing radical pelvic surgery is important for several reasons.

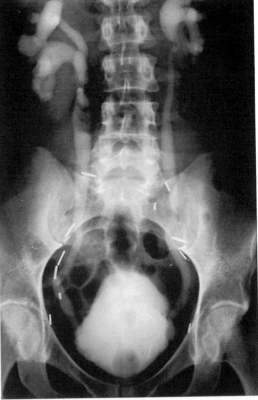

Figure 6-5. *Intravenous urography in 45-year-old woman 7 months after radical hysterectomy showing upper tract dilatation. Note the indwelling catheter is occluded by a clamp.*

1. If the urodynamic studies, symptoms, and physical examination before surgery show no bladder outlet obstruction, it is unlikely to be a reason for voiding dysfunction after surgery.

2. It is important preoperatively to estimate the extent of the infiltration of a tumor, if any, into the pelvic neuroplexus.

3. The pattern of voiding dysfunction may change markedly postoperatively or even resolve.

It is important in the immediate postoperative period to avoid any irreversible surgical in-

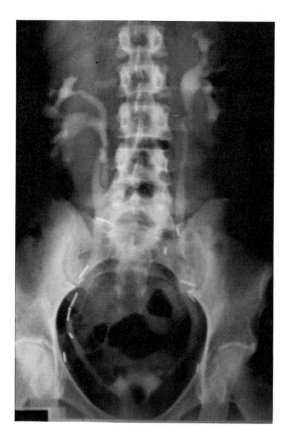

Figure 6-6. Intravenous urography of the same patient in Fig. 6-5, immediately after draining the bladder. Note that the patient did not have vesicoureteral reflux.

tervention until stable function of the lower urinary tract is achieved. Patients may be placed on an intermittent catheterization program and undergo periodic urodynamic evaluation to determine if the dysfunction is permanent or will resolve over time.

After radical pelvic surgery, the bladder should be drained immediately either with a Foley catheter or with clean intermittent catheterization. This period of drainage should continue for 2 to 4 weeks. If the patient suffers bladder dysfunction, urodynamic studies should be performed. In a male patient, if the studies reveal abnormalities consistent with injury of the parasympathetic, sympathetic, and pudendal nerves, there is a high risk of incontinence if prostatectomy is performed.

BLADDER OUTLET OBSTRUCTION AND INSTABILITY

Strips of rabbit bladder tested in physiologic organ bath showed significant compliance decrease in response to bladder outlet obstruction.[55] Histologic studies showed increased collagen content and both muscular hypertrophy and hyperplasia. Such hypertrophied detrusor may be less amenable to stretch (*i.e.,* become less compliant and capable only of sluggish, weak, or dissociated contraction).[56]

Elbadawi summarized five structural changes leading to such dysfunction.[57] First, the branching processes of hypertrophied muscle cells become interlocked, rendering their containing fascicle more resistant to stretch (*i.e.,* less compliant) and less capable of effective shortening (*i.e.,* less contractile). Second, the individual muscle cells become widely separated, interfering with coupling to propagate a contraction. Third, considerable deposits of collagen and elastin occur between muscle cells and between fascicles. Fourth, the neural complement is reduced. Fifth, there is an exproportionate increase of a component of the neural compartment, creating imbalance of bladder contraction.

Clinically bladder instability, as a result of outlet obstruction, can lead to low compliance. In patients with benign prostatic hyperplasia, bladder compliance was significantly decreased when compared with those patients with no instability.[58]

DEFUNCTIONALIZED BLADDER

In patients with urinary diversion or patients on dialysis, a low or no urinary output usually suggests a defunctionalized bladder, characterized by low compliance and small capacity. This low compliance and low capacity can be altered by bladder cycling in a clinical setting with the patient admitted to the hospital with a small indwelling catheter. Gradual filling of the bladder is done maintaining a pressure below 80 cm H_2O (to avoid exceeding systolic blood pressure). The bladder is filled every hour for 15 minutes and then drained while the patient is awake. Treatment with anticholinergic agents can help to accelerate the process. Most patients with normal bladders respond to this regimen of treatment.

Hydrodistention of a small-capacity bladder with low compliance can also be achieved using a Helmstein balloon. This is a specially designed balloon catheter filled in the bladder under high epidural anesthesia. The balloon is inflated for 4 hours, up to a pressure equal to the systolic blood pressure, during which time fluid is added or removed as necessary to maintain the desired pressure. Blaivas has reported that it is effective in about 60% of cases but also reported 5% of the patients had bladder rupture as a complication.[59] Because bladder rupture occurs retroperitoneally, the patient should be treated with antibiotics, and an indwelling catheter should remain for 7 to 10 days.

If no significant response to either technique is noted, permanent bladder changes should be considered. In this situation, augmentation cystoplasty at the time of undiversion could be performed. In patients who are candidates for renal transplantation, augmentation cystoplasty should be performed before kidney transplantation.[60] Large bowel is preferred for two reasons. First, using the sigmoid colon allows preservation of the retropubic anterior bladder surface and iliac fossa region, thus facilitating the subsequent transplant procedure. Second, a nonrefluxing ureteral anastomosis is easier to perform in the large bowel if there is not enough bladder wall available.

AGING

As rats age, the bladder weight increases by 20%, whereas total body weight and bladder compliance diminish.[61] During maturation, rabbits showed decrease of both compliance and active tension.[62]

In humans, biochemical evidence suggests significant connective tissue changes in the aging bladder wall. In women, collagen content increases by 10% with age.[63] In addition, elastin content increases by 30% with age.[64] In the submucosa, collagen fibers are bound into fascicles with arborizing intercollagenous channels. With age, the collagen fascicles separate into individual fibers, and there is a proportional widening of the intercollagenous channels. In addition, the channels progressively fill with an electron-dense fine particulate matter of unknown origin.[65] These changes are thought to alter the permeability and compliance of the submucosa and to encroach on the neurovascular bundle. Accordingly it seems that bladder compliance changes with age, being highest in infancy and lowest in the elderly population.

Clinically the resultant *impaired contractility* is more important than the low compliance. Resnick and Yalla found a large percentage of elderly nursing home patients with impaired bladder contractility that led to high residual urine and incontinence.[66]

LOCAL IRRITATIVE FACTORS

Indwelling urethral catheters, bladder stones, or urinary tract infections can cause low bladder compliance. This compliance change is usually temporary and usually disappears after treatment of the offending problem.

LESS COMMON CAUSES

Interstitial cystitis, accidental injection of a caustic liquid into the bladder, and pelvic radiation therapy may result in low compliance. In the latter, it is probably due to devascularization and induction of bladder collagenosis.

Specific chronic infections such as tuberculosis or schistosomiasis produce low compliant bladders secondary to extensive fibrosis. Extremely low compliant, small bladder capacity and severe vesicoureteral reflux is the full-blown picture in schistosomiasis[67] (Fig. 6-7).

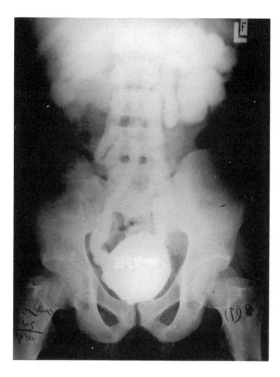

Figure 6-7. *Cystogram in 52-year-old man with schistosomiasis. Small-capacity, low-compliant bladder caused severe bilateral vesicoureteral reflux. Scarring of the ureterovesical area is a contributing factor.*

Conclusion

The degree of bladder compliance is due to both viscoelastic and neuromuscular components. Standardization of methodology is needed to reach a more objective description of compliance. Abnormal bladder compliance (low) leads to upper tract deterioration or urinary incontinence. Research to define the different components more accurately will lead to better and less invasive methods to control abnormal compliance.

References

1. McGuire EJ, Ghoniem GM. Detrusor compliance. Neurourol Urodynam 1986;5:124.

2. Nesbit R, Lapides J. Tonus of the bladder during spinal shock. Arch Surg 1948;56:138.
3. Ruch TC, Tang PC. The higher control of the bladder. In: Boyarsky S, ed. The neurogenic bladder. Baltimore: Williams & Wilkins, 1969:34.
4. Coolsaet B. Bladder compliance and detrusor activity during the collection phase. Neurourol Urodynam 1985;4:263.
5. Landowne M, Stacy RW. Glossary of terms. In: Remington JW, ed. Tissue Elasticity. Washington, DC, American Physiological Society, 1957:191.
6. Abrams P, Blaivas JG, Stanton SL, Andersen JT. Standardization of terminology of lower urinary tract function. Neurourol Urodynam 1988; 7:403.
7. Ghoniem GM, Bloom DA, McGuire EJ, Stewart KL. Bladder compliance in meningomyeolocele children. J Urol 1989;141:1404.
8. Ghoniem GM, Shoukry MS, Cerniglia FR Jr. Detrusor properties in meningomyelocele patients: In vitro study (abstr). Neurourol Urodynam 1991;10:209.
9. Klevmark B. Motility of the urinary bladder in cats during filling at physiologic rates. I. Intravesical pressure patterns by a new method of cystometry. Acta Physiol Scand 1974;90:565.
10. Ghoniem GM, Shoukry MS. Effect of time interval and bladder overdistension on repeated urodynamic studies: Animal study (abstr). Neurourol Urodynam 1990;9:367.
11. Woodside JR, Borden TA. Determination of true intravesical filling pressure in patients with vesicoureteral reflux by Fogarty catheter occlusion of ureters. J Urol 1982;127:1149.
12. Woodside JR, McGuire EJ. Technique for detection of detrusor hypertonia in the presence of urethral sphincteric incompetence. J Urol 1982; 127:740.
13. Wang SC, McGuire EJ, Bloom DA. Urethral dilatation in the management of urological complications of myelodysplasia. J Urol 1989;142:1054.
14. McGuire EJ: Clinical evaluation and treatment of neurogenic vesical dysfunction. In: Libertino J, ed. International Perspectives in Urology. Vol 2. Baltimore: Williams & Wilkins, 1984:1.
15. McGuire EJ. Experimental observations on the integration of bladder and urethral function. Invest Urol 1978;15:303.
16. McGuire EJ. Physiology of the lower urinary tract. Am J Kidney Dis 1983;2:402.
17. Kock N, Pompeius R. Inhibition of vesical motor activity induced by anal stimulation. Acta Clin Scand 1963;126:244.
18. Sundin, T, Carlsson CA, Kock NA. Detrusor inhibition induced from mechanical stimulation of the anal region and from electrical stimulation of

pudendal nerve afferents. An experimental study in cats. Invest Urol 1974:11:374.

19. Ghoniem GM, Cherry RJ, Thomas R. Efficacy of transurethral balloon dilatation of the prostate (TUDP) in treating patients with benign prostatic hyperplasia (BPH) (abstr). Neurourol Urodynam, 1991;10:202.

20. Smith ED. Urinary prognosis in spina bifida. J Urol 1972;108:815.

21. McGuire EJ, Woodside JR, Borden TA, Weiss RM. Prognostic value of urodynamic testing in myelodysplastic patients. J Urol 1981;126:205.

22. McGuire EJ, Woodside JR, Borden TA. Upper urinary tract deterioration in patients with myelodysplasia and detrusor hypertonia: A followup study. J Urol 1983;129:823.

23. McLorie GA, Perez-Marero R, Csima A, Churchill BM. Determinants of hydronephrosis and renal injury in patients with myelomeningocele. J Urol 1988;140:1289.

24. Sidi AA, Dykstra DD, Gonzalez R. The value of urodynamic testing in the management of neonates with myelodysplasia: A prospective study. J Urol 1986;135:90.

25. Bauer SB, Hallett M, Khoshbin S, et al. Predictive value of urodynamic evaluation in newborns with myelodysplasia. JAMA 1984;252:650.

26. Ghoniem GM, Roach MB, Lewis VH, Harmon EP. The value of leak pressure and bladder compliance in the urodynamic evaluation of meningomyelocele patients. J Urol 1990;144:1440.

27. Wang SC, McGuire EJ, Bloom DA. A bladder pressure management system for myelodysplasia—clinical outcome. J Urol 1988;140:1499.

28. Weston PMT, Robinson LQ, Williams S, Thomas M, Stephenson TP: Poor compliance early in filling in the neuropathic bladder. Br J Urol 1989; 63:28.

29. Elbadawi A, Atta MA, Frank JI. Intrinsic neuromuscular defects in the neurogenic bladder. I. Short term ultrastructural changes in muscular innervation of the decentralized feline bladder base following unilateral sacral ventral rhizotomy. Neurourol Urodynam 1984;3:93.

30. Ghoniem GM, Regnier CH, Biancani P, et al. Effect of bilateral sacral decentralization on detrusor contractility and passive properties in dog. Neurourol Urodynam 1984;3:23.

31. Torrens MJ. The role of denervation in the treatment of detrusor instability. Neurourol Urodynam 1985;4:353.

32. McGuire EF, Morrissey SG. The development of neurogenic vesical dysfunction after experimental spinal cord injury or sacral rhizotomy in nonhuman primates. J Urol 1982;128:1390.

33. Sundin T, Dahlstrom A. The sympathetic innervation of the urinary bladder and the urethra in the normal state and after parasympathetic denervation at the spinal root level. An experimental study in cats. Scand J Urol Nephrol 1977; 7:131.

34. Sundin T, Dahlstrom A, Norlen L, Svedmyr N. The sympathetic innervation and adrenoreceptor function of the human lower urinary tract in the normal state and after parasympathetic denervation. Invest Urol 1977;14:322.

35. Hanno AG-E, Atta MA, Elbadawi A. Intrinsic neuromuscular defects in the neurogenic bladder: IX. Effects of combined parasympathetic decentralization and hypogastric neurectomy on neuromuscular ultrastructure of the feline bladder base. Neurourol Urodynam 1988;7:93.

36. McGuire EJ, Savastano JA. Effect of alpha-adrenergic blockade and anticholinergic agents on the decentralized primate bladder. Neurourol Urodynam 1985;4:139.

37. McGuire EJ, Wagner FC. The effects of sacral denervation on bladder and urethral function. Surg Gynecol Obstet 1977;144:343.

38. Koyanagi T. Denervation supersensitivity of the urethra to alpha adrenergics in the chronic neurogenic bladder. Urol Res 1978;6:89.

39. Mundy AR. An anatomical explanation for bladder dysfunction following rectal and uterine surgery. Br J Urol 1982;54:501.

40. Gerstenberg TC, Nielsen ML, Clausen S, et al. Bladder function after abdominoperineal resection of the rectum for anorectal cancer. Urodynamic investigation before and after operation in a consecutive series. Ann Surg 1980; 191:81.

41. Blaivas JG, Barbalias GA. Characteristics of neural injury after abdominoperineal resection. J Urol 1983;129:84.

42. Low JA, Mauger GM, Carmichael JA. The effect of Wertheim hysterectomy upon bladder and urethral function. Am J Obstet Gynecol 1981; 139:826.

43. Sislow JG, Mayo ME. Reduction in human bladder wall compliance following decentralization. J Urol 1990;144:945.

44. Roman-Lopez JJ, Barclay DL. Bladder dysfunction following Schanta hysterectomy. Am J Obstet Gynecol 1973;115:81.

45. Fraser AC. The late effects of Wertheim's hysterectomy on the urinary tract. Br J Obstet Gynaecol 1966;73:1002.

46. Woodside JR, McGuire EJ. Detrusor hypertonicity as a late complication of a Wertheim hysterectomy. J Urol 1982;127:1143.

47. Forney JP. The effect of radical hysterectomy on

bladder physiology. Am J Obstet Gynecol 1980;
138:374.

48. Yalla SV, Andriole GL. Vesicourethral dysfunction following pelvic visceral ablative surgery. J Urol 1984;132:503.

49. Seski JC, Diokno AC. Bladder dysfunction after radical abdominal hysterectomy. Am J Obstet Gynecol 1977;128:643.

50. Campbell MF. Urologic complications of anorectal and colon surgery. Am J Proctol 1961;12:43.

51. Barbaric ZL, Daniel EW, Segal JS. Urinary tract after abdominoperineal resection. Radiology 1978;128:345.

52. Baumrucker GO, Shaw JW. Urologic complications following abdomino-perineal resection of the rectum. Arch Surg 1953;67:502.

53. Kontturi M, Larmi TKI, Tuononen S. Bladder dysfunction and its manifestations following abdominal-perineal extirpation of the rectum. Am Surg 1974;179;179.

54. Fowler JW, Bremner DN, Moffat LEF. The incidence and consequences of damage to the parasympathetic nerve supply to the bladder after abdomino-perineal resection of the rectum for carcinoma. Br J Urol 1978;50:95.

55. Ghoniem GM, Regnier CH, Biancani P, et al. Effect of vesical outlet obstruction on detrusor contractility and passive properties in rabbits. J Urol 1985;135:1284.

56. Elbadawi A, Meyer S, Malkowicz SB, et al. Atta MA. Effects of short-term partial bladder outlet obstruction of the rabbit detrusor: An ultrastructural study. Neurourol Urodynam 1989;8:89.

57. Elbadawi A. Microstructural basis of detrusor contractility: The MIN approach to its understanding and study. Neurourol Urodynam 1991;10:77.

58. Ghoniem GM. Impaired bladder contractility in association with detrusor instability: Underestimated occurrence in benign prostatic hyperplasia. Neurourol Urodynam 1991;10:111.

59. Blaivas JG. Pathophysiology of lower urinary tract dysfunction. Urol Clin North Am 1985; 12:215.

60. Thomalla JV. Augmentation of the bladder in preparation for renal transplantation. Surg Gynecol Obstet 1990;170:349.

61. Chun AL, Wallace LJ, Gerald MC, et al. Effect of age on in vivo urinary bladder function in the rat. J Urol 1988;139:625.

62. Zderic SA, Duckett JW, Snyder HM III, et al. Ontogeny of bladder compliance. Neurourol Urodynam 1990;9:595.

63. Susset JG, Servot-Viguier D, Lamy F, et al. Collagen in 155 human bladders. Invest Urol 1978;16:204.

64. Cortivo R, Pagano F, Passerini G, et al. Elastin and collagen in the normal and obstructed urinary bladder. Br J Urol 1981;53:134.

65. Levy BJ, Wight TN. Structural changes in the aging submucosa: New morphologic criteria for the evaluation of the unstable human bladder. J Urol 1990;144:1044.

66. Resnick NM, Yalla SV. Detrusor hyperactivity with impaired contractile function. An unrecognized but common cause of incontinence in elderly patients. JAMA 1987;257:3076.

67. Ghoniem GM. Vesico-ureteral reflux in urinary bilharziasis. Master's thesis, Faculty of Medicine, University of Alexandria, 1978.

7

Idiopathic Bladder Instability

Edward J. McGuire

Incontinence resulting from an uncontrolled or unanticipated detrusor contraction may be related to common urologic conditions. A search for these can improve results of therapy, which, lacking any possible contributing cause, is simply empiric. These conditions include, but are not limited to, stress incontinence associated with urethral hypermobility or poor function; obstructive uropathy, most commonly due to a prior stress incontinence operation; and neural disease or injury involving the spinal cord or the spinal centers concerned with lower urinary tract function. As a rule, the character of the cystometric response to bladder filling, the presence or absence of residual urine, and the other findings on historical or physical examination point the examiner in the right direction.

Cystometry in Evaluating Bladder Instability

Idiopathic bladder instability is called that because the exact cause of the problem is not easily determined. As with every kind of bladder instability, by convention the condition can be diagnosed only by a cystometrogram (CMG). When the International Continence Society (ICS) in a very worthwhile effort attempted to standardize urodynamic terminology, one of the criteria advanced for the diagnosis of bladder instability was a rise in bladder pressure of 15 cm/H_2O during filling.[1] It was later recognized that a pressure elevation alone was not necessarily the result of a reflex bladder contraction, and the definition was changed to include phasic activity of any pressure.[2] The definition is restrictive, in that a provocative CMG is the only method sanctioned by the ICS to establish the diagnosis. To be certain that a measured rise in pressure was in fact the result of bladder activity, rectal subtraction cystometry has been advocated.[3] This ensures that abdominal pressure is not interpreted as bladder contractile activity. Subtracted abdominal pressure introduces another source of artifact because it requires a continuous monitor of intrarectal pressure, and it does not provide information that permits the precise differentiation of autonomous from reflex detrusor contractile activity. Indeed, the literature is replete with examples of autonomous bladder responses to filling labeled as detrusor instability when in fact the measured pressure rise is not a reflex contraction at all.[4-6] There are definite urodynamic findings that are associated with detrusor reflex contractility and with autonomous contractility, but rectal subtraction cystometry does not measure these. The constant

Female Urology, edited by Elroy D. Kursh and Edward McGuire. J. B. Lippincott, Philadelphia, © 1994.

subtraction of intrarectal pressure from bladder pressure is used to differentiate true detrusor contractile activity from abdominal straining or alternatively to allow the examiner to pick out detrusor contractile activity from the abdominal pressure increase associated with a cough during stress testing, an event that is both extremely rare and without clinical significance. In contrast to a urodynamic search for a problem that is not of clinical import, the differentiation of reflex from autonomous causes of poor bladder storage behavior is essential to the selection of a method of treatment that will actually work. Despite this, rectal subtraction cystometry is the standard sanctioned urodynamic examination.

The concept of an unstable bladder evolved from some accurate observations made in the urodynamics laboratory of the Middlesex Hospital in London.[7] Workers in that laboratory noted that a normal detrusor did not contract despite overfilling to the point of an intense sensation of urgency. Thus, a detrusor that contracted during the filling part of a CMG was "unstable." Although the original workers noted that only an abnormal bladder contracted during filling, they did not establish (nor did they claim to) that a bladder that did not contract was normal or had a normal control mechanism. Parenthetically the urodynamics community has never demonstrated the percentage of hyperactive or poorly controlled bladders that are discoverable by a provocative rectal subtraction cystometric study. In other words, there is no study regarding the specificity or sensitivity of a CMG. Despite a lack of specific information on exactly what a CMG, positive or negative, actually meant, the concept of the unstable detrusor became merged with a clinical condition, *urge incontinence*. In effect we mixed a clinical diagnosis with a laboratory finding based on the assumption that the two were identical conditions. The urodynamics community may argue that it did no such thing, and officially it did not; however, accepting the diagnosis of urge incontinence only if the CMG is positive amounts to the same thing.

Urge incontinence became a symptom but not a diagnosis until the cystometric study confirmed the fact of motor urge incontinence. We forgot Yeates' description of sudden incontinence that occurred in patients who noted urine passing at the very time of the initial feeling of urgency.[8] Yeates called the condition *hypesthetic urgency*, meaning that there was a lack of recognition of detrusor contractile activity until it was already in progress and then it was too late. Neurosurgeons also described the same phenomenon in various clinical settings.[9] These descriptions included the observation that the individuals afflicted did not recognize the event, urinary incontinence, until it was underway. It is now clear that some of the patients described by Yeates and the neurosurgeons do not necessarily manifest an unstable detrusor at the time of cystometry. According to modern urodynamic theory and practice, we can make a firm diagnosis in patients complaining of urge incontinence only by a CMG. That study either will or will not demonstrate an unstable contraction. If the CMG is positive, the patient has an unstable bladder and motor urge incontinence. If it is negative, the patient's bladder is normal or suffers from *sensory urge incontinence*. The latter term suggests that the cause of the wetting is something other than a bladder contraction. That is a major error. Bladder instability is a cystometric diagnosis of uncertain significance, with both false-positive and false-negative findings. Although false-positive results are probably not rare, we have little information on how often this occurs, or more to the point we have no information on how often a urodynamic diagnosis is accepted as the explanation for a patient's symptoms when in fact it is not.

As Blaivas points out, unless a urodynamic finding actually duplicates the patient's symptoms, it cannot be considered the explanation for those symptoms.[10] Because the results of urodynamic testing are sometimes negative, particularly in a substantial percentage of incontinent patients, they are not reported. To reflect reality, a survey of incontinent elderly patients, for example, would have to include some number of patients documented to be incontinent by some acceptable means whose provocative rectal subtraction CMG was negative for a contractile response. The negative response to filling, however, is not the same as normal. In the urodynamics facility at the University of Michigan, at least 40% of patients complaining of urge incontinence show a stable detrusor by cystometry. It might be argued that this is related to the manner in which CMGs are done at the University of Michigan, but continuous monitoring of bladder pressures while patients go about their daily tasks reveals that most patients who complain of urge incontinence do suffer from sudden uncontrolled detrusor contractility despite a negative provocative CMG.[11–13] Although strictly speaking this cannot be considered detrusor instability, that is in fact what it is. It is possible that overt, cystometrically demonstrable bladder contractility is a different condition than detrusor contractile activity demonstrable only by continuous monitoring but that has not been established. It is moreover not likely to be established because we ignore CMG-negative urge incontinence because we cannot diagnose it using the standard, approved test for that condition.

One of the problems with provocative cystometry is the inability of the examiner to ascertain how much the test itself, which focuses the attention of the subject on the bladder, has to do with the outcome. The usual pattern of incontinence associated with provocative CMG-negative urge incontinence is no pattern. The incontinence is neither related to time nor to volume, occurring sometimes immediately after urination in very small amounts or hours afterward in large amounts in the same patient.[14] Urinary incontinence in such individuals may occur during sleep, when behavioral factors are not operable. Available evidence suggests that these disorders are less a problem of an unruly, hyperactive bladder than a defective warning and modulating system. Unfortunately for urologists, one of the times that the control mechanism is likely to work is during a CMG. If the CMG is negative, that means nothing regarding the problem except perhaps that it will be resist-

ant to standard therapy. A "normal" CMG, or one that does not show bladder contractility during filling, is not the same thing as a normal bladder or a normal bladder control mechanism.

This is conceptually something of a problem because the test is generally accepted as the definitive diagnostic measurement of a problem of urinary loss associated with bladder contractile activity. Patients with normal cystometric findings but a strong history of urge incontinence have been regarded as normal or excluded from populations selected for the evaluation of the treatment of incontinence by one method or another. Exclusion of such patients results in the selection of others who may or may not have detrusor-related incontinence, while eliminating some who certainly do suffer from incontinence related to uncontrolled detrusor contractility. Often patients with a subtle problem of detrusor control are more difficult to treat than those with a hyperactive bladder that contracts repeatedly at very low volumes. The latter almost always respond to treatment even if the treatment is not always associated with perfect continence, whereas the former cannot be precisely defined, and the response to treatment is often poor. For that reason alone, these patients should be included in study groups for the determination of the epidemiology and incidence of incontinence as well as the determination of the efficacy of a particular treatment. In passing we accept as truthful statements by control subjects that they are continent, but we are unwilling to accept a statement from an incontinent patient who claims to be wet without further testing. If that testing is a CMG or a urethral pressure profile, in any of its various forms, static, dynamic, and "other," we fail to identify approximately 40% to 50% of the population that we should study. No matter how carefully done, a study based on selection criteria that are as poor as those we commonly use will not be very useful.

False-positive cystometric results are equally troublesome in at least one clinical setting. Patients incontinent as a result of poor urethral sphincteric function often suffer from problems with detrusor control or bladder compliance.

These are abnormalities that in this particular circumstance may not respond to anticholinergic agents.[15] This is an area where conventional wisdom is simply irrational. Consider for instance that as many as 65% of women with severe stress incontinence also complain of urge incontinence.[16] Half of these women show on provocative cystometry a positive response. Most of the remaining women, although demonstrating a stable detrusor by cystometry, also suffer from sudden uncontrolled detrusor contractility even if we cannot easily prove that. Conventional wisdom requires that those patients with a positive CMG be treated by anticholinergic agents before an operation for stress incontinence is even contemplated. Despite that recommendation, it has been established in just this circumstance that approximately 85% of women are relieved of urge incontinence by an operation that cures the stress incontinence.[17] Moreover, the results of treatment of patients with both stress and urge incontinence with medication alone are not good and could be described as very bad. In fact, the results are so bad that conventional wisdom allows an operation to be performed for such patients after the institution of anticholinergic therapy in tacit admission that failure is common. Conventional wisdom holds that operative results in such patients will be poor, but in fact the results are good with respect to both stress and urge incontinence.

The observation that operative correction of stress incontinence was associated with resolution of urge incontinence has been made by several workers.[19,20] These results suggest that stress incontinence can be causally related to motor urge incontinence and often is. This relationship is identical for both CMG-positive and CMG-negative varieties of urge incontinence. Conventional wisdom does not require that women with urge incontinence and a negative CMG be treated medically before operation even though they have basically the same condition as those with a positive CMG. The CMG is accepted as a definitive study as if it were a chest film when it is nothing of the kind. The standard evaluation of women with stress incontinence

symptoms is directed at the bladder in an effort to ferret out those women with urge incontinence and consists of retrograde filling cystometry. A false impression of causality with respect to the symptom *incontinence* may result from abnormal detrusor behavior that is in fact the result of urethral dysfunction. This occurs in any population with poor function of the urethra, including men with postprostatectomy incontinence. Moreover, treatment of the urethral problem often relieves the problem of bladder control. Thus, it would be more sensible to establish first whether a sphincteric abnormality exists. If a sphincteric insufficiency exists and is severe enough to require treatment or repair, that should be done. One compelling reason to do this is the fact that the results of treatment of urge incontinence associated with sphincteric deficiency by correction of the urethral problem are as good or better than standard therapy for urge incontinence as an isolated primary condition. Further, a positive CMG does not rule out stress incontinence, and neither does it have a bearing on whether the stress incontinence will respond to operative therapy. That depends on the type and character of the stress incontinence and the operation selected to fix it but not on the results of a CMG.

Nevertheless, the CMG has been used to make a diagnosis of genuine stress incontinence, as illogical as that seems. Stanton at the ICS meeting in Oslo referred to patients selected for a needle suspension procedure as having "genuine stress incontinence" by virtue of a "negative rectal subtraction CMG." Taking that argument to its logical absurdity would bring us to a situation in which stress incontinence and detrusor instability could not, in the same patient, exist together. Further, the diagnosis of stress incontinence, which is a definite condition quantifiable as to incidence, severity, and causality, could be made only by a negative provocative CMG. That is simply not a tenable position, nor does it have any relationship to reality. What Stanton meant was that a group of women with symptoms of stress incontinence and some other clinical data that more or less confirmed that diagnosis were selected as suitable candidates for a stress incontinence operation as a result of a provocative CMG that was normal. The selection of patients in that manner for a particular operation is not useful, but that is another matter.

Most urodynamics experts would admit that some patients with sensory urge incontinence suffer from uncontrolled detrusor contractility as the basis for the incontinence. Sensory urgency, which used to mean the inappropriate desire to urinate at low bladder volumes, is almost never associated with incontinence. Indeed, that is an important differential point in the history: whether there is incontinence associated with the urgency. If there is, a workup for motor urge incontinence is appropriate. If there is no incontinence, a standard urologic workup, including culture, cystoscopy, and cytology, is in order rather than an evaluation of bladder storage and expulsive function.

Subtypes of Instability

In enuretic children, a standard CMG frequently shows no contractile activity, but if the study is done while the child is asleep, the bladder is shown to contract.[21] The basis of the problem is, at least when the child is asleep, uninhibited vesical activity and a lack of the arousal response to a certain degree of bladder filling that is seen in normal children. The reason for the lack of arousal response is not known, but it is not dependent on the sleep phase. Deep rapid eye movement sleep is not a prerequisite for a lack of arousal, which can occur even during very light sleep. When these children are awake, we have no information regarding how they compensate for the abnormality, or even if they do, because our ability to measure responses is dependent on the end result, a bladder contraction. If some subtle adjustment is required on the part of such children to compensate, for example, for an altered brain stem reflex center threshold for a contractile bladder response, we simply cannot measure that.

Idiopathic urge incontinence strictly speaking includes all those syndromes of incontinence characterized by urinary loss, which is both involuntary and due to a detrusor contraction. We know from the results of continuous monitoring studies that a patient who tells us that she is surprised by sudden urgency and incontinence—when she gets up from a chair, or returns home from shopping and attempts to unlock the door, or when her feet hit the floor in the morning—suffers from motor urgency related to a bladder contraction. Of 100 women who present with urge incontinence, how many will have CMG-negative urge incontinence and how many a positive CMG is at present unknown. It is possible that the CMG does differentiate at least two groups of patients with detrusor incontinence. In the first place are those patients with a neural or obstructive basis for the uninhibited detrusor contractility, in whom the CMG is always positive and at roughly the same volume. These patients can be treated by anticholinergic agents and, if required, intermittent catheterization. At the other end of the spectrum are those patients with urge incontinence, a negative CMG, and no apparent underlying problem that contributes to the urge incontinence other than possibly age or some equally tenuous cause. These patients generally do not respond well to anticholinergic agents without some ancillary measures. The most effective of these in my hands is the discussion with the patient of the effect of the lack of cerebral appreciation of bladder events, which results in situations in which they are surprised by sudden bladder contractility and wetting. A simple explanation that the sign the individual has used all her life that urination was required no longer functions and that her bladder can do as it wishes in some circumstances without her permission is sufficient to provide a background for timed voiding and a voiding log, both of which effect a change in behavior. In addition to these rather discrete groups of patients are those in whom the CMG is positive but only at very large volumes, or the urethral pressure tracing shows instability during filling, in whom treatment is complicated by the imprecision of our diagnostic tests.

Some of these individuals, who are frequently elderly or very young, may have significant amounts of residual urine on occasion, but the amount varies just as does the pattern of the uninhibited response. In this regard, there may be a variant of the *nonneurogenic-neurogenic bladder* in the elderly. Although many elderly individuals have trouble with incontinence, the problem is not unique to the elderly, and age does not seem to be a determining feature. Neither is dementia related in an absolute sense to uninhibited detrusor activity. There are many demented patients who are never incontinent and many nondemented patients who are. Admittedly if incontinence occurs in a patient with dementia, it may be untreatable, but the incontinence itself is not identifiable as a specific type related to dementia. A curious kind of incontinence, however, does occur in demented patients, which might be described as social urinary loss because the event appears to have the full volitional approval of the subject concerned, but it occurs in a totally inappropriate setting, such as the waiting room, in the wastebasket, or in another patient's water pitcher. As far as I know there is no treatment for this "incontinence," which is a behavioral problem and not in a physiologic sense a loss of detrusor control.

CMG-negative urge incontinence is a problem because the usual treatment agents, anticholinergic agents, do not often work. We found pelvic floor exercises effective for this problem but were unable to document clearly what the exercises did because the CMG was as negative before treatment as it was afterward. In keeping with these results, however, other techniques that focus the attention of the patient on the bladder, by voiding logs or diaries or a bladder drill, seem to work better than drugs and with fewer side-effects. Some patients will fail any treatment and continue to be wet despite timed voiding logs, diaries, pelvic floor exercises, and drugs. In this circumstance, documentation of the fact and degree of incontinence is probably warranted because the next steps in treatment are surgical. The easiest way to do this is a pad test, either using phenazopyridine hydrochloride (Pyridium) for staining of the pad or an actual standardized pad weighing after a period of standardized physical activity.

Once the fact of urinary incontinence has been documented as well as the resistance of the condition to standard therapy, we inject 10 ml of a local anesthetic beneath the vaginal epithelium to block the perivesical neural plexus. If that provides 6 to 10 hours of absolute freedom from incontinence, the patient is advised that an Ingleman-Sundberg transvaginal denervation operative procedure has an approximately 70% chance of effecting permanent relief from the urge incontinence. Unfortunately, although transcutaneous electrical stimulation has an approximately equal efficacy, none of our patients have ever persisted in the long-term use of the technique. Some patients stopped the treatment after a time and reported long-term benefit, but these instances were rare and not well documented. If the injection of a local anesthetic fails to relieve the problem, or after the transvaginal operation there is a gradual recurrence of incontinence, the only two options remaining are direct neural stimulation and augmentation cystoplasty. Both of these are rather extreme measures, but either may be required in a small group of 10% to 12% of patients with idiopathic detrusor instability who fail all other treatment methods. Of course, because a considerable number of these patients are elderly, augmentation cystoplasty may be precluded by other medical conditions.

References

1. Bates CP, Bradley WE, Glenn E, Griffiths D, Melchiov H, Rowan D, Sterling A, Zinner N, Hald T. The standardization of terminology of the lower urinary tract. J Urol 1979;121:551.
2. Woodside JR, McGuire EJ. Detrusor hypertonicity after Wevtheim hysterectomy. J Urol 1979;121:783.
3. Whiteside G, Bates P. Synchronous video pressure flow cystourethrography. Urol Clin North Am 1979;6:93.
4. Stark G. Pathophysiology of the bladder in meningomyelocele and its correlation with the neuro-

logical picture. Dev Med Child Neurol 1968; 16:76.

5. Mayo ME, Chapman WH, Shirtleff DB. Bladder function in children with mingomyelocele. Comparison of fluoroscopy and urodynamics. J Urol 1979;121:458.

6. Godec CJ, Cass AS. Electrical stimulation for incontinence in myelomingocele. J Urol 1979;120:728.

7. Turner-Warwick RTW. Observations on the function and dysfunction of the sphincter and detrusor mechanisms. Urol Clin North Am 1979;6:13.

8. Yeates WK. Disorders of bladder function. Ann R Coll Surg 1972;50:335.

9. Nathan PW, Smith MC. The centripetal pathway for the bladder and urethra within the spinal cord. J Neurol Neurosurg Psychiatry 1951;14:262.

10. Blaivas JG. Techniques of evaluation. In Yalla S, McGuire E, Elbadawi A, Blaivas J (eds). Neurourology and Urodynamics, pp 155–198. New York, Macmillan, 1988:155.

11. Bradley WE, Bhatia N, Haldeman S. 24-hour continuous monitoring. Proc AUA abstract 113, 1982.

12. James D. Continuous monitoring. Urol Clin North Am 1979;6:125.

13. Kulseng-Hanssen S, Klevmark B. Ambulatory urethro-cysto-rectometry a new technique. Neurourol Urodyn 1988;7:119.

14. O'Donnell PD, Sutton L, Beck C, Finkbeiner A. Urinary incontinence detection in elderly impatient men. Neurourol Urodyn 1987;6:101.

15. McGuire EJ, Lytton B, Pepe V, Kohorn EJ. Stress urinary incontinence. Obstet Gynecol 1976;47:255.

16. Cardozo L, Stanton S. Genuine stress incontinence and detrusor instability. A clinical and urodynamic review of 200 cases. Br J Obstet Gynaecol 1989;87:184.

17. McGuire EJ. Bladder instability and stress incontinence. Neurourol Urodyn 1988;7:563.

18. Hodgekinson CP, Ayers MA, Drukker BH. Dyssynergic detrusor dysfunction in the apparently normal female. Am J Obstet Gynecol 1963;87:717.

19. Blaivas JG, Saulinas J. Type III stress urinary incontinence. The importance of proper diagnosis and treatment. Surg Forum 1974;35:472.

20. Awad SA, Flood HD, Acker KL. The significance of prior anti-incontinence surgery in women who present with urinary incontinence. J Urol 1988;140:514.

21. Norgaard JR. Urodynamics in enuretics. Neurourol Urodyn 1989;8:199.

8

Medical Therapy for Detrusor Incontinence

Alan J. Wein

Most drugs that affect lower urinary tract function do so by initially combining with specialized functional components of cells known as receptors. The drug receptor interaction alters the function of a cell component and initiates the series of biochemical, physiologic, and urodynamic changes that we associate with the use of that agent. Many such drugs affect accepted neurotransmitter mechanisms by affecting the synthesis, transport, storage, or release of neurotransmitter; the combination of the neurotransmitter with postjunctional receptors; or the inactivation, degradation, or reuptake of neurotransmitter. Other drugs affect receptor mechanisms that are not universally accepted as a part of the normal physiology of bladder filling and urine storage or lower urinary tract emptying. In any case, the complex physiologic and biochemical changes that occur after receptor activation are what are ultimately responsible for the contraction, relaxation, facilitation, or inhibition that occurs. These mechanisms, *metabolically distal* to receptor stimulation and blockade, are also potential sites of pharmacologic stimulation, inhibition, or modulation. This chapter includes the relevant data on which drug therapy for detrusor incontinence is based and summarizes current data and opinion on the efficacy of various drugs.

Despite disagreements on some details, all "experts" would doubtless agree that, for the purposes of description and teaching, the filling and storage phase of micturition can be conceptually summarized as follows.[1,2] Bladder filling and urine storage require:

1. Accommodation of increasing volumes of urine at a low intravesical pressure and with appropriate sensation.
2. A bladder outlet that is closed at rest and remains so during increases in intra-abdominal pressure.
3. Absence of involuntary bladder contractions (detrusor instability or detrusor hyperreflexia).

This very simple but acceptable overview implies that any type of voiding dysfunction must result from an abnormality of one or more of the factors listed. This description, with its implied subdivisions under each category, provides a logical framework for the discussion and classification of all types of incontinence. Some types of voiding dysfunction do indeed represent a combination of filling/storage and emptying abnormalities. Within this scheme, however, these become readily understandable and their detection and treatment can be logically described. All aspects of urodynamic, radiologic, and video-urodynamic evaluation can be con-

Female Urology, edited by Elroy D. Kursh and Edward McGuire. J. B. Lippincott, Philadelphia, © 1994.

ceptualized as to exactly what they evaluate in terms of either bladder or outlet activity during filling/storage or emptying. Likewise, one can easily classify all known treatments for incontinence under the broad categories of whether they facilitate filling/storage by an action that is primarily on the bladder or on one or more of the components of the bladder outlet (Table 8-1). This classification (Table 8-1) will be used as the framework for discussion for this chapter.

The pathophysiology of failure of the lower urinary tract to fill with or store urine adequately may be secondary to reasons related to the bladder, to the outlet, or both.[68] Hyperactivity of the bladder during filling can be expressed as discrete involuntary contractions or as low compliance with or without phasic contraction. Involuntary contractions are most commonly seen in association with neurological disease or following neurological injury, but may also be associated with inflammatory or irritative processes in the bladder wall or with bladder outlet obstruction, or they may be idiopathic. Decreased compliance during filling may be secondary to the sequelae of neurological injury or disease, but may also result from any process that destroys the viscoelastic properties of the bladder wall. Purely sensory urgency can also account for storage failure, and this can be on an inflammatory, infectious, neurologic, psychological, or idiopathic basis. Treatment of detrusor incontinence is directed toward inhibiting bladder contractility, increasing bladder capacity, or decreasing sensory input during filling.

Decreasing Bladder Contractility

ANTICHOLINERGIC AGENTS

The major portion of the neurohumoral stimulus for physiologic bladder contraction is acetylcholine-induced stimulation of postganglionic parasympathetic cholinergic receptor sites on bladder smooth muscle.[2] Atropine and atropinelike agents therefore depress normal bladder contractions and contractions (IVC, involuntary bladder contraction) of any cause.[3,4] The volume to the first

Table 8-1. *Therapy to Facilitate Bladder Filling/ Urine Storage*

A. Inhibiting bladder contractility/decreasing sensory input/increasing bladder capacity
  1. Timed bladder emptying
  2. Pharmacologic therapy
    a. Anticholinergic agents
    b. Musculotropic relaxants
    c. Calcium antagonists
    d. Potassium channel openers
    e. Prostaglandin inhibitors
    f. Beta adrenergic agonists
    g. Tricyclic antidepressants
    h. Dimethyl sulfoxide
    i. Polysynaptic inhibitors
  3. Biofeedback, bladder retraining
  4. Bladder overdistention
  5. Electrical stimulation (reflex inhibition)
  6. Acupuncture
  7. Interruption of innervation
    a. Central (subarachnoid block)
    b. Peripheral (sacral rhizotomy, selective sacral rhizotomy)
    c. Perivesical (peripheral bladder denervation)
  8. Augmentation cystoplasty
B. Increasing outlet resistance
  1. Physiotherapy, biofeedback
  2. Electrical stimulation of the pelvic floor
  3. Pharmacologic therapy
    a. Alpha adrenergic agonists
    b. Tricyclic antidepressants
    c. Beta adrenergic antagonists
    d. Estrogens
  4. Vesicourethral suspension (SUI)
  5. Bladder outlet reconstruction
  6. Surgical mechanical compression
    a. Sling procedures
    b. Artificial sphincter
  7. Nonsurgical mechanical compression
    a. Periurethral Polytef
    b. Periurethral collagen
    c. Occlusive devices
C. Circumventing problem
  1. Antidiuretic hormone-like agents
  2. Intermittent catheterization
  3. Continuous catheterization
  4. Urinary diversion
  5. External collecting devices
  6. Absorbent products

IVC is generally increased, the amplitude of the contraction is decreased, and the total bladder capacity is increased. Although the volume/pressure threshold at which an IVC is elicited may increase, the *warning time* and the ability to suppress an IVC are not changed. Thus, urgency and incontinence still occur unless such therapy is combined with a timed voiding or toileting regimen. Bladder compliance in normal individuals and in those with detrusor hyperreflexia, in whom the initial slope of the filling curve on cystometry is normal before the involuntary contraction, does not seem to be significantly altered.[3] McGuire and Savastano reported that atropine increased the compliance and increased the capacity of the decentralized primate bladder and that both of these effects were additive to those produced by phenoxybenzamine (see subsequent discussion on inhibition of bladder contractility by alpha-adrenergic blocking agents).[5] The effect, however, of antimuscarinics in patients who exhibit only decreased compliance has not been well studied. Outlet resistance, as reflected by urethral pressure measurements, does not seem to be clinically affected by anticholinergic therapy.[6]

Although the antimuscarinic agents generally produce significant clinical improvement in patients with involuntary bladder contractions and symptoms consequent to these, only partial inhibition *in vivo* results. In many animal models, atropine only partially antagonizes the response of the whole bladder to pelvic nerve stimulation and of bladder strips to field stimulation, although it does completely inhibit the response of bladder smooth muscle to exogenous cholinergic stimulation. Of the theories proposed to explain this phenomenon, called *atropine resistance*, the most attractive and most commonly cited is that a major portion of the neurotransmission involved in the final common pathway of bladder contraction is nonadrenergic and noncholinergic (NANC)—secondary to release of a transmitter other than acetylcholine or norepinephrine. Although the existence of atropine resistance in human bladder muscle is by no means agreed on, this concept is the most common theory invoked to explain clinical difficulty in abolishing involuntary bladder contractions with anticholinergic agents alone, and it is also invoked to support the rationale of treatment of such types of bladder activity with agents with different mechanisms of action. Brading, however, has presented and summarized evidence that seems to show that atropine resistance, although it does exist in the guinea pig and rabbit bladder, does not exist in normal pig and human detrusor.[7] Whether it is a factor in detrusor hyperactivity secondary to various causes has not been completely settled.[4]

It should be noted that, as Andersson points out, there are good and bad results reported regarding the efficacy of anticholinergic drugs given orally to patients with detrusor hyperactivity.[4] Zorzitto and colleagues concluded that 30 mg four times per day of propantheline bromide administered to a group of institutionalized incontinent geriatric patients had a marginal clinical benefit, which was outweighed by side-effects.[8] Blaivas, increasing the dose of propantheline until incontinence was eliminated or side-effects precluded further use, obtained a complete response in 25 out of 26 patients with involuntary contractions.[9] The doses ranged up to 60 mg four times per day. It is unclear to what extent such disparate results are due to differences in bioavailability or susceptibility to dose-limiting side-effects, differences in pathophysiology, or the presence of atropine resistance.

Atropine sulfate is no longer available as a tablet form according to our hospital pharmacy. That is unfortunate because it and all related belladonna alkaloids are well absorbed from the gastrointestinal tract. Atropine has almost no detectable central nervous system effects at clinically used doses; it has a half-life of about 4 hours.[10] A lack of selectivity is a major problem with all the antimuscarinic compounds because they tend to affect parasympathetically innervated organs in the same order, with generally larger doses required to depress bladder activity than to affect salivary, bronchial, nasopharyngeal, and sweat secretions. Scopolamine (hyoscine) is another belladonna alkaloid marketed as a soluble salt. It has prominent central depressive effects at low doses probably as a result of greater penetration (than atropine) through the blood-brain barrier.

Propantheline bromide (Pro-Banthine, others) is probably the oral agent most commonly used to produce an antimuscarinic effect in the lower urinary tract. The usual adult oral dosage is 15 to 30 mg every 4 to 6 hours, although higher doses are often necessary. Propantheline is a quarternary ammonium compound. All of these are poorly absorbed after oral administration.[10] Oral administration in the fasting state rather than with or after meals is preferable from the standpoint of bioavailability. There seems to be little difference between the antimuscarinic effects of propantheline on bladder smooth muscle and those of other antimuscarinic agents, such as glycopyrrolate, isopropamide, anisotropine, methylbromide, methscopolamine, homatropine, and others. Some of these agents, such as glycopyrrolate, have a more convenient dosage schedule (two or three times daily), but their clinical effects on the lower urinary tract seem to be indistinguishable. Although there are obviously many other considerations to account for the activity of a given dose of drug at its site of action, there is no oral drug available whose direct *in vitro* antimuscarinic binding potential approximates that of atropine better than the long available and relatively inexpensive propantheline bromide.[11] The problems are bioavailability and selective delivery.

It would seem that an anticholinergic agent with a significant ganglionic blocking action as well as such action at the peripheral receptor level might be more effective in suppressing bladder contractility. Although methantheline (Banthine) has a higher ratio of ganglionic blocking to antimuscarinic activity than does propantheline, the latter drug seems to be at least as potent in each respect, clinical dose for dose. Methantheline does have similar effects on the lower urinary tract, and some clinicians still prefer it over other anticholinergic agents.

The potential side-effects of all antimuscarinic agents include inhibition of salivary secretion (dry mouth), blockade of the ciliary muscle of the lens to cholinergic stimulation (blurred vision for near objects), tachycardia, drowsiness, and inhibition of gut motility. Those agents that possess some ganglionic blocking activity may also cause orthostatic hypotension and impotence at high doses. Antimuscarinic agents are generally contraindicated in patients with narrow-angle glaucoma and should be used with caution in patients with significant bladder outlet obstruction because complete urinary retention may be precipitated.

MUSCULOTROPIC RELAXANTS

These agents fall under the general heading of direct-acting smooth muscle depressants, whose *antispasmodic activity* reportedly is directly on smooth muscle at a site that is metabolically distal to the cholinergic receptor mechanism. Although all three of the agents discussed do relax smooth muscle *in vitro* by a papavarinelike activity, all have been found in addition to possess variable anticholinergic and local anesthetic properties. There is still a question as to how much of their clinical efficacy is due simply to their atropinelike effect. If in fact any of these agents do exert a clinically significant inhibitory effect that is independent of antimuscarinic action, there exists a therapeutic rationale for combining their use with that of a relatively pure anticholinergic agent.

Oxybutynin chloride (Ditropan) is a moderately potent anticholinergic agent with a strong independent musculotropic relaxant activity as well as local anesthetic activity. This agent has been used successfully to depress detrusor hyperreflexia in patients with neurogenic bladder dysfunction and to depress other types of bladder hyperactivity.[4,12] A randomized double-blind, placebo-controlled study in 30 patients with detrusor instability comparing oxybutynin, 5 mg three times daily, and placebo was carried out by Moisey and co-workers.[13] Seventeen of 23 patients had symptomatic improvement, and 9 had evidence of urodynamic improvement—mainly an increase in total bladder capacity. Hehir and Fitzpatrick found that 16 of 24 patients with neuropathic voiding dysfunction secondary to myelomeningocele were cured or improved (17% dry, 50% improved) with oxybutynin.[14] In a prospective, randomized study of 34 patients with voiding dysfunction secondary to multiple sclerosis, Gajewski and Awad found that 5 mg of oral oxybutynin three times a day produced a good response more frequently than 15 mg of propantheline three times a day.[15] They concluded that oxybutynin was more effective than propantheline in the treatment of detrusor hyperreflexia secondary to multiple sclerosis. Holmes and colleagues compared oxybutynin and Pro-Banthine in a small group of women with detrusor instability.[16] The experimental design was a randomized crossover trial with a patient-regulated, variable-dose regimen. Of the 23 women in the trial, 14 reported subjective improvement with oxybutynin, 11 with Pro-Banthine. Both drugs significantly increased the maximum cystometric capacity and reduced the maximum detrusor pressure on filling. The only significant objective difference was a greater increase in the maximum cystometric capacity with oxybutynin. The mean total daily dose of oxybutynin tolerated was 15 mg (range 7.5 to 30), and that of propantheline was 90 mg (range 45–145). Thuroff and associates compared oxybutynin versus propantheline versus placebo in a group of patients with symptoms of instability and either instability or hyperreflexia. Oxybutynin (5 mg three times per day) performed best, but propantheline did have a beneficial effect, even at the relatively low dose used—15 mg three times per day. The rate of side-effects was higher for oxybutynin at just about the level of the clinical and urodynamic improvement.

There are negative reports with oxybutynin as well. Zorzitto and colleagues came to conclusions similar to those regarding propantheline (see previously) in a double-blind, placebo-controlled trial in incontinent geriatric institutionalized patients—that oxybutynin was no more effective than placebo with scheduled toileting in treating this incontinence in this type of population with detrusor hyperactivity.[18] The recommended adult oral dose of oxybutynin is 5 mg, three to four times daily. The potential side-effects are antimuscarinic ones. Topical application of oxybutynin to normal or intestinal bladders has been mentioned. This conceptually attractive form of alternative drug delivery, by periodic intravesical instillation of either liquid or timed-release pellets, awaits further clinical trials and the development of a preparation specifically formulated for that purpose. Madersbacher and Jilg reviewed such usage and presented data on 13 patients with complete suprasacral cord lesions on CIC.[19] One 5-mg tablet was dissolved in distilled water and the solution instilled intravesically. Of the 10 who were incontinent, 9 remained dry for 6 hours. For the group, the changes in bladder capacity and maximal detrusor pressure were significant. Plasma oxybutynin levels were reported in a group of patients in whom administration was intravesical or oral. The level following an oral dose rose to 7.3 ng/ml within 2 hours and then precipitously dropped to slightly less than 2 ng/ml at 4 hours. Following intravesical administration, the level rose gradually to a peak of about 6.2 ng/ml at 3.5 hours, but the level at 6 hours was still greater than 4 and at 9 hours was still between 3 and 4. Does the intravesically applied drug act locally or systemically?

Dicyclonine hydrochloride is also reported to possess a direct relaxant effect on smooth muscle in addition to an antimuscarinic action.[20] An oral dose of 20 mg three times daily in adults has been reported to increase bladder capacity in patients with detrusor hyperreflexia.[21] Beck and colleagues compared the use of 10 mg dicyclonine, 15 mg propantheline, and placebo three times daily in patients with detrusor hyperactivity.[22] The cure or improved rates were 62% for dicyclonine, 73% for propantheline, and 20% for placebo. Awad and co-workers reported that 20 mg dicyclonine three times daily caused resolution or significant improvement in 24 of 27 patients with involuntary bladder contractions.[23]

Flavoxate hydrochloride is a compound that has a direct inhibitory action on smooth muscle but very weak anticholinergic properties.[4,24] Favorable clinical effects have been noted in patients with frequency, urgency, and incontinence and in patients with urodynamically documented detrusor hyperreflexia.[25,26] Briggs and associates, however, reported essentially no effect on detrusor hyperreflexia in an elderly population, an experience that would coincide with the laboratory effects obtained by Benson and associates.[27, 28] The recommended adult dosage is 100 to 200 mg three to four times daily. As with all agents in this group, a short clinical trial may be worthwhile. Reported side-effects are few.

CALCIUM ANTAGONISTS

The role of calcium as a messenger in linking extracellular stimuli to the intracellular environment is well established, including its involvement in excitation-contraction coupling in striated, cardiac, and smooth muscle. The dependence of contractile activity on changes in cytosolic calcium varies from tissue to tissue, but interference with calcium inflow or intracellular release or contraction is a potential mechanism for bladder smooth muscle relaxation. The calcium antagonist nifedipine has been shown to be an effective inhibitor of contraction induced by several mechanisms in human and guinea pig bladder muscle.[4, 29] It has also been shown to be capable of completely blocking the noncholinergic portion of the contraction produced by electrical field stimulation in rabbit bladder.[30] Nifedipine more effectively inhibited potassium-induced than carbachol-induced contraction in rabbit bladder strips, whereas terodiline, an agent with both calcium antagonistic and anticholinergic properties, had the opposite effect. Terodiline, however, caused complete inhibition of the response of rabbit bladder to electrical field stimulation. At low concentrations, it has mainly an antimuscarinic action, whereas at higher concentrations, a calcium-antagonistic effect becomes evident. *In vitro* experiments appeared to show that these two effects were at least additive with regard to bladder contractility. More recent experiments have confirmed the inhibitory effect of the calcium antagonists nifedipine, verapamil, and diltiazem on a variety of experimental models of spontaneous and induced bladder muscle strip and whole bladder preparation activity.[31, 32] Andersson and associates showed that

nifedipine effectively and with some selectivity inhibited the nonmuscarinic portion of contraction of rabbit detrusor strips, whereas verapamil, diltiazem, flunarizine, and lidoflazine caused a marked depression of both the total and the nonmuscarinic part of the contraction, suggesting differences between various calcium channel blockers with respect to effects on at least electrically induced bladder muscle contraction.[33] These results were used as support for the view that even if *atropine-resistant* contractions in rabbit and human bladder were of a different etiology, combined muscarinic receptor and calcium channel blockade might offer a more effective way of controlling bladder hyperactivity than those presently available with a single type of agent action. There have been a number of clinical studies on the inhibitory action of terodiline on bladder hyperactivity, which have shown clinical effectiveness.[34] In a double-blind, cross-over study of 12 women with motor urge incontinence, Ekman and colleagues reported an increase in bladder capacity and the volume at which sensation of urgency was experienced in all but one of the patients treated with terodiline, whereas placebo treatment had no objective or subjective effect.[35] Peters and others reported the results of a multicenter study that ultimately included data from 89 patients (or an original 128) comparing terodiline and placebo in women with motor urge incontinence.[36] They concluded that terodiline was more effective than placebo. They noted, however, that this improvement was much more apparent on subjective assessment than on objective assessment of cystometric and micturition data. Sixty-three percent of patients in this study preferred terodiline, regardless of treatment sequence. Although statistically significant results were recorded on objective parameters between terodiline and placebo, these were not impressive. Frequency of voluntary micturition decreased from 9.6 to 8.9 per 24 hours on placebo and from 9.9 to 7.3 on terodiline. Involuntary micturitions decreased from 2.3 to 1.7 on placebo and from 2.5 to 1.5 on terodiline. Volume at first desire to void increased on placebo from

159 to 162 ml and on terodiline from 151 to 198 ml, whereas bladder capacity increased from 312 to 318 on placebo and from 320 to 374 on terdiline. The daily dose in this study was 12.5 mg in the morning and 25 mg at night. Tapp and co-workers reported on a double-blind placebo study, using dose titration, of 70 women with urodynamically proven detrusor instability and bladder capacities of less than 400 ml.[37] Sixty-two percent of the 34 women in the terodiline group considered themselves improved, as opposed to 38% unchanged. Of the 36 women in the placebo group, 42% considered themselves improved, 47% unchanged, and 11% worse, a statistically significant response in favor of the terodiline group with regard to the improvement rate. Micturition variables of daytime frequency, daytime incontinence episodes, number of pads used, and average voided volumes were statistically changed in favor of terodiline, but the absolute value changes were small (for instance, a daytime incontinence episode change in placebo from 2.5 to 1.9 per day versus 3.7 to 1.6 for terodiline). Urodynamic data, although showing a trend in favor of terodiline in each parameter, showed no statistically significant differences in any category. Side-effects were noted in a large number and with equal frequency in both groups after the dose titration phase. The incidence of anticholinergic side-effects, however, was higher in the drug group, with 29% of the terodiline patients and 11% of the placebo patients spontaneously complaining of a dry mouth and 20% of the terodiline patients and none of the placebo patients complaining of blurred vision.

Terodiline is almost completely absorbed from the gastrointestinal tract and has a low serum clearance. The recommended dosage in adults is 25 mg twice a day, reduced to an initial dose of 12 mg twice a day in geriatric patients. The half-life is around 60 hours, and Abrams logically proposes, on this basis, a once-daily dose but emphasizes the necessity of dose titration for each patient.[34] The common side-effects seen with calcium antagonists (hypotension, facial flushing, headache, dizziness, abdominal discomfort, constipation, nausea, rash, weakness, and palpitations) have not been reported in the larger clinical studies with terodiline, its side-effects consisting primarily of those consequently to its anticholinergic action. Reports in England, however, of serious cardiotoxicity raised about patients taking terodiline simultaneously with antidepressants or antiarrhythmic drugs have occurred, and the drug has been voluntarily withdrawn by the manufacturer pending the results of further safety studies.[38,39]

Calcium antagonists have been administered intravesically, both experimentally and clinically.[40] Mattiasson and associates reported that verapamil so administered produced a significant increase in bladder capacity in patients with detrusor hyperreflexia but not in patients with instability.[41] Other calcium antagonist drugs (than terodiline) have not been widely used to treat voiding dysfunction. Palmer and co-workers reported a double-blind placebo trial with a single 20-mg daily dose of flunarizine in 14 women with detrusor instability and consequent symptoms.[42] A statistically significant decrease in urgency was produced in the drug-treated group, but there was no change in the frequency of micturition. Although there was a trend toward improvement of cystometric parameters, this was not statistically significant at the 0.05 level. Nifedipine may be used as prophylaxis in high spinal injury patients against the development of autonomic hyperreflexia during endoscopic examination. A dose of 10 mg orally 30 minutes before the procedure has been successful, and a sublingual dose of 10 mg was shown effective in relieving an episode.[43]

ALPHA-ADRENERGIC BLOCKING AGENTS

These agents have also been used to treat bladder abnormalities (and outlet problems as well) in patients with so-called autonomous bladders, such as those with myelodysplasia, sacral spinal cord or infrasacral neural injury, voiding dysfunction following radical pelvic surgery.[44] Parasympathetic decentralization has been reported to lead to a marked increase in adrenergic innervation of the bladder, with a resultant conversion of the usual beta (relaxant) response of the bladder body in response to sympathetic stimulation to an alpha (contractile) effect.[45] Although alterations in innervation have been disputed, the alterations in receptor function have not. Koyanagi showed supersensitivity of the urethra to alpha-adrenergic stimulation in a group of patients with autonomous neurogenic bladders, implying change in adrenergic receptor function in the urethra following parasympathetic decentralization.[46] Parsons and Turton observed a similar phenomenon but ascribed the cause to adrenergic supersensitivity of the urethral smooth muscle caused by sympathetic decentralization.[47] Nordling and associates described a similar phenomenon in women after radical hysterectomy and ascribed this change to damage to sympathetic innervation.[48] Decreased bladder compliance is a common clinical problem in such patients, and this, along with a fixed urethral sphincter tone, results in the paradoxical occurrence of both storage and emptying failure. Norlen has summarized supporting evidence for the success of alpha-adrenolytic treatment in these patients.[44] Such treatment with phenoxybenzamine is capable of increasing bladder compliance (increasing storage) and decreasing urethral resistance (facilitating emptying). McGuire and Savastano reported that phenoxybenzamine decreased filling cystometric pressure in the decentralized primate bladder.[5] Anderson and associates used prazosin in such patients and found maximum urethral pressure during filling was decreased, with *autonomous waves* being reduced.[49]

There is another mechanism whereby alpha-adrenergic blockade can decrease bladder contractility in patients with voiding dysfunction. Jensen reported an increased alpha-adrenergic effect in bladders he characterized as "uninhibited."[3,50,51] Short-term and long-term prazosin administration increased capacity and decreased the amplitude of contractions in such patients. Thomas and colleagues found that intravenous phentolamine produced a significant reduction in the maximum voiding detrusor pressure, voided volumes, and peak flow rates in patients

with suprasacral spinal cord injury, with no reduction of outflow obstruction.[52] Rohner and co-workers found that, after bladder outlet obstruction, the normal beta response of canine bladder body smooth musculature was changed to an alpha response.[53] Perlberg and Caine studied bladder dome muscle from patients with obstructive prostatic hypertrophy and found an alpha-adrenergic response to noradrenalin stimulation (instead of the usual beta response) in 23% of 47 patients.[54] They speculated a potential relationship between the irritative symptoms of prostatism, and this altered adrenergic response. They further theorized that at least some of the symptomatic improvement in irritative symptoms in such patients treated with alpha-adrenergic antagonists is due to a direct effect on bladder muscle, rather than on outflow resistance.

POTASSIUM CHANNEL OPENERS

Potassium channel openers efficiently relax various types of smooth muscle by increasing potassium efflux, resulting in membrane hyperpolarization.[4] There are some suggestions that the bladder instability associated at least with infravesical obstruction and detrusor hypertrophy might be secondary to supersensitivity to depolarizing stimuli. Theoretically the potassium channel openers might be an attractive alternative for the treatment of detrusor instability in such circumstances without decreasing contractile ability produced in response to a voluntary initiation of micturition.[55] Pinacidil is such a compound whose concentration dependently inhibits not only spontaneous myogenic contractions but also contractile responses induced by electrical field stimulation and carbachol in isolated human detrusor and in normal and hypertrophied rat detrusor.[56] Unfortunately, a preliminary study with this agent in a double-blind crossover format has shown no effect, administered orally in a dose sufficient to decrease both standing systolic and diastolic blood pressure, on symptom status in nine patients with detrusor instability and bladder outlet obstruction.[57] Nurse and colleagues reported on the use of cromkalin, another potassium channel opener, in 17 patients with refractory detrusor instability or hyperreflexia or who had stopped other drug therapy because of intolerable side-effects.[58] Six of 16 patients who completed the study showed a decrease in frequency and an increase in voided volume. Long-term observation was not possible because the drug was withdrawn owing to reported adverse effects of high doses in animal toxicologic studies. Further experimental and clinical trials with potassium channel openers for various detrusor hyperactivity states are awaited.

PROSTAGLANDIN INHIBITORS

Prostaglandins are ubiquitous compounds that have been mentioned as having a potential role in excitatory neurotransmission to the bladder, in the development of bladder contractility or tension occurring during filling, in the emptying contractile response of bladder smooth muscle to neural stimulation, and even in the maintenance of urethral tone during the storage phase of micturition as well as in the release of this tone during the emptying phase.[2] Downie and Carmazyn suggest a different type of contractile influence of prostaglandins on detrusor muscle.[59] They found that mechanical irritation of the epithelium of rabbit bladder increased basal tension and spontaneous activity in response to electrical stimulation and that these responses were related to the intensity of the irritative trauma, mimicked by prostaglandins, and that the effect was significantly reduced by pretreatment of the epithelium, but not the muscle, with prostaglandin synthetase inhibitors. Andersson suggests possible sensitization of sensory afferent nerves by prostaglandins, increasing afferent input at a given degree of bladder filling and contributing to the triggering of IVC at a small bladder volume.[4] Thus there exists multiple mechanisms whereby prostaglandin synthesis inhibitors might decrease bladder contractility in response to various stimuli. Objective evidence that such can occur, however, is scant. Cardozo and co-workers reported on the effects of 50 mg three times daily of flurbiprofen, a prostaglandin synthetase inhibitor, on 30 women with detrusor instability.[60] In a double-blind placebo study, it was concluded that the drug did not abolish involuntary bladder contractions or abnormal bladder activity but delayed the intravesical pressure rise to a greater degree of distention. Forty-three percent of the patients experienced side-effects, primarily nausea, vomiting, headache, indigestion, gastric distress, constipation, and rash. Cardozo and associates reported symptomatic improvement in patients with detrusor instability given indomethacin in doses of 50 to 200 mg daily.[60] This was a short-term study with no cystometric data, and the drug was compared only with bromocriptine. The incidence of side-effects was high (19 out of 32), although no patient had to stop treatment because of these. Prostaglandin synthetase inhibitors have proved useful in the treatment of primary dysmenorrhea, a condition that is thought to be related to a high level of menstrual endometrial prostaglandin synthesis.[61] Numerous prostaglandin inhibitors exist, most of which fall under the heading of nonsteroidal anti-inflammatory drugs, and every clinician has a "favorite." It should be remembered that these drugs can interfere with platelet function and contribute to excess bleeding in surgical patients, and some may have adverse renal effects.[62]

BETA-ADRENERGIC AGONISTS

The presence of beta-adrenergic receptors in human bladder muscle has prompted attempts to increase bladder capacity with beta-adrenergic stimulation. Such stimulation can cause significant increases in the capacity of animal bladders, which contain a moderate density of beta-adrenergic receptors.[2] *In vitro* studies show a strong dose-related relaxant effect of $beta_2$ agonists on the bladder body of rabbits but little effect on the bladder base or proximal urethra. Terbutaline, in oral doses of 5 mg three times daily, has been reported to have a "good clinical effect" in some patients with urgency and urgency incontinence but no significant effect on the bladders of neurologically normal humans without voiding difficulty.[63] Although these results are compatible with those in other organ systems (beta-adrenergic stimulation causes no acute change in total lung capacity in normal humans, whereas it does favorably affect patients with bronchial asthma), few adequate studies are available on the effects of beta-adrenergic stimulation in patients with detrusor hyperactivity. Lindholm and Lose used 5 mg three times daily of terbutaline in eight women with motor and seven with sensory urge incontinence.[64] After 3 months of treatment, 14 patients claimed beneficial effects, and 12 became subjectively continent. In six of eight cases, the detrusor became stable on cystometry. Interestingly the volume of the first desire to void increased in the patients with originally unstable bladders from a mean of 200 to 302 ml, but the maximum cystometric capacity did not change. Nine patients had transient side-effects, including palpitations, tachycardia, hand tremor, and in three of these, side-effects continued but were acceptable. In one patient, the drug was discontinued because of severe adverse symptoms. Gruneberger reported that in a double-blind study, clerbuterol, 0.01 mg three times daily, had a good therapeutic effect in 15 of 20 women with motor urge incontinence.[65] Unfavorable results on beta-agonist usage for bladder hyperactivity were published by Castleden and Morgan and Naglo and associates.[66,67]

TRICYCLIC ANTIDEPRESSANTS

Many clinicians, including ourselves, have found tricyclic antidepressants, particularly imipramine hydrochloride, to be especially useful agents for facilitating urine storage, by both decreasing bladder contractility and increasing outlet resistance.[68] These agents have been the subject of a voluminous amount of highly sophisticated pharmacologic investigation to determine the mechanisms of action responsible for their varied effects.[69-71] Most data have been accumulated as a result of trying to explain the antidepressant properties of these agents and

consequently have been accumulated primarily from central nervous system tissue. The results, conclusions, and speculations inferred from the data are extremely interesting, but it should be emphasized that it is essentially unknown whether they apply to or have relevance for the lower urinary tract. All of these agents possess varying degrees of at least three major pharmacologic actions. They have central and peripheral anticholinergic effects at some, but not all, sites; they block the active transport system in the presynaptic nerve ending, which is responsible for the reuptake of the released amine neurotransmitters noradrenaline and serotonin; and they are sedatives, an action that occurs presumably on a central basis but is perhaps related to antihistaminic properties (at H_1 receptors, although they also antagonize H_2 receptors to some extent). There is also evidence that they desensitize at least some $alpha_2$ adrenoceptors and some beta adrenoceptors. Paradoxically they also have been shown to block some alpha and serotonin$_1$ receptors. Imipramine has prominent systemic anticholinergic effects but has only a weak antimuscarinic effect on bladder smooth muscle.[72,73] A strong direct inhibitory effect on bladder smooth muscle does exist, however, which is neither anticholinergic nor adrenergic.[28,72,74] This may be due to a local anestheticlike action at the nerve terminals in the adjacent effector membrane, an effect that seems to occur also in cardiac muscle[75] or to an inhibition of the participation of calcium in the excitation-contraction coupling process.[72,76] Akah has provided supportive evidence in the rat bladder that desipramine, the active metabolite of imipramine, depresses the response to electrical field stimulation by interfering with calcium movement (perhaps not only extracellular calcium movement, but also internal translocation and binding).[77] Clinically imipramine seems to be effective in decreasing bladder contractility and in increasing outlet resistance.[78-82] Attempting to correlate the clinical effects with mechanisms of action, besides the direct nonanticholinergic inhibitory effect on bladder smooth muscle, one might also postulate a beta receptor to induced decrease in bladder body contractility if peripheral blockade of norepinephrine reuptake does occur there, owing to the increased concentration of beta-adrenergic over alpha-adrenergic receptors in that area. An enhanced alpha-adrenergic effect in the smooth muscle of the bladder base and proximal urethra, where alpha receptors outnumber beta receptors, is generally considered to be the mechanism whereby imipramine increases outlet resistance.

Castleden and colleagues began therapy in elderly patients with detrusor instability with a single 25-mg nighttime dose of imipramine, which was increased every third day by 25 mg until the patient was continent, the patient had side-effects, or a dose of 150 mg was reached.[82] Six of 10 patients became continent, and in those who underwent repeated cystometry, bladder capacity increased by a mean of 105 ml, and bladder pressure at capacity decreased by a mean of 18 cm H_2O. Maximum urethral pressure increased by a mean of 30 cm H_2O. Although our subjective impression was that the bladder effects become evident only after days of treatment, some patients in this series became continent after only 3 to 5 days of therapy.[80] Our usual adult dose for voiding dysfunction is 25 mg four times daily; half that dose is given in elderly patients in whom the drug half-life may be prolonged. In our experience, the effects of imipramine on the lower urinary tract are often additive to those of the atropinelike agents, and consequently a combination of imipramine and an antimuscarinic or an antispasmodic is sometimes especially useful for decreasing bladder contractility.[80] If imipramine is used in conjunction with an atropinelike agent, it should be noted that the anticholinergic side-effects of the drugs may be additive. It has been known for many years that imipramine is relatively effective in the treatment of childhood nocturnal enuresis. Doses range from 10 to 50 mg daily. Whether the mechanisms of action in the situation are the same as those for decreasing bladder contractility or increasing outlet resistance or whether the antienuretic effect is more centrally mediated is unknown. Korczyn and Kish have

presented evidence that the antienuretic effect is neither on a peripheral anticholinergic basis nor on the same basis of whatever effects are responsible for the drug's antidepressant action.[83] The antienuretic effect occurs soon after initial administration, whereas the antidepressant effects generally take 2 to 4 weeks to develop.

Doxepin (Sinequan) is another tricyclic antidepressant, which was found to be more potent, using in vitro rabbit bladder strips, than other tricyclic compounds with respect to antimuscarinic and musculotropic relaxant activity.[74] Lose and co-workers, in a randomized, double-blind, crossover study of women with involuntary bladder contractions and frequency, urgency, or urge incontinence, found that this agent caused a significant decrease in nighttime frequency and nighttime incontinence episodes and a near significant decrease in urine loss and in the cystometric parameters of first sensation and maximum capacity.[84] The dosage of doxepin used was either a single 50-mg bedtime dose or such a dose with 25 mg in the morning. The number of daytime incontinence episodes decreased in both doxepin and placebo groups, and the difference was not statistically significant. Doxepin treatment was preferred by 14 patients, whereas 2 preferred placebo. Three patients had no preference. Of the 14 patients who stated a preference for doxepin, 12 claimed that they became continent during treatment, and 2 claimed improvement. The two patients who preferred placebo claimed improvement.

When used in the generally larger doses employed for antidepressant effects, the most frequent side-effects of the tricyclic antidepressants are those attributable to their systemic anticholinergic activity.[70,71] Allergic phenomena, including rash, hepatic dysfunction, obstructive jaundice, and agranulocytosis, may also occur but rarely. Central nervous system side-effects may include weakness, fatigue, parkinsonian effect, a fine tremor noted most in the upper extremities, a manic or schizophrenic picture, and sedation, probably from its antihistaminic effect. Postural hypotension may also be seen, presumably on the basis of selective blockade (a paradoxical effect) of alpha$_1$-adrenergic receptors in some vascular smooth muscle. Tricyclic antidepressants can cause orthostatic hypotension, produce arrhythmias, and interact in deleterious ways with other drugs, and so caution must be observed in their use in patients with cardiac disease.[71] Whether cardiotoxicity will prove to be a legitimate concern in patients receiving smaller doses (than antidepressant ones) for lower urinary tract dysfunction remains to be seen but is a potential matter of concern. Consultation with an individual patient's internist or cardiologist is always helpful before instituting such therapy in questionable situations. Tricyclic antidepressants can also cause excess sweating of obscure cause and a delay of orgasm and orgasmic impotence, the cause of which is likewise unclear. The use of imipramine is contraindicated in patients receiving monoamine oxidase inhibitors because severe central nervous system toxic effects, including hyperpyrexia, seizures, and coma, can be precipitated. The potential side-effects of the antidepressants may be especially significant for elderly persons, specifically weakness, fatigue, and postural hypotension. If imipramine or any of the tricyclic antidepressants is to be prescribed for the treatment of voiding dysfunction, the patient should be thoroughly informed of the fact that this is not the usual indication for this drug and that potential side-effects exist. The onset of significant side-effects (severe abdominal distress, nausea, vomiting, headache, lethargy, and irritability) following abrupt cessation of high doses of imipramine in children would suggest that the drug should be discontinued gradually, especially in patients receiving high doses.

DIMETHYL SULFOXIDE (DMSO)

Dimethyl sulfoxide is a relatively simple, naturally occurring organic compound that has been used as an industrial solvent for many years. It has multiple pharmacologic actions (membrane penetrant, anti-inflammatory, local analgesic, bacteriostatic, diuretic, cholinesterase inhibitor, collagen solvent, vasodilator) and has been used

for the treatment of arthritis and other musculoskeletal disorders, generally in a 70% solution. The formulation for human intravesical use is a 50% solution. Sant has summarized the pharmacology and clinical usage of dimethyl sulfoxide and has tabulated good to excellent results in 50% to 90% of the collected series of patients treated with intravesical instillations for interstitial cystitis.[85] Dimethyl sulfoxide has not been shown, however, to be useful in the treatment of detrusor hyperreflexia or instability or in any patients with urgency or frequency but without interstitial cystitis.

POLYSYNAPTIC INHIBITORS

Baclofen is an agent that can decrease outlet resistance secondary to striated sphincter dyssynergia. It has also been shown to be capable of depressing detrusor hyperreflexia secondary to a spinal cord lesion.[86] Taylor and Bates, in a double-blind crossover study, reported it to be effective also in decreasing daytime and nighttime urinary frequency and incontinence in patients with idiopathic instability.[87] Cystometric changes were not recorded, however, and considerable improvement was also obtained in the placebo group. The intrathecal use of baclofen for treatment of detrusor hyperactivity is a potentially exciting area (see prior discussion), and further reports are awaited.

Increasing Bladder Capacity by Decreasing Sensory (Afferent) Input

The potential clinical implications of being able to defunctionalize at least some primary afferent neurons from the lower urinary tract pharmacologically are extraordinary. Such an action would be ideal for the treatment of sensory urgency. It could also be used to treat instability or hyperreflexia in a bladder with relatively normal viscoelastic properties in which the sensory afferents were the first limb in the abnormal micturition reflex. Maggi and others have written extensively about this type of potential pharmacologic treatment, specifically with reference to the properties of capsaicin.[88,89] Capsaicin is the pungent ingredient in a variety of red peppers and a neurotoxic compound, which causes initial excitation then desensitization of thin type B sensory neurons, depleting their content of certain neuropeptides, including substance P. Although obvious potential problems exist with respect to mode of administration, undesirable sequelae of the initial excitatory effects, and potential adverse long-term sequelae, this is an interesting concept that holds promise of future avenues of drug treatment.

Circumventing the Problem

ANTIDIURETIC HORMONELIKE AGENTS

The synthetic antidiuretic hormone peptide analog DDAVP (1-deamina-9-D-arginine vasopressin) has been used for the symptomatic relief of refractory nocturnal enuresis in both children and adults.[90,91] The drug can conveniently be administered by intranasal spray at bedtime (dose 10 to 40 µg) and effectively suppresses urine production for 7 to 10 hours. Its clinical long-term safety has been established by continued use in patients with diabetes insipidus. Normal water deprivation tests by Rew and Rundle would seem to indicate that long-term use does not cause depression of endogenous antidiuretic hormone secretion at least in patients with nocturnal enuresis. At present, this novel circumventive approach to the treatment of urinary frequency and incontinence has been pretty much restricted to those with nocturnal enuresis and diabetes insipidus. The fact that the drug seems to be much more effective than simple fluid restriction alone for the former condition is perhaps explained by relatively recent reports suggesting a decreased nocturnal secretion of antidiuretic hormone by such patients.[90] Suggestions have been made that DDAVP might be useful in patients with refractory nocturnal frequency and incontinence but who do not fall into the category of primary nocturnal enuresis.

Kinn and Larsson reported that micturition frequency "decreased significantly" in 13 patients with multiple sclerosis and urge incontinence treated with oral tablets or desmopressin and that less leakage occurred.[92] The actual average change in the number of voiding during the 6 hours after drug intake was approximately 3.2 to 2.5. It will be interesting to see whether any drug companies pursue this avenue of treatment for the large number of patients with refractory nocturnal bladder storage problems or for "spot" usage before some important event in patients with urgency and frequency, with and without incontinence.

References

1. Wein AJ. Classification of neurogenic voiding dysfunction. J Urol 1981;125:605.
2. Wein AJ, Levin RM, Barrett DM. Voiding function: Relevant anatomy, physiology and pharmacology. In: Gillenwater JY, Grayhack JT, Howards St, Duckett JW, eds. Adult and pediatric urology. 2nd ed. St. Louis: Mosby-Year Book, 1991:933–999.
3. Jensen D Jr. Pharmacological studies of the uninhibited neurogenic bladder. Acta Neurol Scand 1981;64:175.
4. Andersson KE. Current concepts in the treatment of disorders of micturition. Drugs 1988;35:477.
5. McGuire E, Savastano J. Effect of alpha adrenergic blockade and anticholinergic agents on the decentralized primate bladder. Neurourol Urodynam 1985;4:139.
6. Ulmsten U, Andersson KE, Persson CGA. Diagnostic and therapeutic aspects of urge urinary incontinence in women. Urol Int 1977;32:88.
7. Brading A. Physiology of bladder smooth muscle. In: Torrens M, Morrison JFB, eds. The physiology of the lower urinary tract. London: Springer Verlag, 1987:161–192.
8. Zorzitto ML, Jewett MA, Fernie GR, et al. Effectiveness of propantheline bromide in the treatment of geriatric patients with detrusor instability. Neurourol Urodynam 1986;5:133.
9. Blaivas JG. Management of bladder dysfunction in multiple sclerosis. Neurology 1980;30:12.
10. Brown JH. Atropine, scopolamine and related antimuscarinic drugs. In: Gilman AG, Rall TW, Nies AS, Taylor P, eds. Goodman and Gilman's

the pharmacological basis of therapeutics. 8th ed. New York: Pergamon Press, 1990:150–165.

11. Levin RM, Staskin D, Wein AJ. The muscarinic cholinergic binding kinetics of the human urinary bladder. Neurourol Urodynam 1982;1:221.

12. Thompson I, Lauvetz R. Oxybutynin in bladder spasm, neurogenic bladder and enuresis. Urology 1976;8:452.

13. Moisey C, Stephenson T, Brendler C. The urodynamic and subjective results of treatment of detrusor instability with oxybutynin chloride. Br J Urol 1980;52:472.

14. Hehir M, Fitzpatrick JM. Oxybutynin and the prevention of urinary incontinence in spina bifida. Eur Urol 1985;11:254.

15. Gajewski JB, Awad JA. Oxybutynin versus propantheline in patients with multiple sclerosis and detrusor hyperreflexia. J Urol 1986;135:966.

16. Holmes DM, Monty FJ, Stanton SL. Oxybutynin versus propantheline in the management of detrusor instability. A patient regulated variable dose trial. B J Obstet Gynaecol 1989;96:607.

17. Thuroff J, Bunke B, Ebner A, et al. Randomized double-blind multicenter trial on treatment of frequency, urgency and incontinence related to detrusor hyperactivity: Oxybutynin vs. propantheline vs. placebo. J Urol 1991;145:813.

18. Zorzitto ML, Holliday PJ, Jewett MA, et al. Oxybutynin for geriatric urinary dysfunction: A double-blind placebo controlled study. Age Aging 1989;18:195.

19. Madersbacher H, Jilg G. Control of detrusor hyperreflexia by the intravesical instillation of oxybutynin hydrochloride. Paraplegia 1991;19:84.

20. Downie J, Twiddy D, Awad S. Antimuscarinic and non-competitive antagonist properties of dicyclomine hydrochloride in isolated human and rabbit bladder muscle. J Pharmacol Exp Ther 1977;201:662.

21. Fischer C, Diokno A, Lapides J. The anticholinergic effects of dicyclomine hydrochloride in uninhibited neurogenic bladder dysfunction. J Urol 1978;120:328.

22. Beck RP, Amausch T, King C. Results in testing 210 patients with detrusor overactivity incontinence of urine. Am J Obstet Gynecol 1976;125:593.

23. Awad S, Downie J, Kiruluta H. Alpha adrenergic agents in urinary disorders of the proximal urethra: I. Stress incontinence. Br J Urol 1978;50:332.

24. Ruffman R. A review of flavoxate hydrochloride in the treatment of urge incontinence. J Int Med Res 1988;16:317.

25. Delaere Michiels HGE, Debruyne FMJ, Moonen WA. Flavoxate hydrochloride in the treatment of detrusor instability. Urol Int 1977;32:377.

26. Jonas U, Petri E, Kissal J. The effect of flavoxate on hyperactive detrusor muscle. Eur Urol 1979;5:106.

27. Briggs R, Castleden C, Asher M: The effect of flavoxate on uninhibited detrusor contractions and urinary incontinence in the elderly. J Urol 1980;123:665.

28. Benson GS, Sarshik SA, Raezer DM, Wein AJ. Bladder muscle contractility: Comparative effects and mechanisms of action of atropine, propantheline, flavoxate, and imipramine. Urology 1977;9:31.

29. Forman A, Andersson K, Henriksson L, et al. Effects of nifedipine on the smooth muscle of the human urinary tract in vitro and in vivo. Acta Pharmacol Toxicol 1978;43:111.

30. Husted S, Andersson KE, Sommer L, et al. Anticholinergic and calcium antagonistic effects of terodilene in rabbit urinary bladder. Acta Pharmacol Toxicol 1980;146:20.

31. Finkbeiner AE. Effect of extracellular calcium and calcium blocking agents on detrusor contractility: An in vitro study. Neurourol Urodynam 1983;2:245.

32. Malkowicz SB, Wein AJ, Brendler K, Levin RM. Effect of diltiazem on in vitro rabbit bladder function. Pharmacology 1985;31:24.

33. Andersson KE, Fovaeus M, Morgan E, et al. Comparative effects of five different calcium channel blockers on the atropine resistant contraction in electrically stimulated rabbit urinary bladder. Neurourol Urodynam 1986;5:579.

34. Abrams P. Terodiline in clinical practice. Urology 1990;36(suppl):60.

35. Ekman G, Andersson KE, Rud T, Ulmsten K. A double-blind crossover study of the effects of terodiline in women with unstable bladder. Acta Pharmacol Toxicol 1980;46(suppl):39.

36. Peters D, Multicentre Study Group: Terodilene in the treatment of urinary frequency and motor urge incontinence, a controlled multicentre trial. Scand J Urol Nephrol 1984;87(suppl):21.

37. Tapp A, Fall M, Norgaard J, et al. Terodiline: A dose titrated, multicenter study of the treatment of idiopathic detrusor instability in women. J Urol 1989;142:1027.

38. Veldhuis GJ, Inman WHW: Terodilene and torsades de pointes (letter). BMJ 1991;303:519.

39. Connolly MJ, Astridge PS, White EG, et al. Torsades de pointes ventricular tachycardia and terodilene. Lancet 1991;338:344.

40. Kato K, Kitada S, Chun A, et al. In vitro intravesical instillation of anticholinergic antispasmodic and calcium blocking agents in rabbit whole bladder model. J Urol 1989;141:1471.

41. Mattiasson A, Ekstrom B, Andersson KE. Effects

of intravesical instillation of verapamil in patients with detrusor hyperactivity. J Urol 1989;141:174.

42. Palmer J, Worth P, Exton-Smith A: Flunarizine: A once daily therapy for urinary incontinence. Lancet 1981;2:279.

43. Dykstra D, Sidi A, Anderson L. The effect of nifedipine on cystoscopy induced autonomic hyperreflexia in patients with high spinal cord injuries. J Urol 1987;138:1155.

44. Norlen L. Influence of the sympathetic nervous system on the lower urinary tract and its clinical implications. Neurourol Urodynam 1982; 1:129.

45. Sundin T, Dahlstrom A, Norlen L, Svedmyr N. The sympathetic innervation and adrenoreceptor function of the human lower urinary tract in the normal state and after parasympathetic denervation. Invest Urol 1977;14:322.

46. Koyanagi T. Further observation on the denervation supersensitivity of the urethra in patients with chronic neurogenic bladders. J Urol 1979; 122:348.

47. Parsons K, Turton M. Urethral supersensitivity and occult urethral neuropathy. Br J Urol 1980; 52:131.

48. Nordling J, Meyhoff H, Hald T. Urethral denervation supersensitivity to noradrenaline after radical hysterectomy. Scand J Urol Nephrol 1981;15:21.

49. Andersson K, Ek A, Hedlung H, et al. Effects of prazosin on isolated human urethra and in patients with lower neuron lesions. Invest Urol 1981;19:39.

50. Jensen D Jr. Altered adrenergic innervation in the uninhibited neurogenic bladder. Scand J Urol Nephrol 1981;60:61.

51. Jensen D Jr. Uninhibited neurogenic bladder treated with prazosin. Scand J Urol Nephrol 1982;15:229.

52. Thomas DG, Philp NH, McDermott TE. The use of urodynamic studies to assess the effect of pharmacological agents with particular references to alpha adrenergic blockade. Paraplegia 1984; 22:162.

53. Rohner T, Hannigan J, Sanford E. Altered in vitro adrenergic responses of dog detrusor muscle after chronic bladder outlet obstruction. Urology 1978;11:357.

54. Perlberg S, Caine M. Adrenergic response of bladder muscle in prostatic obstruction. Urology 1982;10:524.

55. Malmgren A, Andersson KE, Fovaeus M, Sjogren C. Effects of cromkalin and pinacidil on normal and hypertrophied rat detrusor in vitro. J Urol 1990;143:828.

56. Fovaeus M, Andersson KE, Hedlund H. The ac-

tion of pinacidil in the isolated human bladder. J Urol 1989;141:637.

57. Hedlund H, Mattiasson A, Andersson KE. Lack of effect of pinacidil on detrusor instability in men with bladder outlet obstruction. J Urol 1990; 143:369A.

58. Nurse D, Restorick J, Mundy A. The effect of cromkalin on the normal and hyperreflexic human detrusor muscle. Br J Urol 1991;68:27.

59. Downie JW, Carmazyn M. Mechanical trauma to bladder epithelium liberates prostanoids which modulate neurotransmission in rabbit detrusor muscle. J Pharmacol Exp Ther 1984;230:445.

60. Cardozo L, Stanton S, Robinson H, Hale D. Evaluation of flurbiprofen in detrusor instability. BMJ 1980;1180:281.

61. Chan WY. Prostaglandins and nonsteroidal anti-inflammatory drugs in dysmennorrhea. Am Rev Pharmacol Toxicol 1983;23:131.

62. Brooks PM, Day RO. Non-steroidal anti-inflammatory drugs—differences and similarities. N Engl J Med 1991;324:1716.

63. Norlen L, Sundin T, Waagstein F. Beta-adrenoceptor stimulation of the human urinary bladder in vivo. Acta Pharmacol Toxicol 1978;43:5.

64. Lindholm P, Lose G. Terbutaline (Bricanyl) in the treatment of female urge incontinence. Urol Int 1986;41:158.

65. Gruneberger A. Treatment of motor urge incontinence with clerbuterol and flavoxate hydrochloride. Br J Obstet Gynaecol 1984;91:275.

66. Castleden CM, Morgan B. The effect of beta adrenoceptor agonists on urinary incontinence in the elderly. Br J Clin Pharmacol 1980;10:619.

67. Naglo AS, Nergardh A, Boreus LO. Influence of atropine and isoprenoline on detrusor hyperactivity in children with neurogenic bladder. Scand J Urol Nephrol 1981;15:97.

68. Barrett D, Wein AJ. Voiding dysfunction: Diagnosis, classification and management. In: Gillenwater JY, Grayhack JT, Howards ST, Duckett JW, eds. Adult and pediatric urology. 2nd ed. St. Louis: Mosby-Year Book, 1991:1001–1099.

69. Hollister LE. Current antidepressants. Ann Rev Pharmacol Toxicol 1986;26:23.

70. Richelson E. Antidepressants and brain neurochemistry. Mayo Clin Proc 1990;65:1227.

71. Baldessarini RJ. Drugs and the treatment of psychiatric disorders. In: Gilman AG, Rall TW, Nies AS, Taylor P, eds. Goodman and Gilman's the pharmacological basis of therapeutics. 8th ed. New York: Pergamon Press, 1990:383–435.

72. Olubadewo J. The effect of imipramine on rat detrusor muscle contractility. Arch Int Pharmacodyn Ther 1980;145:84.

73. Levin RM, Staskin DR, Wein AJ. Analysis of the

anticholinergic and musculotropic effects of des-methylimipramine on the rabbit urinary bladder. Urol Res 1983;11:259.

74. Levin RM, Wein AJ. Comparative effects of five tricyclic compounds on the rabbit urinary bladder. Neurourol Urodynam 1984;3:127.

75. Bigger J, Giardino E, Perel J, et al. Cardiac antiar-rhythmic effect of imipramine hydrochloride. N Engl J Med 1977;296:206.

76. Malkowicz SB, Wein AJ, Ruggieri MR, Levin RM. Comparison of calcium antagonist proper-ties of antispasmodic agents. J Urol 1987;138:667.

77. Akah PA. Tricyclic antidepressant inhibition of the electrical evoked responses of the rat urinary bladder strip effect of variation in extracellular Ca concentration. Arch Int Pharmacodyn 1986; 284:231.

78. Cole A, Fried F. Favorable experiences with imi-pramine in the treatment of neurogenic bladder. J Urol 1972;107:44.

79. Mahony D, Laferte F, Mahoney J. Observations on sphincter augmenting effect of imipramine in children with urinary incontinence. Urology 1973;2:317.

80. Raezer DM, Benson GS, Wein AJ, et al. The func-tional approach to the management of the pedi-atric neuropathic bladder. A clinical study. J Urol 1977;117:649.

81. Tulloch AGS, Creed KE. A comparison between propantheline and imipramine on bladder and salivary gland function. Br J Urol 1979;51:359.

82. Castleden CM, George CF, Renwick AG, Asher MJ. Imipramine—a possible alternative to cur-rent therapy for urinary incontinence in the el-derly. J Urol 1981;125:218.

83. Korczyn AD, Kish I. The mechanism of imipra-mine in enuresis nocturna. Clin Exp Pharmacol Physiol 1979;6:31.

84. Lose G, Jorgensen L, Thunedborg P. Doxepin in the treatment of female detrusor overactivity: A randomized double-blind crossover study. J Urol 1989;142:1024.

85. Sant G. Intravesical 50% dimethylsulfoxide in the treatment of interstitial cystitis. Urology 1987;4(suppl):17.

86. Kiesswetter H, Schober W. Lioresal in the treat-ment of neurogenic bladder dysfunction. Urol Int 1975;30:63.

87. Taylor MC, Bates CP. A double-blind crossover trial of baclofen: A new treatment for the unstable bladder syndrome. Br J Urol 1979;51:505.

88. Maggi CA, Barbank G, Santicoli P, et al. Cys-tometric evidence that capsaicin sensitive nerves modulate the afferent branch of micturition reflex on humans. J Urol 1989;142:150.

89. Maggi CA. Capsaicin and primary afferent neu-rons: From basic science to human therapy? J Auton Neurol Syst 1991;33:1.

90. Norgaard JP, Rillig S, Djurhuus JC. Nocturnal enuresis: An approach to treatment based on pathogenesis. J Pediatr 1989;114:705.

91. Rew DA, Rundle JSH. Assessment of the safety of regular DDAVP therapy on primary nocturnal enuresis. Br J Urol 1989;63:352.

92. Kinn AC, Larsson PO. Desmopressin: A new principle for symptomatic treatment of urgency and incontinence in patients with multiple scle-rosis. Scand J Urol Nephrol 1990;24:109.

9

Surgical Therapy of Uncontrollable Detrusor Contractility

Edward J. McGuire

Michael L. Ritchey

Julian H. Wan

Surgical therapy is relatively limited in scope but effective if the underlying problem is accurately identified and the surgery planned to deal with that problem.

Relief of Obstructive Uropathy

Obstructive uropathy is commonly associated with detrusor instability and detrusor hyper-reflexia with resultant incontinence. In women, this is most commonly encountered after operative procedures for the relief of stress incontinence, but infrequently primary bladder neck obstruction or distal urethral stenosis and stricture formation are associated with uninhibited bladder contractility and incontinence as well. For accurate diagnosis, a videourodynamic study that demonstrates high intravesical pressures, full relaxation of the external urethral sphincter, and a poor flow rate is required. In the absence of videourodynamics, a poor flow rate in association with a high bladder pressure and perfect sphincter relaxation is consistent with the diagnosis of bladder outlet obstruction. Residual urine is not always present, but if so it helps to make the diagnosis in association with the other findings. Residual urine by itself is not sufficient evidence to permit the certain diagnosis of obstructive uropathy.

Most patients who develop obstructive uropathy as a result of operative procedures for the relief of stress incontinence have experienced the problem of an unstable bladder for at least 1 year and often much longer than that. On physical examination, the urethra is in a high retropubic position, which makes endoscopy somewhat difficult. Trabeculation of the bladder and residual urine are almost always present. Patients clearly relate the development of their symptoms to the immediate postoperative period. Cystoscopy with both a 30- and 70-degree lens is essential to search for suture erosion into the bladder and urethra, which are occasional unpleasant surprises necessitating a suprapubic search for both right and left sutures and any bolster material, at the time of a procedure to correct urethral obstruction.

The operative procedure of choice for the relief of outlet obstruction associated with prior stress incontinence surgery is a transvaginal urethrolysis, which employs the first, mobilization, steps of a Raz type urethral suspension operation. This involves first determining the degree of urethral fixation, which is usually total, by gentle traction on the indwelling Foley catheter. Traction on the catheter results in absolutely no motion of the urethra into the potential space of the vagina. At this point, an up-and-down vaginal incision is made over the urethra.

Female Urology, edited by Elroy D. Kursh and Edward McGuire. J. B. Lippincott, Philadelphia, © 1994.

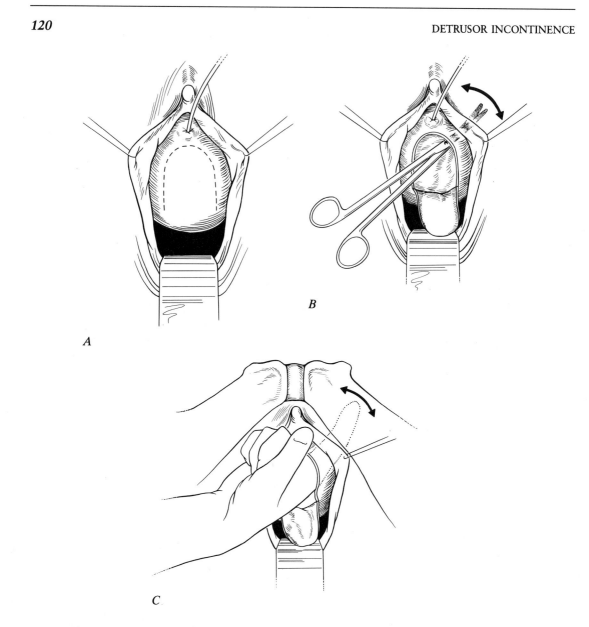

Figure 9-1. *Transvaginal urethrolysis for relief of urethral hypersuspension after needle suspension or pubovaginal sling and retropubic procedures. (A) Vaginal approach incision—can be vertical or U-shaped variety. (B) Sharp entry into the retropubic space, well lateral to the urethra—as for a Raz type urethral suspension. (C) Blunt mobilization of the urethra and bladder base to achieve adequate urethral mobility.*

The incision is medial to the area of the suspension sutures, sling, Birch, or Marshall-Marchetti-Krantz sutures, which are usually visible or palpable on the anterior vaginal wall well lateral to the urethra. The vaginal epithelium is lifted off the underlying white glistening periurethral fascia. Care taken at the beginning of the procedure to stay superficial to the periurethral fascia pays great dividends in terms of freedom from injury to the bladder or urethra. The dissection is continued laterally until the junction of the endopelvic fascia with the ischium is reached. An opening, with the scissors directed 90 degrees away from the urethra, is then made into the retropubic space, as one would do for the first part of a Raz procedure (Fig. 9-1). This maneuver on both sides is usually all that is required to free the urethra and thereby to gain urethral mobility. We do not routinely do a suspension procedure. The extent of urethral dissection is somewhat less than that described by Raz and associates, who sharply mobilize the urethra circumferentially and then perform a lateral neourethral suspension procedure. Recurrent obstruction has been a problem in 2 of our 21 patients after a period of complete freedom from symptoms for 1 to 3 months. When re-examined, the urethra was again suspended in a high retropubic position as it had been before the urethrolysis.

The degree of mobility induced by the operative procedure is judged during the procedure by traction on the Foley catheter and determining the amount of mobility conferred by the dissection. Typically 30 to 40 degrees angular motion into the potential space of the vagina with traction on the urethral catheter is sufficient and is associated with good postoperative result (Fig. 9-2).

Urethral Strictures and Bladder Neck Obstruction

These conditions are rare but when present can be associated with unstable detrusor dysfunc-

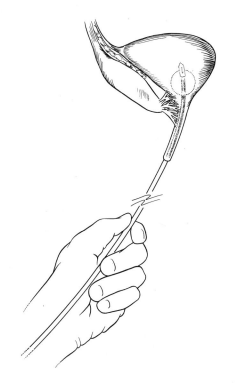

Figure 9-2. *Method of traction on the Foley catheter to determine mobility of the proximal urethra, judged by palpation intravaginally behind the urethra.*

tion. The entire University of Michigan experience with these entities in the past 10 years involves seven patients.

Isolated idiopathic vesical outlet obstruction occurred in five patients and was treated successfully by endoscopic incision of the bladder neck on one side and long-term self-obturation thereafter. Urethral strictures involving the distal urethra or the area immediately distal to the external sphincter, with retention of 200 to 300 ml postvoid volumes, were treated by U-shaped vaginal inlay flap on three occasions. We also used self-obturation after that procedure. Long-term results have been excellent (Fig. 9-3).

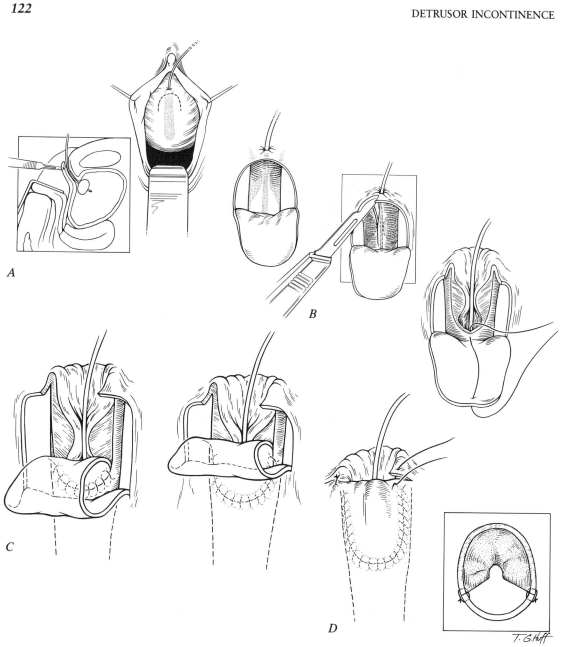

Figure 9-3. *Vaginal inlay flap for repair of a distal urethral stricture in a woman. (A) A filiform catheter is placed in the urethra. The urethra can be dilated to accept a small (8 French) Foley or the procedure done with the filiform in place. A U-shaped flap of vaginal epithelium is developed. (B) The strictured area is incised. The incision should be carried well into the normal urethra. The strictured area is obvious, having a thick scarred wall. The flap is turned into the opened urethra to prevent recurrent urethral cicatricial narrowing. The first suture is shown. (C) The flap is rolled into the open urethra. (D) Completed flap—urethral closure. The adjacent vaginal epithelium is easily closed over the flap and urethra without additional mobilization.*

Neurogenic Incontinence Due to Uncontrollable Bladder Contractility

This occurs in spinal cord–injured patients and in those with multiple sclerosis and is particularly likely to be a problem in patients treated for protracted periods by Foley catheter or suprapubic tube drainage. When attempts to control reflex vesical activity with drugs and intermittent catheterization fail, some surgical option is usually chosen. There are four basic approaches, which are each applicable in certain circumstances. A simple procedure, which is used primarily for high quadriplegics or for patients who are virtually quadriplegic as a result of multiple sclerosis, involves a short segment of ilium employed as a kind of suprapubic tube. This uses a right lower quadrant stoma for continuous urinary drainage. The procedure spares the trigone, requires only about 60 minutes of operating time, and can be done most expeditiously by way of a Gibson incision. The latter is particularly useful for massively obese patients or those with long-term suprapubic tube sinuses or multiple prior operative procedures by way of the midline route. The lateral approach avoids the suprapubic tube and brings the operator to the lower right bladder wall in an extraperitoneal location quickly. Access to the peritoneal contents adjacent to the cecum is also easy and quickly accomplished (Fig. 9-4). The small bowel to bladder anastomosis should be as large as practicable. Long-term experience with the procedure at the University of Michigan has been excellent, with the first individuals treated now reaching 30 years since operation with preservation of normal upper urinary tracts. Upper urinary tract function measured by intravenous urography and creatinine clearance has remained normal in all of these patients.

More recently, we have used a determination of the pressure required to drive urine out of the conduit as an index of efficacy. Determined pressures less than 20 cm H_2O for leakage of urine from the bladder across the conduit into the drainage bag are indicative of excellent function. The procedure preserves bladder reservoir function, which in turn is associated with maintenance of normal upper tracts. If the urethra has been destroyed or injured by indwelling Foley catheters of progressively larger sizes, deliberate urethral closure may be required or some other procedure used to augment urethral closing function. Urethral closure is more difficult to achieve in women than in men. The operation can be done transvesically or by way of a vaginal approach. The vaginal approach gives better results, but occasionally we use the transvesical procedure as a matter of operative expediency.

Transvesical Approach

The anterior bladder is incised to the bladder outlet, and circumferentially from that point, the bladder neck is transected from the urethra. Each is grasped with a long Allis clamp. The bladder outlet is closed in two layers, the urethra in two layers, and some perivesical fat interposed between the two structures (Fig. 9-5).

An alternative method involves injection of saline beneath the bladder mucosal surface circumferentially and then a circular incision around the vesical neck with mobilization of the mucosal segments. The denuded bladder neck is then closed with large Vicryl pursestring sutures, and the mucosal edges are approximated over the closed bladder outlet (Fig. 9-6).

Transvaginal Closure

The transvaginal approach involves mobilization of the urethra circumferentially, including detachment of the urethra anteriorly from the symphysis. Once the urethra is fully mobilized, it can be transected and the distal segment closed with a running large suture. The proximal end should be closed in three layers so the mucosal surface is inverted into the lumen of the bladder. The fascial covering of the urethra posteriorly is reclosed over the bladder neck closure. Failure of the urethral closure occurs in up to 10% of these cases, although the provision for a low pressure *(text continues on page 127)*

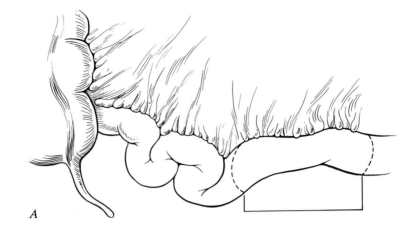

A

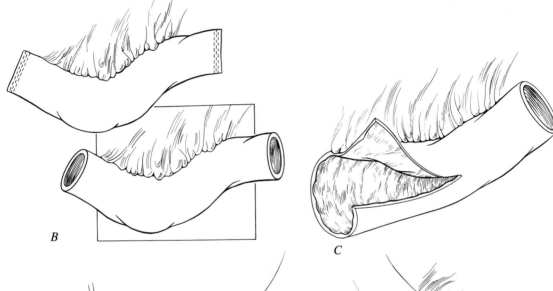

B

C

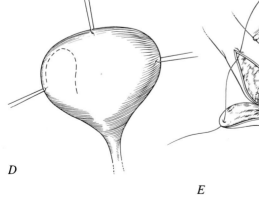

D

E

F

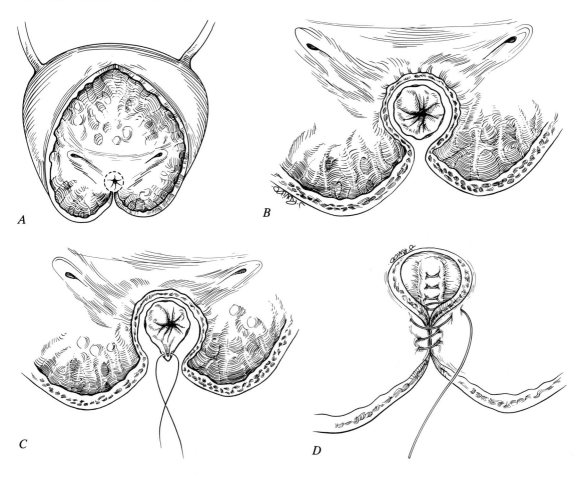

A

B

C

D

Figure 9-5. *Transvesical closure of the urethra. (A) The anterior bladder incision (with the electrocautery) is carried to the vesical neck and then circumscribes that structure. (B) Completed transection of the bladder neck from the proximal urethra. (C) Initial sutures in closure of the urethral stump. (D) Closure of the vesical neck proper. Adjacent perivesical fat is interposed between the two suture lines.*

Figure 9-4. *(opposite) Ileovesicostomy procedure. (A) Small bowel segments chosen at some distance from the ileocecal valve. (B) Isolated segment—varies in length to accommodate the abdominal wall girth and distance from bladder to the skin site chosen. (C) The proximal ileum is spatulated to enlarge the bladder-ileal anastomosis as much as possible. (D) Incision in the bladder to create a U-shaped flap—an extraperitoneal location is best, with the loop directed toward the right lower quadrant usually. (E) Detail of anastomosis—the posterior wall is done first. (F) Completed ileovesicostomy. We drain the bladder through a 22 French catheter placed through the stoma into the bladder for 3 weeks before removal.*

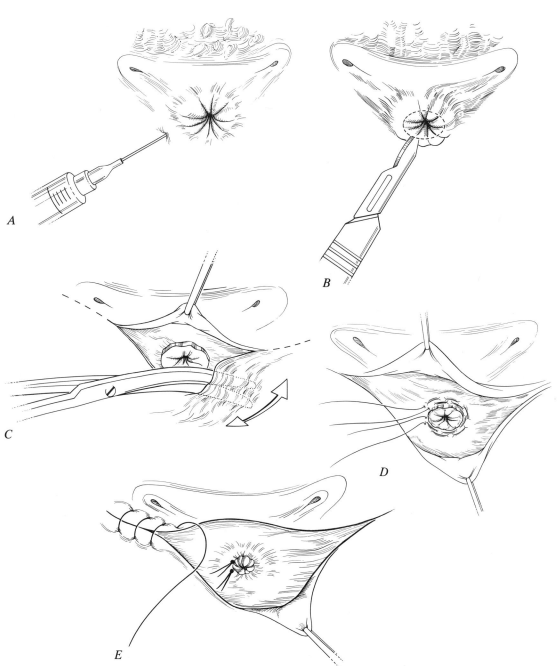

Figure 9-6. *Transvesical submucosal closure of the urethra. (A) Injection with 0.9% saline of the mucosa of the vesical neck to facilitate dissection. (B) Incision circumscribing the urethra, with denudation of the mucosa surrounding the urethral meatus. (C) Elevation of mucosal flaps circumferentially around the denuded urethral meatus. (D) Pursestring closure (two sutures) of the urethral stump. (E) Closure of the bladder mucosal flaps over the urethral (pursestring) closure.*

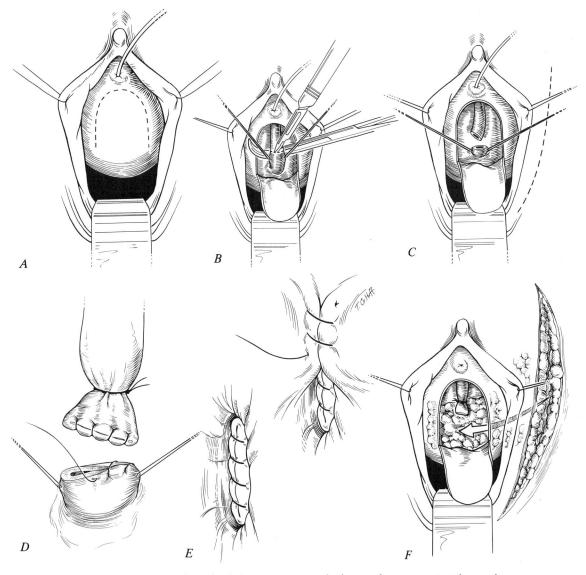

Figure 9-7. *Transvaginal urethral closure. (A) Detail of vaginal incision. (B) The urethra has been mobilized circumferentially and is then transected. (C) Completed transection— the proximal urethra and bladder neck are closed in three layers so as to place the urethral mucosal suture line inside the bladder. (D) First closure layer of proximal urethra. The distal urethra is closed in two layers and tied as well. (E) Third layer of periurethral fascia completes the closure of the proximal urethra. (F) A Martius labial fat pad graft can be used for additional security.*

urinary reservoir as described earlier aids healing of the urethral closure. We leave a multiple eyelet catheter held in place by an adjacent 8 French Foley balloon catheter through the incontinent conduit for at least 3 weeks after urethral closure to protect the closure from the opening mechanism that occurs with reflex bladder contractility (Fig. 9-7).

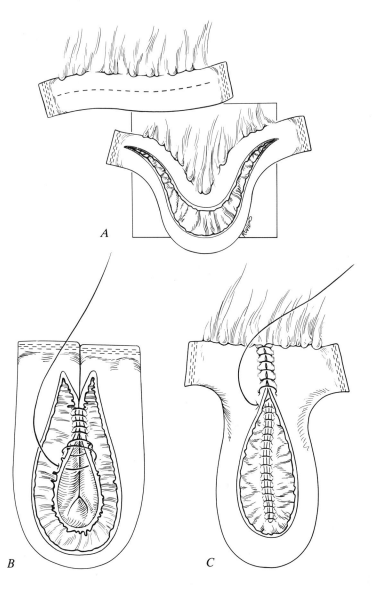

Figure 9-8

Augmentation Cystoplasty

This procedure (Fig. 9-8) can be used in circumstances in which the bladder is hypercontractile, uncontrollable with respect to pressure gain during filling, or fibrotic. A fibrotic bladder is generally related to prolonged catheter drainage or radiation therapy. We usually use detubularized ileum as the segment for augmentation and do not employ partial or subtotal detrusor resection. The operative procedure requires approx-

imately 2 hours, even in difficult cases, and the basic objective is the interposition of a large low pressure bowel reservoir between the trigone and the major mass of the detrusor muscle. These procedures require intermittent catheterization in almost every instance, and patients offered treatment by bladder augmentation for neurogenic incontinence should be cautioned that intermittent catheterization on a lifelong basis is a reasonable possibility.

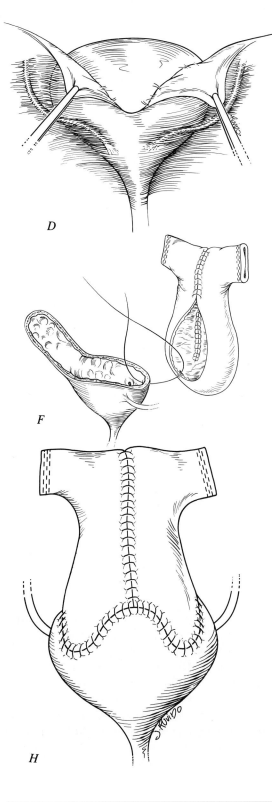

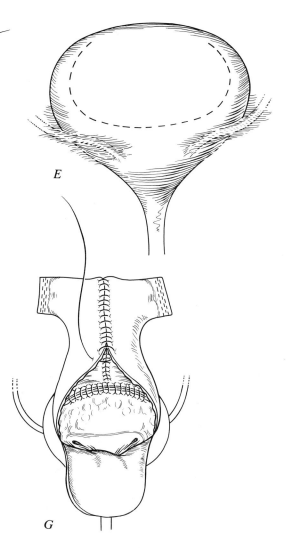

Figure 9-8. *Augmentation cystoplasty—with ileum. (A) Segment of ileum opened along its antemesenteric border. (B) Closure of the posterior wall of the opened folded segment to create a reservoir— as for a Koch pouch. (C) Partial closure of the anterior wall. (D) Dissection of the peritoneum off the posterior bladder to the level of the trigone. (E) Plan of incision in the bladder. The transverse incision lies just superior to the trigone, and the anterior-superior levels come up toward the superior pole of the bladder. (F) Detail of placement of the initial sutures for the enterocystoplasty. Note the open bladder and the open small bowel reservoir. (G) Closure of the anterior aspect of the enterocystoplasty. (H) Completed enterocystoplasty.*

Continent Urinary Reservoir

In some instances, catheterization per urethra may be difficult or impossible, and construction of a continent abdominal urinary stoma as part of the augmentation cystoplasty is useful (Fig. 9-9). This can, in some cases, be combined with a pubovaginal sling procedure or deliberate closure of the urethra to obviate urethral urinary loss.

Denervation Procedures

These procedures can be done within the sacral vertebral canal or beneath the bladder as described by Ingleman-Sundberg.[1] Procedures involving transection of the bladder have been abandoned because of the lack of long-term efficacy. Partial sacral root section used in the 1960s and 1970s has likewise been abandoned because of a lack of long-term efficacy. Section of the S-2–4 dorsal roots in either an intradural location or as the root becomes extradural, incorporating removal of the dorsal root ganglion, leaving intact the anterior motor root, induces detrusor areflexia. Long-term outcome studies in patients subjected to dorsal root ganglionectomy or section of the dorsal roots show preservation of detrusor areflexia provided that all roots subserving vesical function are severed. The areflexic bladder induced, in contrast to that resulting from combined anterior and posterior root section, does not gradually lose compliance. These procedures have more recently been largely supplemented by augmentation cystoplasty. The development, however, of effective intradural and extradural electrical stimulation techniques for bladder control and for electrical micturition has brought about a renewed interest in selective sensory decentralization that has some definite advantages over augmentation cystoplasty. The procedure can be done under local anesthesia, involves minimal dissection, and obviates some major problems encountered in patients who must undergo augmentation cystoplasty. These include mucus production, the risk of carcinoma in a bowel segment exposed to urine, the risk of spontaneous perforation, and the usual complications of any intraperitoneal operative procedure involving a bowel resection. These relatively serious potential complications of augmentation cystoplasty are important in patients with virtually complete neural lesions only in that the disadvantages of total sacral deafferentation in patients with a normal neuraxis preclude their use in that circumstance.

Electrical neural stimulation can be effective in the control of unwanted hyperreflexic detrusor contractility. Certain types of periodic electrical stimulation applied to the sacral roots or the pudendal nerve result in active inhibition of the detrusor reflex with preservation of the storage mode of lower urinary tract function as long as the stimulation continues to be applied. These techniques are currently under study at a number of centers in the United States, Canada, and Europe. The basic physiologic mechanisms on which these techniques depend are reasonably well known and understood. Predictable responses remain somewhat of a problem, but available instruments enable the urologist to try stimulation for several days or weeks using percutaneous systems before proceeding to fully implantable devices.

Ingleman-Sundberg Denervation

This procedure (Fig. 9-10), described some years ago in Sweden, has been used in the United States only occasionally and at one or two centers.[1] As described, a vaginal approach is used to locate and transect the pelvic nerve branches as they approach the bladder base. Patients with urge incontinence unresponsive to medication and timed voiding can be tested by injecting some 10 to 15 ml of lidocaine (Xylocaine) or bupivacaine (Marcaine) beneath the trigone transvaginally. The position of the trigone is determined by palpation of an indwelling Foley catheter balloon filled with 10 ml of solution, which is pulled down gently at the bladder neck. If the patient reports, after the trial injection, a 6- to 24-hour period of complete freedom from any urge incontinence, an Ingleman-Sundberg operation has a 70% chance of effecting symptomatic im-

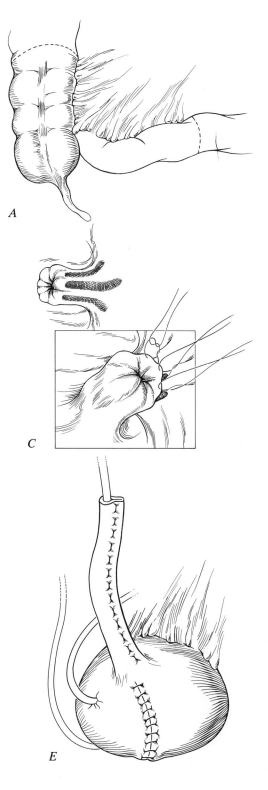

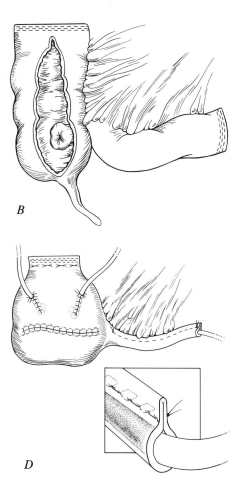

Figure 9-9. *Continent bladder replacement, or ileocecal segment construction for an augmentation enterocystoplasty with a continent abdominal stoma. (A) Selection of the ileocecal segment. (B) Completely open cecum with visible ileocecal valve leaflets. (C) Detail of valvuloplasty to hold the ileal valve in an intraluminal position. The cecal mucosa is dissected off the underlying bowel muscularis, and the valve leaflets are sutured to the muscularis. (D) Detail of the ileal segment suture to create a narrowed straight passageway for the catheter used intermittently to empty the bladder. (E) Completed free reservoir. The ileal segment can be brought to the skin anywhere or sutured to the urethra.*

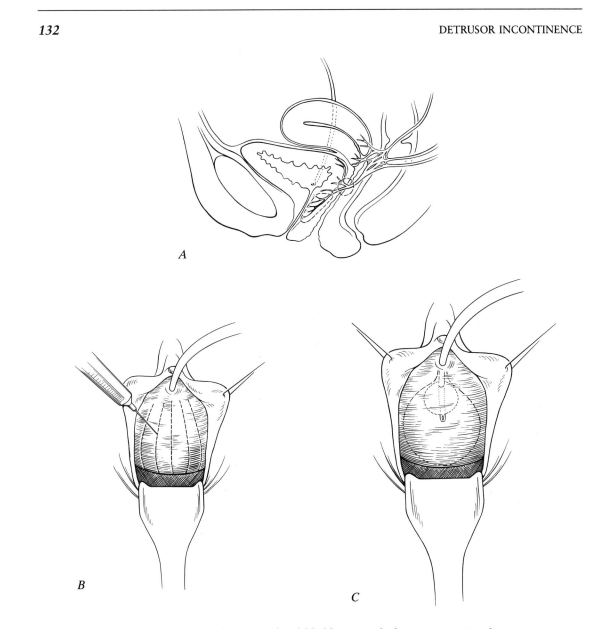

Figure 9-10. Ingleman-Sundberg peripheral bladder (partial) denervation. (A) Pelvic nerve branches approach and enter the bladder at the trigone. (B) Injection of 0.9% saline solution to facilitate dissection of the vaginal epithelium off the bladder. (C) Position of trigone—outlined by a catheter balloon filled to 30 ml. (D) Incision. (E) Transection of the vaginal epithelium off the bladder. (F) Completed dissection.

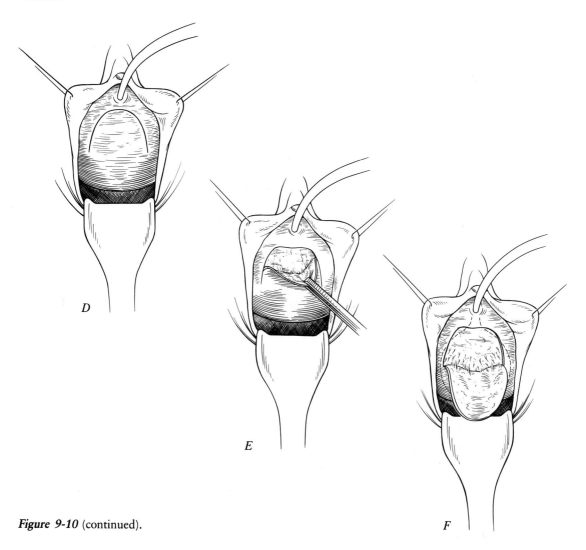

D

E

Figure 9-10 (continued).

F

provement for at least 1 year.[1] If the procedure fails, early or late, a repeat operative procedure usually does not work, and we no longer do secondary Ingleman-Sundberg procedures. Using a slightly modified operative approach involving less dissection but basically selecting patients in the same way as that described by Ingleman-Sundberg and Hodgekinson, we achieved the same late operative results (70% dry rate).[1,2] We have not restricted the procedure to those patients with a positive cystometrogram, however, and have performed the lidocaine injection test and subsequent surgery in patients with urge incontinence but a negative cystometrogram and clear videourodynamic evidence that stress incontinence was not present. Results in the latter group are the same as those recorded following Ingleman-Sundberg denervation in those patients with easily demonstrable cystometrogram-positive bladder instability.[2,3] These results are consistent with the observations made by several workers during the continuous monitoring of intravesical pressure in patients with negative provocative cystometry, which showed that uninhibited detrusor contractility was the underlying problem responsible for their incontinence.

References

1. Ingleman-Sundberg A. Partial bladder denervation for detrusor dysnergia. Obstet Gynecol 1978; 21:797.
2. Wan J, McGuire EJ, Wang JC, Cerny JC, Hodgkinson CP. Ingleman-Sundberg denervation for detrusor instability. J Urol 1991;145:Abstr. #81.
3. Wang SC, McGuire EJ, Management of severe bladder instability by Ingleman-Sundberg bladder dennervation. J Urol 1988;139:Abstr. #137, 272A.

10

Neurostimulation in Urology

Richard Schmidt

The neural control of bladder function is spatially unique in the nervous system. There is a diffuse neural network linking bladder function to almost every level of the central nervous system (CNS). There is no other visceral or somatic parallel among the body's various systems. It is this complexity of regulatory control that places the lower urinary tract at high risk for dysfunction with virtually any neurologic disturbance within the CNS. Micturition problems may secondary to functionally driven instabilities in central reflex behavior or more obviously linked to a wide variety of neural pathologies. It can be extremely difficult, if not impossible, to differentiate between the two in many clinical situations. Neurostimulation has been shown to have a useful role in managing many voiding disorders regardless of their causes or the fact that they may appear to have totally opposite natures: incontinence versus retention.

The rationale and motivation for therapeutic use of neural stimulation have arisen from the following observations:

1. Many dysfunctional voiding syndromes are associated with instability in sacral reflex behavior. Dampening of this sacral nerve reflex excitability, by way of neural stimulation, is associated with a therapeutic benefit.

2. Many voiding syndromes occur because of functional disconnection between higher center regulation and bladder function. Neural stimulation helps restore higher center awareness of bladder behavior and improves central coordination of bladder function.

3. Direct stimulation of motor nerves has the ability to bypass the CNS regulation and restore bladder function in an otherwise permanently compromised CNS.[1-4]

The clinical goals of sacral nerve pathway stimulation can thus be divided into one of two categories: (1) a direct cause and effect (*e.g.*, evacuation of the paraplegic bladder) or (2) an indirect (*i.e.*, modulatory) effect on a behavior, for example, detrusor instability.

The aim of this chapter is to discuss the present-day role of neuroprosthetics in urology.

Neuromodulation

CANDIDATES FOR FUNCTIONAL ELECTRICAL STIMULATION (FES)

This approach has been used extensively to manage patients with urge frequency disorders, pelvic pain, and urinary incontinence. It is a simple

Female Urology, edited by Elroy D. Kursh and Edward McGuire. J. B. Lippincott, Philadelphia, © 1994.

approach with few if any side-effects, and the literature is strongly supportive of its role as a viable therapy.[5] The approach has been used extensively in Europe but has had limited exposure in the United States. The same support mechanisms to provide an outlet for this therapy are not operable in the United States, and a device that is acceptable to patients is not available. Surface stimulation, using a greatly improved device, is presently being reassessed in clinical trials in this country.

Even when the approach works well, however, patients may not be good candidates over the long term for this approach for a variety of reasons. Because of lifestyle demands, patients may not be able to use the devices for sufficient time periods during the day or at regular enough intervals to maintain benefit. There may be a psychological aversion to an anal or vaginal device. A patient may be too sensitive to insert the device or may simply grow tired of the format. Reimbursement for the medical services needed to support the use of this approach has not yet been established or may be insufficient to provide incentive for the physician to become involved with the treatment format.

CANDIDATES FOR SACRAL FORAMEN PROSTHESIS

This approach can be used as the primary treatment for patients with urge-related incontinence, pelvic pain syndromes, urinary retention of a functional nature, or urge frequency syndromes. It has its appeal in that the sacral nerves are stimulated directly, and hence an efficient contraction of the pelvic muscle is achieved.

Many patients with hypersensitive perineal tissues do not like instrumentation, whether it is per urethra, per vagina, or per rectum. These same patients will tolerate insertion of a needle into the sacral foramen because it is a site removed from the area of symptoms. A trial of sacral nerve root stimulation can then be carried out as a screen for this approach to modulate symptoms on a more permanent level. A trial therapy can lead to a permanent implant. This gives the patient convenience and discretion for self-therapy under almost all situations and without time constraints. As with functional electrical stimulation, there are pragmatic financial constraints that limit the availability of the technique, and clinical trials are now ongoing.

CANDIDATES FOR INTRAVESICAL THERAPY

There is an increasing interest in the use of this approach to manage spastic neurogenic bladders and areflexic (lazy) bladders.[6–9] The approach works on submucosal receptors in the bladder, which leads over time to enhanced reflex detrusor contractions and improved synergic voids. It has been reported to be useful in the management of the lazy bladder syndrome, to recover synergic voiding in spinal injury patients, and to produce voids in myelomeningocele bladders. Multiple, regular treatments are required to rehabilitate detrusor reflex contractions initially, and ongoing sessions are necessary to maintain the benefit. Often biofeedback is necessary to maximize the benefits of intravesical stimulation. There are technical limits, and there is no device presently available in the United States. For a number of reasons, there are constraints limiting the ability of physicians to offer this approach.

PATIENT SCREENING

Candidates for neuromodulation therapy are asked to complete a 3-day voiding diary and are then given a standardized urodynamic evaluation. This consists of a four-channel catheter, placed into the urethra and positioned for simultaneous recording of bladder and urethral activity. The main purpose of these studies is to obtain a qualitative and quantitative measure of the excitation and coordination of the void reflex. Such tests are not only diagnostic, but also provide an important baseline to gauge the effectiveness of therapy and for future reference. Patients with demonstrable dysfunction in micturition reflex efficiency are considered good candidates for neuromodulation.

Sacral Nerve Test Stimulation

METHOD AND RESULTS

The following technique is used to evaluate response(s) to sacral nerve stimulation:[10] The patient is positioned prone on the cysto table. The skin is prepared as per a sterile minor surgical procedure, and local anesthesia (1% lidocaine) is used to numb the skin and subcutaneous tissues. The sciatic notch and superficial curvature of the sacrum are identified to mark the approximate level of the S-3 foramen. An insulated needle is inserted into this foramen, about one fingerbreadth off the midline. The response to a gradually increasing amplitude of current is tested (using a fixed 200-μsec pulse width and frequency settings of 2 Hz then 15 Hz). The ideal response consists of a visible bellowslike contraction of the pelvic floor, along with plantar flexion of the large toe. The patient feels a throb at 2 Hz and a pulling sensation at 15 Hz. Sensation refers to the rectum but extends forward toward the scrotum or labia. If necessary, on completion of the study at S-3, other sacral roots can then be identified and similarly tested.

The perineal response obtained with stimulation of the S-2 root is either none or that of a clamplike contraction of the perineum.[10] Lower limb responses consist of an outward rotation of the leg (*i.e.*, medial rotation of the heel), a plantar flexion of the entire foot with visible contraction of the calf, or plantar flexion of just the distal foot and toes.

A well-defined clamplike sphincter contraction is readily obtained under circumstances when pain is not an issue—for example, spinal injury. Also, stimulation of the pudendal nerve, which originates primarily from S-2, produces an evident, clamplike perineal response. Activity in the perineum, however, is not commonly seen with stimulation of S-2. Because of the disproportionate contribution of S-2 to the sciatic nerve, a stimulating current required to elicit perineal activity exceeds the pain threshold.

S-4 stimulation produces a strong contraction of the levator, but patient perception often, but not exclusively, is limited to a pulling in the rectum. Forward referral into the anterior perineum was not as much a given as with the S-3.

Test stimulation of the various sacral nerves is helpful in understanding the degree of dysfunction in the pelvic musculature. One can compare stimulation-induced pelvic muscle activity with that of the patient's own efforts. The comparison often underscores a distinct lack of understanding by the patient in voluntary use of the pelvic muscles. One can often identify components of pelvic floor activity that are missing or inefficient (*e.g.*, bellowslike S-3 or a viselike clamp S-2). The possibility therefore exists that long-standing inefficiency in perineal muscle use precedes or predisposes patients to various conditions, such as urge-frequency syndromes, prostatism, pelvic pain, incontinence, interstitial cystitis, and even bowel dysfunctions. A high percentage of these patients lack proper control and use of their pelvic musculature.

Percutaneous testing of the sacral nerve roots appears to be benign. Although there are a number of potential risks associated with the technique, no significant difficulties have been reported. The testing also helps to establish whether neurostimulation has a therapeutic role.

TRIAL STIMULATION

A test/trial period of stimulation has proved to be an effective way to assess the therapeutic potential of chronic sacral nerve stimulation.[11] The S-3 nerve is most frequently used, the S-4 infrequently, and the S-2 rarely. The aim is to achieve a comfortable and complete response in the perineum, with as little foot or toe recruitment as possible. Without consistent, good muscular recruitment, the value of therapeutic stimulation is generally limited.

After screening the response obtained with stimulation, a thin wire electrode (3–0 flexon pacer wire) is inserted into the foramen by way of the angiocatheter guide, coiled in place, and secured with Tegaderm for 3 to 7 days. It is then coupled to a pulse generator (Medtronic, Inc.). The electrode has been left for up to 4 weeks, but care must be given to the skin puncture site and

the wire removed at the first sign of skin irritation. Should the wire move, steps should be taken
to re-establish contact. If inserted too deeply, it
can be pulled back carefully, or if too superficial,
it should be withdrawn and reinserted. Conclusions regarding therapeutic benefit of stimulation cannot be made without a 2- to 3-day period
of consistent perineal muscle stimulation. Thus
daily monitoring of both technical and physiologic results is necessary for proper conclusions
regarding the test to be made.

The location and number of temporary wires
inserted can vary from patient to patient. Variables that determine the number and location of
wires inserted include (1) the neurologic and
mental status of a patient, (2) the laterality and
location of pelvic pain, (3) the severity of the
voiding dysfunction, (4) patient anatomy and
habitus, (5) the time available for the evaluation,
(6) available technical support, and, most importantly, (7) the skill of the treating urologist.

If the initial trial fails despite achieving the
appropriate muscle response with stimulation of
one nerve, consideration is given to testing another or a combination of nerves (e.g., in the case
of a partial control of symptoms). Alternatively,
one excludes further testing of this modality.

If the trial is successful, a patient may not
need further testing, can be considered for a
second trial at another date, or elect to have a
permanently implanted device. The choice varies
with the effectiveness of stimulation to modulate
symptoms, both during the trial and after the
cessation of stimulation.

EVOKED POTENTIAL MONITORING

A useful aid in assessing the effectiveness and
efficiency of sacral nerve stimulation is to monitor the motor-evoked activity of the pelvic floor.
An electromyographic signal from the deep and
superficial anal sphincter provides a sensitive
monitor of any contractile activity in the levator
(S-3) or superficial anal sphincter (S-2 or pudendal). There is a clear separation in these responses with stimulation of the various sacral
nerves (Fig. 10-1). Levator responses are restricted to stimulation of S-3 and S-4. Superficial
anal sphincter responses are restricted to the S-2
and pudendal. There are diagnostic and therapeutic advantages to this information. The motor-evoked potential (MEP) quantitates the
amount of muscle recruitment, providing information as to the integrity of the perineal muscle

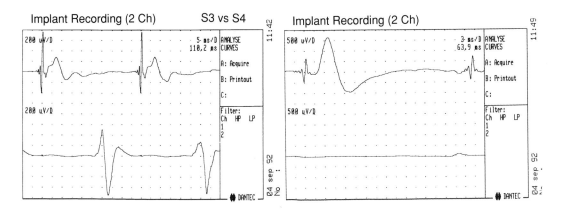

Figure 10-1. *Motor-evoked responses recorded from the levator muscle. The responses are normal. The S-3 response shows a weak contraction of the levator with strong plantar flexion of the large toe. S-4 stimulation produces a strong contraction of the levator but no contraction of the toe.*

makeup and the position of the stimulating needle (or electrode) relative to the nerve being stimulated. This is helpful in patients with a suspected nerve injury from spine surgery or patchy neural deficits associated with neural disease.

On a technical level, it can be difficult to appreciate the efficiency of pelvic floor stimulation in patients who are obese or just apprehensive and tense. At the time of a permanent implant, the MEP can be used as a guide to duplicate the same type of stimulation response known to have had a beneficial effect on symptoms. After implant of a permanent neuroprosthesis, the MEP is helpful in selecting the ideal parameters of stimulation. The threshold response and the point of maximum recruitment can be defined. The peak MEP response below the pain threshold, yet as close to the maximum response as possible, can be accurately selected. Overstimulation, with pain or wasted energy, is therefore avoided, and battery life with the permanent implants is optimized.

The recording provides a clear documentation of a response, which can be correlated with clinical benefit. The MEP can be used as a marker of nerve integrity over time and to facilitate a decision as to whether there will be a need to revise the electrode owing to malfunction or positioning problems.

Advantages to Pelvic Floor Monitoring in Foramen Implant Candidates

Advantages to monitoring are as follows:
1. Quantitates amount of muscle contraction.
2. Identifies muscles and area being stimulated.
3. Allows comparisons of response over time.
4. Gives clinician an objective documentation of stimulation result. This helps in the following circumstances:
   a. When it is difficult to appreciate pelvic floor movement to stimulation visually (obese or tense individuals).
   b. To compare a percutaneous retest post-implant with the implanted electrode response in cases in which a revision seems needed.

Responses to Nerve Stimulation

SURGICAL IMPLANTS

Once a decision has been made to implant a permanent neural prosthesis, one has an option of placing an electrode either at the foramen level, usually one of the S-3 nerves (Figs. 10-2*A* and *B*), or at the ischial level, on one of the pudendal nerves. The actual site chosen varies and depends somewhat on the response obtained with the temporary trial. The S-3 foramen is attractive in that it is technically easier to implant an electrode at this site than through exposure of the pudendal nerve. A foramen electrode should always be the first choice in those patients who do extremely well with the outpatient trial.

As a rule, one electrode implant is sufficient to produce the desired effect. The modulation principle works quite well for patients with milder degrees of symptomatic voiding dysfunction (pelvic pain, recurrent urinary tract infections, urgency or frequency, dribbling, incontinence, or intermittent retention). There are occasional patients (*e.g.*, those with incontinence, secondary detrusor instability, or bilateral pelvic pain), however, who stand to benefit from two or more electrode implants. Technically this is not difficult and certainly feasible. From a cost-effectiveness standpoint, however, and with present technology, it is impractical. Also, it is not always apparent who requires a dual implant until several weeks or months after use of the first implant. Eventually as pulse generators are programmed to control more than one electrode site and as electrode designs simplify the surgical implant, this will become a more realistic possibility.

SAFETY

The experience noted in these patients is consistent with reports concerned with the safety of long-term stimulation.[12,13] There has been no instance of reported change in sensation or behavior of the sphincter or bladder as a result of long-term stimulation. There have been instances of decline in perineal muscle recruitment

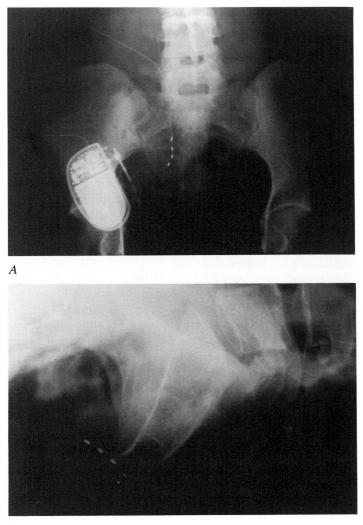

A

B

Figure 10-2. *(A and B) X-ray views of quad leads implanted in the sacral foramen.*

as a response to stimulation, but these have not been associated with any change in sensorium or in micturition physiology. Animal experiments have shown that a 50-Hz rectangular pulse, applied to a peripheral nerve continuously for a period as short as 16 hours, results in a loss of large-diameter axons. Such a change is not seen at frequencies of 20 Hz or less. Presumably there is a progressive risk of nerve injury as the frequency increases above 20 Hz, but by how much and over what length of time is as yet undetermined. Physiologically electromyograph monitoring of neuromuscular behavior demonstrates a low-frequency background behavior with intermittent bursts of more intense activity. Nerve damage may occur as a result of overdrive of the

Table 10-1. *Advantages of 10-Hz Stimulation Parameter*

Effective fused contraction of perineal muscles.

Inhibition of labile sphincter behavior contributing to voiding dysfunction.

Safety of long-term stimulation.

Maximum patient comfort.

Minimal fatigue of stimulated muscle.

Preserved sense of muscle activity and awareness of stimulation effect.

Effective conversion of fast-twitch muscle to slow-twitch muscle.

peripheral nerve, rather than from direct harm from the current delivered. Lower frequency stimulation parameters would therefore be safer from the aspect that they more closely mimic neuromuscular physiology (Table 10-1). Nevertheless, a maximum current density should not exceed 45 $\mu C/cm^2$.

Patients implanted as far back as 1982 have accumulated in excess of 30,000 hours of stimulation time without harm. There are occasions wherein the stimulation effect is lost or poorly sustained. But in all instances, there is no associated change in bladder function. Patients at risk for this difficulty are the elderly and those with a previously compromised nervous system (*e.g.*, myelomeningocele). The ability to maintain a muscular response to stimulation may reflect on the integrity of the underlying neural metabolism more than on physical effects of the current delivered to the tissues. Healthy neuromuscular units have not shown any predisposition to response deterioration. These points suggest that screening procedures for neuroprosthesis implants should be more rigid (*i.e.*, a longer trial) for patients who do not demonstrate a strong contraction of the perineum with initial stimulation.

The therapeutic benefit obtained with stimulation is closely tied to the contraction of muscle fibers. There is a much higher tolerance level for stimulation when muscle contracts than when it does not. A pure sensory effect, without visually apparent muscle contraction, does not effectively modulate voiding dysfunction and is asso-

ciated with a narrow patient tolerance level. This observation suggests that direct stimulation of afferent nerves results only in pain and is not therapeutic. It does not, however, negate the possible indirect influence the muscle afferents may have as a result of the muscle stimulation. Thus a patient should be able to tolerate the effect of stimulation for long periods, without annoying distraction or discomfort. Patient tolerance for stimulation declines precipitously above 15 Hz. Fortunately, a healthy fused recruitment of muscle contraction is seen at 15 Hz, and a therapeutically acceptable one is seen at 10 Hz. These ranges are also those safest for long-term stimulation. Frequency adjustments can be made for any one patient between 2 and 15 Hz. The initial setting should be 10 Hz because it is sufficiently therapeutic, is the most comfortable frequency range, and prolongs battery life of the implanted generator.

It is important to keep in mind that the therapeutic effectiveness of the stimulation is that of a modulatory influence on the reflexes controlling micturition and the related dysfunction. Such similar parameters of stimulation can be applied to seemingly paradoxical clinical problems, for example, a urinary retention disorder as well as one of urinary incontinence. Both can be secondary to a dysfunction of neural reflexes and as such respond to the same modulation input to the CNS obtained from neurostimulation.

The exact pattern of stimulation and time of use vary from patient to patient. In the absence of any deleterious effect of neurostimulation on tissue, patients are left free to determine the amount of "on" time they think is necessary to keep symptoms under control. As such, they may elect to use the stimulation unit 24 hours a day, a few hours a day, or intermittently throughout the day. Because experimental data suggest that damage from neurostimulation is greater with continuous stimulation than from intermittent patterns of use, a cycle pattern is used at the onset of stimulation. The pulse generator unit offers a choice between continuous stimulation and cycled delivery of stimulation. A cycle of 15 seconds on and 5 seconds off is selected with the initiation of stimulation. The cycle pattern can be varied to accommodate patient comfort. Some patients may find a shorter "off" interval less distracting (*e.g.*, 10 seconds on and 2 seconds off), or some may prefer to use the implant in the continuous mode intermittently throughout the day. There is no magic formula. The goal is to provide sufficient "on" time of the stimulation for a modulation effect. This "on" time should be therapeutic, within the parameter ranges that have been shown to be safe, and comfortable so as not to inhibit the patient from using the implant. Nor should the implant be abused by excessive use. As a general rule, patients require less "on" time of the unit 6 months from the time of their implant than in the initial months. Patients need to be monitored periodically and encouraged to use their implant only as is necessary to control symptoms.

Surgical Nerve Injury

Damage to a nerve is far more likely to occur during placement of an electrode than it is during stimulation. Excessive pressure on the nerve, either during or after placement of an electrode, is obviously detrimental. Chronic pressure on the nerve can result from tension on the lead wires from an electrode. Great care must be taken to fix the electrodes and leads to minimize this risk. Sufficient lead length should be left wherever possible to allow for strain relief.

Patients Who Benefit

Table 10-2 reflects the experience obtained with a variety of patient categories. Patients were considered cured if symptoms improved better than 90% and considered significantly improved if the symptoms diminished 50% or more. Certain problems responded to the effect of stimulation with more predictability. Thus, urge incontinence tended to have a much higher success ratio than patients with pelvic pain. Given all types of problems—urge incontinence, stress incontinence, retention syndromes, pelvic pain, and urge/frequency disorders—the best results followed the principles outlined earlier. It is therapeutically more rewarding to manage symptoms associated with identifiable muscle function than symptoms that are mostly sensory in nature.

These results suggest that the therapy can be effective in a variety of circumstances apart from just treating urinary incontinence. Also, the data suggest that one can improve results if indeed a more stringent screening maneuver is undertaken. A patient should not be offered permanent implantation unless there has been a clear-cut demonstration of improvement of symptoms during the trial therapy. More than one trial therapy should be undertaken if there is any ambiguity in the response to the trial, any decision hesitation on the part of the patient, or any question as to the technical success achieved with the initial outpatient trial.

The results also support the view that the therapeutic benefit is a result of modulation of neural reflex excitability rather than there being a direct change in muscle behavior (the effect is immediate) or in the integrity of neural conduction (voluntary muscle contraction is not inhibited by the stimulation). Thus therapeutic responses are found that would appear to be clinically contradictory.

All patients must be carefully screened before consideration is given to a permanent implant. There should be a clear-cut demonstration of consistency in the ability of neurostimulation to restore or improve the bladder functions of storage and evacuation. More than one evaluation may be necessary if there is any doubt in the mind of the patient or physician as to the result of the trial.

SYNDROMES OF VOIDING DYSFUNCTION

Urge Incontinence/Urge Frequency Syndromes

Neurostimulation can be beneficial to these patients. Precipitate urge can result from either sphincter instability or detrusor instability. Modulation of sphincter instability results in an apparent dampening of the precipitate urge and

Table 10-2. Results Obtained with Neuroprosthetic Foramen Implants

DIAGNOSIS	NO. PTS.	BENEFIT		
		<50%	50–75%	75–100%
Voiding dysfunction	33	10	6	17
Incontinence	24	4	5	15
Urge	20	3	5	12
Stress	4	1	0	3
Totals	57	14 (25%)	11 (19%)	32 (56%)

This table reflects results obtained with neuroprosthetic foramen implants (57 patients) between 1987 and 1989. Seventy-five percent of patients implanted for symptomatic voiding dysfunction experienced greater than a 50% benefit when followed for a period of two years.

triggering of inappropriate detrusor activity. Bladder capacity also proved to be a good selection criterion. Patients in whom strong sphincter control could be demonstrated (≥ 80 cm H_2O) and who had a bladder capacity of greater than 200 ml before experiencing spontaneous detrusor contractions did much better than other patients. Others who did well were those with an innate tendency to overrelax their perineum. The combined use of anticholinergics and neurostimulation may broaden the patient selection criteria in the future. Careful screening of these patients is time-consuming but necessary because therapeutic responses to stimulation can be highly variable from individual to individual.

Prostatodynia

This is the male equivalent of the urethral syndrome seen in women. One interesting observation is that pudendal nerve stimulation refers directly to the testicle. This helps the physician to understand testicular pains that do not respond to cord blocks or that cannot be explained by inguinal or scrotal pathology. As a group, these patients are more difficult to cure, regardless of the modality used. Treatment is most effective in patients with scrotal symptoms that are associated with pelvic myalgia (demonstrated on rectal examination) and in modulation was effective in decreasing symptoms.

Pelvic Pain

Patients with pelvic floor myalgias often do quite well with S-3 stimulation. Patients with discomfort more localized to the urethral area do not do as well. Occasionally pudendal nerve stimulation is more effective for these patients than the S-3 location. Each patient needs to be evaluated individually. Regardless of similarities in symptoms, there is no guarantee that two patients will respond the same.

Postprostatectomy Incontinence

Patients suffering from this type of incontinence who obtained the greatest benefit tended to be less symptomatic than those who did not. This is the logical outcome of a healthier muscle state, better muscular integrity, and better reflexogenic excitability. The stronger the sphincter contraction elicited with stimulation, the better the retentive capability in the case of weakness and the better suppression of detrusor instability. Sphincter stimulation was effective in suppressing milder levels of hyperreflexia but was ineffective in the treatment of higher spastic bladders.

Stimulation of the pudendal nerve is more exact than that of the S-3 nerve because a cuff can be placed around the pudendal nerve that reliably couples the stimulus to the nerve. Also, stimulation of the pudendal nerve more frequently leads to discomfort. The therapeutic window (*i.e.*, the difference in threshold between stimulation of muscle and pain), however, is narrower with it than the S-3 nerve. This is because the pudendal nerve has a much greater afferent component. The stimulation site should be below the dorsal nerve of the penis so no feelings are referred to the penis. Such a stimulation site also results in the pudendal nerve being excluded from the stimulus field.

Complications of Sacral Foramen Implants

Revisions were required for the following:

A. Technical problems.
 1. Lead fixation failure (*i.e.*, migration of lead).
 2. Addition of an electrode on another nerve needed.
 3. Conversion of receiver (*i.e.*, modernization).
 4. Receiver removal, replacement, relocation secondary to pain at receiver site, failure to relieve symptoms, battery failure.
 5. Electrode failure.
  a. Lead wire fracture.
  b. Lead wire pain.
  c. Cable tension with displacement of electrode from nerve.
  d. Connection failure.
  e. Erosion of lead through skin.
B. Biological problems.
 1. Suspected metal allergy.
 2. Infection.
 3. Lack of sustained therapeutic effect.

Problems with the implant are to be expected. As an overview, most of the reoperations were performed because of technical failures. Leads became displaced, lead wires fractured, and positioning errors were encountered. Revisions performed because of loss or deterioration of response with stimulation were less common. In part, these occurred because of poor selection criteria, for example, radiated tissue. There were patients, however, who had successful trial responses but failed to achieve relief with the permanent implant. These patients can be screened out in the selection criteria by restricting the technique to those who achieve clear-cut thera-

peutic benefit of measurable objective criteria. Reliance on subjective criteria can lead to long-term response failures. Finally, there were patients who achieved relief, but an efficient couple with the nerve could not be maintained or a second implant was required to complete the therapy. Generally, if the stimulus amplitudes went above 4 volts (PW 200, 10 to 15 Hz), there was in all probability either an intrinsic deficiency in the nerve or a less than optimal orientation of the lead to the nerve. Patients in the latter circumstance could be retested on an outpatient basis. If the responses obtained on retest were beneficial, the patient could be returned to surgery to reposition the lead in the same foramen, change to a new foramen location, or implant a second electrode. On occasion, an electrode was placed on the pudendal nerve to augment or replace the modulation effect obtained at the S-3 foramen site.

Bladder Pacemaker

Implanted neuroprosthetics were developed primarily to benefit the spinal cord injury patient. Electrodes are placed around the ventral root of the S-3 nerves, coupled with a simultaneous division of the S2-4 dorsal roots.[14-16] With the attenuation of all micturition reflex behavior, an efficient contraction of the bladder with stimulation is possible. The sphincter relaxes immediately after the stimulation is stopped, allowing for detrusor emptying. It is important to divide all of the sacral dorsal roots to stabilize both the sphincter and the urinary bladder. This then restores continence and minimizes dyssynergic sphincter behavior to permit efficient emptying. The dorsal rhizotomy by itself is beneficial to patients with highly spastic bladders. Not only is continence restored, but also the risks of a high-pressure bladder to the upper tracts is greatly diminished. Erection and bowel evacuation patterns are affected but, surprisingly, often preserved. Only the lability with which sacral reflexes govern these varied functions is affected. On occasion, they may even improve, as if there were too much reflex inhibition of visceral behavior before the dorsal rhizotomy.

CANDIDATES FOR A BLADDER PACEMAKER

The primary candidates for this technology are patients with spinal cord injuries (Table 10-3). Patients with neurologic disabilities, such as multiple sclerosis or transverse myelitis, may be considered. There are two main limitations for bladder stimulation, pain from the levels of current required to stimulate the bladder and the responsivity of the bladder. There are many factors to consider before a patient can be considered a good candidate. These can be summarized as follows:

1. Completeness of injury. Complete cord injury patients do better than incomplete cord injury patients for two reasons.
2. Level of injury. Spinal injury patients between the levels T10-L2 are often the most ideal candidates for bladder pacemaker. Detrusor responsivity to stimulation may be insufficient to empty the bladder in the high Quad or in Cauda Equina patients.
3. Psychological status. Patients must be emotionally prepared to interact with their device and the treating physician.
4. General medical health. Serious medical problems, for example, decubitus ulcers, kidney stones, or pulmonary difficulties, need to be addressed before consideration of an implant.
5. Age. The limits as to age are those of available technology and degenerative age-related changes in the nervous system.
6. Time from injury. Although there is no time exclusion, the experience to date suggests that patients would be better served over the long run by having an implant early, even within the first year of injury.
7. Mobility. Patients must be able to achieve suitable and convenient collection of the voided urine. Female patients thus must be able to transfer to a toilet facility. Male patients can opt to void into a condom catheter and leg bag.

UROLOGIC CONSIDERATIONS

Detrusor Reflex Contractility

For successful electromicturition, a detrusor contraction associated with 75 to 100 cm H_2O must be achieved. Hence the integrity of detrusor contractility needs to be assessed before an implant. This can be done by a simple cystometrogram, obstructing the urethra of the bladder temporarily to measure peak detrusor pressure as a measurement of the maximal contractile force. If intravesicular pressures remain low, that is, less than 50 cm H_2O, direct stimulation of the sacral roots can be performed to assess the potential for voiding.

Competence of Urethral Sphincter

Implant patients must have the potential for continence. Female patients incontinent secondary to an intrinsically weak urethral sphincter are not good candidates, but men with partial incontinence from failed sphincterotomies are good candidates.

Detrusor Morphology

Bladders that are mildly hypertrophic secondary to unstable behavior respond much better than thin-walled bladders to stimulation. Contracted, poorly compliant bladders do not have the potential for sufficient storage.

Status of Upper Tracts

Upper tract pathology, principally stones, should be ruled out or treated before considering the patient for an implant. Urinary reflux may improve or disappear after dorsal rhizotomy. Renal parenchymal loss, unless the patient is left with marginal kidney function, does not disqualify a patient from an implant.

Functional Status of Erections

Approximately 50% of patients retain the ability to have a reflex erection after dorsal rhizotomy.

Table 10-3. Neuroprosthesis Implant Results

PATIENT NAME	INJURY LEVEL	DATE OF IMPLANT	S2 DR	S-3	S-4	PREOPERATIVE CONTINENCE	POSTOPERATIVE CONTINENCE	VOID STATUS	LEFT SOMATIC	RIGHT SOMATIC	COMMENT
NA	SI—T-10	6-19-81	Intact	Split	Intact	No	<25%	<25%			Incomplete rhizotomies
KS	SI—C5-6	3-3-82	Intact	Rt S-3vr Lt S-3 intact	Intact	No	<50%	<25%		Rt Ureth Br	Incomplete rhizotomies
RH	SI—C5-6	8-23-83	Rt split	Split	Intact	No	50-75%	50-75%	Pud + lev	Rt Ureth Br	Incomplete rhizotomy, good detrusor
RD	SI—C5-6	9-22-83	Lt S-2	LT S-3, Split Rt S-3	Intact	No	75-90%	<25%	Pud		Incompetent detrusor contractions, capacity >1000 ml
BM	SI—C5-6	1-1-84	Intact	Intact	Intact	No	>90%	<25%			Incomplete rhizotomy, autonomic dysreflexia, too unstable for stimulation of incomplete rhizotomies
DP	SI—T-6	11-12-84	Intact	Split	Intact	No	<50%	<25%		Pud + lev	
DH	SI—C6-7	3-18-85	Intact	Split	Intact	No	<25%	<25%			Incomplete rhizotomy
KN	SI—T-6	6-13-85	Intact	Rt S-3, Lt S-3 separation	Intact	No	>90%	>90%	U + lev	A + lev	Voids fine with residuals of 50-75 ml
MG	SI—T-10	12-10-85	Lt S-2	Lt S-3, Rt S-3 separation	Intact	No	<50%	<25%			Incomplete rhizotomy
FM	SI—C5-6	12-12-85	Rt S-2	Lt S-3	Intact	No	<25%	<25%			Incomplete rhizotomy infection led to removal of leads
RF	SI—C6-7	3-4-86	Bil S-2	Rt S-3, lt S-3 split	Lt S-4	No	>90%	>90%	U + lev	lev	Voids fine
JB	SI—T9-10	6-5-86	Bil S-2	Bil S-3	Bil S-4	No	>90%	<25%	Pud	U + lev	Requires anticholinergics for continence, negating voids

Patient	Date	SI level	S-2	S-3	S-4	S-3vr			Pud + lev	Pud	Comments
LL	7–3–86	SI—L-2	Bil S-2	Bil S-3	Intact	No	>90%	>90%		Intact	Voids fine
WW	8–19–86	SI—T-10	Bil S-2	Bil S-3	Intact	No	>90%	<25%	Pud + lev		Incomplete rhizotomies, but continent, prefers SIC
JD	9–4–86	SI—T-12	Bil S-2	Rt S-3, Lt separation	Rt S-4 (Lt atrophic)	No	>90%	75–90%		Pud (alc)	Voids fine, residuals consistently ~100 ml, SIC 1/day
CB	11–18–86	SI (tubercular meningitis)	Bil S-2	Bil S-3	Bil S-4	No	<25%	<25%			Incompetent urethra with persisting incontinence
LW	12–2–86	SI—T-3	Intact	Bil S-3	Bil S-4	No	<25%	<25%			Incompetent urethra with persisting incontinence
RW	1–12–87	SI—C-6	Bil S-2	Bil S-3	Intact	No	>90%	>90%	Intact	Intact	Complete rhizotomies, good capacity, good voids
MF	1–30–87	SI—T10-11	Bil S-2	Bil S-3	Intact	No	<25%	<25%			Sphincteric incompetence with incontinence
LL	7–9–87	SI—T-5	Bil S-2	Bil S-3	Intact	No	75–90%	<25%			Incomplete rhizotomy, requires anticholinergics for continence
JV	12–18–87	SI—T-12	Intact	Bil S-3	Bil S-4	No	>90%	75–90%			Voiding
FB	9–29–88	SI—T12-L1	S-2	Bil S-3	Intact	No	>90%	>90%			Voids fine
FG	12–1–88	SI—T-12	Bil S-2	Bil S-3	Intact	No	75–90%	<25%			Inadequate detrusor, preoperatively and postoperatively
JF	1–19–89	SI—C6-7	Intact	Bil S-3	Intact	No	>90%	<25%			Ventral root damaged
MG	1–25–89	SI—T-10	Bil S-2	Lt S-3, rt S-3 Split	Intact	No	<50%	<25%			Incomplete rhizotomies with dependence on anticholinergics
SS	6–16–89	SI—T4-5	Bil S-2	Bil S-3	Intact	No	>90%	>90%			Voids fine
JM	9–25–90	SI—T-4	Bil S-2	Bil S-3	Bil S-4	No	>90%	100%			

Alc, alcohol block; A, anal; Bil, bilateral; Lt, left; Lev, levator nerve; Pud, pudendal nerve; Rt, right; SI, spinal injury level; S-3vr, third sacral ventral root; U, urethral (pud) nerves.

Brindley and colleagues report a 60% success in producing an erection through stimulation.[16]

Bowel Evacuation Program

As with erection, sacral rhizotomies have a variable dampening effect on the use of trigger techniques for achieving bowel movement. Bowel evacuation routines on the whole, however, do not otherwise significantly change after rhizotomy. Spontaneous movements can be induced or coaxed with suppositories and aided by electrostimulation.

TECHNIQUE

A sacral laminectomy is performed using a curved sacral incision designed to avoid any skin areas prone to pressure breakdown. The dorsal lamina is opened, exposing the various sacral nerves. Neurostimulation is used to identify the nerves capable of producing a detrusor contraction. The S-3 roots are virtually always the principal nerves concerned with the innervation of the bladder. With the aid of magnification lenses, the dorsal roots are separated from the ventral roots and the dorsal roots divided. This has been carried out extradurally to avoid the risks of cerebrospinal fluid leak or infection. Intradural separation, however, has been performed by way of a small incision in the terminal dura and combined with extradural electrode placement. As an alternative, both steps can be performed intradurally. Careful closure of the dura must then be carried out to minimize risks of cerebrospinal fluid–related complications.

Generally electrodes are placed on each of the S-3 nerves' ventral roots as well as on any additional nerve roots that were found to give significant bladder activity with stimulation. Lead wires are then tunneled subcutaneously to a pulse generator (Itrel, Medtronic, Inc.) located conveniently for patient comfort and access. This step may require a separate incision after the patient has been turned and reprepped. Table 10-2 provides an overview of experience. Of note is that the dorsal rhizotomies in themselves produce significant enhancement of continence.

There does not appear to be a significant downside to the procedure as long as the dorsal rhizotomies are performed from S-2 through S-4. These patients are continent, experience a much lower incidence of urinary tract infections, have dramatically lower intravesical pressures, and are often able to empty their bladders in a timed fashion without instrumentation. As long as a bladder contraction above 80 cm H_2O is achieved, the patient has an excellent chance of achieving evacuation control over the bladder.

Case Histories

A 35-year-old man suffered a traumatic injury to the spinal cord at the T-4 level, resulting in complete motor paralysis and a mixed sensory defect.[17] The patient attempted to manage his bladder with crede maneuvers and spontaneous voiding. Four years after the injury, the patient developed renal failure with a creatinine level of 9.0 mg/dl and sepsis. He was treated with an indwelling urethral catheter and intravenous antibiotics. His sepsis cleared, and nadir creatinine fell to 3.8 mg/dl. Urodynamic and radiographic evaluation revealed a small noncompliant bladder with severe bilateral vesicourethral reflux. Attempts at managing the patient with intermittent catheterization and anticholinergic medication failed secondary to an abrupt increase in serum creatinine when the urethral catheter was removed. Long-term management with the indwelling urethral catheter led to recurrent episodes of urosepsis.

Because the patient was not considered a good candidate for augmentation or diversion, bilateral selective dorsal root rhizotomy of sacral roots S-2, S-3, and S-4 was performed. Concurrently neural prosthesis electrodes were attached to the ventral roots of S-3 and S-4 for subsequent direct electrical bladder stimulation and emptying.

Postoperatively the patient's bladder changed from a small-capacity, high-pressure reservoir to a large-capacity (400 ml), low-pressure reservoir with almost complete resolution of severe bilateral reflux. Urodynamic studies confirm a decrease in bladder pressures from greater than 40 cm H_2O preoperatively to a maximum of 15 cm H_2O postoperatively. The patient voids by initiating a bladder contraction through the neuroprosthesis, which is activated by a magnetic transcutaneous signal. He typically voids six times per day and once in the middle of the night, the impetus being a feeling of lower abdominal fullness or timed voiding. His postvoid residuals remain less than 30 ml, his creatinine level has been stable at 3.4, and he remains free from infection. The patient's erectile function actually improved postimplant.

A 47-year-old man presented with a problem of recurrent urinary tract infections. He had developed a spastic neurogenic bladder 10 years previously from encephalitis that left him a T-4 paraplegic and wheelchair dependent. He had received two previous sphincterotomies in an attempt to control infections. He continued to carry large residuals, however, putting him at risk for recurrent urinary tract infections, and became incontinent. He tried an indwelling Foley catheter but continued experiencing recurrent episodes of urosepsis. He then became leg bag dependent because of incontinence. In 1987, he underwent evaluation and subsequently implant of an S-3 ventral root electrodes and bilateral S-3 and S-4 dorsal rhizotomies. He is now 5 years' postimplant and doing well. He is continent and able to void himself completely by the pacemaker four to six times per day. He has been virtually infection free.

These cases are examples of the remarkable clinical benefit this approach can have on spinal injury patients. In these situations, there were no other good choices that offered a chance to stabilize the patients' renal status for the long term.

Conclusions

The experience with neuroprosthetic implants has shown that electrical stimulation can be used on a long-term basis to treat problems of voiding dysfunction. In patients who have been followed for several years, consistency of response to stimulation was observed. Even after use of the stimulator for several months or years, symptoms often return as soon as the stimulation ceases because of a malfunction or electrode migration.

Neurostimulation is no panacea: Patients must be carefully selected for their willingness to cooperate in their care and for their having specific muscle dysfunction as determined urodynamically. Test stimulation of the sacral nerves has provided invaluable insight into the neuromusculature responses mediated by the S2-4 nerves and has thus helped to identify dysfunction that is specifically associated with each of these nerves. It has also helped to discern differences between the potential function of pelvic muscles and the capability of the patient to use these muscles. This information allows the urologist to focus on a specific muscle dysfunction and re-educate the patient to use the pelvic musculature properly or, failing this, to use neurostimulation by way of an implant to modulate the dysfunction.

There must be a real commitment on the part of the physician. No two patients are alike. Patient symptoms, the pattern of muscle dysfunction found in the pelvis, the responses to test stimulation, the urodynamic findings with and without stimulation, and the underlying anxieties of patients that can contribute to symptoms are all important considerations.

Neurostimulation is an exciting and fascinating addition to the urologist's armamentarium. Most important, urologists are now able to test for the functional integrity of the pelvic musculature and to identify weakness and dysfunction with specificity. Therapy can now be based on an assessment of the functional capabilities of the nervous system concerned with micturition control.

References

1. Bradley WE, Timm GW, Chou SN. A decade of experience with electronic stimulation of the micturition reflex. Urol Int 1971;26:283.

2. Hald T. Neurogenic dysfunction of the urinary bladder. An experimental and clinical study with special reference to the ability of electrical stimulation to establish voluntary micturition. Danish Med Bull 1969;16(suppl 5):1.

3. Jonas U, Tanagho EA. Studies on the feasibility of urinary bladder evacuation by direct stimulation of the spinal cord. II. Post stimulus voiding: A way to overcome outflow resistance. Invest Urol 1975;13:151.

4. Jonas U, Honefellner R. Late results of bladder stimulation in 11 patients: Follow up to 4 years. J Urol 1978;120:565.

5. Fall M. Does electrostimulation cure urinary incontinence. J Urol 1984;131:664.

6. Ebner A, Lindstrom S, Jiang CH. Intravesical electrostimulation: How does it work? An experimental study. J Neurourol Urodynam 1991; 10:281.

7. Katona F. Stages of vegetative afferentation in reorganization of bladder control during electrotherapy. Urol Int 1975;30:192.

8. Kaplan WE, Richards I. Intravesical transurethral electrotherapy for the neurogenic bladder. J Urol 1986;136:243.

9. Madesbacher H, Pauer W, Reiner E. Rehabilitation of micturition by transurethral electrostimulation of the bladder in patients with incomplete spinal cord lesions. Paraplegia 1982;20:191.

10. Schmidt RA. Advances in genitourinary neurostimulation. Neurosurgery 1986;18:1041.

11. Juenemann KP, Lue TF, Schmidt RA, Tanagho EA. Clinical significance of sacral and pudendal nerve anatomy. J Urol 1988;139:74.

12. McCreery D, Agnew WF. Mechanisms of stimulation induced neural damage and their relation to guidelines for safe stimulation. In: Agnew, McCreery, eds. Neural prosthesis fundamental studies. Biophysics and Bioengineering Series. Englewood Cliffs, NJ: Prentice-Hall, 1990:298–315.

13. Mortimer JT. Electrical excitability: The basis for applied neural control. Eng Med Biol 1983;2:12.

14. Thuroff JW, Schmidt RA, Tanagho EA. Chronic stimulation of the sacral roots in dogs. Eur Urol 1983;9:102.

15. Schmidt RA, Tanagho EA. Extradural approach to bladder pacemaker. World J Urol 1991;9:109.

16. Brindley GS, Polky CE, Rushton DN, Cardozo L. Sacral anterior root stimulators for bladder control in paraplegia. The first 50 cases. J Neurol Neurosurg. Psychiatry 1986;49:1104.

17. Baskin LS, Schmidt RA. The severe neurogenic bladder: An alternative approach to management. Paraplegia 1992;30(11):787.

III   *Urethral Incontinence*

11

Disorders
of Urethral Support

Steven W. Siegel

Stress incontinence related to weakened bladder outlet resistance is the most common form of incontinence among women and the most often treated surgically by urologists and gynecologists.[1] The mechanism of stress incontinence can be further defined as due to either anatomic displacement of a functional vesicoureteral sphincter or intrinsic sphincteric dysfunction.[2] This chapter focuses on disorders of urethral support that are associated with anatomic displacement of the urethra (hypermobility) during stress maneuvers.

Pathophysiology

Genuine *stress incontinence* is defined as urethral leakage during periods of increased abdominal pressure in the absence of a detrusor contraction.[3] The bladder neck and proximal urethra function as the continence zone in the female.[4] When functioning normally, pressure in the continence zone remains higher than that of the bladder at all times except during normal voiding.[5] If pressure in the bladder exceeds maximal urethral pressure, leakage of urine occurs. When the pelvic floor structures responsible for urethral support have been impaired, descent of the bladder and proximal urethra into the vagina

may occur during stress maneuvers. This situation allows increased abdominal pressure to be distributed unevenly, and if the intravesical pressure, augmented by abdominal straining, exceeds the maximal urethral pressure, leakage occurs. Factors that tend to prevent or limit the degree of leakage associated with loss of urethral support include the degree of competency of the intrinsic sphincteric mechanism, the guarding response of the somatically innervated external sphincter, which occurs during stress maneuver, and possible blunting of increased intravesical pressures by a large dependent cystocele.[6] Although it is clear that leakage does not always result from weakness of the pelvic supporting structures, genuine stress urinary incontinence associated with urethral hypermobility is the cardinal symptom of disorders of urethral support.[7]

Etiology of the Lack of Support

Impaired urethral support can result from many causes, generally falling under three main categories: anatomic, hormonal, and neurologic[8] (Table 11-1).

Anatomic causes may be congenital or acquired from trauma, inflammatory disease, or chronically increased intra-abdominal pressure.

Female Urology, edited by Elroy D. Kursh and Edward McGuire. J. B. Lippincott, Philadelphia, © 1994.

Table 11-1. Causes of Pelvic Floor Weakness

Anatomic
  Congenital
  Traumatic
    Labor
    Pelvic surgery
    Pelvic fracture
  Inflammatory
  Chronic increased intra-abdominal pressure
    Chronic obstructive pulmonary disease
    Ascites
Hormonal
  Menopause
Neurologic
  Congenital
  Cord lesion
  Pelvic surgery
  Pelvic fracture

A congenital weakness implies a genetic or fascial predisposition toward herniation of the pelvic floor. Traumatic injuries, such as those arising during the second stage of labor, pelvic surgery (*i.e.*, hysterectomy without reconstruction of pelvic supports), or pelvic fracture, may lead to urethral hypermobility. Inflammatory disease, such as pelvic inflammatory disease, may cause fibrotic scarring and dysfunction of the pelvic supports. Lastly, severe physical exertion or diseases associated with chronically increased intra-abdominal pressure, such as ascites or chronic obstructive pulmonary disease, can weaken pelvic support over time.

Hormonal withdrawal, which accompanies aging, is responsible for atrophy of the muscular and connective supporting tissues of the urethra.[9] There may also be thinning of the suburethral vascular cushion and impaired mucosal apposition or seal.[10] This component of intrinsic urethral dysfunction tends to accentuate the degree of leakage associated with urethral hypermobility.

Any lesion that affects the somatic innervation of the pelvic floor can be responsible for weakness, or diastasis, of the associated pelvic floor muscles. Such injuries include those from trauma, pelvic surgeries, and prolonged labor as well as congenital and acquired neurologic diseases, such as myelomeningocele or a cauda equina lesion of the spinal cord.

Presentation

Stress incontinence is the principal symptom of impaired urethral support and is most often the presenting complaint to urologists. Impaired urethral support without associated stress incontinence may occur with a prominent cystocele, and therefore patients may present to the gynecologist with other symptoms related to pelvic prolapse. The history is important to define the type or types of incontinence present, precipitating activities, degree of leakage, chronicity of the complaint, and degree of distress perceived by the patient related to these symptoms. The history is also helpful by providing a meaningful basis to plan and interpret an evaluation of a given patient's complaints. Other important aspects of the history include those present in a general urologic history, with special emphasis on prior pelvic or anti-incontinence surgeries and results, medications that might affect bladder or urethral function, and review of systems with special emphasis on disorders that are known to affect voiding function.

Genuine stress urinary incontinence occurs during periods of increased abdominal pressure. It is important to find out what activity the patient engages in that causes her the most leakage. A rare episode of stress urinary incontinence occurring only during a very severe cough or sneeze or only with strenuous physical activity, such as weight lifting, implies a mild degree of stress incontinence. More severe degrees of leakage require less of an increase in intra-abdominal pressure to precipitate leakage and may occur with common activities, such as walking or bending over. The type of activity that produces leakage may need to be duplicated in the laboratory to demonstrate the mechanism of incontinence objectively.

The pattern of leakage is also important. A squirt or brief gush of incontinence associated with a stress maneuver is characteristic of weakened urethral support, whereas a stream of incontinence that cannot be stopped is usually due to the bladder. Continuous incontinence may represent an extreme form of stress incontinence, such as that due to an intrinsic sphincteric defect, or this symptom may represent extra-urethral leakage caused by a fistula or ectopic ureter.

Symptoms of urgency and urge incontinence should be elicited and distinguished from stress urinary incontinence if possible. Approximately 30% of patients with stress incontinence also complain of urge incontinence at the time of presentation.[11] The history may not always be successful in distinguishing these because patients can be vague about the circumstances of incontinence. This could be because they are not comfortable exploring the details of such a personal complaint, which may have been dealt with by neglect or denial in the past. A patient who experiences a small amount of leakage associated with repetitive physical activity may simply know that she is wet but not be able to pinpoint the exact nature of activity that brings this symptom on. Physical stress, such as getting up out of a chair, can precipitate detrusor instability in some patients (stress hyperreflexia). Overflow incontinence, although less common among women than men, mimics stress incontinence but can readily be distinguished by determining the postvoid residual.

The degree of incontinence is implied by the precipitating circumstances and also by the number and type of padding material used to maintain patient comfort. The need for padding is certainly an indirect measure of severity because it can be affected by patient education, financial resources, or personal habit or hygienic standards. Some patients change pads frequently even if they are only minimally damp, whereas others wait until the pads are saturated because of the expense of the product. It is also useful to note if pads are required at night because this implies either a severe degree of incontinence or another mechanism of leakage other than urethral incompetence.

The chronicity of the complaint is also important to establish. A gradual worsening of

degree of leakage over many years is entirely consistent with anatomic stress urinary incontinence, whereas sudden severe incontinence associated with a precipitating event, such as a pelvic fracture or trauma with labor, implies an intrinsic sphincteric defect. In a similar way, the age at presentation may reflect the causes, as postmenopausal, multiparous women are more likely to experience stress incontinence secondary to weakness of the pelvic floor than young nulliparous women.[12]

It is a mistake to conclude that a patient's symptoms of stress incontinence are insignificant solely on the basis of the frequency or volume of the incontinent episodes. Although stress urinary incontinence is a common condition, several studies have shown that women tend to underreport the incontinence symptoms to their physicians.[13-15] This underlines the fact that when a patient does report incontinence, it is likely to be perceived as a significant problem that requires evaluation and treatment. It is not uncommon to find that patients alter their social interactions, limit their excursions outside the home, and have a more negative impression of their overall health as a result of symptoms of stress incontinence.[16] Some individuals are not distressed by large amounts of leakage, whereas others may be devastated by even one drop of leakage at an inappropriate moment. It is important to assess how bothersome symptoms are to a given patient because this is the ultimate determining factor for treatment goals. Similarly, it is also necessary to determine which component of mixed incontinence is most bothersome to a given patient. For example, a patient who experiences both stress and urge incontinence and is most bothered by the urge component of her symptoms might be satisfied with medical treatment aimed at correcting bladder instability.

Etiologic factors should be sought, such as multiparity with prolonged or traumatic labor, previous pelvic surgeries, or operations for incontinence, including whether a vaginal or transabdominal approach was used. Although the most common cause of a failed anti-incontinence procedure is recurrence of the anatomic defect predisposing to stress incontinence, the risk of intrinsic or urethral injury increases with multiple anti-incontinence procedures or pelvic surgeries.[17–20]

Because stress incontinence is mainly a symptom of pelvic prolapse, there are often other symptoms associated with pelvic floor defects. Patients may report a fullness or painful vaginal mass with intercourse, a feeling as if something is "out of place," or, as with a third-degree cystocele, they may actually see a protruding mass or feel as if they are "sitting on a beach ball." Patients with large cystoceles often complain of obstructive symptoms, including difficulty initiating and maintaining a urinary stream, and occasionally may volunteer that manual correction of the cystocele improves voiding function. If a symptomatic rectocele is present, the patient may complain of chronic constipation or the feeling of difficult or incomplete bowel evacuation.

In addition to those aspects of the history that are related to pelvic floor weakness, a general urologic history should be obtained. A medication history is also important to look for drugs that affect bladder or urethral function. These might include tricyclic antidepressants, alpha agonists or alpha blockers, and estrogens or antiestrogens.

PHYSICAL EXAMINATION

The pelvic examination is the most critical aspect of the physical examination concerning stress incontinence. With the patient in a modified lithotomy position, the perineum is inspected for evidence of excoriation, estrogen effect, and obvious pelvic prolapse. The bottom blade of a speculum, or Sims retractor, is then placed into the vagina to displace gently the posterior vaginal wall inferiorly. The anterior wall is inspected for estrogen effect and general position of the urethra and bladder in the resting and stressed state. An isolated defect of pelvic support leading to protrusion of the area anterior to the trigone is known as an anterior cystocele or urethrocele. Isolated protrusion of the area posterior to the bladder neck is termed a *posterior cystocele*, or cystocele. Combined defects, which are most commonly found, are termed *cystourethrocele*. These defects can be graded I to IV, depending on the degree of bladder descent found in the resting state:

Grade I—minimal bladder descent.
Grade II—descent to introitus with stress.
Grade III—descent to introitus at rest.
Grade IV—descent beyond introitus.

Although an isolated urethral defect is uncommon, it may occur following vaginal delivery in women with a wide pubic arch.[21] It is more common to see an isolated posterior cystocele, which results from previous urethropexy without simultaneous management of the cystocele.

The patient should be examined with a moderately full bladder in the supine and upright positions. We routinely examine the patient supine and view the bladder with a voiding cystourethrogram (VCUG) in the upright position. Stress incontinence can be induced by coughing or straining, and a note should be made as to whether the degree of leakage is small or large and how much effort was required to produce this result. Minimal leakage with maximal effort represents mild stress urinary incontinence and might adequately be managed with conservative measures. Maximal leakage with minimal stress suggests an intrinsic urethral defect and deserves careful evaluation with a videourodynamic study. The degree of motion of the vaginal wall is also assessed. When stress incontinence is associated with minimal hypermobility, there should be concern about intrinsic urethral function. Urethral hypermobility can be judged by the degree of downward and outward protrusion of the urethra during the stress maneuver. When there is evidence of urethral hypermobility associated with a stress maneuver but stress incontinence cannot be demonstrated in the supine position, we generally stand the patient up and have her squat and cough while observing the anterior vaginal wall for evidence of stress incontinence. If stress incontinence does not occur in this position, it is possible that the leakage is being prevented by conscious guarding of the external sphincter (Type 0 incontinence), and a video-urodynamics study will need to be performed to document opening of the bladder neck with urethral hypermobility.[20]

Additional examination is needed to assess for coexisting defects. The speculum blade is repositioned to retract the anterior vaginal wall upward, and the posterior wall is inspected for evidence of enterocele or rectocele. When a prominent rectocele has been found, it may be necessary to use a second speculum blade to retract the anterior and posterior walls simultaneously, to inspect for evidence of an enterocele or uterine prolapse. It must be emphasized that in most cases, stress incontinence is merely a symptom of the overall problem of pelvic floor prolapse. To address the problem satisfactorily, coexisting defects must be identified, and if they are of sufficient degree, they should be repaired at the time that surgical correction of stress urinary incontinence is undertaken.

Evaluation

URINALYSIS

A urinalysis and urine culture, when appropriate, are always done at the time of initial examination. Every attempt should be made to resolve a urinary tract infection and reassess incontinence symptoms before a more elaborate evaluation.

VOIDING CYSTOURETHROGRAPHY

A VCUG is an essential tool for evaluation of stress incontinence and may almost be considered an extension of the physical examination. Our technique is similar to that described by Zimmern.[22] The study is performed with the patient in a standing position. After voiding, a small radiopaque catheter is placed into the bladder, and a postvoid residual is measured. The study is monitored under fluoroscopy with spot films taken to limit patient radiation exposure. Rest and stressed views are taken with the bladder filled to a comfortable level for the pa-

tient in the anteroposterior, oblique, and lateral projections. The presence of the radiopaque catheter allows definition of the position of the urethra and bladder neck. In the lateral projection, with catheter in place, the angle of intersection of the urethra with the vertical plane, or angle of inclination, is normally less than 30 degrees in rest and stressed states. An angle greater than this is consistent with weakened support. Therefore, a urethra that appears parallel to the vertical axis is well supported or even oversupported, whereas a urethra that intersects the vertical axis at a 90-degree angle is poorly supported. The catheter is removed, and rest, straining, and voiding films are obtained in the oblique and anteroposterior positions. This allows for better assessment of bladder neck function and also provides a mechanism to document stress urinary incontinence in many cases. Under normal circumstances, the bladder neck remains closed at rest and with stress. The base of the bladder remains at or above the level of the symphysis pubis with the patient upright and in a resting state. Normally there is less than 2 cm of descent of the bladder base relative to the symphysis, with the bladder neck remaining closed during stress maneuvers.[20] If the bladder neck is closed at rest but descends and opens with a stress maneuver, this is consistent with stress urinary incontinence. If the bladder neck appears opened at rest, the patient either has intrinsic damage to the vesical neck or is undergoing an uninhibited contraction. During the voiding phase of this study, coexisting urethral defects, such as urethrovaginal fistula or urethral diverticuli, can be ruled out. In addition, descent of the base of the bladder can be assessed. A grade I cystocele represents descent of the bladder base just below the symphysis. A grade II cystocele represents descent 2 to 5 cm below the symphysis pubis, and a grade III cystocele represents descent greater than 5 cm. The degree of cystocele noted on radiographic examination should correlate with that seen on physical examination. It is clear, however, that physical examination in the modified lithotomy position tends to underestimate the prominence of the cystocele noted radiographically in the upright position. Additionally, at the time of physical examination, it is often impossible to distinguish a cystocele from a large enterocele, or vaginal vault prolapse, and thus the VCUG becomes the most accurate means of determining the degree of bladder and urethral support preoperatively in this circumstance.

The VCUG provides an excellent means of determining the position and configuration of the urethra during the rest and stress states. It allows documentation of the presence of a cystocele and the ability to assess the degree of urethral hypermobility with or without a cystocele. It also provides an additional opportunity to document stress urinary incontinence as the event associated with the patient's presenting complaint. It has great value in the routine preoperative evaluations of patients undergoing treatment for stress incontinence. It may also serve as a baseline test in prospective clinical studies and as a useful tool in evaluating the cause of failure of a prior suspension because the resultant degree of urethral support, or discrepancy between urethral and bladder base support, can easily be judged. It is also valuable in differentiating between complex symptomatic complaints when the patient cannot clearly distinguish between stress or urge incontinence. In these circumstances, and when intrinsic sphincteric damage is suspected, we find it more useful to perform the VCUG in conjunction with urodynamic monitoring as is discussed later.

VOIDING DIARY

A 2 or 3 consecutive day voiding diary is helpful in evaluating incontinence. It guides the patient to focus her attention on her true urinary frequency, presence or absence of urgency with voiding or incontinence episodes, activity during leakage episodes, degree of leakage episode, and number of pads used. It may also be helpful to gauge fluid intake. During a urodynamic assessment, basic information from the voiding diary is helpful to perform an accurate urodynamic assessment tailored to a particular patient. The largest voided volume on a voiding chart represents the patient's functional capacity and, if there is no significant residual volume, the true capacity. With this information, a target range of bladder filling relevant for a particular patient can be chosen, and this, in turn, reduces the chance of producing an artifact in the laboratory.

URODYNAMIC EVALUATION OF STRESS INCONTINENCE

Urodynamic evaluation of the lower urinary tract allows us to witness an episode of urinary incontinence, confirm that this is indeed the type of incontinence that is bothersome to the patient, define the mechanism of an incontinence episode, rule out other coexisting conditions, and predict the success of treatment for stress incontinence. Our routine urodynamic assessment includes voiding flowmetry, determination of postvoid residual, and a bedside or "eyeball" urodynamic assessment in uncomplicated cases, in which medical management may be instituted as a first form of treatment. In more complex cases, in which the history is ambiguous, there has been a failed previous surgical attempt to correct the incontinence, or an intrinsic sphincteric defect is suspected, multichannel urodynamic studies, with or without simultaneous fluoroscopy, are employed.

VOIDING FLOWMETRY

A simple voiding flow rate can act as a general screen for normal bladder function. At capacity, a characteristic flow pattern with a minimal residual indicates the high likelihood of normal bladder function. High flow rates may be associated with diminished outlet resistance or abdominal straining, and intermittent flow patterns with a diminished flow rate and incomplete evacuation may be associated with bladder outlet obstruction, impaired detrusor contractility, or inefficient bladder evacuation secondary to a large cystourethrocele. To distinguish between bladder outlet obstruction and diminished bladder contractility, it is necessary to measure detrusor pressure and urinary flow simultaneously.

We think that voiding flowmetry is helpful in assessing which patients may have difficulty voiding after a bladder neck suspension owing to impaired detrusor contractility. If the flow rate is significantly diminished, the uninstrumented or free flow analysis can be compared with invasive flow studies, which are also necessary to evaluate this condition properly.

BEDSIDE OR "EYEBALL" URODYNAMICS

As has been emphasized by Blaivas, much can be gained by a routine urodynamic assessment of the patient, during the physical examination, simply by placing a catheter.[23] A postvoid residual is obtained. An increased residual may be associated with bladder outlet obstruction or impaired detrusor contractility. It is always important to catheterize the patient shortly after bladder evacuation and to confirm with the patient that the void was a normal, uninhibited one. This does not always occur in the physician's office, and the patient usually can recognize the difference. With the catheter in place and the patient in the dorsolithotomy position, the catheter can be filled gradually with sterile irrigating solution through an open irrigating syringe. As filling occurs at a slow and steady rate, the patient is asked to indicate the first sensation of fullness as well as the perceived volitional capacity. Volumes at which these events occur are recorded. The meniscus at the top of the water column can be observed through the irrigating syringe. In a normally compliant bladder, the meniscus remains constant until the bladder capacity is reached, at which time it may rise slowly. In a poorly compliant bladder, the meniscus rises in direct proportion to the volume of filling. When an unstable bladder is present, the meniscus rises suddenly at a constant rate of filling. The patient may volunteer that she is experiencing a sense of urgency associated with this event. Leakage of urine around the catheter can also be observed with an uninhibited contraction. The patient must be questioned carefully to confirm that this feeling or type of leakage is present during her normal daily activities.

With the bladder at a comfortable capacity, the catheter can be removed. The patient is asked to perform a stress maneuver by coughing, and the urethral meatus is observed for urinary leakage. The degree of hypermobility of the bladder neck is also judged at this time, as mentioned earlier in discussion of the physical examination. If the patient's history is consistent with stress incontinence but no evidence of stress incontinence is seen in the dorsolithotomy position, the patient is asked to stand, and with one foot elevated on a stool, the patient is asked to squat and cough. The urethra is observed during this augmented stress maneuver for evidence of leakage.

MULTICHANNEL URODYNAMICS EVALUATION

This rudimentary examination may be the only urodynamics study required to confirm stress incontinence in an unambiguous patient, such as a middle-aged woman with progressively worsening symptoms of stress incontinence, without complaint of urgency or urge incontinence, who demonstrates evidence of urethral hypermobility on physical examination. In less clear-cut situations, when there may be a strong component of urge or urge incontinence, when the patient cannot help to distinguish between types of incontinence by history, or when findings of bedside urodynamics do not seem to agree with the examiner's impression garnered by other means, a multichannel urodynamics study is required.[24] We also find such a study helpful in clinical evaluation of patients for prospective study. As part of a multichannel study, a small-caliber, double-lumen catheter is placed transurethrally to allow filling of liquid medium at a specified rate by an infusion pump. The catheter is left in place during the voiding phase of the study to determine detrusor pressure. A transvaginal or transrectal balloon catheter is also used to determine abdominal pressure, and the subtracted product of the abdominal plus detrusor pressures measured by the intravesical catheter, minus the abdominal pressures measured by the vaginal or rectal catheter, is equal to the true detrusor pressure. During the filling phase of such a study, a more accurate assessment of bladder compliance and capacity can be determined. This study is also more sensitive in determining the presence of uninhibited detrusor activity. Flow can also be measured during the storage phase, and leakage associated with stress incontinence can be documented. Similarly, leakage associated with an uninhibited contraction can also be measured. During the voiding phase of the study, a more accurate determination of detrusor contractility can be made and used to predict the ability to void after a bladder neck suspension. Such a urodynamics study, in conjunction with a VCUG, provides an adequate means of evaluating stress urinary incontinence in the majority of patients.

VIDEOURODYNAMICS STUDY

A videourodynamic study, wherein simultaneous urodynamic and radiographic information is obtained, may be needed in a minority of patients. Such studies are useful in patients who complain of stress urinary incontinence yet cannot demonstrate leakage on physical examination or urodynamics study. Such a patient may have type 0 stress urinary incontinence, which is defined as opening and descent of the bladder neck on stress maneuver without associated leakage.[20] These individuals are unconsciously guarding against an incontinence episode by contracting the external sphincter during the testing circumstances and may experience stress incontinence only when they "let down their guard" in a nontesting environment. Patients who have a strong component of urge and urge incontinence, in addition to their complaint of stress urinary incontinence, also benefit from a videourodynamics study. These patients frequently display evidence of an open bladder neck during the rest phase of a VCUG. Without simultaneous urodynamic monitoring, it is impossible to determine why the bladder neck is open. During a videourodynamic study, the bladder neck is observed during early phases of filling, and detrusor pressure can be monitored to confirm the presence or absence of an associated uninhibited detrusor contraction. In such a patient, it is important to determine which aspect of the incontinence is most disturbing because medical therapy may be more advantageous for patients whose most bothersome complaint is due to detrusor instability. Patients who have had multiple surgical failures deserve the most careful preoperative assessment before any further interventions for stress urinary incontinence. The configuration and degree of support of the urethra and bladder neck, with reference to intravesical activity, can best be determined with a videourodynamic study.

CYSTOSCOPY

Cystoscopy with a 20 French female urethroscope and 0-degree lens is useful to rule out a urethral fistula, diverticulum, or Skene's gland absence. It is also another means of assessing bladder neck hypermobility and urethral function, as the patient can be asked to cough and strain while viewing the vesical neck directly from the midurethra with the water flowing slowly. Cystoscopy should be performed preoperatively in any patient who has undergone a previous bladder neck suspension to determine the presence of foreign body or suture material. It is also necessary under special circumstances, such as presence of hematuria or recurrent infection.

References

1. Siegel SW, Montague DK. Surgery for stress urinary incontinence. In: Novick AC, Streem SB, Pontes JE, eds. Stewart's operative urology. Baltimore: Williams & Wilkins, 1989:715–725.
2. Bates P, Bradley WE, Glen E, et al. The standardization of terminology of lower urinary tract function. J Urol 1979;121:551.
3. Staskin DR, Zimmern PE, Hadley HR, Raz S. The pathophysiology of stress incontinence. Urol Clin North Am 1985;12:271.
4. Fosling JA. The structure of the female lower urinary tract and pelvic floor. Urol Clin North Am 1985;12:207.
5. Blaivas JG. Pathophysiology of lower urinary

tract dysfunction. Urol Clin North Am 1985; 12:215.

6. Wein AJ, Barrett DM. In: Marshall DK, ed. Voiding function and dysfunction: A logical and practical approach. Chicago: Yearbook Medical Publishers, 1988:109–112.

7. McGuire EJ. Urinary incontinence—clinical correlations. AUA Update Series 1990;9:290.

8. Staskin DR, Hadley HR, Leach GE, et al. Anatomy for vaginal surgery. Sem Urol 1986;4:2.

9. Bavendam TG. Geriatric female incontinence. Prob Urol 1991;5:42.

10. Klutke CG, Little NA, Raz S. The anatomy of stress incontinence. AUA Update Series 1990; 9:306.

11. McGuire EJ, Lytton B, Kohorn EL, Pepe V. The value of urodynamic testing in stress urinary incontinence. J Urol 1980;124:256.

12. Wolin LH. Stress incontinence in young, healthy, multiparous female subjects. J Urol 1969;101:545.

13. Jeter KF. Incontinence in the American home: Facts, not myths. Union, SC: HIP, Inc, 1985.

14. Diokno AC, Brock BM, Brown MB, Herzog AR. Prevalence of urinary incontinence and other urological symptoms in the noninstitutionalized elderly. J Urol 1986;136:1022.

15. Nygaard I, DeLancey JO, Arnsdorf L, Murphy E. Exercise and incontinence. Obstet Gynecol 1990; 75:848.

16. Urinary incontinence in adults. National Institutes of Health Consensus Development Conference Statement 1988;7:5.

17. Killing MJ, Leach GE. Long-term results of bladder neck suspension procedures. Prob Urol 1991; 5:94.

18. Stanton SL. Stress incontinence: Why and how operations work. Urol Clin North Am 1985; 12:279.

19. McGuire E. Urodynamic findings in patients after failure of stress incontinence operations. In: Zimmer NR, Sterling AM, eds. Female incontinence. New York: Alan R. Liss, 1980:351–360.

20. Blaivas JG, Olsson CA. Stress incontinence: Classification and surgical approach. J Urol 1988; 139:727.

21. Snyder JA, Westmacott R. Treatment of mild, moderate, and severe cystoceles. Prob Urol 1991;5:85.

22. Zimmern PE. The role of voiding cystourethrography in the evaluation of the female lower urinary tract. Prob Urol 1991;5:23.

23. Blaivas JG. A modest proposal for the diagnosis and treatment of urinary incontinence in women. J Urol 1987;138:597.

24. Wein AJ, Barrett DM. In: Marshall DK, ed. Voiding function and dysfunction: A logical and practical approach. Chicago: Yearbook Medical Publishers, 1988:173.

12

Urethral Dysfunction

Edward J. McGuire

Disorders of Urethral Function

Incontinence, which results either from urethral hypermobility or a lack of normal urethral closure, is the result of a disorder of urethral function. In this chapter, we are concerned with abnormal urethral closure as a cause of urinary symptoms in women, rather than disorders of the urethral supporting structures. Although loss of normal function of the supporting structures of the urethra can often be associated with stress incontinence, there need not be any loss of intrinsic urethral closing function for the incontinence to occur. Loss of proximal urethral closing function can be associated with severe incontinence with no abnormality of the urethral supporting structures.[1]

Mechanisms Involved in Urethral Closure

The urethral lumen is normally closed by muscular activity, and this active contractility is aided by the structure and composition of the urethra as well as its anatomic position vis a vis the bladder and the abdominal cavity.[2] In the first place, the urethra functions as an organ of continence because the bladder, despite filling continuously, maintains a very low pressure. The pres-

sure advantage of the internal sphincter of the urethra over that of the bladder is not great in normal circumstances and may be low in some circumstances, but provided that the bladder pressure remains low, only a little pressure advantage on the part of the urethra over the bladder is sufficient for passive continence to be maintained.[3] There are two active components of urethral closure: smooth and skeletal muscle.

The skeletal muscle of the urethra proper is composed primarily of slow twitch fibers capable of maintaining considerable tension for protracted periods of time. These fibers more or less surround the midurethra, but they are entirely within the urethral wall.[4] The fast twitch fibers of the pelvic floor musculature also partly surround the urethra, but these fibers do not insert on or take origin from the urethra itself. The activity of the fast twitch musculature is most notable in the midurethra, and it can be registered, during a fluoroscopically guided urodynamic study, beginning approximately 1 to 1.5 cm distal to the anatomic bladder neck. The skeletal sphincter, under volitional control, exerts an influence on urethral closure for a distance of about 1 cm. Active contraction of the muscles of the pelvic floor increases midurethral pressure, results in radiographically visible hyperclosure of the midurethra, and lifts the urethra and bladder upward, an effect that can

163

Female Urology, edited by Elroy D. Kursh and Edward McGuire. J. B. Lippincott, Philadelphia, © 1994.

be easily seen radiographically (Fig. 12-1). Separating activity of the intrinsic skeletal muscle from the extrinsic or the intrinsic smooth muscle clinically, even with very good urodynamic systems, is virtually impossible.[5]

There are circumstances in which one component or another of the innervation of the various muscles that close the urethra has been lost, and some determination of the effect of a given muscle group can be made by urodynamic testing. If we (urologists, basic scientists, and gynecologists) could agree on the innervation of the various muscular groups that close the urethra, perhaps some progress could be made, but we cannot agree at present. As an illustration, the innervation of the *smooth (muscle) sphincter* of the urethra, which closes all the urethra not closed by skeletal muscle and contributes to closure in the skeletal muscle area as well, is said by some to be parasympathetic, derived from the pelvic nerve.[6] Others are convinced the innervation is sympathetic and derived from the thoracolumbar sympathetic outflow by way of the hypogastric nerves. Anatomic studies document a paucity of sympathetic fibers and receptors in the smooth muscle of the female urethra, which supports the contention that the motor innervation of the urethra is parasympathetic. Functional studies, however, appear to support the idea that the urethra is closed by sympathetic motor activity. On a clinical level, the arguments do not matter a great deal as long as some relatively fundamental findings are kept in mind. In the first place, alpha-blocking agents can diminish urethral closing pressure enough to cause stress incontinence in women. Some cases of stress incontinence do respond to alpha-stimulating agents. Tricyclic antidepressant agents, in combination with estrogens, can improve urethral closing function enough to double the amount of abdominal pressure required to cause urine to leak from the urethra in selected elderly, estrogen-deficient women. Normally the proximal smooth muscle area and the more distal area of the urethra closed by skeletal muscle maintain a perfectly reciprocal relationship with the bladder.[7] Although the external sphincter can voli-

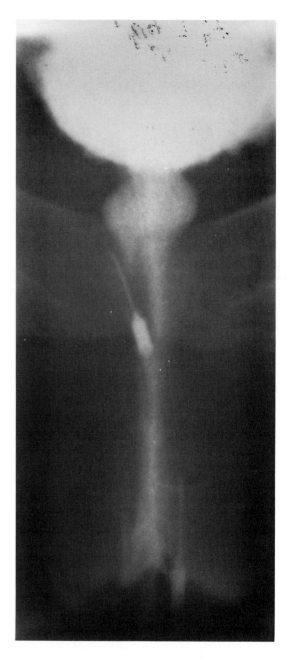

Figure 12-1. *Simultaneous detrusor: external sphincter contraction in a 34-year-old woman attempting to stop reflex bladder contractility. The EMG needle is located in the area of maximal skeletal muscular electrical activity. The smooth muscle sphincter is open; the distal sphincter is closed.*

tionally be made to act in a manner that is antagonistic to bladder contractility, the smooth sphincter area of the urethra maintains its reciprocal relationship with the bladder in virtually every clinical circumstance except when its function is lost or the bladder no longer displays reflex function. If the urethra is really closed by parasympathetic activity, a complicated neural system would be required to maintain neural silence to the bladder during filling but supply a continuous motor input to the urethra. With a bladder contraction, the reverse would have to occur. Because available clinical and experimental evidence indicates that control of both bladder and urethral function requires vesical ganglionic activity, it is more likely that both parasympathetic and sympathetic systems interact to close and open the urethra and that the dominant neural force during the storage mode of lower urinary tract function is sympathetic and norepinephrine mediated.[8]

Clinical Correlates

Many different workers made the observation using fluoroscopically guided urodynamic techniques that a nonfunctional bladder neck and proximal urethra are associated with severe incontinence. Indeed, the abdominal pressure required to induce a urethra with a nonfunctional internal sphincter to leak is less than peak urethral closing pressure registered in the mid-urethral high pressure zone. In contrast, a urethra deprived of most, if not all, of its skeletal muscle closure by a total sacral rhizotomy continues to resist excursions in abdominal pressure normally if the resting internal urethral sphincter pressure is greater than about 10 cm H_2O. These findings suggest that it is not the magnitude of urethral closing pressure that determines function but where a relatively low pressure is exerted.

Myelodysplastic children constitute a case in point because 85% show a congenital absence of closure of the proximal urethra (Fig. 12-2). External sphincter pressures are, however, main-

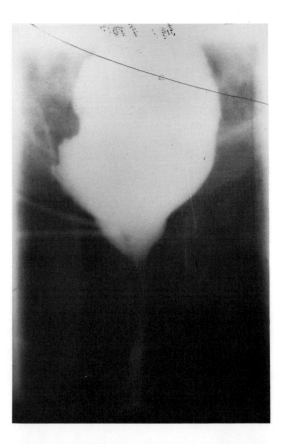

Figure 12-2. Upright cystogram from a 9-year-old myelodysplastic child. The bladder neck and proximal sphincter are widely patulous. Leakage of contrast resistance across the closed "external sphincter" is visible.

tained. Indeed, in approximately 40% of these children, external sphincter pressures are high enough to produce back pressure effects on the ureters and thereby destroy the upper urinary tracts. Nevertheless, myelodysplastic children are incontinent, including those who damage their upper tracts, more incontinent than any other group of patients suffering from neurogenic bladder dysfunction, worse than those with spinal cord injury or multiple sclerosis. The reason for this lies in the nonfunction of the internal sphincter. Active continence is related to activity of the fast twitch musculature of the pelvic floor and perhaps the intrinsic external

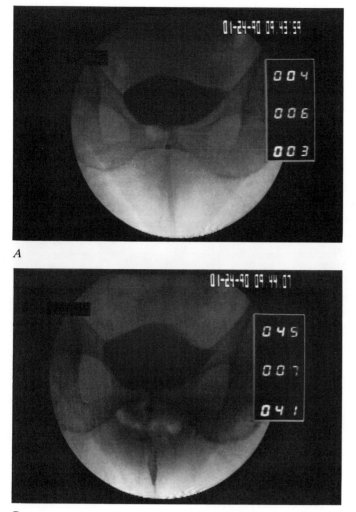

A

B

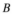

Figure 12-3. (A) *Resting bladder pressure is 4, and midurethral pressure has fallen from 48 to 3, the initial event in a reflex bladder contraction. The patient is unaware that this is happening.* (B) *The bladder contracts (45 cm H_2O); the patient recognizes this and the leakage and contracts the "external sphincter" (pressure 41). Note the compression of the midurethral "high pressure zone."*

sphincter but in a surprisingly indirect way. When an alert individual wishes to stop a bladder contraction in progress, he or she contracts the external sphincter. When a child with a non-neurogenic-neurogenic bladder is bothered by bladder activity, he or she contracts the external sphincter. When an elderly adult is surprised by sudden unanticipated detrusor activity, he or she contracts the external sphincter (Fig. 12-3). The effect of this activity is a sudden elevation in midurethral pressure, but that by itself is not enough to control leakage, which is instead the result of the rapid inhibition of detrusor activity that is also a consequence of external sphincter contractility. Patients with spinal cord injury or multiple sclerosis are incontinent despite a high pressure external sphincter because the bladder inhibitory effect, similar to the sphincter contraction, is poorly phased, out of sequence, and nonsustained.[9]

Unfortunately, we (urodynamic practitioners) made an early mistake when we began to use urethral pressure profiles to evaluate urethral function. The assumption was made that intraurethral pressures measured by the profile technique were related to continence function.[10] In effect, the working theory of measurable urethral function (which made perfect sense) was that if the urethral pressure is, at any place in the urethra, higher than bladder pressure, at that time no leakage is possible. Urethral pressure profile values were expressed in terms of the maximum pressure advantage over the bladder, by convention, so all workers were describing the same measurement. Several workers in several countries made the observation that urethral pressure profile values did not by themselves allow the diagnosis of stress incontinence and noted that urethral pressure profile values did not change in patients successfully cured of stress incontinence by an operation. Despite these observations and the fluoroscopically guided urodynamic studies that demonstrated that proximal urethral closing pressures were related to the ability of the urethra to resist changes in intra-abdominal pressure, whereas midurethral or maximum urethral closing pressures were not, we continued to investigate urethral function using pressure profiles. We also continued to conceptualize urethral function vis a vis the ability of the urethra to resist changes in intra-abdominal pressure as related to maximum urethral pressure profile values. In fact, there is no urethral pressure value, however derived, static or dynamic, that by itself will provide definitive information on the strength of the urethral continence mechanism in terms of resistance to excursions in intra-abdominal pressure. In the absence of fluoroscopy, one can evaluate urethral continence function best by a measurement of the amount of intra-abdominal pressure required to drive urine across the sphincter mechanism. One can show by this technique as well as by full videourodynamic studies that many patients with poor urethral function leak urine at pressures substantially less than peak urethral closing pressure, static or dynamic (Fig. 12-4). These findings indicate that the part of the urethra that is the most important in terms of resistance to abdominal pressures is not the midurethral high pressure zone but the much lower pressure area of the urethra above the area of skeletal sphincter influence.

In addition to the observations regarding an open bladder outlet in neurogenic conditions, many surgeons noted that poor or absent function of the proximal urethra was present in patients who failed operations for the relief of stress incontinence (Fig. 12-5). One early study reported that patients presenting with primary stress incontinence had a low (6%) incidence of poor urethral function, but patients who failed one operation had a higher incidence (25% to 30%), whereas those who failed two or more operations had a high rate of urethral failure (75%).[12] The lack of proximal urethral function in these women was radiographically and by direct intraurethral pressure measurements identical to that encountered in patients with myelodysplasia and patients who suffer neural injury at the time of pelvic extirpative surgery or pelvic fracture. Patients treated successfully by radiotherapy for cervical malignancy also develop urethral dysfunction apparently as a late result of the radiation.[13]

In addition, elderly women who develop new-onset stress incontinence after age 70 often show poor proximal urethral closing function. Valsalva-generated leak point pressures in these patients are low: in the 30 to 60 cm H_2O range. Patients who develop urinary incontinence after transurethral bladder neck incision, internal urethrotomy, or urethral diverticulectomy also show abnormal proximal urethral closure.

The importance of these sometimes subtle, and sometimes not so subtle, findings has been

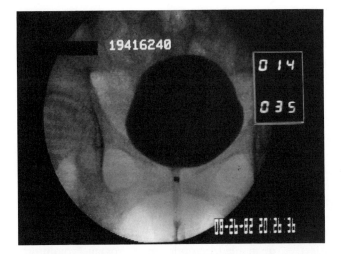

Figure 12-4. *Upright cystogram from a 56-year-old woman after four prior operations for stress incontinence. Leakage of urine is visible at a bladder pressure of 14, across a sphincter registering a pressure of 35 cm H₂O. This is type III stress incontinence. This is a Valsalva leak point pressure—the "bladder" pressure reflects the patient's volitional increase in intra-abdominal pressure and not intrinsic ("subtracted") bladder pressure.*

known for some time. Virtually every American urologist and gynecologist interested in the treatment of severe incontinence recognized the more overt expression of the disease, and fascia slings, synthetic material slings, round ligament slings, and artificial sphincters have been described as treatment for the severe incontinence that is associated with proximal urethral dysfunction.[14–17] Although the operative procedures to treat the problem were developed long ago, a uniform method of diagnosis is still not available, and most patients are diagnosed and selected for a particular operation on purely clinical grounds, often no more exact than the finding of severe incontinence in a patient who has already had two or more procedures for incontinence. Although there is nothing wrong with that clinical diagnosis, it would be better if such patients could be diagnosed before their first, second, or subsequent operations. It is unfortunate that we have been unwilling to

use fluoroscopy routinely in the diagnosis of urethral dysfunction, but that is the situation. With the advent of improved injectable materials for the treatment of incontinence, precise assessment of the function of the internal sphincter will become even more important. In this respect, it appears that the determination of Valsalva leak point pressure may be a reasonable substitute for fluoroscopically guided urodynamics.

Valsalva Leak Point Pressure

The objective of the test is to determine the abdominal pressure required to drive urine across the urethral sphincter mechanism and cause leakage. A normal internal sphincter, regardless of whether or not the external sphincter works, will not leak at any attainable physiologic pressure. Stress incontinence associated with urethral hypermobility is associated with Valsalva

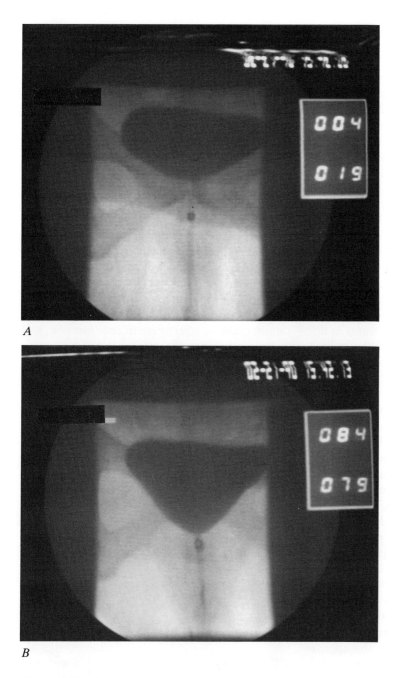

A

B

Figure 12-5. *(A) Resting cystogram. Bladder and abdominal pressure is 4; sphincter pressure (at marker) is 19. (B) A Valsalva maneuver generates an intra-abdominal pressure of 84, and leakage occurs in conjunction with mobility of the bladder base and urethra.*

leak point pressures greater than 60 and ranging up to 120 to 130 cm H_2O. Watching the process of leakage generated by straining in patients with urethral hypermobility, considerable pressure is required first to induce urethral motion and still more to induce leakage (see Figs. 12-4 and 12-5). On the contrary, in patients with poor internal sphincter function, no pressure is required to make the urethra move; it simply leaks as the intra-abdominal pressure overcomes it. This occurs at pressures as low as 5 cm H_2O and ranges up toward 30 or 40 cm H_2O. In the middle range are patients with features of both conditions: hypermobility and poor function.

If these somewhat tortuous constructions and explanations are correct, sealing the urethra as close to the vesical neck as possible at a pressure just slightly greater than intravesical pressure should cure incontinence related to urethral dysfunction. Because normally pressures in this area are not very high and because the smooth muscle cannot respond to sudden increases in abdominal pressure, the sphincter mechanism must in good measure function mechanically. That is, abdominal pressure must be transmitted to the urethra just as it is to the bladder and just as completely; otherwise stress incontinence would be pretty universal. Indeed, a study of precisely what happens when collagen is injected into a nonfunctional internal sphincter confirms most of the earlier observations. There is no measurable change in the urethral closing pressure, either maximum pressure or pressure measured with fluoroscopic control, just where the collagen was injected. The increased urethral closure is lost in the greater pressure of the high pressure zone, and yet there is a dramatic improvement in the efficiency with which the urethra resists intra-abdominal pressure and a radiographically visible change in the appearance of the urethra (Fig. 12-6).

Although the findings after successful collagen injection are more dramatic than after sling procedures, essentially the same phenomenon has been described in patients cured of total incontinence by a sling procedure. Slings increase resting intraurethral closing pressure di-

rectly beneath the sling very little, the average being on the order of 6 to 10 cm H_2O. When distal or midurethral sphincter pressures are, before treatment, in the 60 to 70 cm H_2O range, an increase of 6 to 10 cm H_2O does not seem like much, yet these procedures have been shown over time to be exceedingly effective in the treatment of incontinence associated with failure of the proximal urethral closing mechanism.[18] Slings can be shown to increase the efficiency with which the urethra opposes changes in abdominal pressure enormously, rendering a totally incompetent internal sphincter in a myelodysplastic girl capable of resisting intra-abdominal pressure excursions of well over 180 cm H_2O. These findings taken together indicate that the assumptions on which one of our most cherished urodynamic tests is based are faulty and further that the midurethra is not important in regard to antigravity continence function, presumably because of a mechanical disadvantage conferred by the position of this part of the urethra, which is on the boundary of the abdominal cavity. Although pelvic floor musculature pretty clearly has a role in the support of the urethral sphincter mechanism, which keeps the urethra within the abdominal cavity where it is exposed to the same pressure as the bladder, that role is not the same as that related to closure of the proximal urethra. Unfortunately, we failed to separate the components of urethral closure by their function, and we have used a measure of pelvic floor strength in the urethral pressure profile as an indication of what is, in fact, a proximal urethral function.

Medical Therapy for Urethral Dysfunction

The nonfunctional urethra associated with myelodysplasia does not respond to alpha-stimulating agents nor to tricyclic antidepressants. It is not clear why this is the case. There is some experimental evidence in a naturally occurring model of the disease in the cat that the problem involves failure of the local urethral receptors to

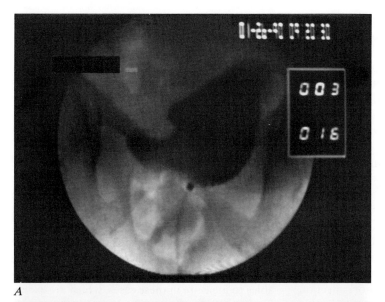

A

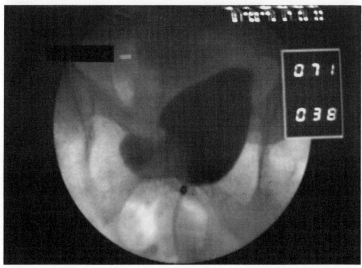

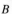

B

Figure 12-6. (A) Resting cystourethrogram from an 83-year-old woman 12 months after collagen injection. Intra-abdominal pressure is 3; urethral pressure is 16. (B) Straining Valsalva maneuver results in an intra-abdominal pressure of 71 but no leakage despite a peak urethral closing pressure of only 38.

develop.[19] This might occur because there is no neural input to the urethral receptors to generate their development or for some other reason.

In general, the lack of response seen in myelodysplasia is duplicated in patients with loss of urethral function related to central spinal cord lesions and peripheral neural lesions, although an occasional patient may respond.[20] In this regard, to be certain that a response did or did not occur, a Valsalva leak point pressure is required.

Elderly women with weakness of the urethral sphincter, manifested by a low leak point pressure, and signs of estrogen deficiency on physical examination or low peripheral estrogen blood levels often (68%) respond to a combination of estrogen vaginal cream and a tricyclic antidepressant.[21] A trial of these medications is often worthwhile before surgery or injection therapy is contemplated. Most patients in this category also respond to alpha-stimulating agents, but the side-effects of these agents in the elderly, including hypertension and other symptoms, are not worth the therapeutic effect. One of the problems with the prior studies on the effect of estrogen or various drugs on the function of the urethra is the way patients were selected. If, for example, a group of incontinent postmenopausal women is selected for treatment by estrogen, even the inclusion of a control group does not obviate the central problem, which is unless patients selected show a low proximal urethral closing pressure or a low leak point pressure, unless estrogen is given with a tricyclic antidepressant, and unless the patients are actually estrogen deficient, the drugs will have no effect. Not surprisingly, that is exactly what has been reported. Unfortunately, we continue to select patients for study using inaccurate methods or on the basis of assumptions that are in error. The conclusions drawn from studies done in patients so selected are suspect no matter how carefully the studies are done.

In certain circumstances, there is a linkage between proximal urethral and bladder dysfunction, which is important to understand before treatment is undertaken. The best illustration of this phenomenon occurs in patients with myelodysplasia, but the relationships are almost always the same after sacral level spinal cord or root injury, or after peripheral neural injury sustained as a result of intrapelvic trauma, surgical or otherwise. This relationship involves a link between detrusor storage behavior and urethral closing pressure. In this case, the maximum closing pressure is the important variable. In longitudinally studied myelodysplastic children, detrusor compliance was found to be directly related to the amount of pressure required for the intrinsic bladder pressure response to filling to overcome urethral resistance. In other words, the storage ability of the bladder was related to the magnitude of urethral closure, in a reciprocal way.[22] As urethral closing pressure increased, compliance deteriorated. There are two variables to measure in these cases, which are examples of detrusor decentralization. In a decentralized bladder, filling is not accompanied by changes in urethral behavior because these are normally driven by pelvic nerve afferent activity, generated in the bladder as it fills. The urethral closing mechanism then is fixed or nearly so. Intrinsic bladder pressure must rise to a pressure equal to peak urethral closing pressure to generate leakage. When urethral closing pressure is higher than a relatively low value, over time bladder compliance can be documented to deteriorate, or the volume required to achieve expulsion pressure becomes progressively less.[23] As long as the expulsion pressure is less than 40 cm H_2O, the upper urinary tract seems to be able to continue to deliver urine into the bladder. When the expulsion pressure is 40 or higher, ureteral dilation, vesicoureteral reflux, and upper tract disease, including pyelonephritis, stone formation, and renal parenchymal loss, become common.

These developments are related to sustained intravesical pressure of storage and are not the result of brief or momentary elevations in intravesical pressure. They result ultimately from poor compliance and elevated bladder pressures at low volumes. One way to resolve the problem is to decrease sphincter resistance, which allows low pressure leakage. This does nothing for continence, but it does surprisingly often result in a dramatic and substantial improvement in bladder compliance.[24] That observation led to the establishment of a direct link between detrusor behavior and outlet resistance. That in turn has a powerful influence on what we ultimately choose for a surgical treatment to close nonfunctional proximal urethra because the magnitude of the pressure increase will have an effect on compliance in patients with decentralized bladders. The compressive effect of an artificial sphincter in this circumstance could raise urethral pressure so effectively that a gradual loss of bladder storage function would occur, with a risk to upper tract function as well as recurrent incontinence. Although some increase in outlet resistance is measurable after a sling procedure or collagen injection, neither of these raises outlet resistance enough to risk upper tract function. Thus, where an increase in urethral resistance is needed, artificial sphincters are best not used in cases in which the bladder is decentralized, and collagen or slings are a safer choice.

Dysfunction of Urethral Conduit Function

In addition to function as an organ of continence, the urethra also, during micturition, functions as a conduit. The bladder does work to pump urine across the urethra, but in females, as compared with males, bladder work is minimal, provided that the urethra opens normally. The amount of stream pressure loss in males is normally about 20 to 25 cm H_2O across the area of the membranous urethra. In females, the stream energy loss is less, and measured as pressure drop, it amounts to only 5 cm H_2O. The early studies of Gleason and coworkers found that most of the stream energy loss in females occurred in the sphincter inactive urethral segment distal to the pelvic floor, which acted as a nozzle, or a *flow control zone*.[24] There are naturally occurring bladder outlet obstructions in females involving the bladder neck and the distal urethra, even though these are rare. The most

common cause of bladder outlet obstruction in females currently is a stress incontinence operation. To make the diagnosis of urethral dysfunction and associated obstruction, one needs to demonstrate diminished flow for a given pressure. Although that seems simple enough, the parameters that would allow us to define female urethral obstruction are not yet established, and we do not have good normative data for women in various age groups. Nevertheless, it is reasonably well established that whatever urethral dilation does in females, it does not affect the energy balance of micturition. In other words, the effect of urethral dilation does not appear to unburden the bladder and make its work less arduous. There was a study done by Susset and Biancani in Rhode Island in which they attempted to define the elasticity and compliance of the female urethra, which they found often diminished with age.[25] They were able to show in some women that urethral dilation influenced the compliance characteristics of the urethra and that this sometimes correlated with an improvement in symptoms. Presently there is no clinically applicable technique to define subtle abnormalities in urethral behavior, and we are left with only empiric methodology.

External, extrinsic skeletal sphincter muscular activity can have an obstructive character, and there are two basic situations in which this occurs. In the first, a suprasacral spinal cord injury or lesion interferes with the proper sequencing and phasing of bladder and urethral behavior during filling and bladder contraction.[9] There is no urethral guarding response during filling as there is normally, but there is instead a burst of external sphincter activity that occurs simultaneously with the bladder contraction. This abnormality is called detrusor sphincter dyssynergia, and although it has the same characteristics as it does when it occurs in males, in females urethral and therefore bladder pressures are not nearly as high, and upper tract disease in females with spinal cord injury, treated by diapers, is exceedingly rare.

In the second variety, there is sphincter activity that is, in a sense, inappropriate. The owner of the sphincter, however, is basically responsible for the activity, for whatever reason. In children, this may be learned but unconscious behavior. In adults, perhaps this also occurs, but it must be rare. If a bladder is filled during a cystometrogram, the urethral sphincter increases its activity and the EMG recording becomes very active. However, the bladder pressure is flat, and even though the patient complains about fullness and the need to urinate, the urodynamic findings are still normal. These are the events recorded when an individual with a normal neuraxis declines to urinate. That urodynamic information does not suggest a diagnosis of external sphincter misbehavior, nor is the flat pressure volume curve in the face of sphincter activity abnormal; indeed, that is precisely what should happen during bladder filling and the volitional hold maneuver, even if we did not ask the patient to perform that maneuver. Most often these findings reflect psychological influences during the study, but because the findings are basically normal, they do not constitute a diagnosis.

References

1. McGuire EJ, Woodside JR. Diagnostic advantages of fluoroscopic monitoring during urodynamic evaluation. J Urol 1981;125:830.
2. McGuire EJ, Herlihy E. The influence of urethral position on urinary continence. Invest Urol 1977;15:205.
3. McGuire EJ, Wagner FC Jr. The effect of sacral denervation on bladder and urethral function. Surg Gynecol Obstet 1977;144:343.
4. Gosling JA. Structure of the lower urinary tract and pelvic floor. Clin Obstet Gynecol 1985;12:285.
5. McGuire EJ. Combined radiographic and manometric assessment of urethral sphincter function. J Urol 1977;118:631.
6. Ek A, Alm P, Anderson KE, Perssom CGA. Adrenergic and cholinergic nerves of the human urethra and urinary bladder: A histochemical study. Acta Physiol Scand 1977;99:345.
7. McGuire EJ. Mechanisms of urethral continence and their clinical application. World J Urol 1984;2:272.
8. McGuire EJ, Herlihy E. Bladder and urethral responses to isolated sacral motor root stimulation. Invest Urol 1978;16:219.
9. McGuire EJ, Brady S. Detrusor sphincter dyssynergia. J Urol 1979;121:774.
10. Massey A, Abrams P. Urodynamics of lower urinary tract. Clin Obstet Gynecol 1985:12;319.
11. McGuire EJ. Urethral pressure profiles: Techniques and applications. In: Barrett D, Wein A, eds. Controversies in neurourology. New York: Churchill Livingstone, 1984:313–337.
12. McGuire EJ. Urodynamic findings in patients after failure of stress incontinence operations. In: Zinner N, Sterling A, eds. Female incontinence. New York: Alan R. Liss, 1981:351–360.
13. Zoubek J, McGuire EJ, Noll F, DeLancey JOL. Late effects of radiation therapy on the lower urinary tract. J Urol 1989;141:1347.
14. McGuire EJ. Pubovaginal sling. Urol Rounds 1980;1:90.
15. Hadley HR, Zimmern PE, Staskin PR, Raz S. Transvaginal middle bladder neck suspension. Clin Obstet Gynecol 1985;12:497.
16. Scott FB. Use of the artificial sphincter in the treatment of urinary incontinence. Clin Obstet Gynecol 1985;12:415.
17. Hilton P, Stanton SL. Clinical and urodynamic evaluation of the polypropylene (Marlex) sling for genuine stress incontinence. Neurourol Urodynam 1983;2:145.
18. McGuire EJ, Lytton B. The pubovaginal sling in stress urinary incontinence. J Urol 1978;119:82.
19. Woodside JR, Dail WG, McGuire EJ, Wagner FC Jr. The Manx cat as an animal model for neurogenic vesical dysfunction associated with myelodysplasia. J Urol 1982;127:180.
20. McGuire EJ. Neurovesical dysfunction after abdomino-perineal resection. Surg Clin North Am 1980;60:1207.
21. McGuire EJ. Identifying and managing stress incontinence in the elderly. Geriatrics 1990;45:44.
22. Ghoniem EM, Bloom DA, McGuire EJ, Stewart KL. Bladder compliance in meningomyelocelic children. J Urol 1989;141:1404.
23. Bloom DA, Knechtel JM, McGuire EJ. Urethral dilation improves bladder compliance in children with meningomyelocele and high leak point pressures. J Urol 1990;144:430.
24. Gleason D, Bottaccini MR. The vital role of the distal urethral segment in the control of urinary flow rate. J Urol 1968;100:167.
25. Susset JG, Regnier CH, Ghoniem GM. Abnormal urethral compliance in females: Diagnosis, results and treatment. J Urol 1983;129:1063.

13

Goals of Therapy and Mechanisms of Urethral Incontinence

Pat O'Donnell

In defining goals of therapy for urinary incontinence, it is important to consider the scope of the problem of urinary incontinence in our society. Urinary incontinence is a problem that causes immense personal distress for millions of people who suffer from the disorder. At least 20 million people in the United States suffer from urinary incontinence.[1] For a person in our society who has urinary incontinence, it is a problem that separates them from the quality of life that they are capable of living. Not only are daily activities of the person limited, but also the interaction among friends and relatives is limited in people who suffer from urinary incontinence. The self-imposed restrictions of daily activities by the incontinent person represent an attempt to minimize the impact of incontinence in daily life. The self-imposed social isolation by the incontinent person represents an effort to avoid the social embarrassment of incontinence. These restrictions in daily activities of the person cause a loss of self-esteem as well as changes in the psychological and social attitudes of the individual.

Although the psychosocial impact of incontinence on the individual is immense, urinary incontinence in women is not a fatal disease, and it does not represent a serious threat to long-term survival. Although the effects of urinary incontinence on the life of the individual are enormous, the actual changes that occur involve the quality of life of the person. The quality of life changes affecting the person who suffers from incontinence are changes that touch every aspect of life. In considering the treatment of urinary incontinence for people suffering from this problem, the treatment goals involve rehabilitation of a functionally disabled person in our society. The goal is to restore the patient to a quality of life that is the best possible for that person to experience regarding the effects of urinary incontinence in daily life.

The amount of personal distress suffered by the individual with incontinence and the major alterations in the quality of life resulting from urinary incontinence are sometimes greatly underestimated by both the physician and the patient and often can be appreciated only after successful treatment has occurred. Patients may have extreme embarrassment owing to incontinence, and it is important to make the patient aware that many other women suffer the same problem and that she is not alone in dealing with the problem.

Patients who present with urinary incontinence have a wide range of social environments in which they live as well as personal perceptions of the problem. The perception of the problem of incontinence by the individual and the perceived alteration in the quality of life by that person resulting from incontinence represent major

175

Female Urology, edited by Elroy D. Kursh and Edward McGuire. J. B. Lippincott, Philadelphia, © 1994.

considerations in defining the goals of therapy. For example, in our society, incontinence affects physically active young women who are unwilling to modify their strenuous physical activities or accept urinary incontinence as a consequence. In contrast, incontinence also affects elderly women, whose final incapacitating event is the onset of urinary incontinence. There is a wide range of problems related to functional status to consider in establishing the management goals of the individual patient with incontinence, which include age of the patient, living environment of the patient, occupation, and personal perception of the problem of incontinence by the individual. The restrictions imposed by the presence and severity of urinary incontinence in the daily life of people are different. The perceived impact of incontinence on the quality of life of an individual often can be misleading because extreme personal discomfort resulting from incontinence may be tolerated without complaints. Once incontinence has been treated, many of these patients often express a deep personal regret for having tolerated the condition for so long.

In considering the aims and goals of incontinence therapy, it is important to recognize that incontinence management and treatment outcome are major quality of life issues for the individual affected and that the goal of therapy is to restore to that individual the best quality of life that is possible for that person. This represents a health care problem in which surgical and non-surgical treatment alone and in combination are used to achieve a major change in quality of life for the patient. The decision to manage stress incontinence surgically is not one to prolong survival of the patient but rather to rehabilitate the individual to a functional status level that enables her to be an active and productive member of society.

Assessment in Treatment Goals

The characteristics and complexity of the anatomy and physiology of urinary incontinence are not uniform among people and vary considerably among individual patients. The physician needs to be able to assess the complexity of the problem for a particular patient to advise the patient regarding treatment. One of the goals of the physician is to provide the patient with a reasonably accurate expectation of the outcome of treatment. One cannot always predict with certainty the treatment outcome, but it is possible to assess an individual patient with urinary incontinence and advise the patient of the degree of complexity of the problem as well as predict with reasonable accuracy the outcome of treatment so that the expectations of the patient are realistic and appropriate. In this way, a decision regarding treatment can be made by the patient that allows the patient to take into consideration the complexity of the problem, the treatment options, the expectations of outcome, and how the management interfaces with the life situation of the individual. In advising the patient of the complexity of the problem and the treatment options, the physician needs to be able to identify patients with complicated incontinence. The role of incontinence assessment is important in achieving the treatment goals.[2]

FAVORABLE AND UNFAVORABLE CHARACTERISTICS OF INCONTINENCE

A careful and thorough history is always essential to the clinician in advising the patient of the status of her condition as well as of clinical decisions regarding further evaluation and the approach to therapy.[3] Although all of the information obtained from the urologic history is important in the assessment of the patient, there are certain aspects of the history that have special significance related to complexity and treatment outcome. For example, a patient who has failed previous incontinence operative procedures has a particularly unfavorable characteristic in the incontinence history for successful treatment outcome.[4-6] One can consider these patient characteristics to have either a favorable or an unfavorable influence on the incontinence status of the patient and the expected outcome of treatment. Other issues to consider include the age of the patient because elderly women tend to have less favorable results than younger women.[4,7–9]

Also, nocturnal enuresis, severe incontinence requiring more than six pads per day, marked obesity, severe urgency with urgency incontinence, and recurrent urinary tract infections are additional unfavorable characteristics in the history of patients being evaluated for urinary incontinence. The history of the patient is important to the clinician in the initial formulation of a clinical opinion of the incontinence status and complexity of the problem. The ability of the physician to achieve treatment goals as well as advise the patient regarding options and expectations of outcome depends on assessment of the incontinence status of the patient.

On physical examination of the anterior vaginal wall, the finding of mobility of the urethra and base of the bladder is a favorable physical observation.[10] A well-vascularized vaginal epithelium and the objective demonstration of urine leaking with straining represent additional favorable physical findings. A fixed urethra with scarring of the vaginal wall due to previous surgery along with an atrophic vaginal mucosa represent unfavorable physical findings. As the clinician completes each part of the evaluation process, more clinical data are provided that allow the formulation of an opinion related to the functional status of the bladder and urethra that allows a treatment approach that can best achieve the functional goals of incontinence therapy.

A favorable radiographic evaluation of the bladder and urethra using a lateral view would include mobility of the proximal urethra during straining, an incompetent bladder neck during straining, rotation of the urethral axis during straining, and a dependent position of the proximal urethra relative to the bladder. Radiographic studies that show a fixed urethra during straining, an anteriorly positioned urethra with no rotation of the urethral axis on straining, and an open bladder neck at rest represent unfavorable radiographic findings.

In addition, an endoscopic evaluation that shows mobility of the urethra during straining, a well-vascularized urethral mucosa, coaptation of the urethral mucosa at rest, and a nontrabeculated bladder is favorable. An endoscopic examination that shows a fixed proximal urethra during straining, an atrophic appearance of the urethra mucosa, loss of coaptation of the urethral mucosa at the bladder neck level at rest, and marked bladder trabeculation is unfavorable.

Finally, favorable urodynamic findings would include a patient having no postvoid residual urine volume, a maximum urinary flow rate greater than 25 ml/sec with no abdominal straining during voiding, a maximum bladder capacity of 300 to 500 ml, a maximum urethral pressure greater than 20 cm H_2O, a negative bladder-urethra pressure gradient on stress urethral pressure profile, normal bladder sensation during filling, and normal bladder compliance.[11] A patient having a residual urine volume greater than 50 ml, a maximum urinary flow rate less than 10 ml/sec with abdominal straining during voiding, a maximum bladder capacity less than 150 ml, a maximum urethral pressure less than 10 cm H_2O, loss of bladder compliance, and involuntary detrusor contractions during filling would be considered to have an unfavorable urodynamic evaluation regarding treatment for stress urinary incontinence.

In the evaluation of patients for incontinence, some are very favorable, whereas others are very unfavorable. Most patients have various combinations of both, which characterizes the complexity of clinical decisions involved in the treatment of incontinence. In the evaluation of a patient who presents with stress urinary incontinence having every aspect of the evaluation favorable, the likelihood of that patient being restored to a normal lifestyle by incontinence surgery is extremely high. This not only means that it is unlikely that the patient will have persistent stress incontinence, but also it is unlikely that she will have prolonged urinary retention or significant voiding dysfunctions following surgery. The patient who has most of the unfavorable characteristics described presents a complex problem in management and is less likely to have a continent outcome and more likely to have persistent postoperative voiding dysfunctions. Although a complete evaluation of a patient will not allow a clinician to predict with certainty the outcome of surgery, there clearly are many factors associated with favorable and unfavorable surgical outcomes.

If the patient is being considered for surgical treatment of incontinence, that patient needs to know what she personally can expect from incontinence treatment. For example, although 90% of patients with stress urinary incontinence can be cured of their incontinence with surgery, one should be careful in advising every patient regarding surgical outcome based on those results.[12-16] For example, a patient who has failed multiple previous operative procedures for stress urinary incontinence, has a maximum urethral closure pressure of 5cm H_2O, and has a small-capacity, poor-compliant bladder has almost no chance for surgical success using a conventional urethral suspension procedure. It is important that the patient is not only aware of the overall results of surgical treatment, but also how those results particularly apply to her.

Because urinary incontinence has such a major impact on the psychosocial aspects of the patient's life and the incontinence status related to the complexity of pathophysiology varies among patients, the relationship between the physician and the patient regarding the discussion of treatment options and management decisions is an especially important one. Assessment of a patient with stress urinary incontinence to determine the complexity of the problem allows the clinician to communicate to the patient the characteristics of the problem and to advise the patient regarding how it should be approached. Although the results of surgical treatment of incontinence are excellent in most patients, postoperative problems related to surgical therapy can reduce significantly the functional outcome of treatment. This is apparent in the occasional patient who has severe irritative syndromes following surgical correction of sphincteric incompetence. Even though sphincteric incompetence

is surgically corrected, it is possible that the quality of life of the patient can continue to be significantly compromised by postoperative voiding dysfunctions. In these cases, an aggressive and persistent approach to these problems is needed to achieve the goal of the highest quality of life possible for that patient.

Nonsurgical Treatment Goals

Many patients may elect an initial conservative approach or may have specific reasons for nonsurgical treatment. Also, nonsurgical treatment can provide important adjunctive therapy for patients following incontinence surgery who have persistent incontinence or postoperative voiding dysfunctions. A nonsurgical approach to incontinence generally includes pharmacologic or behavioral therapy. These types of nonsurgical therapy may be used in patients whose urinary incontinence severity is relatively mild. Patients who present initially with stress urinary incontinence may have an associated component of urgency that also can be managed with nonsurgical therapy.

PHARMACOLOGIC THERAPY

In patients who present with stress urinary incontinence, the most commonly used medications are those having an effect of increasing bladder outlet resistance. The frequently used medications in this group are the alpha-adrenergic agonists, including ephredine, pseudoephedrine, and phenylpropanolamine hydrochloride. Phenylpropanolamine hydrochloride can be purchased without a prescription as a component of many medications used for appetite suppression. By careful examination of the contents of the numerous proprietary mixtures marketed as appetite suppressants, one can identify products that are free of other drugs such as stimulants and have the advantage of time-released capsules. The oral use of timed-release products containing phenylpropanolamine hydrochloride, 75 mg twice daily, has the effect of increasing maximal urethral closing pressure and significantly improving symptoms of stress urinary incontinence.[17,18] Another commonly used drug that has been shown to improve urinary incontinence subjectively in women is imipramine.[19]

Estrogen supplements are also commonly used for treatment of stress urinary incontinence. The urethral mucosa responds to estrogen therapy with increased vascularity, increased urethral closure pressure, improved abdominal pressure transmission to the proximal urethra, and improvement in the symptoms of stress urinary incontinence.[20] As is often the case with pharmacologic therapy, these medications may have side effects. Phenylpropanolamine and imipramine primarily have cardiac side-effects. Estrogen has a potential for increased risk of breast cancer and endometrial carcinoma.

Pharmacologic therapy of stress urinary incontinence can be used initially to determine the response of the patient and to assess the willingness of the patient to use long-term pharmacologic therapy. In patients who are likely to have an excellent outcome of surgical treatment, the option for surgical management may be more suitable to the individual than long-term pharmacologic therapy. Again it is important to integrate the treatment approach with the needs of the individual patient. Even though the patient may have significant improvement in the symptoms of stress urinary incontinence with pharmacologic therapy, the side-effects of medications and the long-term use are significant considerations, especially in patients who have a favorable outcome for surgical therapy.

BEHAVIORAL THERAPY

The most common form of behavioral therapy used is pelvic muscle exercises. Pelvic muscle exercises were popularized by Kegel, who used a perineometer to teach patients voluntary contraction of the levator ani muscle complex.[21–23] Since that time, pelvic muscle exercises for women have been commonly used both with and without the aid of a perineometer. Improvement in symptoms of stress urinary incontinence has occurred in a high percentage of women using pelvic muscle exercises. Pelvic muscle exercises may be used in younger women with mild symptoms of stress incontinence, although they have also been used in elderly women with significant improvement in symptoms of stress incontinence.[24] In patients who have irritative symptoms associated with stress urinary incontinence, bladder drill techniques have been effective in reducing the symptoms of frequency and urgency. The bladder drill technique involves a schedule of gradually increasing the interval between voluntary voiding by the patient.[25–27]

Biofeedback treatment of stress urinary incontinence is another nonsurgical behavioral treatment that has shown improvement in a high percentage of patients with stress urinary incontinence.[24,28] Biofeedback therapy usually involves the training of the patient to contract the external anal sphincter muscles voluntarily.[29] The external sphincter muscles are anatomically superficial to the deeper levator ani muscles used in the original pelvic muscle exercise programs. The exact mechanism of action of pelvic muscle exercises and biofeedback therapy is unclear. Increases in resting urethral pressure and urethral closure pressure do not appear to be involved in the changes that result in improvement in symptoms of incontinence.

Prompted voiding in the elderly and timed voiding in younger patients represent another form of behavioral therapy that can significantly improve incontinence.[30] The mechanism involved in symptomatic improvement following timed voiding and prompted voiding is unclear, but the technique appears to teach the patient the ability to initiate voiding voluntarily. In both young patients and elderly patients, symptoms of urgency are often associated with an inability to initiate voiding voluntarily in a normal way.

Behavioral therapy involves a structured training program of incontinence treatment for the patient and requires persistence as well as active involvement by the patient in the program.

For patients who have limited treatment options, behavioral therapy can improve the quality of life by significantly reducing the severity of incontinence. Behavioral therapy may have an important role in incontinence therapy when used in conjunction with surgery in patients who have complex incontinence problems. Behavioral therapy programs offer a treatment option that has minimal side-effects and does not alter the future treatment options for the patient. For many patients, behavioral therapy is an ideal choice based on a personal positive attitude about behavioral therapy as well as attitudes of uncertainty about the alternative treatment options. In these cases, the goal of incontinence therapy may be realized in many patients, without complete continence being the outcome of treatment. Again the quality of life of the individual as perceived by the individual relative to the problem of incontinence is a major issue involved in incontinence management. Subjective and objective outcome of therapy are usually but not always the same. For patients who are likely to have a continent outcome with surgical treatment, however, the decision to elect surgical therapy over long-term behavioral programs is often more suitable for the patient.

Surgical Treatment Goals

The surgical treatment of patients with stress urinary incontinence has an excellent continence outcome for a very high percentage of patients. Also, the quality of life of the patient is excellent following surgery in most cases because there are no behavioral regimens or drug side-effects after surgical treatment. The surgical management of stress urinary incontinence, however, must be approached carefully in every case because both short-term and long-term surgical failures can occur. There appear to be many factors that can contribute to surgical failures. Some of these factors can be identified preoperatively and some cannot. Those factors affecting outcome of surgery that can be identified should be evaluated during the initial assessment and addressed at the time of the initial operative procedure. The best chance for long-term success for surgical treatment is the first operative procedure. Each subsequent operative procedure is more difficult to perform and more difficult to obtain the desired outcome. The goal of surgical therapy is not only urinary continence, but also urinary continence with normal voiding. Urinary continence with normal voiding following surgery provides the patient with the best quality of life possible as an outcome of incontinence treatment.

The issue of what causes stress incontinence and how best to correct it still has many unanswered questions. There are numerous interesting and important observations that have been made regarding the cause of incontinence and the factors that affect surgical correction of incontinence.

URETHRAL LENGTH

Lapides and colleagues believed that the cause of stress incontinence was a functional shortening of the urethra to a length of less than 30 mm, and they thought that cure of the condition depended on lengthening the urethra to greater than 30 mm.[31] Hodgkinson and associates, however, found that only 12% of patients with stress incontinence had a urethra measuring less than 30 mm, and in patients without stress incontinence, 10% had a urethral length less than 30 mm long.[32] Although all of the patients described in that series were subjectively cured following surgery, 46% demonstrated no significant lengthening of the urethra. Since that time, many studies have been done measuring the functional urethral length following surgery for stress urinary incontinence, and there has been little evidence to support changes in urethral length as being a significant factor in the success of surgical treatment.[33,34] The concept of a short functional urethral length as a cause of stress incontinence and the role of increased functional length of the urethra in the success of surgical treatment of incontinence have not been supported by clinical observations. Therefore, it appears that the surgical goal in the treatment of stress urinary incontinence is not one of increasing the functional length of the urethra.

URETHRAL VESICAL ANGLE

Studies by Jeffcoate and Roberts emphasize the importance of the urethral vesical angle as an underlying factor in stress urinary incontinence.[2] Greenwald and colleagues found that the urethral vesical relationship of continent patients did not differ from that of incontinent patients.[36] It appears that these anatomic alterations of the bladder and urethra may not necessarily be the cause of stress incontinence, but the changes represent an anatomic displacement that is commonly associated with stress incontinence. The loss of the urethral vesical angle appears to represent prolapse of the posterior urethra and bladder neck. Although prolapse of the posterior urethra and bladder neck does not result in stress urinary incontinence in all patients, it is a radiographic finding that appears to be associated with stress urinary incontinence.[35, 37] When the anatomic defect is identified, however, the surgical correction of the anatomic abnormality results in a continence outcome in a high percentage of patients. The loss of the posterior urethral vesical angle without change in the urethral axis was initially described by Green as type I incontinence, which in his experience responded favorably to an anterior colporrhaphy.[38]

URETHRAL AXIS

The urethral axis refers to the perpendicular position of the urethra determined by a radiographic evaluation. Normally the angle of inclination of the urethra is approximately 30 degrees from a perpendicular line. During straining, this should remain relatively unchanged. In women with stress urinary incontinence, however, there is often an increase in the urethral axis of inclination varying from 45 to 120 degrees depending on the amount of rotational descent of the urethra. Usually there is also loss of the posterior urethral vesical angle in this group. This was described as type II stress incontinence by Green. In these patients, a urethral suspension procedure, which places the bladder neck in a high retropubic position with fixation of the bladder neck in the high retropubic position during stress maneuvers, results in an excellent continence outcome following surgery.

Radiographic studies of continent patients have also been done that show that many patients who are completely continent also have loss of the posterior urethral vesical angle and a loss of the angle of inclination of the urethra.[35, 36] In addition, an incompetent bladder neck during straining has been found in 25% of continent subjects.[39, 40] Therefore, loss of the angle of inclination of the urethra and loss of the posterior urethral vesical angle, which indicate prolapse of the proximal urethra and base of the bladder during straining, do not always result in stress urinary incontinence. The role of the loss of support of the urethra and base of the bladder in the cause of stress urinary incontinence is not completely clear. What is of critical importance, however, relative to the anatomy of the urethra regarding surgery for stress incontinence is that regardless of the role of these anatomic abnormalities in incontinence, the successful surgical correction of these anatomic abnormalities results in the restoration of continence and normal voiding in most patients. The surgical success appears to be related to the high retropubic fixation of the bladder neck.[16, 41]

Another observation that has been made is the occurrence of stress incontinence in patients whose bladder neck is located at the most dependent position of the bladder. In these patients, it appears that a continence outcome of surgery is dependent on repositioning of the bladder neck to a nondependent position relative to the bladder.[15] Whatever the physiologic basis of these surgical results, the success of a urethral suspension procedure for correction of type I and type II stress urinary incontinence as described by Green and co-workers is excellent following the surgical high retropubic fixation of the bladder neck and the repositioning of the bladder neck from a dependent position relative to the bladder[13, 15, 16] (Figs. 13-1 through 13-3).

(*continued on page 188*)

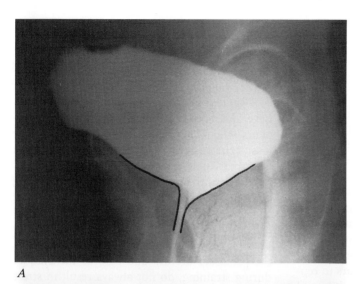

A

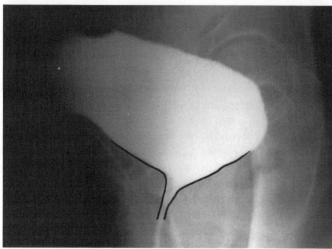

B

Figure 13-1. Lateral cystogram series performed on a patient who became incontinent following a previous Marshall-Marchetti-Krantz procedure. (A) The resting lateral cystogram shows the urethra in the most dependent portion of the bladder with loss of the posterior urethral vesical angle. The urethral axis is normal. (B) During straining, there is minimal change in the urethral axis. There is evidence of sphincteric incompetence at the bladder neck level.

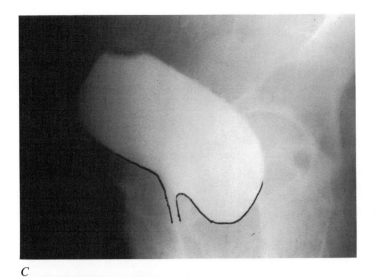

C

D

Figure 13-1. (continued) *(C) Following a Raz procedure, which allows mobilization of the urethra and base of the bladder, the urethra has been repositioned relative to the bladder. The resting position of the urethra is in a high retropubic position with a perpendicular urethral axis. Also, there is restoration of the posterior urethral vesical angle. (D) During straining, there is no change in the urethral axis, posterior urethral vesical angle, or bladder neck. Although the patient had failed a previous operative procedure, the Raz procedure achieved the goal of incontinence management, which is urinary continence with normal voiding.*

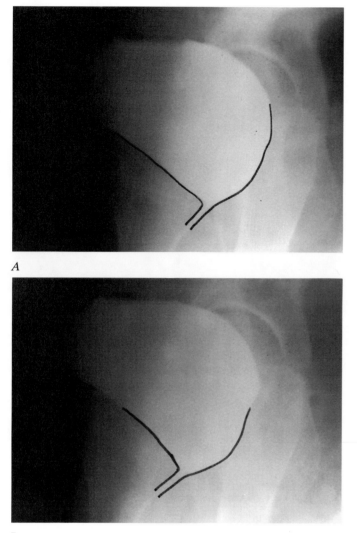

A

B

Figure 13-2. *This lateral cystogram series was performed on a woman who had failed a previous anterior repair. The patient was undergoing colon surgery, and a modified Burch procedure was performed in conjunction with the colon procedure. (A) At rest, there is loss of the posterior urethral vesical angle, the urethral axis is abnormal, and the bladder neck is located in the most dependent part of the bladder. (B) During straining, there is little change in the posterior urethral vesical angle or the urethral axis.*

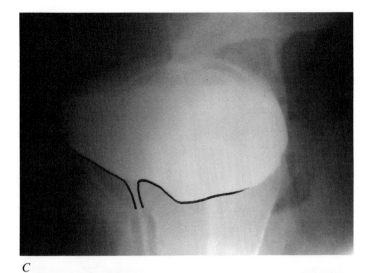

C

D

Figure 13-2. (continued) (C) Following a Burch suprapubic vesicourethropexy, the posterior urethral vesical angle was restored,
the axis of the urethra was corrected, and the bladder neck was
no longer positioned in the most dependent part of the bladder.
(D) During straining, there is little change in the posterior
urethral vesical angle and the urethral axis. Although the patient
had failed one previous operative procedure, she was restored to
continence with normal voiding following the modified Burch
procedure.

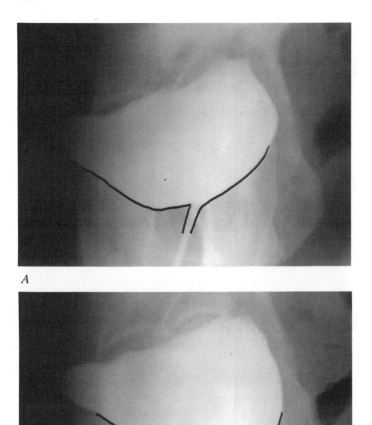

A

B

Figure 13-3. *This lateral cystogram series was performed on a woman who had failed four previous operative procedures. (A) The resting cystogram shows loss of the posterior urethral vesical angle and an abnormal urethral axis. (B) During straining, there is further loss of the posterior urethra vesical angle, change in the urethral axis, and evidence of sphincteric incompetence at the bladder neck level.*

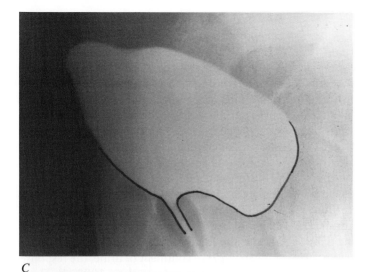

C

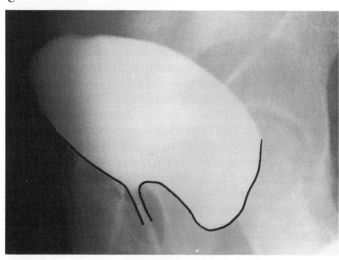

D

Figure 13-3. (continued) *(C) The maximum urethral closure pressure was less than 10 cm H_2O. A Raz urethral suspension procedure was combined with a McGuire sling procedure. Postoperatively the axis of the urethra is accentuated in an anterior position at rest. (D) During straining, there is minimal change in the urethral position. Although the patient experienced a period of postoperative urinary retention, this outcome of the procedure resulted in urinary continence with normal voiding.*

Physiologic Treatment Goals

URETHRAL PRESSURE PROFILE

The measurement of the urethral pressure profile has provided important information in the understanding of the functional characteristics of the urethra. The measurement of the urethral pressure profile is an assessment of pressure characteristics of the urethra. It is important to recognize that the urethral pressure profile is not an assessment of continence. Many of the characteristics of the urethral pressure profile, however, appear to contribute to continence function. The physiologic events involved in urinary continence that occur involuntarily during daily activities of the individual are complex events with many parameters that cannot be measured completely by currently available assessment techniques. Nevertheless, the measurement of the urethral pressure profile has made significant contributions to our understanding of some of the mechanisms involved in stress urinary incontinence.

In comparing the resting urethral pressure profile of incontinent women with the resting urethral pressure profile of women suffering from stress urinary incontinence, the maximum urethral pressure is significantly lower in women who have urinary incontinence.[15,42,43] There is no significant difference, however, in functional urethral length.

The use of microtipped urethral pressure profile catheters or catheter mounted transducers has allowed a more accurate technique for measurement of urethral pressure. By using a catheter that has a transducer in the bladder as well as a transducer in the urethra, it is possible to measure the difference between the pressure in the bladder and the pressure in the urethra. The subtraction of intravesical pressure from urethral pressure results in the urethral closure pressure. Because stress urinary incontinence occurs during episodes of increased intra-abdominal pressure, it is at those times that the pressure inside the bladder exceeds the resistance to outflow of urine provided by the urethra, and urinary leakage occurs.[42,44] Therefore, a commonly used technique for evaluating urethral pressure is a stress urethral pressure profile. This involves the measurement of urethral closure pressure during episodes of stress, which include coughing and straining. It is important to recognize that although the urethral pressure profile measurement provides information regarding the pressure characteristics of the urethra, it is not a measure of continence during stress maneuvers.

In the measurement of the stress urethral pressure profile in continent women, it has been shown that the pressure response in the urethra during coughing and straining is equal to or exceeds the increased pressure that occurs within the bladder. In fact, in most young women who are continent of urine, the response of the urethra is greater than 100%.[45] These observations have led to the concept that an active reflex mechanism is involved in the continence mechanism of normal women. Additional studies have shown that the increase in intra-urethral pressure in response to an increase in intra-abdominal pressure actually precedes in time the change in intra-abdominal pressure.[46,47] These observations further support the concept that an active reflex mechanism in the urethra is involved in the continence mechanism during stress. Other studies have indicated that a passive mechanism of transmission of intra-abdominal pressure to the urethra is a major component of continence during stress. At present, there is evidence that supports both an active and a passive mechanism involved in normal continence.

Additional studies in the measurement of the urethral pressure profile have investigated pressure responses in the anterior and posterior segment of the urethra. The pressure response in the anterior segment of the urethra is higher than that of the posterior segment of the urethra in patients who have stress incontinence.[15,48,49] This suggests the possibility of an anatomic defect involving the posterior aspect of the urethra. These physiologic findings are consistent with radiographic findings of loss of the posterior urethral vesical angle during stress. Also, these findings are consistent with the proposed anatomic defect of an attenuated posterior peri-urethral fascia as a cause of stress incontinence.[50,51]

There have been many studies of the urethral pressure profile in women with stress urinary incontinence before and after urethral suspension procedures. Although the data are extensive, the urethral pressure measurements show common observations. First, the functional urethral length following urethral suspension procedures is not significantly different from the functional urethral length before surgery.[52–55] There is no evidence to support the concept that increased functional urethral length is a significant factor in the continence outcome of a urethral suspension procedure.[33] Second, the maximum urethral closure pressure at rest before surgery is not significantly different from the maximum urethral closure pressure at rest after surgery.[33,39,52–57] Therefore, there is little evidence to support the concept that the long-term outcome of continence is related to significant changes in resting urethral closure pressure following surgery.

The single urethral pressure parameter that uniformly has been shown to change following successful surgical procedures for stress urinary incontinence is the maximum urethral closure pressure during stress, or the stress urethral pressure profile.[9,33,34,39,52,54–58] A urethral suspension procedure that successfully repositions the bladder neck to a high retropubic position with fixation of the bladder neck in that position during increased intra-abdominal pressure appears to result in a change in the urethral pressure response to increases in intra-abdominal pressure. The mechanism by which the change in urethral pressure response to intra-abdominal pressure occurs is unclear. It has been proposed that the urethra and bladder neck are repositioned to an intra-abdominal position, which allows the transmission of intra-abdominal pressure to the urethra and thereby provides a positive urethral closure pressure during increased intra-abdominal pressure episodes. Another proposed explanation is that retropubic positioning of the urethra and bladder neck may

produce a stretching effect on the urethra, which enhances the efficiency of the smooth muscle activity of the urethra and allows the active reflex mechanism of the urethra to become more efficient in compensating for increased intra-abdominal pressure.[12,60,62] It is also possible that there may be a kinking effect of the urethra at the bladder neck following a successful urethral suspension procedure owing to the change in position of the urethra relative to the bladder.[17,58] Another important possibility is that the mechanism of accentuated pressure transmission following surgery may not be the same as that in the symptom-free woman and that an alternative mechanical event results in continence following urethral suspension procedures.[39,56,61]

Whatever the mechanism involved in the changes of the pressure response of the urethra, the successful repositioning of the bladder neck to a high retropubic position with fixation of the bladder neck in that position during straining results in functional pressure changes that occur in the urethra, which produce a positive urethral closure pressure during episodes of increased intra-abdominal pressure and results in the clinical outcome of continence. Therefore, the goal of improvement in quality of life is achieved by altering the physiology of the urethra through successfully achieving the anatomic goals of surgery.

The mechanism by which surgical success or failure occurs, however, is still not completely clear. Fortunately, achievement of the anatomic goals of surgery, which include the high retropubic fixation of the bladder neck, results in physiologic changes of the urethra and a continence outcome in a high percentage of patients (Figs. 13-4 through 13-6).

INTRINSIC URETHRAL INCONTINENCE

The value of staging or categorizing any disorder is the value of that classification in selecting treatment of the disorder according to the classification. One of the most important categorizations of patients with stress urinary incontinence has been one introduced by McGuire and col-

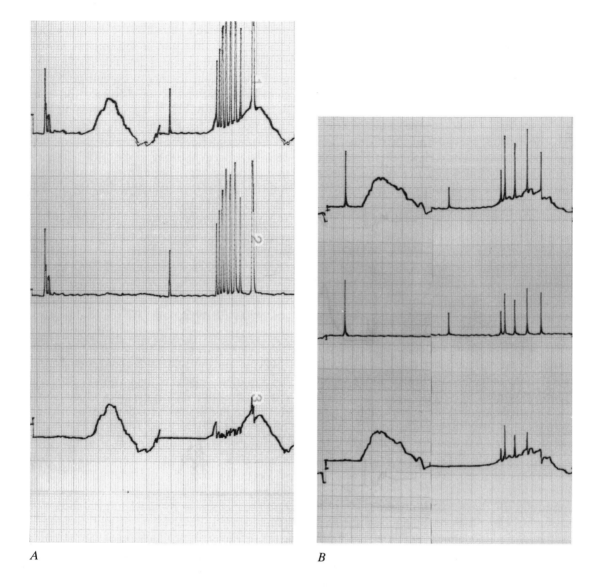

A   B

Figure 13-4. *Resting and stress urethral pressure profile of the patient whose lateral cysto-gram is shown in Fig. 13-1. This was performed with a Millar dual channel microtip cath-eter with a chart speed and catheter advancement of 1 mm/sec. The full-scale range of the strip chart is 100 cm H_2O with each division equal to 10 cm H_2O. The urethral pressure profile was performed in the supine position. (A) Preoperative urethral pressure profile, which shows a resting maximum closure pressure of 22 cm H_2O and a functional urethral length of 2.2 cm. The stress urethral pressure profile shows negative pressure gradients throughout the proximal urethra. (B) Postoperative urethral pressure profile in the same patient as shown in Figs. 13-1 and 13-4A. The postoperative stress urethral pressure pro-file shows positive pressure gradients throughout the proximal urethra. The Raz procedure restored the positive pressure gradient between the bladder and urethra.*

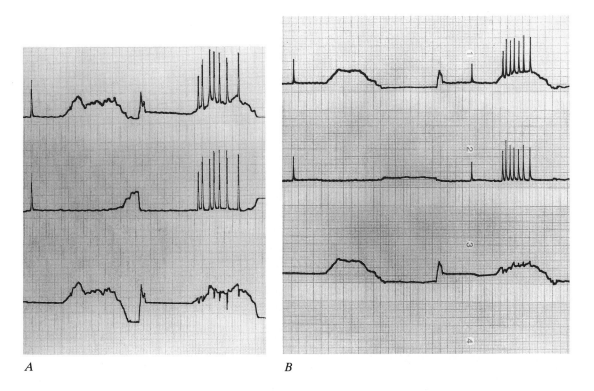

A   *B*

Figure 13-5. *Urethral pressure profile of the patient whose lateral cystogram is shown in Fig. 13-2. The urethral pressure profile was performed in the same way as the studies shown in Fig. 13-4. (A) As can be seen in the preoperative stress urethral profile, there is a loss of transmission of intra-abdominal pressure to the urethra. (B) Following a Burch anterior vesicourethropexy, the pressure transmission is significantly improved.*

leagues.[63] Along with the definition of type I and type II incontinence in this description was the introduction of the concept of type III incontinence. The type III category represents a group of patients with a sphincter dysfunction characterized by a low resting urethral pressure of less than 20 cm H_2O with or without urethral hypermobility. The value of the clinical identification of this group of patients is the extremely high failure rate of conventional urethral suspension procedures in this group.[9, 12, 62, 64] Patients with type III incontinence often have a history of having failed previous surgical procedures for incontinence. In fact, failure of multiple previous operations is associated with a 75% incidence of type III incontinence.[65]

This group of patients appears to represent a special problem in the surgical management of urinary incontinence. Failure to recognize this particular patient preoperatively usually results in an operative failure using conventional urethral suspension procedures. There is still much that is unclear about this group of patients. *Sphincteric dysfunction, intrinsic urethral abnormality,* and *poor urethral function* are common terms applied to this entity. Because many of these patients have failed previous operative procedures, it is unclear whether the previous operative procedures are a factor in the cause of the type III abnormality or whether the surgical procedure selected patients who were destined to fail the operative procedures owing to the pre-

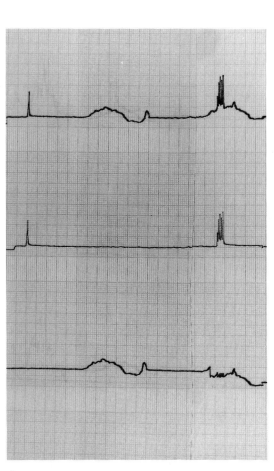

A

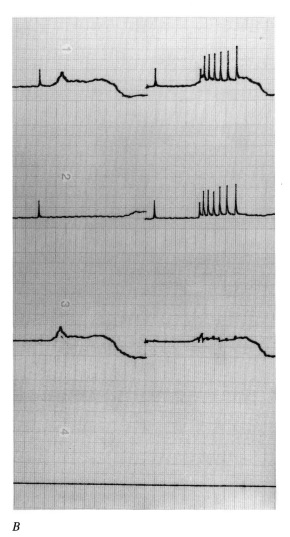

B

Figure 13-6. *Urethral pressure profile of the patient whose lateral cystogram is shown in Fig. 13-3. (A) The preoperative resting pressure profile has a maximum urethral closure pressure of less than 10 cm H_2O. There is complete loss of urethral closure pressure during stress maneuvers. (B) Following a combined Raz suspension procedure with placement of a McGuire fascial sling, there is little change in the resting urethral pressure. The surgical procedure resulted in minimal increase in urethral closure pressure during stress. This patient was totally incontinent before surgery. Following surgery, she experienced urinary retention for 4 weeks and subsequently has been completely continent and voids normally.*

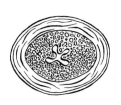
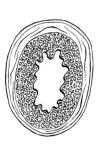
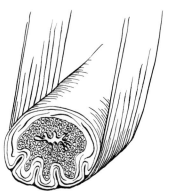

Normal urethra   Incontinent urethra   Fascia sling to support urethra

Figure 13-7. The McGuire sling procedure. The mechanism by which continence occurs following a pubovaginal sling procedure is not completely understood. In patients with stress incontinence, there appears to be loss of support of the posterior segment of the urethra and loss of coaptation of the mucosa, which is important in the normal continence mechanism. The pubovaginal sling appears to restore support to the posterior urethra and to bring the urethral mucosa into a position of coaptation, which is an important part of continence. The pubovaginal sling also supports the urethral position during episodes of stress, which allows the abdominal pressure to be transmitted to the urethra and urinary continence to be maintained.

existing urethral abnormality and were further selected by repeated failures.

In evaluating a population of patients who have stress urinary incontinence using the urethral pressure profile measurement, as with any population, there is variation over a wide range of measurements from a low value to a high value. It is unclear whether the type III group represents the extreme of a spectrum of urethral dysfunction that includes all patients with stress urinary incontinence or whether type III represents a unique group of patients with a particular urethral dysfunction. Whatever the clinical condition in this group of patients, the awareness of the existence of this group of patients and the identification of these patients preoperatively is essential to the successful management of patients with incontinence.

Because the major functional treatment goal of surgery is urinary continence, it is essential that this group of patients be identified preoperatively and the treatment approach modified to

address the severity of the sphincteric dysfunction. The only operative procedure that consistently provides good results for this difficult group of patients is the pubovaginal sling procedure[66] (Fig. 13-7). It also appears that intraurethral collagen may have some role in the management of this group of patients in the future. In patients who have intrinsic urethral dysfunction with a urethral position that is anatomically fixed in a dependent position at the bladder neck owing to previous operative procedures, a combined procedure may be considered. In these patients, a Raz urethral suspension procedure repositions the urethra in a high retropubic position, and a McGuire fascial sling corrects the intrinsic urethral dysfunction (see Figs. 13-3 and 13-6). A technique for the combined procedure has been described with excellent results in this particular group of patients.[67] The most important aspect of the type III incontinent patient is that the urologist must identify that individual preoperatively and avoid considering a conventional urethral suspension procedure for that patient because the failure rate of a urethral suspension procedure in that group is high.[68]

Another important aspect of this group is the need to convey to the patient accurately the magnitude of the problem. The patient who has type III incontinence needs to be well informed of the nature of the problem because this is a particularly difficult group to achieve a continence outcome following surgery.

LEAK POINT PRESSURES

As described previously, the anatomic and physiologic changes that result from surgical intervention in the disorder of stress urinary incontinence that change the daily life of the individual from one of episodes of involuntary loss of urine to complete voluntary control of micturition are complex and unclear. Our assessments involve radiographic evaluation of the anatomic status and urodynamic assessment of the physiologic status of the bladder and urethra. In 1977, McGuire described a technique of combined radiographic and manometric assessment of urethral sphincter function.[69] This technique allows the simultaneous evaluation of the anatomic and physiologic characteristics of urethral dysfunction, which enables the clinician to identify the effects of changes in urethral position on urethral function. The intravesical pressure at which the urethra becomes incompetent can be seen radiographically and measured manometrically. The intravesical pressure at which the urethra becomes incompetent has been described by McGuire as the *leak point pressure* of the urethra. This combined technique allows a much more direct measurement of the functional status of the urethra as well as the bladder. Preoperatively the videourodynamic studies show the changes in urethral position and pressure during increases in abdominal pressure. This measurement method provides the most complete assessment of urethral function that is currently available. Other measurement methods require the clinician to integrate information from static radiographic studies and urethral

pressure measurements to assess urethral function. The leak point pressure determined on videourodynamic studies before surgery demonstrate the anatomic and functional status of the urethra at the point that the urethra is incompetent (Fig. 13-8). Postoperatively the "leak point pressure" can be used to determine changes in the continence function of the urethra resulting from the surgical intervention (Fig. 13-8). The leak point pressure as measured by McGuire represents the most accurate method of identifying intrinsic urethral dysfunction or the type III stress incontinence entity as described by McGuire.

DETRUSOR INSTABILITY

The unstable detrusor is one that is shown objectively to contract, spontaneously or on provocation, during the filling phase while the patient is attempting to inhibit micturition. Detrusor instability is a measured response of the bladder to filling, but similar to urethral pressure profile responses, detrusor instability is not a measure of continence. Detrusor instability is associated with irritative bladder symptoms consisting of frequency, urgency, and nocturia. Symptoms of stress urinary incontinence are often associated to some degree with irritative bladder symptoms. In the clinical evaluation of patients with stress urinary incontinence, there appears to be a spectrum of severity of associated irritative bladder symptoms. In many cases, stress incontinence and irritative bladder symptoms seem to be components of the same disorder.

The presence of irritative bladder symptoms associated with stress urinary incontinence and the urodynamic finding of detrusor instability are important issues to address with the patient regarding the outcome of a surgical procedure. The presence of detrusor instability has caused a reluctance of surgeons to consider the patient for incontinent surgery because of the concern that detrusor instability would represent a source of incontinence during the postoperative period. As pointed out by McGuire and colleagues, how-

(*continued on page 198*)

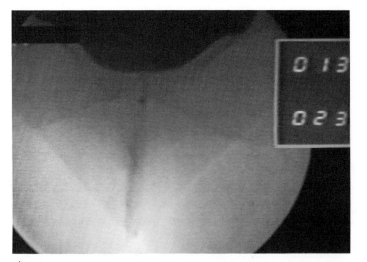

A

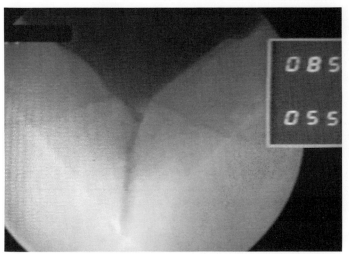

B

Figure 13-8. *The combined radiographic and manometric measurements of bladder and urethral function described by McGuire. The* leak point pressure *represents the pressure point at which the increase in intravesical pressure owing to abdominal straining exceeds the outlet resistance of the urethra and the urethra becomes incompetent. When the urethra becomes functionally incompetent, the contrast material can be seen fluoroscopically to escape from the bladder through the urethra. (A) The resting state of this patient shows no contrast material escaping from the bladder. The urethral pressure is seen in the digital display below and the bladder pressure above. (B) During abdominal straining, contrast material can be seen escaping from the bladder, and the associated pressures of the urethra and bladder were measured (same patient as Fig. 13-7A). (Figure continued on next page.)*

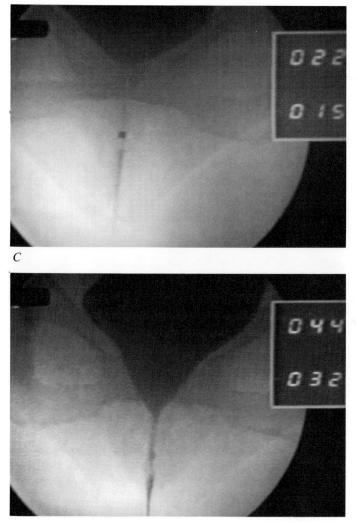

C

D

Figure 13-8. (continued) (C) In this patient, mild straining shows a lower urethral pressure than the intravesical pressure without loss of contrast material fluoroscopically. (D) With further increase in intra-abdominal pressure, the urethra is incompetent with loss of contrast material through the urethra at a low leak point pressure (same patient as Fig. 13-7C).

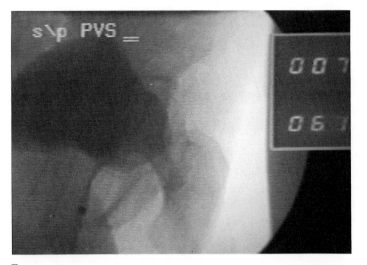

E

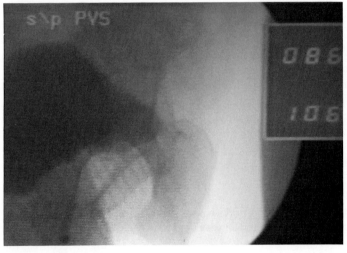

F

Figure 13-8. (continued) (E) This patient has had a pubovaginal sling procedure for stress urinary incontinence. This lateral view shows excellent position of the urethra and no abnormality of the bladder neck. (F) During straining, the urethral pressure has a dynamic increase that exceeds the intravesical pressure and maintains a positive pressure gradient regardless of the intravesical pressure. There is no point of intravesical pressure in this patient at which leaking of contrast material occurs. This anatomic observation, which is made radiographically, is supported by the pressure measurements made manometrically. (Courtesy of Dr. E. J. McGuire.)

ever, most patients who have stress urinary incontinence and detrusor instability have a resolution of both incontinence and detrusor instability following successful incontinent surgery.[70,71] Other investigators have also found that the problem of detrusor instability resolves in most cases following successful incontinent surgery.[72,73] It is possible, however, that patients who have detrusor instability preoperatively may be at a slightly higher risk for persistent detrusor instability following surgery.[73,74]

Perhaps the most difficult problem related to detrusor instability is the fact that it can occur in a small number of patients following surgery for stress urinary incontinence regardless of the preoperative findings.[8,73–75] A difficult problem in the surgical management of stress urinary incontinence is the unexpected occurrence of persistent irritative bladder syndromes associated with detrusor instability in the postoperative period, which does not seem to be predictable by any preoperative studies. The treatment goals of restoring urinary continence and improving the quality of life of the patient are greatly compromised in this small segment of patients owing to persistent irritative symptoms. The fact that the operative procedure was successful in correction of genuine stress incontinence may not be appreciated by the patient who has significant residual irritative symptoms. Fortunately, postoperative irritative symptoms improve over time, and a small number of patients have a significant functional impairment over a long period of time either in the continence outcome or quality of life owing to persistent irritative symptoms. It is important during the postoperative course of these patients to consider aggressive treatment with pharmacologic therapy, biofeedback therapy, bladder training, pelvic floor exercises, timed voiding, electrical stimulation, and supportive management in every way possible. An aggressive approach to these uncommon postoperative problems can allow one to achieve the treatment goals of continence with minimal associated postoperative voiding disturbances to achieve the highest quality of life possible for the many people who suffer from urinary incontinence.

Summary

Stress urinary incontinence results from an abnormal function of the urethra. Although vesicourethral prolapse can occur in continent women, the anatomic displacement of the urethra and base of the bladder appears to be associated with the occurrence of stress urinary incontinence. Prolapse of the posterior urethra results in the anatomic loss of the posterior urethral vesical angle. Prolapse of the base of the bladder and urethra results in changes in the urethral axis. Patients having these anatomic abnormalities and stress urinary incontinence who have no particularly unfavorable outcome characteristics can be restored to normal bladder function, which includes continence and normal voiding in approximately 90% of patients, by surgically repositioning the bladder neck to a high retropubic position. Patients who have failed previous operative procedures represent a different group clinically and require complete evaluation of bladder and urethral function because these patients may be at risk for failure of additional operative procedures. An important group of patients to identify preoperatively are those with the type III classification of McGuire because the continence outcome of conventional urethral suspension procedures in this group is extremely poor. Although these patients may present with no previous history of surgical failure, many patients have failed one or more previous operative procedures. A pubovaginal sling procedure is the preferred surgical approach for this group of patients. It must be recognized that this is an extremely difficult group of patients to manage. Although a successful surgical continence outcome in this group is difficult to achieve, an appropriately placed pubovaginal sling can restore continence in a high percentage of these patients. The pubovaginal sling procedure is an operative procedure that can be applied to all types of sphincteric incompetence with an expected continence outcome in a high percentage of patients. Identification of the incontinence status of the patient by assessment of the anatomic and functional characteristics with the appropriate application of surgical and nonsurgical treatment to patients with urinary incontinence result in the rehabilitation of most patients to a continence status and restore patients to an active role in their environment and in society.

References

1. Blaivas JG. A modest proposal for the diagnosis and treatment of urinary incontinence in women. J of Urol 1987;138:597–598.
2. Jeffcoate TNA, Roberts H. Observations on stress incontinence of urine. Am J Obstet Gynecol 1952;64:721–738.
3. Lee RA. Recurrent stress incontinence of urine: Preoperative assessment and surgical management. Clin Obstet Gynecol 1976;19:661–671.
4. Stanton SL, Cardozo L, Williams JE, et al. Clinical and urodynamic features of failed incontinence surgery in the female. J Obstet Gynecol 1978;51:515–520.
5. McGuire EJ, Lytton B, Pepe V, et al. Stress urinary incontinence. J Obstet Gynecol 1976;47:255–264.
6. Arnold EP, Webster JR, Loose H, et al. Urodynamics of female incontinence: Factors influencing the results of surgery. Am J Obstet Gynecol 1973;117:805–813.
7. McGuire EJ. Identifying and managing stress incontinence in the elderly. Geriatrics 1990;45:44–52.
8. Hilton P. A clinical and urodynamic study comparing the Stamey bladder neck suspension and suburethral sling procedures in the treatment of genuine stress incontinence. Bri J Obstet Gynaecol 1989;96:213–220.
9. Langer, R, Golan A, Ron-El R, et al. Colposuspension for urinary stress incontinence in premenopausal and postmenopausal women. Surgery Gynecol Obstet 1990;171:13–16.
10. O'Donnell P. Pitfalls of urodynamic testing. Urol Clin North Am 1991;18:257–268.
11. Bhatia NN, Bergman A. Urodynamic predictability of voiding following incontinence surgery. Obstet Gynecol 1984;63:85–91.
12. Francis LN, Sand PK, Hamrang K, Ostergard DR. A urodynamic appraisal of success and failure after retropubic urethropexy. J Reprod Med 1987;32:693–696.
13. Green DF, McGuire EJ, Lytton B. A comparison of endoscopic suspension of the vesical neck versus anterior urethropexy for the treatment of stress urinary incontinence. J Urol 1986;136:1205–1207.
14. Stamey TA. Endoscopic suspension of the vesical neck for urinary incontinence in females. Ann Surg 1980;192:465–471.
15. Schaeffer AJ, Stamey TA. Endoscopic suspension of vesical neck for urinary incontinence. Urology 1984;23:484–494.
16. Hodgkinson CP. "Recurrent" stress urinary incontinence. Am J Obstet Gynecol 1978;132:844–860.
17. Awad SA, Downie JW, Kiruluta HG. Alpha-adrenergic agents in urinary disorders of the proximal urethra. Part 1. Sphincteric incontinence. Br J Urol 1978;50:332–335.
18. Collste L, Lindskog M. Phenylpropanolamine in treatment of female stress urinary incontinence. Urology 1987;30:398–403.
19. Gilja I, Radej M, Kovacic M, Parazajder J. Conservative treatment of female stress incontinence with imipramine. J Urol 1984;132:909–911.
20. Bhatia NN, Bergman A, Karram MM. Effects of estrogen on urethral function in women with urinary incontinence. Am J Obstet Gynecol 1989;160:176–181.
21. Kegel AH. Progressive resistance exercise in the functional restoration of the perineal muscles. Am J Obstet Gynecol 1948;56:238–248.
22. Kegel AH. Stress incontinence of urine in women: Physiologic treatment. J Int Coll Surg 1956;25:487–499.
23. Kegel AH. Physiologic therapy for urinary stress incontinence. JAMA 1951;146:915–917.
24. Burns PA, Pranikoff K, Nochajski T, et al. Treatment of stress incontinence with pelvic floor exercises and biofeedback. J Am Ger Soc 1990;38:341–344.
25. Elder DD, Stephenson TP. An assessment of the Frewen regime in the treatment of detrusor dysfunction in females. Br J Urol 1980;52:467–471.
26. Frewen WK. A reassessment of bladder training in detrusor dysfunction in the female. Br J Urol 1982;54:372–373.
27. Jarvis GJ. A controlled trial of bladder drill and drug therapy in the management of detrusor instability. Br J Urol 1981;53:565–566.
28. Burgio KL, Robinson JC, Engel BT. The role of biofeedback in Kegel exercise training for stress urinary incontinence. Am J Obstet Gynecol 1986;154:58–64.
29. O'Donnell PD, Doyle R. Biofeedback therapy technique for treatment of urinary incontinence. Urology 1991;37:432–436.
30. Creason NS, Grybowski JA, Burgener S, et al. Prompted voiding therapy of urinary incontinence in aged female nursing home residents. J Adv Nurs 1989;14:120–126.
31. Lapides J, Ajemian EP, Stewart BH, et al. Physi-

opathology of stress incontinence. Surg Gynecol Obstet 1960;111:224–231.

32. Hodgkinson CP, Ayers MA, Drukker BH. Dyssynergic dtrusor dysfunction in the apparently normal female. Am J Obstet Gynecol 1963;87:717.

33. Henriksson L, Ulmsten U. A urodynamic evaluation of the effects of abdominal urethrocystopexy and vaginal sling urethroplasty in women with stress incontinence. Am J Obstet Gynecol 1978;131:77–82.

34. Tenaillon M, Toppercer A, Elhilali M. Clinical and urodynamic evaluation of urethrocystopexy for stress urinary incontinence. Urology 1981;28:527–530.

35. Bergman A, McKenzie C, Ballard CA, Richmond J. Role of cystourethrography in the preoperative evaluation of stress urinary incontinence in women. J Reprod Med 1988;33:372–376.

36. Greenwald SW, Thornbury JR, Dunn LJ. Cystourethrography as a diagnostic aid in stress incontinence. Obstet Gynecol 1967;29:324–327.

37. Kujansuu E, Kauppila A, Lahde S. Correlation between urethrovesical anatomy and urethral closure function in female stress urinary incontinence before and after operation: Urethrocystographic and urethrocystometric evaluation. Urol Int 1983;38:19–24.

38. Green TH Jr. Urinary stress incontinence: Differential diagnosis, pathophysiology, and management. Am J Obstet Gynecol 1975;122:368–400.

39. Hilton P, Stanton SL. Urethral pressure measurement by microtransducer: The results in symptom-free women and in those with genuine stress incontinence. Br J Obstet Gynecol 1983;90:919–933.

40. Versi E, Cardozo LD, Studd JWW, et al. Internal urinary sphincter in maintenance of female continence. BMJ 1986;292:166–167.

41. Addison WA, Haygood V, Parker RT. Recurrent stress urinary incontinence. Obstet Gynecol Ann 1985;14:252–265.

42. Kauppila A, Penttinen J, Haggman V. Six-microtransducer catheter connected to computer in evaluation of urethral closure function of women. Urology 1989;33:159–164.

43. Faysal MH, Constantinou CE, Rother LF, Govan DE. The impact of bladder neck suspension on the resting and stress urethral pressure profile: A prospective study comparing controls with incontinent patients preoperatively and postoperatively. J Urol 1981;125:55–60.

44. Bump RC, Copeland WE Jr, Hurt WG, Fantl JA. Dynamic urethral pressure/profilometry pressure transmission ratio determinations in stress-incon-

tinent and stress-continent subjects. Am J Obstet Gynecol 1988;159:749–755.

45. Heidler H, Wolk H, Jonas U. Urethral closure mechanism under stress conditions. Eur Urol 1979;5:110–112.

46. Van Der Kooi JB, Wanroy V, De Jonge MC, Kornelis JA. Time separation between cough pulses in bladder rectum and urethra in women. J Urol 1984;132:1275–1278.

47. Constantinou CE, Govan DE. Spatial distribution and timing of transmitted and reflexly generated urethral pressures in healthy women. J Urol 1982;127:964–969.

48. Vereecken RL, Cornelissen M. Rotational differences in urethral pressure in incontinent women. Urol Int 1985;40:201–205.

49. Constantinou CE. Resting and stress urethral pressures as a clinical guide to the mechanism of continence in the female patient. Urol Clin North Am 1985;12:247–258.

50. Leach GE, Raz S. Modified Pereyra bladder neck suspension after previously failed anti-incontinence surgery. Urology 1984;23:359–362.

51. Klutke C, Golomb J, Barbaric Z, Raz S. The anatomy of stress incontinence: Magnetic resonance imaging of the female bladder neck and urethra. J Urol 1990;143:563–566.

52. Koonings PP, Bergman A, Ballard CA. Low urethral pressure and stress urinary incontinence in women: risk factor for failed retropubic surgical procedure. Urology 1990;36:245–248.

53. Leach GE, Yip C, Donovan BJ. Mechanism of continence after modified Pereyra bladder neck suspension. Urology 1987;29:328–331.

54. Constantinou CE, Faysal MH, Rother L, Govan DE. The impact of bladder neck suspension on the mode of distribution of abdominal pressure along the female urethra. In: NR Zinner, AM Sterling, eds. Female incontinence. New York: Alan R. Liss, 1981:121–132.

55. Rottenberg RD, Weil A, Brioschi PA, et al. Urodynamic and clinical assessment of the Lyodura sling operation for urinary stress incontinence. Br J Obstet Gynaecol 1985;92:829–834.

56. Penttinen J, Kaar K, Kauppila A. Effect of suprapubic operation on urethral closure—evaluation by single cough urethrocystometry. Br J Urol 1989;63:389–391.

57. Beisland Ho, Fossberg E, Sander S, Moer A. Urodynamic studies before and after retropubic urethropexy for stress incontinence in females. Oslo: Aker University, 1982: 333–336.

58. Beck RP, McCormick FS, Nordstrom L. Intra-urethral-intravesical cough-pressure spike differ-

ence in 267 patients surgically cured of genuine stress incontinence of urine. Obstet Gynecol 1988;72:302.

59. Massey JA, Anderson RS, Abrams P. Mechanisms of continence during raised intra-abdominal pressure. Br J Urol 1987;60:529–531.

60. Bruschini H, Schmidt RA, Tanagho EA. Effect of urethral stretch on urethral pressure profile. Invest Urol 1977;15:107–111.

61. Hilton P, Stanton SL. A clinical and urodynamic assessment of the Burch colposuspension for genuine stress incontinence. Br J Obstet Gynecol 1983;90:934–939.

62. Sand PK, Bowen LW, Panganiban R, Ostergard DR. The low pressure urethra as a factor in failed retropubic urethropexy. Obstet Gynecol 1987; 69:399–402.

63. McGuire EJ, Lytton B, Kohorn EI, Pepe V. The value of urodynamic testing in stress urinary incontinence. J Urol 1980;124:256–258.

64. Bowen LW, Sand PK, Ostergard DR, Franti CE. Unsuccessful Burch retropubic urethropexy: A case-controlled urodynamic study. Am J Obstet Gynecol 1989;160:452–458.

65. McGuire EJ. Urodynamic findings in patients after failure of stress incontinence operations. In: NR Zinner, AM Sterling, eds. Female incontinence. New York: Alan R Liss, 1981:351–360.

66. McGuire EJ, Bennett CJ, Konnak JA, et al. Experience with pubovaginal slings for urinary incontinence at the University of Michigan. J Urol 1987;138:525–526.

67. O'Donnell PD. Combined Raz urethral suspension and McGuire pubovaginal sling for treatment of complicated stress urinary incontinence. J Ark Med Soc J 1992;88:389–392.

68. Horbach NS, Blanco JS, Ostergard DR, et al. Instruments and methods. Obstet Gynecol 1988; 71:648–652.

69. McGuire EJ. Combined radiographic and manometric assessment of urethral sphincter function. J Urol 1977;118:632–635.

70. McGuire EJ, Lytton B. Pubovaginal sling procedure for stress incontinence. J Urol 1978;119: 82–84.

71. McGuire EJ, Savastano JA. Stress incontinence and detrusor instability/urge incontinence. Neurol Urodynam 1985;4:313–316.

72. Koonings P, Bergman A, Ballard CA. Combined detrusor instability and stress urinary incontinence: Where is the primary pathology? Gynecol Obstet Invest 1988;26:250–256.

73. Eriksen BC, Hagen B, Eik-Nes SH, et al. Long-term effectiveness of the Burch colposuspension in female urinary stress incontinence. Acta Obstet Gynecol Scand 1990;69:45–50.

74. Langer R, Ron-El R, Newman M, et al. Detrusor instability following colposuspension for urinary stress incontinence. Br J Obstet Gynecol 1988; 95:607–610.

75. Sand PK, Bowen LW, Ostergard DR, et al. The effect of retropubic urethropexy on detrusor stability. Obstet Gynecol 1988;71:818–822.

14

Retropubic Repair of Urethral Incontinence

Mark D. Walters

Since 1949, when Marshall and co-workers first described retropubic urethrovesical suspension for the treatment of stress urinary incontinence, retropubic procedures have emerged as consistently curative for that disease.[1] Although numerous terms for and variations of retropubic repairs have been described, the basic concept remains the same: to suspend and to stabilize the bladder neck and proximal urethra in a retropubic position to avoid excessive mobility during increases in intra-abdominal pressure. Selection of a retropubic approach (versus a vaginal approach) depends on many factors, such as the need for laparotomy for other pelvic disease, the amount of pelvic relaxation, the age and health status of the patient, and the preference and expertise of the surgeon.

Few data exist to differentiate one retropubic procedure from another, although advantages and disadvantages exist for each. This chapter describes the surgical techniques for the three most studied and popular retropubic procedures: the Marshall-Marchetti-Krantz (MMK) procedure, the Burch colposuspension, and the vagino-obturator shelf (VOS) and paravaginal repairs. The surgical techniques described herein are contemporary modifications of the original operations: The MMK technique has been described by Krantz, and the modified Burch colposuspension has been described by Tanagho.[2,3]

The VOS and paravaginal repairs are similar procedures; the techniques have been described by Turner-Warwick and Webster and Kreder (VOS repair) and by Richardson and colleagues and Shull and Baden (paravaginal repair).[4–7] Although less critically studied, these techniques are regionally popular and widely performed in the United States and Great Britain. It is understood that the operations described do not represent one correct technique but a commonly used and proven method.

Indications for Retropubic Procedures

Retropubic urethrovesical suspension procedures are indicated for women with the diagnosis of genuine stress incontinence and a hypermobile proximal urethra and bladder neck. These procedures yield the best results when the urethral sphincter is capable of maintaining a watertight seal at rest but cannot withstand the unequal transmission of abdominal pressure to the proximal urethra, relative to the bladder, with straining. This corresponds to type I and type II genuine stress incontinence as described by McGuire.[8,9] Although retropubic procedures can be used for type III stress urinary incontinence (open vesical neck and proximal urethra at rest, with or without urethral mobility), other

Female Urology, edited by Elroy D. Kursh and Edward McGuire. J. B. Lippincott, Philadelphia, © 1994.

more obstructive operations probably yield better long-term results.[9, 10]

To diagnose genuine stress incontinence, clinical and urodynamic (simple or complex) tests must be done to evaluate bladder filling, storage, and emptying. Clinically the urethra is shown to be incompetent by observing loss of urine simultaneous with increases in intra-abdominal pressure. Urodynamic or radiologic methods may also be used for diagnosis. Abnormalities of bladder-filling function, such as detrusor instability, can coexist with urethral sphincter incompetence but may be associated with lower cure rates after retropubic surgery.[11]

Women with genuine stress incontinence should generally have a trial of conservative therapy before corrective surgery is offered. Conservative treatment comes in the form of pelvic floor exercises, bladder retraining, pharmacologic therapy, functional electrical stimulation, and mechanical devices, such as pessaries. Eligible postmenopausal patients with atrophic urogenital changes should be prescribed estrogen before surgery is considered.

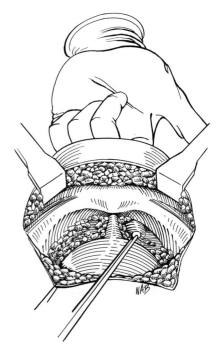

Figure 14-1. *Dissection of the lateral retropubic space. After forceful elevation of the surgeon's vaginal finger, the fat overlying the glistening white periurethral fascia is cleared, in preparation for suture placement.*

Surgical Techniques

OPERATIVE SETUP AND GENERAL ENTRY INTO THE RETROPUBIC SPACE

The patient is supine, with the legs supported in a slightly abducted position, allowing the surgeon to operate with one hand in the vagina and the other in the retropubic space (Fig. 14-1). The vagina, perineum, and abdomen are sterilely prepared and draped in a fashion permitting easy access to the lower abdomen and to the vagina. A three-way, 16 or 20 French Foley catheter with a 20- to 30-ml balloon is inserted sterilely into the bladder and kept in the sterile field. The drainage port of the catheter is left to gravity drainage, and the irrigation port is connected to a dilute methylene blue solution. One to three perioperative intravenous doses of an appropriate antibiotic should be given as prophylaxis against infection.[12]

A Pfannenstiel or Cherney incision is made. If intraperitoneal surgery is to be done, the peritoneum is opened, the surgery is completed, and the cul-de-sac is plicated. The retropubic space is then exposed. Staying close to the back of the pubic bone, the surgeon's hand is introduced into the retropubic space and the bladder and urethra gently moved downward. Sharp dissection is not usually necessary in primary cases. To aid visualization of the bladder, 100 ml of sterile water with methylene blue dye may be instilled into the bladder after the catheter drainage port is clamped.

When previous retropubic (especially MMK) procedures have been done, dense adhesions from the anterior bladder wall and urethra to the symphysis pubis are frequently present. These adhesions should be dissected sharply from the pubic bone until the anterior bladder wall, urethra, and vagina are free of adhesions and are mobile. If identification of the urethra or lower border of the bladder is difficult, one may perform a cystotomy and, with a finger inside the bladder, define its lower limits for easier dissection, mobilization, and elevation.

BURCH COLPOSUSPENSION

Once the retropubic space is entered, the urethra and anterior vaginal wall are depressed downward. No dissection should be done in the midline over the urethra or at the urethrovesical junction, thus protecting the delicate musculature of the urethra from surgical trauma. Attention is directed to the tissue on either side of the urethra. Most of the overlying fat should be cleared away, using a swab mounted on a curved forceps. This dissection is done with forceful elevation of the surgeon's vaginal finger (or a Deaver retractor in the vagina) until glistening white periurethral fascia and vaginal wall are seen.[13] This area is extremely vascular, with a rich, thin-walled venous plexus that should be avoided, if possible. The position of the urethra and the lower edge of the bladder should be determined by palpating the Foley balloon and by partially distending the bladder to define the rounded lower margin of the bladder as it meets the anterior vaginal wall.

Once dissection lateral to the urethra is completed and vaginal mobility is judged to be adequate by using the vaginal fingers to lift the anterior vaginal wall upward and forward, it is time for placement of the sutures. Number 0 or 1 delayed absorbable or nonabsorbable sutures are placed as far laterally in the anterior vaginal wall as is technically possible. We apply two sutures bilaterally, using double bites for each suture. The distal suture is placed approximately 2 cm lateral to the midurethra. The proximal suture is placed approximately 2 cm lateral to the reflection of the anterior bladder wall at, or slightly proximal to, the level of the urethrovesical junction.

In placing the sutures, one should take a full thickness of vaginal wall, excluding the epithe-

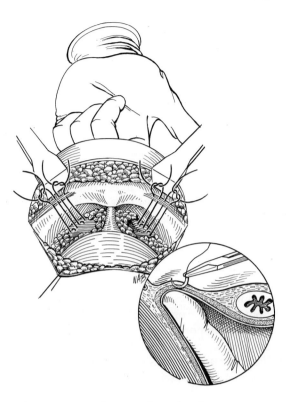

Figure 14-2. *Technique of Burch colposuspension. After the two sutures are placed on each side, they are passed through the pectineal (Cooper's) ligament, so that all four suture ends exit above the ligament to facilitate knot tying. (Inset) In placing the sutures, one should take a full thickness of vaginal wall, excluding the epithelium, with the needle parallel to the urethra. This is best done by suturing over the vaginal finger.*

lium, with the needle parallel to the urethra (Fig. 14-2 [inset]). This is best done by suturing over the vaginal finger at the appropriate selected sites. On each side, after the two sutures are placed, they are then passed through the pectineal (Cooper's) ligament, so that all four suture ends exit above the ligament (Fig. 14-2). Before tying the sutures, a 1 cm × 4 cm strip of Gelfoam may be placed between the vagina and obturator fascia below Cooper's ligament to aid adherence and hemostasis.[14]

As noted previously, this area is extremely

vascular, and visible vessels should be avoided if at all possible. When excessive bleeding occurs, it can be controlled by direct pressure, sutures, or vascular clips. Less severe bleeding usually stops once the fixation sutures are tied.

Once all four sutures are placed in the vagina and through the Cooper's ligaments, the assistant ties first the distal sutures and then the proximal ones, while the surgeon elevates the vagina with the vaginal hand. In tying the sutures, one does not have to be concerned about whether the vaginal wall meets Cooper's ligament, so one should not overdo the tension on the vaginal wall. A suture bridge between the two points is of no disadvantage. After the sutures are tied, one can easily insert two fingers between the pubic bone and the urethra, thus avoiding compression of the urethra against the pubic bone. Continued vaginal fixation and urethral support are dependent on fibrosis and scarring of periurethral and vaginal tissues over the obturator internus fascia rather than on the suture material itself.

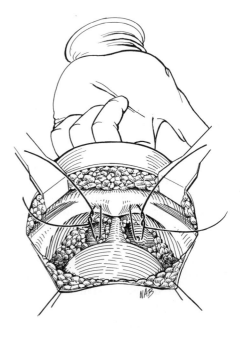

Figure 14-3. *Technique of Marshall-Marchetti-Krantz procedure. One suture is placed bilaterally at the level of the bladder neck and then into the periosteum of the pubic symphysis.*

MARSHALL-MARCHETTI-KRANTZ PROCEDURE

The retropubic space is exposed and the urethra and bladder base palpated with the Foley catheter in place. The surgeon's left hand is placed into the vagina, and the index and middle fingers are placed at the urethrovesical neck on either side of the urethra. Gentle dissection of periurethral fat is made at the urethrovesical junction on each side over the vaginal fingers. This area is extremely vascular, having a rich, thin-walled venous plexus that should be avoided, if possible.

Delayed absorbable sutures are usually used and are placed at right angles to the urethra and parallel to the vesical neck. A single suture is placed bilaterally at the urethrovesical junction. A double bite is taken over the surgeon's finger, incorporating full thickness of the vaginal wall but excluding the vaginal epithelium. Following placement of the sutures, the point of fixation of the urethra to the symphysis pubis can be determined by elevating the two vaginal fingers to the point where the vesical neck comes in contact with the pubic symphysis and noting the position at which the sutures will be placed into the pubic periosteum. The needle is placed medially to laterally, against the periosteum, and turned with a simple wrist action. It may involve the cartilage in the midline, depending on the width, the thickness, and the availability of the periosteum. The sutures on each side are placed accordingly and tied with the vaginal finger elevating the urethrovesical junction (Fig. 14-3). Venous bleeding is usually controlled after tying the sutures or with direct pressure.

VAGINO-OBTURATOR SHELF AND PARAVAGINAL PROCEDURES

The object of the VOS and paravaginal repairs is to reattach, bilaterally, the anterolateral vaginal sulcus with its overlying pubocervical fascia to the pubococcygeous and obturator internus muscles and fascia at the level of the arcus tendineus fasciae pelvis. The retropubic space is entered, and the bladder and vagina are depressed and pulled medially to allow visualization of the lateral retropubic space, including the obturator internus muscle and the fossa containing the obturator neurovascular bundle. For the VOS repair, three interrupted no. 0 or no. 1 nonabsorbable or delayed absorbable sutures are placed bilaterally at 1-cm intervals through the paravaginal fascia and vaginal wall (excluding the vaginal epithelium), beginning at the urethrovesical junction and continuing proximally toward the bladder base. These sutures are then passed through the adjacent obturator fascia and underlying muscle in a horizontal orientation and tied. To fill the retropubic dead space, the peritoneum is opened, and an omental pedicle is brought down into the retropubic space.

For the paravaginal repair, the lateral retropubic spaces are visualized as noted. Blunt dissection is then carried downward from the obturator fossa for 5 to 6 cm, until the ischial spine is palpated. The arcus tendineus fasciae pelvis is frequently visualized as a white band of tissue running over the pubococcygeus and obturator internus muscles from the back of the lower edge of the symphysis pubis toward the ischial spine. A lateral paravaginal defect representing avulsion of the vagina off the arcus tendineus fasciae pelvis or of the arcus tendineus fasciae pelvis off the obturator internus muscle may be visualized (Fig. 14-4).

The surgeon's left hand is inserted into the vagina. While gently retracting the vagina and bladder medially, the anterolateral vaginal sulcus is elevated. Starting near the vaginal apex, a suture is placed, first through the full thickness of the vagina (excluding the vaginal epithelium) and then into the obturator internus fascia or arcus tendineus fasciae pelvis, 3 to 4 cm below the obturator fossa. After this first stitch is tied, additional (five or six total) sutures are placed through the vaginal wall and overlying fascia and then into the obturator internus at about 1-cm intervals toward the pubic ramus (see Fig.

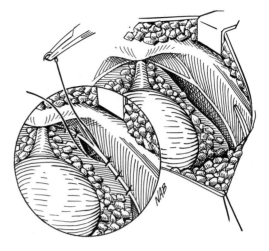

Figure 14-4. *Lateral paravaginal defect and technique of paravaginal repair. Five or six sutures are placed, first through the full thickness of the vagina (excluding the vaginal epithelium) and then into the obturator internus fascia or arcus tendineus fascia pelvis, 3 to 4 cm below the obturator fossa.*

14-4, inset). The most distal suture should be as close as possible to the pubic ramus, into the pubourethral ligament. Number 3–0 nonabsorbable suture on a medium-sized, tapered needle is usually used for the paravaginal repair.

Both procedures leave free space between the symphysis pubis and the proximal urethra but secure support, so descent of the proximal urethra and bladder base are prevented with sudden increases in intra-abdominal pressure. According to Turner-Warwick, they avoid overcorrection and fixation of the paraurethral fascia that might compromise the functional movements of the urethra and bladder base and lead to an element of obstruction and voiding difficulty.[4] This principle may explain why the VOS and paravaginal repairs usually result in spontaneous voiding on the first or second postoperative day.[5,7] In fact, the VOS repair has been used to correct patients with dysfunctional voiding symptoms after previous retropubic surgery.[5]

GENERAL INTRAOPERATIVE AND POSTOPERATIVE PROCEDURES

If the surgeon is concerned that intravesical suture placement or ureteral obstruction may have occurred, cystoscopy—either transurethrally or through the dome of the bladder—or cystotomy may be done to document ureteral patency and absence of intravesical sutures after retropubic procedures.[15-17]

Closed suction drains of the retropubic space are used only as necessary when hemostasis is incomplete and there is concern about postoperative hematoma. The bladder is routinely drained with a suprapubic or transurethral catheter for 2 to 3 days. After that time, the patient is allowed to begin voiding trials, and postvoid residual urine volumes are checked.

Clinical Results

Many studies have reported clinical experiences with retropubic urethral suspension procedures for stress urinary incontinence. Unfortunately, most of these studies are methodologically flawed by modern standards. The major problem with most studies is that objective parameters were not used preoperatively and postoperatively to establish diagnosis and outcome. Few prospective studies are available comparing the results of the various procedures for genuine stress incontinence, and those available compare retropubic procedures with vaginal procedures.

Mainprize and Drutz summarized 56 articles that have reported the results of MMK procedures.[18] Few of these articles employed preoperative diagnostic urodynamic tests, and only Milani and associates reported postoperative urodynamic data after 1 year.[19] Of 2712 cases overall, 2334 (86.1%) were deemed successful, 73 (2.7%) were judged improved, and 305 (11.2%) were considered failures. The success rate of primary MMK procedures was 92.1%; the success rate was 84.5% when the MMK procedure was used for recurrent incontinence.[18] In the study by Milani and associates, the rate of continence confirmed by urodynamic studies was 71% after 1 year.[19] Following MMK procedures, the recurrence of stress incontinence increases over time: The longer the observation period, the more cases of recurrence may be seen. Using a self-reported interview, Park and Miller showed that 86% of patients treated with primary MMK procedures were cured during the first 3 years after surgery, and only 66% were still continent after 3 to 10 years.[20]

The Burch colposuspension is the best studied of the retropubic procedures. From 1980 to 1990, 18 studies have reported using the Burch colposuspension in women with urodynamically proven genuine stress incontinence and with objective measures of cure. Follow-up times range from 3 months to 7 years. A summary of the outcomes is presented in Tables 14-1 and 14-2. At 3 months to 24 months after surgery, 59% to 100% of patients have been reported to be continent, for an overall average cure rate of 84%.[19,21-33] At 3 years to 7 years, continence rates range from 63% to 89%, for an average rate of 76.9%.[28,32,34-37] Although objectively incontinent, a small percentage of additional patients are judged to be improved and satisfied with their surgical results. The overall reported absolute failure rate at 3 months to 24 months is 13.6%, and at 5 years to 7 years it is 14.0%.

In one of the best long-term studies to date, Eriksen and co-workers reported 91 women with urodynamically proven genuine stress incontinence, with or without bladder stability, who had had Burch colposuspension.[34] Urodynamic evaluation was accepted by 76 patients after 5 years. Stress incontinence was cured in 71% of the patients with stable bladders preoperatively and in 57% of those with stress incontinence and detrusor instability, a nonsignificant difference. At the 5-year follow-up, only 52% of the study group were completely dry and free of complications, and about 30% needed further incontinence therapy.

Demographic conditions that increase the risk of surgical failure for retropubic urethropexy are shown in Table 14-3. They include menopause, prior hysterectomy, and prior anti-

Table 14-1. Summary of studies from 1980–1990 in which Burch procedures were used to treat genuine stress incontinence and objective urodynamic outcomes were available after 3 months to 24 months

STUDY	NUMBER OF PATIENTS	NUMBER (%) CURED	FOLLOW-UP TIME (MONTHS)
Bhatia and Ostergard, 1981	12	10 (83.3)	4–12
Walter *et al*, 1982	38	27 (71.0)	12–30
Kujansuu, 1983	29	17 (58.6)	15 (mean)
Hilton and Stanton, 1983	25	22 (88.0)	3
Mundy, 1983	26	22 (84.6)	12
Weil *et al*, 1984	34	31 (91.2)	6
Milani *et al*, 1985	44	35 (79.5)	12
Bhatia and Bergman, 1985	44	43 (97.7)	12
van Geelen *et al*, 1988	34	29 (85.3)	12–24
Bergman *et al*, 1989[30]	38	34 (89.5)	12
Bergman *et al*, 1989[29]	101	88 (87.1)	12
Penttinen *et al*, 1989	29	29 (100)	8–12
Thunedborg *et al*, 1990	17	15 (88.2)	6
Langer *et al*, 1990	122	96 (78.7)	3–6
Total	593	498 (84)	

incontinence procedures.[11,33,38,39] Advanced age does not appear to be associated with lower rates of cure after colposuspension, although one study described a somewhat higher mean age in patients who failed continence surgery.[11,37] Clinical and urodynamic findings that increase the risk of surgical failure include maximum urethral closure pressure less than 20 cm H_2O, abnormal perineal electromyography, and concurrent detrusor instability.[10,11,39–41] The first condition may identify women who are at higher risk of having type III genuine stress incontinence and who are probably better treated with a more obstructive operation, such as a sling.[10]

Women with mixed detrusor instability and genuine stress incontinence who undergo surgical correction have lower postoperative continence rates than do women with pure genuine stress incontinence. Although 60% to 70% of patients with mixed incontinence have resolu-

Table 14-2. Summary of studies from 1980–1990 in which Burch procedures were used to treat genuine stress incontinence and objective urodynamic outcomes were available after 3 years to 7 years

STUDY	NUMBER OF PATIENTS	NUMBER (%) CURED	FOLLOW-UP TIME (YEARS)
van Geelen *et al*, 1988	33	25* (75.8)	5–7
Thunedborg *et al*, 1990	14	11+ (78.6)	6
Eriksen *et al*, 1990	76	48 (63.1)	5
Rydhström and Iosif, 1988	30	26 (86.7)	3 (mean)
Galloway *et al*, 1987	50	42 (84.0)	1–6
Gillon and Stanton, 1984	35	31+ (88.6)	3–5
Total	238	183 (76.9)	

* Determined by questionnaire only.
+ Determined by pad test, urolog only.

Table 14-3. *Conditions that decrease the chance of cure after retropubic urethropexy*

DEMOGRAPHIC

Advanced age(?)
Postmenopausal
Prior hysterectomy
Prior procedures to correct genuine stress incontinence

URODYNAMIC

Concurrent detrusor instability
Urethral closure pressure less than 20 cm H_2O
Abnormal perineal electromyography

From Walters MD. Genuine stress incontinence: Retropubic surgical procedures. In: Walters MD, Karram MM. Clinical Urogynecology. St. Louis: Mosby-Yearbook, 1993.

Table 14-4. *Postoperative complications in 2712 Marshall-Marchetti-Krantz procedures*

TYPE OF COMPLICATION	PERCENT
Wound, total	5.5
Infection or hematoma	3.4
Hernia or dehiscence	1.8
Other	0.3
Urinary tract infection	3.9
Osteitis pubis	2.5
Direct surgical injury to the urinary tract	1.6
Bladder tears	0.7
Urethral obstruction	0.5
Sutures through bladder or urethra with/without catheter sewn in	0.3
Ureteral obstruction or hydronephrosis	0.1
Fistula	0.3
Death	0.2

Modified from Mainprize TC, Drutz HP. The Marshall-Marchetti-Krantz procedure: A critical review. Obstet Gynecol Surv 1988;43:724.

tion of their detrusor instability after urethropexy, residual urgency incontinence often persists and may be interpreted by the patient as surgical failure.[42,43] Although not all authors agree, patients with mixed incontinence should probably receive medical therapy first; surgery is then suggested for those who have continued stress incontinence.[10,43]

Complications

SHORT-TERM POSTOPERATIVE COMPLICATIONS

Of the retropubic procedures, the MMK procedure is the most extensively studied regarding complications. In a thorough review of the literature, Mainprize and Drutz summarized the postoperative complications (excluding urinary retention) of MMK procedures[18] (Table 14-4). Wound complications and urinary infections are the most common surgical complications. Direct surgical injury to the urinary tract is a relatively infrequent, although more severe, occurrence. Bladder lacerations occurred in 0.7% of patients; sutures through the bladder and urethra and catheters sewn into the urethra occurred in 0.3% of patients. Ureteral obstruction occurred in 0.1% of patients. Accidental placement of

sutures into the bladder with the Burch or paravaginal repair, resulting in vesical stone formation, recurrent cystitis, or fistula, may occur but have not been reported.

Ureteral obstruction may occur more commonly after Burch colposuspension.[44,45] This probably results from ureteral kinking after elevation of the vagina and bladder base. One study reported three unilateral ureteral obstructions and three bilateral ureteral obstructions in 483 Burch colposuspensions (1.2%).[45] All cases were treated with removal of sutures and ureteral stenting. No cases of transected ureters have been reported. Eriksen and colleagues found that 1 of 75 patients (1.3%) followed for 5 years after Burch procedures had absent unilateral renal function owing to presumed complete ureteral obstruction.[34] This patient had had only transient postoperative fever. Because of this potential complication, the routine use of cystoscopy, either transurethrally or through the dome of the bladder, or cystotomy should be considered to document ureteral patency and absence of intravesical sutures after retropubic procedures.

Lower urinary tract fistulas are uncommon

after retropubic procedures, with various types occurring after only 0.3% of MMK procedures. Fistulas are probably less common after Burch and paravaginal repairs because the sutures are placed several centimeters lateral to the urethra and bladder base.

POSTOPERATIVE VOIDING DIFFICULTIES

The incidence of voiding difficulties after colposuspension varies widely in the literature, although patients rarely have difficulty voiding after 30 days. Eriksen and co-workers found that only 2 of 91 patients had delayed spontaneous micturition following Burch colposuspension after removal of the catheter the third day postoperatively.[34] Fifteen percent of these patients had residual urine volumes of 100 to 300 ml the fifth day after surgery. In contrast, Korda and associates had a mean postoperative catheter drainage of 10 days (range 5 to 60 days) for 174 patients after colposuspension.[14] Twenty-five percent of these patients required catheter drainage for more than 10 days.

Colposuspension may change the original micturition pattern and introduce an element of obstruction that can disturb the balance between voiding forces and outflow resistance, leading to immediate postoperative as well as late voiding difficulties.[46] Urodynamic findings that may occur after colposuspension include decreased flow rate, increased micturition pressure, and increased urethral resistance.

Urodynamic tests may be used to predict early postoperative voiding difficulties. Bhatia and Bergman found that all patients with adequate detrusor contraction and flow rates preoperatively were able to resume spontaneous voiding by the seventh postoperative day after Burch colposuspension.[47] One third of patients who voided without detrusor contraction needed bladder drainage for 7 days or longer. No patients in their study with decreased flow rates and absent detrusor contraction during voiding were able to void in less than 7 days postoperatively. The use of a Valsalva maneuver during voiding may further lead to postoperative void-

ing difficulties, perhaps by intensifying obstruction at the bladder neck.[48,49] Preoperative uroflowmetry and postvoid residual urine volumes do not appear to be predictive of postoperative voiding difficulties after Burch procedures.[50]

DETRUSOR INSTABILITY

Detrusor instability is a recognized postoperative complication of retropubic procedures. Studies of patients with genuine stress incontinence and stable bladders preoperatively, with follow-up up to 5 years after Burch colposuspension, have reported unstable bladders on cystometrogram in 7% to 27%.[14,25,33,34,51–53] Postoperative detrusor instability is more common in patients with previous bladder neck surgery and in those with mixed detrusor instability and sphincteric incompetence preoperatively. In a study of 148 patients with genuine stress incontinence and stable bladders preoperatively, Steel and co-workers reported that 24 (16.2%) patients had postoperative detrusor instability on cystometrogram 3 to 6 months after surgery.[52] Ten of the 24 patients with detrusor instability were completely asymptomatic. Of the 14 symptomatic patients, 4 were improved with drugs aimed at correcting the instability. The remaining 10 patients (6.8% of total) remained symptomatic with detrusor instability 3 to 5 years after surgery.

The mechanism for this phenomenon is unknown. Cardozo and associates suggested that postoperative onset of detrusor instability may be due to disruption of the autonomic innervation of the bladder, although this has not been proved.[51] Excessive urethral elevation or compression may lead to partial outflow obstruction and resulting detrusor instability. Whatever the mechanism, postoperative detrusor instability predictably occurs in a small but significant number of patients. Patients undergoing retropubic urethropexy should understand the possibility that the operation may cause urinary incontinence owing to detrusor instability, even if it cures their sphincteric incontinence.

OSTEITIS PUBIS

Osteitis pubis is a painful inflammation of the periosteum, bone, cartilage, and ligaments of structures of the anterior pelvic girdle.[54] It is a recognized postoperative complication of urologic and radical gynecologic procedures involving the prostate gland or urinary bladder. Osteitis pubis occurs after 2.5% of MMK procedures.[18] It can also occur, although rarely, after placement of artificial urinary sphincters and after radical pelvic surgery for gynecologic malignancies.[55,56] The cause of osteitis pubis is unclear. In noninfectious cases, it may result from trauma to the periosteum or from impaired circulation in the vessels around the symphysis pubis.[57] Krantz has suggested that osteitis pubis after MMK procedures is caused by using cutting rather than tapered needles.[2]

The onset of the disease occurs 2 to 12 weeks postoperatively. Typically osteitis pubis is characterized by suprapubic pain radiating to the thighs and exacerbated by walking or abduction of the lower extremities, marked tenderness and swelling over the symphysis pubis, and radiographic evidence of bone destruction with separation of the symphysis pubis. The clinical course varies from prolonged, progressive debilitation over several months to spontaneous resolution after several weeks. Suggested treatments include rest, physical therapy, steroids, nonsteroidal anti-inflammatory agents, and wedge resection of the symphysis pubis for recalcitrant cases.[58] Noninfectious osteitis pubis, however, tends to be self-limiting, whatever the therapy.

Osteomyelitis of the symphysis pubis has been documented in a small number of cases.[58–60] Diagnosis is made by bone biopsy and bacterial culture. Treatments are antibiotics and incision and drainage, if abscess formation occurs.

ENTEROCELE

Burch first reported that enteroceles occurred in 7.6% of cases as a late complication following the Burch procedure, but only two thirds of these patients required surgical correction.[61] Langer and colleagues reported that 13.6% of patients who had Burch procedures, but no hysterectomy or cul-de-sac obliteration, developed an enterocele 1 to 2 years postoperatively.[62] It is suggested that, whenever possible, a cul-de-sac obliteration in the form of uterosacral plication, Moschcowitz procedure, or McCall culdoplasty be done at the time of retropubic suspension to prevent enterocele formation.

Role of Hysterectomy in the Treatment of Incontinence

Gynecologists frequently perform hysterectomies at the time of retropubic or vaginal surgery for genuine stress incontinence. The general belief has been that the presence of a uterus somehow contributed to the genesis of sphincteric incompetence. The data supporting this belief, however, are scarce. Langer and co-workers assessed the effect of concomitant hysterectomy during Burch colposuspension on the cure rate of genuine stress incontinence.[62] Forty-five patients were randomly assigned to receive colposuspension only or colposuspension plus abdominal hysterectomy and cul-de-sac obliteration. Using urodynamic investigations 6 months after surgery, the rate of cure for stress incontinence between the two groups did not differ statistically (95.5% and 95.7% for the no-hysterectomy and the hysterectomy groups). This study clearly suggests that hysterectomy adds little to the efficacy of Burch colposuspension in curing genuine stress incontinence. In general, hysterectomies should be done only for specific uterine indications or for the treatment of uterovaginal prolapse.

References

1. Marshall VF, Marchetti AA, Krantz KE. The correction of stress incontinence by simple vesicourethral suspension. Surg Gynecol Obstet 1949; 88:509.
2. Krantz KE. The Marshall-Marchetti-Krantz procedure. In: Stanton SL, Tanagho EA, eds. Surgery

of female incontinence. 2nd ed. New York: Springer-Verlag, 1986:87.

3. Tanagho EA. Colpocystourethropexy: The way we do it. J Urol 1976;116:751.

4. Turner-Warwick R. Turner-Warwick vagino-obturator shelf urethral repositioning procedure. In: Debruyne FMJ, van Kerrebroeck EVA, eds. Practical aspects of urinary incontinence. Dordrecht: Martinus Nejhoff Publishers, 1986:100.

5. Webster GD, Kreder KJ. Voiding dysfunction following cystourethropexy: Its evaluation and management. J Urol 1990;144:670.

6. Richardson AC, Edmonds PB, Williams NL. Treatment of stress urinary incontinence due to paravaginal fascial defect. Obstet Gynecol 1981; 57:357.

7. Shull BL, Baden WF. A six-year experience with paravaginal defect repair for stress urinary incontinence. Am J Obstet Gynecol 1989;160:1432.

8. McGuire EM. Urodynamic findings in patients after failure of stress incontinence operations. In: Zinner NR, Sterling AM, eds. Female incontinence. New York: Alan R. Liss, 1981:351.

9. Blaivas JG, Olsson CA. Stress incontinence: Classification and surgical approach. J Urol 1988; 139:727.

10. McGuire EJ, Lytton B, Pepe V, Kohorn EI. Stress urinary incontinence. Obstet Gynecol 1976;47: 255.

11. Stanton SL, Cordozo L, Williams JE, et al. Clinical and urodynamic features of failed incontinence surgery in the female. Obstet Gynecol 1978;51:515.

12. Bhatia NN, Karram MM, Bergman A. Role of antibiotic prophylaxis in retropubic surgery for stress urinary incontinence. Obstet Gynecol 1989;74:637.

13. Haylen BT, Frazer MI, Golovsky D, McInerney RJF. Elevation of the vagina during colposuspension: The use of a Deaver retractor. Br J Urol 1989;63:220.

14. Korda A, Ferry J, Hunter P. Colposuspension for the treatment of female urinary incontinence. Aust NZ J Obstet Gynaecol 1989;29:146.

15. Linder A, Golomb J, Korczak D. Endoscopic control during colposuspension procedure for the treatment of stress urinary incontinence. Eur Urol 1989;16:372.

16. Timmons MC, Addison WA. Suprapubic teloscopy: Extraperitoneal intraoperative technique to demonstrate ureteral patency. Obstet Gynecol 1990;75:137.

17. Gleason DM, Reilly RJ, Pierce JA. Vesical neck suspension under vision with cystotomy enhances treatment of female incontinence. J Urol 1976; 115:555.

18. Mainprize TC, Drutz HP. The Marshall-Marchetti-Krantz procedure: A critical review. Obstet Gynecol Surv 1988;43:724.

19. Milani R, Scalambrino S, Quadri G, et al. Marshall-Marchetti-Krantz procedure and Burch colposuspension in the surgical treatment of female urinary incontinence. Br J Obstet Gynaecol 1985; 92:1050.

20. Park GS, Miller EJ. Surgical treatment of stress urinary incontinence: A comparison of the Kelly plication, Marshall-Marchetti-Krantz, and Pereyra procedures. Obstet Gynecol 1988;71: 575.

21. Bhatia NN, Ostergard DR. Urodynamic effects of retropubic urethropexy in genuine stress incontinence. Am J Obstet Gynecol 1981;140:936.

22. Walter S, Olesen KP, Hald T, et al. Urodynamic evaluation after vaginal repair and colposuspension. Br J Urol 1982;54:377.

23. Kujansuu E. Urodynamic analysis of successful and failed incontinence surgery. Int J Gynaecol Obstet 1983;21:353.

24. Hilton P, Stanton SL. A clinical and urodynamic assessment of the Burch colposuspension for genuine stress incontinence. Br J Obstet Gynaecol 1983;90:934.

25. Mundy AR. A trial comparing the Stamey bladder neck suspension procedure with colposuspension for the treatment of stress incontinence. Br J Urol 1983;55:687.

26. Weil A, Reyes H, Bischoff P, et al. Modifications of the urethral rest and stress profiles after different types of surgery for urinary stress incontinence. Br J Obstet Gynaecol 1984;91:46.

27. Bhatia NN, Bergman A. Modified Burch versus Pereyra retropubic urethropexy for stress urinary incontinence. Obstet Gynecol 1985;66:255.

28. van Geelen JM, Theeuwes AGM, Eskes TKAB, et al. The clinical and urodynamic effects of anterior vaginal repair and Burch colposuspension. Am J Obstet Gynecol 1988;159:137.

29. Bergman A, Koonings PP, Ballard CA. Primary stress urinary incontinence and pelvic relaxation: Prospective randomized comparison of three different operations. Am J Obstet Gynecol 1989; 161:97.

30. Bergman A, Ballard CA, Koonings PP. Comparison of three different surgical procedures for genuine stress incontinence: Prospective randomized study. Am J Obstet Gynecol 1989;160:1102.

31. Penttinen J, Käär K, Kauppila K. Colposuspension and transvaginal bladder neck suspension in the treatment of stress incontinence. Gynecol Obstet Invest 1989;28:101.

32. Thunedborg P, Fischer-Rasmussen W, Jensen SB. Stress urinary incontinence and posterior bladder

suspension defects. Acta Obstet Gynaecol Scand 1990;69:55.

33. Langer R, Golan A, Ron-El R, et al. Colposuspension for urinary stress incontinence in premenopausal and postmenopausal women. Surg Gynecol Obstet 1990;171:13.

34. Eriksen BC, Hagen B, Eik-Nes SH, et al. Long-term effectiveness of the Burch colposuspension in female urinary stress incontinence. Acta Obstet Gynaecol Scand 1990;69:45.

35. Rydhström H, Iosif CS. Urodynamic studies before and after retropubic colpo-urethrocystopexy in fertile women with stress urinary incontinence. Arch Gynecol Obstet 1988;241:201.

36. Galloway NTM, Davies N, Stephenson TP. The complications of colposuspension. Br J Urol 1987;60:122.

37. Gillon G, Stanton SL. Long-term follow-up of surgery for urinary incontinence in elderly women. Br J Urol 1984;56:478.

38. Sand PK, Bowen LW, Ostergard DR, et al. Hysterectomy and prior incontinence surgery as risk factors for failed retropubic cystourethropexy. J Reprod Med 1988;33:171.

39. Wheelan JB. Long-term results of colposuspension. Br J Urol 1990;65:329.

40. Sand PK, Bowen LW, Panganiban R, et al. The low pressure urethra as a factor in failed retropubic urethropexy. Obstet Gynecol 1987;69:399.

41. Koonings PP, Bergman A, Ballard CA. Low urethral pressure and stress urinary incontinence in women: Risk factor for failed retropubic surgical procedure. Urology 1990;36:245.

42. Langer R, Ron-El R, Newman M, et al. Detrusor instability following colposuspension for urinary stress incontinence. Br J Obstet Gynaecol 1988; 95:607.

43. Karram MM, Bhatia NN. Management of coexistent stress and urge urinary incontinence. Obstet Gynecol 1989;73:4.

44. Maulik TG. Kinked ureter with unilateral obstructive uropathy complicating Burch colposuspension. J Urol 1983;130:135.

45. Ferriani RA, Silva de Sá MF, de Moura MD, et al. Ureteral blockage as a complication of Burch colposuspension: Report of 6 cases. Gynecol Obstet Invest 1990;29:239.

46. Lose G, Jørgensen L, Mortensen SO, et al. Voiding difficulties after colposuspension. Obstet Gynecol 1987;69:33.

47. Bhatia NN, Bergman A. Use of preoperative uroflowmetry and simultaneous urethrocystometry for predicting risk of prolonged postoperative bladder drainage. Urology 1986;28:440.

48. Bhatia NN, Bergman A. Urodynamic predictability of voiding following incontinence surgery. Obstet Gynecol 1984;63:85.

49. Sjöberg B. Hydrodynamics of micturition following Marshall-Marchetti-Krantz procedure for stress urinary incontinence. Scand J Urol Nephrol 1982;16:11.

50. Bergman A, Bhatia N. Uroflowmetry for predicting postoperative voiding difficulties in women with stress urinary incontinence. Br J Obstet Gynaecol 1985;92:835.

51. Cardozo LD, Stanton SL, Williams JE. Detrusor instability following surgery for genuine stress incontinence. Br J Urol 1979;51:204.

52. Steel SA, Cox C, Stanton SL. Long-term follow-up of detrusor instability following the colposuspension operation. Br J Urol 1986;58:138.

53. Sand PK, Bowen LW, Ostergard DR, et al. The effect of retropubic urethropexy on detrusor stability. Obstet Gynecol 1988;71:818.

54. Muschat M. Osteitis pubis following prostatectomy. J Urol 1945;54:447.

55. Bouza E, Winston DJ, Hewitt WL. Infectious osteitis pubis. Urology 1978;12:663.

56. Hoyme OB, Tamimi HK, Eschenbach DA, et al. Osteomyelitis pubis after radical gynecologic operations. Obstet Gynecol 1984;63:47S.

57. Turner-Warwick RT. The pathogenesis and treatment of osteitis pubis. Br J Urol 1960;32:464.

58. Rebenack P, Thompson RJ, Wilf LH. Osteomyelitis pubis following a Burch retropubic urethropexy. J Gynecol Surg 1990;6:205.

59. Burns JR, Gregory JG. Osteomyelitis of the pubic symphysis after urologic surgery. J Urol 1977; 118:803.

60. Rosenthal RE, Spickard WA, Markham RD, et al. Osteomyelitis of the symphysis pubis: A separate disease from osteitis pubis. J Bone Joint Surg 1982;64:123.

61. Burch JC. Cooper's ligament urethrovesical suspension for stress incontinence. Am J Obstet Gynecol 1968;100:764.

62. Langer R, Ron-El R, Neuman N, et al. The value of simultaneous hysterectomy during Burch colposuspension for urinary stress incontinence. Obstet Gynecol 1988;72:866.

15

Endoscopic Urethropexy

Deborah R. Erickson

Ernest M. Sussman

Shlomo Raz

The term *stress urinary incontinence* can describe a symptom, sign, or condition. The symptom is the patient's complaint of urine loss during maneuvers that lead to increases in intra-abdominal pressure. The sign is the observation of urine loss during such maneuvers. The condition of stress urinary incontinence is present when urine is lost through the urethra during increases in intra-abdominal pressure, in the absence of a detrusor contraction.

In women, the condition of stress urinary incontinence can be due to one or both of two main causes. The first is displacement or hypermobility of the bladder neck and proximal urethra (anatomic incontinence). It should be emphasized, however, that not all women with urethral hypermobility have stress urinary incontinence. The second cause is intrinsic deficiency of the urethral sphincter mechanism (intrinsic sphincter deficiency [ISD]). The most common reasons for ISD include urethral scarring from prior surgery, radiation, or trauma; postmenopausal atrophy; and some types of neurologic lesions. However, some women have ISD even without any of these conditions.

The goal of surgery for stress urinary incontinence differs according to which cause is responsible. For anatomic incontinence without ISD, the goal of surgery is to restore the urethral sphincter unit to an appropriate retropubic position, without obstruction. The most commonly used procedures for anatomic incontinence are the anterior repair (Kelly plication), the retropubic suspension procedures (Marshall-Marchetti-Krantz, Burch, and so forth) and the endoscopic (needle) bladder neck suspensions (BNS). If ISD is present, the operation should be one that increases urethral coaptation and resistance. The most commonly used procedures for ISD include periurethral injections, the suburethral sling, or placement of an artificial sphincter.

Among the operations available for treatment of anatomic incontinence, we do not recommend the anterior repair because it has a lower long-term success rate than the other procedures. With the choice between an endoscopic BNS or a retropubic suspension, we prefer the endoscopic procedures, unless the patient has concomitant pathology that requires treatment through an abdominal incision (augmentation enterocystoplasty or ureteral reimplantation). The vaginal approach involves less pain, easier postoperative mobilization, and a shorter hospital stay than the abdominal approach.

Female Urology, edited by Elroy D. Kursh and Edward McGuire. J. B. Lippincott, Philadelphia, © 1994.

Anatomy for Bladder Neck Suspension

The structures relevant for anti-incontinence surgery are described first as seen from above then as seen from a vaginal surgeon's viewpoint. The most important contributions to pelvic support are made by the levator ani muscles and their corresponding fascia. When viewed from above, the levator muscles can be seen to originate from the posterior aspects of the pubic bone and the tendinous arcs bilaterally (Fig. 15-1). The muscle fibers extend posteromedially to unite with the fibers from the contralateral side. A U-shaped hiatus separates these muscles anteriorly, and the urethra, vagina, and rectum pass through it.

The superior fascia of the levator ani (endopelvic fascia) contains several specialized condensations that are important for pelvic support (Fig. 15-2). The condensations that suspend the anterior urethra from the undersurface of the pubic bone are called the pubourethral ligaments. Weakness of these ligaments allows posterior and inferior movement of the distal urethra. They do not appear to provide significant support for the bladder neck and proximal urethra.

A broad condensation of levator fascia passes superior to the anterior vaginal wall, extending from one tendinous arc to the other. In its medial portion, this fascia splits into two layers, which envelop the bladder and urethra. The inferior layer, which is essential for support, is called the periurethral fascia at the level of the urethra and the perivesical fascia at the level of the bladder.

The two layers fuse laterally at the edge of the levator hiatus. The fusion of periurethral fascia with levator (endopelvic) fascia extends to the anterior pubic bone and tendinous arcs, so the urethra is suspended from these structures (Fig. 15-3). This fusion is most appropriately called the *urethropelvic ligament* to emphasize its anatomic course and its role in supporting the urethra from the pelvis. In a similar manner at the level of the bladder, the perivesical fascia fuses with the levator fascia and extends laterally to the tendinous arcs. For this structure, the name *vesicopelvic ligaments* is descriptive of its anatomic course and its role in supporting the bladder.

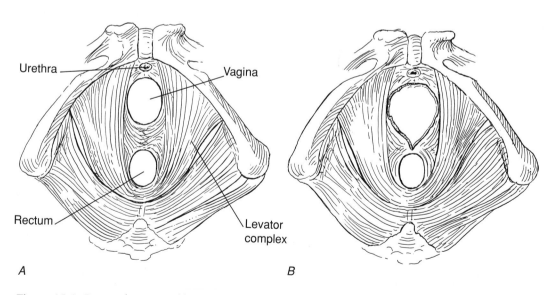

A　　　　　　　　　　　　　　　　*B*

Figure 15-1. *Retropubic view of levator complex providing the major support of the bladder and urethra.*

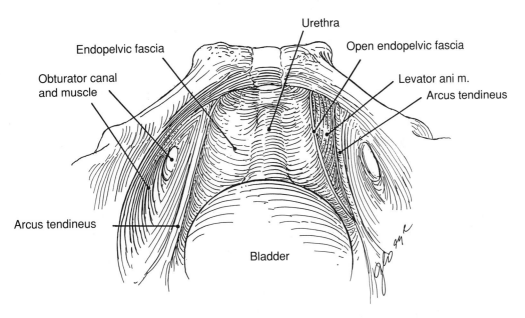

Figure 15-2. *Figure demonstrating specialized condensations of the endopelvic fascia* (Note: *Endopelvic fascia is opened on the right where we enter during the Raz BNS.*)

Other condensations of endopelvic fascia include the cardinal ligaments, which support the cervix from the pelvic side wall, and the uterosacral ligaments, which extend from the posterolateral cervix to the fourth sacral vertebra. Because these ligaments do not provide support to the anterior bladder and urethra, they are not generally used in anti-incontinence surgery. Their strength makes them valuable for repair of cystoceles, enteroceles, and high rectoceles.

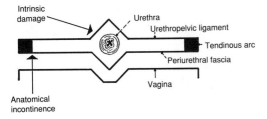

Figure 15-3. *Relationship of periurethral fascia and urethropelvic ligament with its subsequent fusion and insertion to the tendinous arc laterally.*

The vaginal view of pelvic support is best envisioned by considering the anterior vaginal wall after a midline incision is made and the vaginal epithelium is reflected laterally. The urethropelvic ligaments, with their glistening white fascia, extend laterally like two wings to support the urethra. Dissection along these ligaments is stopped by their fusion to the tendinous arcs. More proximally, the vesicopelvic ligaments extend laterally to suspend the bladder from the tendinous arcs. The lateral aspects of the urethropelvic and vesicopelvic ligaments are superior to the levator hiatus. Thus, the vaginal surgeon must reflect the levator muscles laterally to visualize the junctions of these ligaments with the tendinous arcs.

The *pubocervical fascia* is mentioned in some texts, but its exact structure is not always clearly defined. The description most often encountered is that of a condensation of endopelvic fascia that extends from the anterolateral cervix to the back of the pubic bone. From this description, it appears that the pubocervical fascia is a name for the medial portions of the urethropelvic and vesicopelvic ligaments. We prefer to use these anatomic names because pubocervical fascia does not reflect the exact location or supportive function of these structures.

History of Bladder Neck Suspension

The needle BNS was first described by Pereyra in 1959.[1] Since then, several modifications have been developed, both by Pereyra and by others. These modifications have developed in an effort to provide for continued improvement, safety, and efficacy in the performance of these procedures (Fig. 15-4). The highlights of the history of this progression in technique are summarized followed later by a thorough description of our preferred method of BNS, the Raz procedure.

In the original Pereyra procedure, a trocarcannula system was passed from a suprapubic stab incision into the vagina.[1] After the trocar was withdrawn, this brought the ends of the wire loop alongside the urethra to the suprapubic incision. After this procedure was performed bilaterally, the ends of the wire loops were tied over the abdominal fascia.

Two modifications of this procedure were developed by Pereyra and Lebherz, first working independently and then in conjunction for the second one, to address the problem of suture pull-through.[2,3] In the final Pereyra modification, a midline vaginal incision was made to expose the urethropelvic ligaments.[3] The lateral attachments of these ligaments were perforated to allow passage of the trocar through the retropubic space with fingertip guidance and to allow placement of nonabsorbable helical sutures through the entire urethropelvic and pubourethral ligaments.

An important contribution to the advancement of the needle BNS was made by Stamey, who introduced the use of cystoscopy to ensure correct placement of the suspending sutures and to check for bladder or urethral injury.[4] In the Stamey procedure, a long needle is passed from a small suprapubic incision to the vagina at the level of the bladder neck. Correct needle position is verified by cystoscopic visualization of the indentation created by the needle against the bladder neck. Withdrawal of the needle brings one end of a nonabsorbable suture to the suprapubic incision. A second needle pass, lateral to the first, brings the other end, so a loop of suture (often buttressed with a Dacron sleeve) is left alongside the bladder neck. Suspending sutures are placed bilaterally, and the ends are tied over the abdominal fascia.

Cobb and Ragde described the use of a double-pronged needle that created a consistent

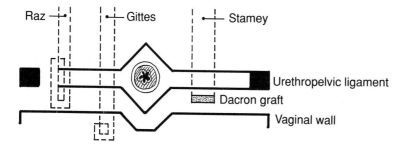

Transvaginal suspensions

Figure 15-4. Transvaginal BNS. (Note: Raz BNS maintains more lateral placement of the suspending sutures.)

1-cm bridge of abdominal fascia between the two suture ends and allowed both ends to be brought to the suprapubic incision with one needle pass.[5] A barrel knot was tied into the center of each nonabsorbable suture to buttress the suspension.

For the Gittes modification, no vaginal or abdominal incisions are used.[6] Bilateral nonabsorbable sutures are placed into the full-thickness vaginal wall at the level of the bladder neck. On each side, a needle is passed into the vagina through a small suprapubic stab puncture. The suture ends are transferred to the suprapubic area and tied independently over the fascia. After a short period, the vaginal sutures are re-epithelialized. An advantage of this procedure is that in most cases it can be performed under local anesthesia.

Raz in 1981 described his version of the original Pereyra procedure, which had essentially two major modifications from the 1978 Pereyra and Lebherz procedure.[7] The first difference was that the incision was made in the form of an inverted U rather than in the midline, so dissection along the periurethral and paraurethral fasciae could take place away from the urethra and bladder neck. The other contribution was the incorporation of the vaginal wall without its epithelium at the level of the bladder neck in addition to the urethropelvic ligament.

Preoperative Preparation

A complete history and physical examination should be performed to determine the type of incontinence present and identify concomitant pathology. Urine infection should be sought and eradicated if present. Laboratory, radiologic, or other preoperative testing should be done as needed according to the patient's medical condition.

The urologic evaluation for endoscopic urethropexy has certain goals, which are described separately. The extent of urologic evaluation required is related to the complexity of the presentation:

1. The first goal is to make the subjective and objective clinical diagnosis of stress urinary incontinence. The subjective diagnosis is made from the patient's history. The objective diagnosis is most commonly made by direct observation of leakage through the urethra during stress maneuvers. Confirmation of leakage can also be made by fluoroscopic examination of the contrast medium–filled bladder during straining maneuvers (videourodynamics). One caveat about these tests is that if the intravesical pressure is not simultaneously monitored (dynamic cystography without urodynamics), incontinence due to stress-induced detrusor instability may be misdiagnosed as "genuine" stress urinary incontinence.

2. The next goal is to determine whether the stress urinary incontinence is due to anatomic incontinence, ISD, or both. It is seldom possible to make a definite decision based on any single test, so the entire clinical picture must be considered. In the history, patients with pure bladder neck hypermobility usually describe mild to moderate stress urinary incontinence, with leakage occurring mainly during vigorous activity. Patients with ISD tend to have severe incontinence and leak with minimal activity. On physical examination, patients with hypermobility have visible descent of the bladder neck and proximal urethra during stress maneuvers, and the leakage stops after the unobstructed elevation of the bladder neck (Marshall test). Demonstration of stress urinary incontinence through a correctly positioned retropubic urethra is diagnostic of ISD.

   Endoscopically urethroscopy in patients with anatomic incontinence reveals hypermobility and funneling when visualizing the proximal urethra while the patient coughs and strains. Urethral coaptation also can be assessed endoscopically; a persistently open, fixed urethra suggests ISD. Radiologically most patients with anatomic incontinence have a closed bladder neck at rest. Patients with ISD have an open bladder neck at rest and may demonstrate leakage while standing still. (*Note*: Detrusor instability also can cause an open bladder neck at rest and leakage of contrast material while standing still.) On the other hand, a closed bladder neck at rest does not rule out ISD.

For these and other complex cases, videourodynamic studies still provide the most accurate information. Continuous monitoring of both the intravesical and intraabdominal pressures provides accurate information about detrusor activity simultaneously with fluoroscopic visualization. Correlation of flow with intravesical pressure (pressure-flow study) also helps to determine the presence or degree of obstruction (most commonly iatrogenic from previous suspension surgery).

Videourodynamics can also be used to determine the Valsalva leak point pressure. The patient is asked to perform a slow Valsalva maneuver in the standing position, with fluoroscopic monitoring. When contrast medium is seen to leak into the proximal urethra, the intravesical pressure is observed. If the pressure is less than 30–60 cm water, this strongly suggests ISD.

3. The third goal of the preoperative evaluation is to determine the degree of anterior vaginal wall prolapse. It is especially important to recognize a cystocele because BNS without concurrent repair of this anterior vaginal wall prolapse can result in obstruction. This is thought to be due to a kinking effect as the cystocele hangs down below the supported bladder neck. A cystocele can be identified as an anterior vaginal bulge during the physical examination. Additional anatomic information defining the degree of descent can best be obtained from the lateral cystogram (the "physical examination in the standing position"). Vaginal techniques for cystocele repair are easily combined with endoscopic bladder neck suspension.

4. The fourth goal is to identify other forms of vaginal wall prolapse, such as rectocele, en-terocele, or uterine prolapse. Vaginal techniques to repair these defects are conveniently performed at the same time as the BNS. The decision for repair should be made according to the findings on examination of the unanesthetized patient. After anesthesia, the degree of prolapse is commonly found to be overestimated or underestimated.

5. The fifth goal is to evaluate for bladder instability because stress urinary incontinence is often accompanied by urgency or urge incontinence. The patient's history does not always correlate with the cystometric findings. Some women have asymptomatic instability, and others with symptoms of urgency and urge incontinence do not demonstrate instability on cystometry. We do perform cystometry in women with symptoms of instability, to look for abnormalities in bladder sensation, capacity, or compliance that may suggest a more serious underlying disorder. The decision to perform BNS for patients who complain of both stress urinary incontinence and urgency incontinence must be made after careful evaluation. If the history, physical examination, cystoscopy, and urodynamic findings confirm that genuine anatomic stress urinary incontinence is present, we perform BNS. However, we do warn the patient that the urge incontinence might not resolve after BNS.

6. The urologic evaluation should ensure adequate bladder emptying. Post-void residuals should be measured before performing anti-incontinence surgery. Patients with a high residual or those complaining of obstructive symptoms require further investigation to evaluate for obstruction or poor bladder contractility.

Technique of Raz Bladder Neck Suspension

PREOPERATIVE CONSIDERATIONS

For the simple BNS without simultaneous repair of other vaginal prolapse, preparation begins the evening before surgery with tap water enemas until clear and povidone-iodine douches. Intravenous antibiotics (aminoglycoside and cefazolin) are started preoperatively and continued for 24 hours after surgery. General or spinal anesthesia can be used. The patient is placed in the high lithotomy position using candy cane stirrups, with the feet protected in foam boots. The lower abdomen and perineum are prepared and draped in the usual sterile manner.

Several options can be used to treat the occasional patient with temporary postoperative urinary retention. One is to leave an indwelling urethral catheter and perform intermittent voiding trials. Another is to have the patient learn self-catheterization. A third option is to place a suprapubic tube during the anti-incontinence procedure. We believe that a suprapubic tube is more comfortable for the patient than the other alternatives. Either a percutaneous insertion or an open procedure can be used. To avoid the difficulties with dislodgment and leakage associated with some percutaneous tubes, yet maintain the ease of percutaneous tube placement, we have devised a method for placing a Foley suprapubic tube using a Lowsley tractor.[8]

The Lowsley tractor is inserted through the urethra and pointed against the anterior bladder and abdominal wall 3 cm superior to the symphysis pubis. A stab incision is made over the palpable tip of the tractor. The tractor emerges through the stab incision and grasps the end of a 16 French Foley catheter. The tractor then brings the end of the catheter out through the urethra. A tonsil clamp is then placed on the tip of the catheter to push it back into the bladder. The tonsil clamp is pressed against the posterior bladder (anterior vaginal) wall to indicate intravesical placement, and the balloon is inflated. Irrigation of the catheter reconfirms intravesical position before the tonsil clamp is released. The catheter is pulled with traction against the anterior bladder and abdominal wall to achieve hemostasis and prevent leakage during the procedure.

STEP 1 (FIG. 15-5)

Another 16 French Foley catheter is inserted per urethra, and an Allis clamp is placed on the anterior vaginal wall in the midline, halfway between the external meatus and the bladder neck. Bilateral oblique incisions are made (1 cm medial to the lateral vaginal walls), from the level of the Allis clamp extending 3 to 4 cm posterior to the bladder neck. The anterior vaginal wall is infiltrated with saline just before this to facilitate dissection.

STEP 2

The dissection is begun very superficially, staying right along the glistening surface of the urethropelvic ligaments. The lateral aspects of the urethropelvic ligaments are covered by fibers of the levator muscle (Fig. 15-6). Thus, the scissors must proceed between the glistening fascia and

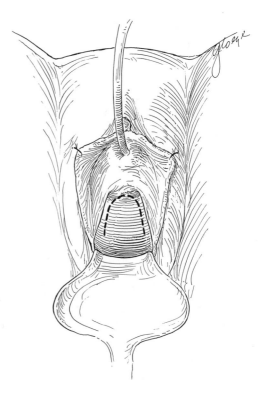

Figure 15-5. *Inverted-U incision in vaginal wall.*

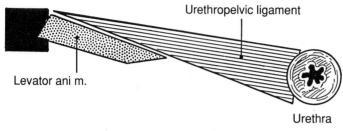

Tendinous arc

Urethropelvic ligament

Levator ani m.

Urethra

Figure 15-6. *Relationship of urethropelvic ligament with the levator complex being intimately associated anterolaterally as the dissection proceeds toward the tendinous arc.*

the levator fibers. Dissection continues toward the juncture of the urethropelvic ligament with the tendinous arc.

STEP 3 (FIG. 15-7)

Closed scissors are used to perforate this junction, aiming toward the ipsilateral shoulder. Through this opening, the retropubic space is entered, and blunt finger dissection is used to mobilize the lateral edge of the urethropelvic ligament from the pubic bone and tendinous arc. If the patient has had prior anti-incontinence surgery, sharp dissection may be necessary.

STEP 4 (FIG. 15-8)

Number 1 polypropylene sutures (Ethicon special order MO-5 or MO-6) are placed through two structures, both at the level of the bladder neck. First, several helical passes are made through the anterior vaginal wall, excluding the epithelium but including the underlying vesicopelvic ligaments. Inclusion of these ligaments adds to the support and provides for correction of concomitant small or mild cystoceles. For the second step, long (Russian) forceps are extended into the retropubic space, opened, and pushed medially to expose the freed lateral edge of the previously freed urethropelvic ligament. Several passes are made through this strong anchoring tissue

("good stuff"), again at the level of the bladder neck. Care is taken to include only the lateral edge and to remain at the level of the bladder neck, so urethral injury or obstruction can be avoided. The strength of the anchoring tissues is tested by placing traction on these sutures.

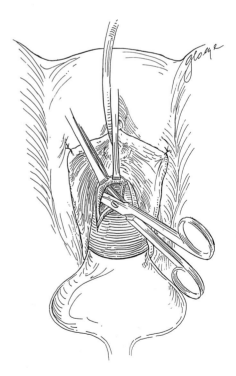

Figure 15-7. *Entrance into the retropubic space.*

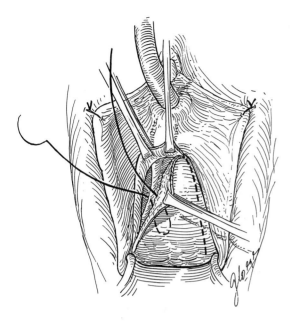

Figure 15-8. *Prolene suture incorporating both the urethropelvic ligament and the anterior vaginal wall without its epithelium.*

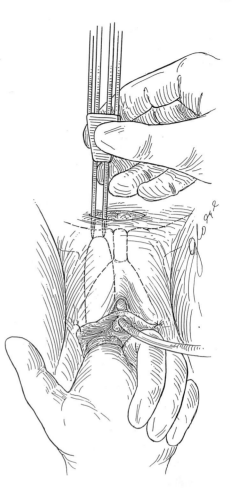

Figure 15-9. *Double-pronged ligature carrier being passed with finger guidance.*

STEP 5

A small transverse suprapubic incision is carried sharply to the level of the anterior rectus fascia. The double-pronged needle is passed from this incision out through the vagina with a retropubically placed finger providing constant guidance (Fig. 15-9). Correct needle placement is important to avoid injury and to prevent postoperative pain from traction on the suspending sutures. The needle should be placed through an immobile portion of the abdominal fascia, close to the midline and as close to the pubic bone as possible. The needle tips literally scratch the periosteum. The ends of the suspending sutures are placed through the needles, which are withdrawn, transferring the suture ends to the suprapubic incision.

STEP 6

After a previous intravenous injection of indigo carmine, cystoscopy is performed to (1) check

for suprapubic tube placement, (2) exclude bladder or urethral injury, (3) rule out ureteral injury by observing for blue efflux from each orifice, and (4) ensure that the proximal urethra and bladder neck are well elevated when the suspending sutures are pulled upward.

STEP 7

The vaginal incisions are closed with a running locked no. 2–0 braided absorbable suture before the suspending sutures are tied over the abdominal fascia (Fig. 15-10). The suprapubic incision

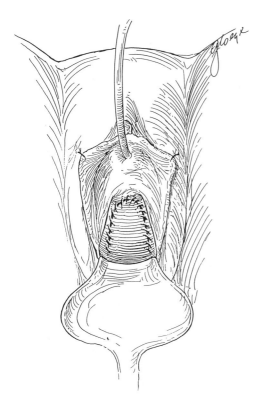

Figure 15-10. Completed closure of anterior vaginal wall.

is then closed subcuticularly. An antibiotic-soaked vaginal pack is placed. The urethral and suprapubic catheters are left to gravity drainage.

POSTOPERATIVE CONSIDERATIONS

On the first postoperative day, the patient ambulates and is placed on a regular diet. The urethral catheter and vaginal pack are removed. The suprapubic tube is plugged, and voiding trials are instituted. If the patient cannot void, the tube is unplugged every 3 hours (or sooner if the bladder is uncomfortably full) to drain the bladder. Discharge with the suprapubic tube in place is usually on the second postoperative day. The tube is removed later on during the first postoperative week or when the residuals are consistently less than 60 ml.

Results

We recently reported on a long-term retrospective review covering 225 patients who underwent the Raz BNS between 1984 and June of 1990 for the condition of stress urinary incontinence.[9] A total of 206 patients were available for follow-up, with a mean of 15 months and a median of 8 months. Overall, 171 (83%) women were cured (no stress incontinence) with an additional 15 (7.3%) patients receiving significant improvement (rare stress incontinence), giving successful results in 90.3% of this study population.

None of the following demographic parameters were found to be statistically significant with regard to predicting the success of our procedure: age, number and type of prior anti-incontinence procedures, hysterectomy, menopause, or presence of urgency incontinence preoperatively. Only the preoperative subjective severity of stress urinary incontinence was found to be predictive ($P < 0.001$). Of the 23 patients with severe stress urinary incontinence before surgery, a 35% failure rate was encountered.

For the 20 of 206 (9.7%) patients who failed, the median time to recurrent stress incontinence was 5 months. Complications included de novo urgency incontinence (11%), secondary prolapse (6%), prolonged retention (2.5%), and suprapubic pain (3%). We are pleased with the results of our procedure for the correction of stress urinary incontinence. In addition, urethrolysis for the correction of concomitant obstruction along with the reduction of other forms of vaginal prolapse can be simultaneously performed.

References

1. Pereyra AJ. A simplified surgical procedure for the correction of stress incontinence in women. West J Surg 1959;67:223.
2. Pereyra AJ, Lebherz TB. Combined urethral vesical suspension vaginal urethroplasty for correction of urinary stress incontinence. Obstet Gynecol 1967;30:537.
3. Pereyra AJ, Lebherz TB. The revised Pereyra procedure. In: Buchsbaum H, Schmidt JD, eds. *Gyne-*

cologic and obstetric urology. 1st ed. Philadelphia: WB Saunders, 1978:208–222.

4. Stamey TA. Endoscopic suspension of the vesical neck for urinary incontinence. Surg Gynecol Obstet 1973;136:547.

5. Cobb OE, Ragde H. Simplified correction of female stress incontinence. J Urol 1978;120:418.

6. Gittes RF, Loughlin KR. No-incision pubovaginal sling suspension for stress incontinence. J Urol 1987;138:568.

7. Raz S. Modified bladder neck suspension for female stress incontinence. Urology 1981;17:82.

8. Zeidman EJ, Chiang H, Alarcon A, Raz S. Suprapubic cystostomy using Lowsley retractor. Urology 1988;32:54.

9. Raz S, Sussman EM, Erickson DR, Bregg KJ, Nitti VW. The Raz bladder neck suspension results in 206 patients. J Urol 1992;148:845.

16

No-Incision Endoscopic Urethropexy

Elroy D. Kursh

Endoscopic urethropexy has been popularized as an effective means of correcting stress urinary incontinence.[1,2] The procedure for performing endoscopic urethropexy continues to evolve, and a number of modifications have been described, the most recent being the no-incision technique described by Gittes and Loughlin in 1987.[3] The technique is based on their laboratory observation in rats and guinea pigs that monofilament mattress sutures placed through the outside of the abdominal skin and tied under tension cut through the skin and become internalized and accepted without any residual inflammation if the knot is buried initially. This principle was used to simplify the endoscopic approach to urethropexy further by eliminating the vaginal incision, whereby the knot becomes buried in the submucosa of the vagina to provide support of the urethra.

Based on their laboratory investigations, the authors described how the suspensory sutures provide support. As the mattress sutures cut through the vaginal wall, a band or curtain of scar tissue is formed to link the tough thick vaginal wall with the inferior loop of the suspending suture. Superiorly the suspending suture presumably remains well anchored to the rectus fascia and muscle. Therefore a two-link chain is formed on each side that connects the vaginal wall to the rectus fascia. When the patient coughs, the chain links hold and prevent urethral descent and leakage.[3]

Preoperative Assessment and Patient Selection

When selecting a particular surgical technique for correction of stress incontinence, it is essential to obtain an accurate menstrual history, ascertain if the patient is taking estrogen replacement therapy, and examine the condition of the vagina to gage the strength of the mucosa and degree of atrophy if it is present. In my review of patients undergoing the no-incision technique, it is noteworthy that there were no failures in premenopausal women, and the cure rate was significantly better in the premenopausal patients compared with the postmenopausal group ($P < 0.001$).[4] Therefore, when employing the no-incision technique, a successful outcome appears to depend on the strength and integrity of the vaginal mucosa. Excellent results can be expected in premenopausal women, but patients with weak atrophic vaginal mucosa are less likely to have a successful outcome.

A significant correlation between the success rate and grade of incontinence was also observed

Female Urology, edited by Elroy D. Kursh and Edward McGuire. J. B. Lippincott, Philadelphia, © 1994.

$(P < 0.001)$.[4] Therefore it is important to take an accurate history regarding the causes, frequency, and volume of incontinence. I prefer to grade the incontinence using the method described by Stamey.[5] Grade 1 incontinence refers to that which occurs with severe stress only, such as during coughing, sneezing, straining, or aerobic exercise. Grade 2 stress incontinence is the designation used for incontinence that occurs during the course of an individual's daily activities, such as walking, getting out of a chair, or climbing stairs. Patients with grade 3 stress incontinence experience total or almost total incontinence. Because fewer than 50% of the patients with grade 3 stress incontinence had a favorable outcome using the no-incision approach, my current practice is to use other surgical techniques for correction of patients with high-grade (grade 3) stress incontinence, unless the patients are premenopausal or clearly have strong vaginal mucosa.

I do not advocate a standardized evaluation for all patients with stress urinary incontinence. Patients with symptoms of bladder irritability undergo cystoscopy to rule out an underlying cause. Stress urinary incontinence is documented in all patients during a vaginal examination with a full bladder or at the time of cystoscopy after bladder filling. Urodynamics are obtained in those patients with symptoms of detrusor instability or recurrent stress incontinence or for complex cases of incontinence and are done in approximately 50% of patients. Radiologic investigation is used only for complex cases of recurrent stress incontinence. Although urethral profilometry has been shown to have limited merit,[6] I think that it is helpful in defining patients with type III stress incontinence (intrinsic sphincter deficiency) along with a careful physical examination and radiographic studies to assess the degree of urethral hypermobility.

Because of the high incidence of urinary retention, patients should be informed preoperatively to anticipate using a suprapubic cystostomy tube for a varying period of time after surgery.[3,4,7]

Preoperative Preparation

In view of the data presented regarding the superior results noted in premenopausal women, when it is anticipated using a no-incision endoscopic technique in postmenopausal patients, they are started on estrogen replacement therapy approximately 1 month before surgery is scheduled.[4] Patients are instructed to use an application of vaginal estrogen cream daily starting 1 month preoperatively, and this is continued for 6 weeks postoperatively. Vaginal estrogens are also given even if the patients are taking another form of estrogen replacement therapy because the strength of the vagina may be dose dependent.

Care is taken to insure sterilization of the urine preoperatively. If there is evidence of a urinary tract infection, it is treated according to the culture and sensitivity data before surgery is performed. Patients are admitted to the hospital on the day of surgery. Prophylactic intravenous antibiotics are administered, usually a cephalosporin.

Surgical Technique

Although others have emphasized that local anesthesia can be used, I prefer to employ other forms of anesthesia if at all possible.[3] The few patients who had local anesthesia experienced modest pain during the operation, and it was somewhat difficult to maintain the lithotomy position or gain adequate vaginal exposure to suture the anterior vaginal mucosa when creating the autologous pledget. In my series, general anesthesia was used in 80% of the patients, spinal in 16%, and epidural and local anesthesia in the remaining patients.[4]

In an attempt to reduce postoperative pain, many patients who underwent general or spinal anesthesia had injection of bupivacaine hydrochloride (Marcaine) into the suprapubic incisions and retropubic space. Because the injection of local anesthetic did not appear to alter the postoperative course, it is no longer administered.

The patient is placed in the lithotomy position with legs suspended in Allen universal stirrups. These stirrups are particularly easy to manipulate to facilitate proper positioning. An exaggerated lithotomy position is avoided to keep the abdomen relatively flat. It is important to position the buttocks low enough on the operating table to provide good vaginal exposure.

The vaginal, genital, and abdominal area is prepared with povidone-iodine. The patient is draped to afford exposure to the vaginal and suprapubic areas. Care is taken to drape off the rectum well to prevent contamination from this area. A 20 French Foley catheter is placed in the urethra, and the balloon is inflated with approximately 10 ml of air. If the surgeon desires, he or she can measure urethral length by holding the catheter firmly against the bladder neck while a hemostat is placed on the catheter at the urethral meatus. The balloon is deflated, the catheter is removed, and measurement from the hemostat to the Foley balloon provides the approximate urethral length. Generally in patients with significant stress urinary incontinence, the urethra is quite short, measuring between 2 and 3 cm.

Three stab incisions are made in the suprapubic area using a no. 15 blade. The initial incision is a longitudinal stab in the midline made approximately a fingerbreadth above the symphysis pubis for later placement of the suprapubic cystostomy tube. Two transverse stab incisions are made at the level of the upper border of the symphysis pubis, each being about 1.5 cm from the midline stab (Fig. 16-1). It is emphasized that the stab incision should not be made much more lateral than this because the rectus fascia is stronger medially, and a better suspension can be achieved medially rather than run the risk of holding the bladder neck in an open position by sutures suspending in a lateral direction.

A standard Stamey needle is passed on the medial aspect of one of the suprapubic stab sites. Generally it is preferable to use a 30-degree needle for the no-incision technique. The needle

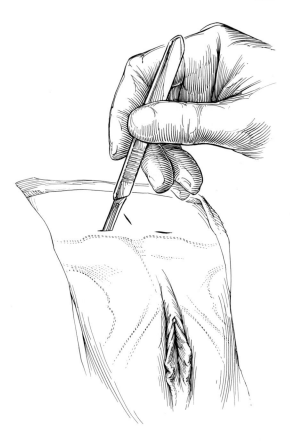

Figure 16-1. Three stab incisions are made in the suprapubic area. A longitudinal incision is made in the midline just above the symphysis, and two transverse stab incisions are made at the upper border of the symphysis pubis. (From Kursh ED. No-incision endoscopic urethropexy. Cont Urol 1991;3:50.)

is held perpendicular to the rectus fascia and is passed through it. The surgeon must exercise care in maintaining good control of the tip of the needle so it passes just through the fascia and not much further. The distal tip of the needle is pushed down on the abdomen so the proximal end scapes the posterior surface of the symphysis pubis as the needle is advanced approximately 1 cm. It is at this point only that the surgeon places the examining left hand in the vagina. The

Foley catheter is draped over the palm of the left hand as the Stamey needle is rotated upward from the abdominal position. The needle is teased up and down in an anterior-posterior direction so the surgeon can palpate its tip. Slight traction on the Foley catheter facilitates palpation of the bladder neck area. The Stamey needle tip is advanced to a position just lateral to the bladder neck. It is emphasized that it is unnecessary to place the needle close or immediately adjacent to the bladder neck because there is a much greater risk of entering the bladder or bladder neck area with the needle. Additionally, excellent support can be achieved with supporting sutures placed slightly lateral to the bladder neck without running the risk of injuring the bladder or urethra. An excellent way of determining the proper position for the needle tip is to walk the needle from lateral to medial at the bladder neck area. As the surgeon walks the needle tip medially, the amount of tissue between the tip of the needle and the vagina becomes thicker, indicating that the needle is positioned too close to the bladder neck. The needle can be rotated slightly more lateral to the location where the amount of tissue thins out again. This is the proper site for placement of the initial pass of the needle. The needle is pushed through the supporting urethral fascia and vaginal mucosa between the index and long fingers (Fig. 16-2).

Now that the first pass of the Stamey needle is completed, cystoscopy is performed using a 70-degree lens to confirm that the needle has not penetrated the bladder or bladder neck (Fig. 16-3). Because the needle is most likely to enter the anterior surface of the bladder, this area is inspected carefully. By rotating the top of the Stamey needle in an anterior and posterior direction, the surgeon can often observe the indentation in the bladder wall that marks the track of the needle. The approximate placement of the needle site can be verified by bobbing the upper end of the needle in and out in an anterior to posterior direction; movement of the bladder neck indicates proper positioning.

A no. 2 polypropylene suture is passed through the eye of the needle, and the needle is withdrawn to deliver one end of the suture from the vaginal area to the suprapubic area (Fig. 16-4). Hemostats are placed on both sides of the suture.

A second pass of the Stamey needle is carried out in the same manner approximately 1 to 1.5 cm lateral to the initial pass. This is achieved by moving the lateral end of the stab incision as far lateral as possible before penetrating the rectus fascia. Before the second pass of the needle is advanced through the vaginal mucosa, it is helpful to have an assistant keep the suture that has already been passed taut by holding each end so the site of perforation in the vagina can be easily palpated. The laterally passed needle must not be passed more than a centimeter or so lateral to the initial supporting suture to prevent tenting up so much vaginal mucosa that the supporting suture lacks a good site of fixation. With each pass of the needle, repeat cystoscopy is done to ensure that the bladder has not been entered and that the needle has been properly positioned.

After the second pass of the Stamey needle, the needle remains in place while a weighted vaginal speculum provides exposure of the vagina. The vaginal end of the no. 2 polypropylene suture is threaded onto a Mayo needle and three to four deep bites of vaginal mucosa are taken in several different directions but generally entering the vaginal mucosa near the exit site of the Stamey needle to exit near the previously placed suture (Fig. 16-5). It is helpful to grasp the vaginal mucosa just lateral to the exit site of the second Stamey needle pass or medial to the previously passed suture with a long Allis clamp, which an assistant holds to facilitate vaginal exposure. A lateral vaginal retractor may also enhance exposure. After several good bites of vaginal mucosa are obtained, the free vaginal end of the suture is passed through the eye of the Stamey needle and delivered to the suprapubic area. This completes placement of the supporting suture on one side of the bladder neck. The vaginal speculum is removed, and the procedure is repeated on the other side of the bladder neck.

After both supporting sutures are placed, cystoscopy and urethroscopy are done with a

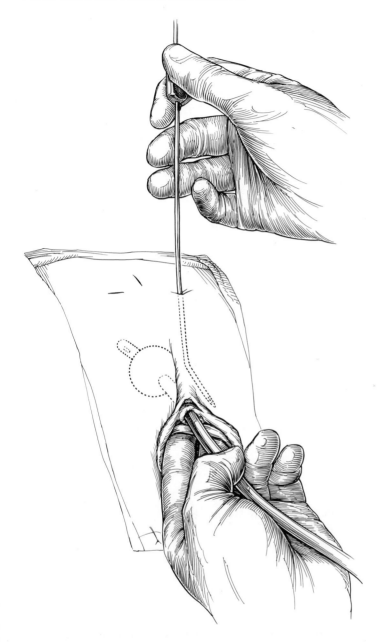

Figure 16-2. *The Stamey needle is advanced through the supporting urethral fascia and vaginal mucosa between the index and long fingers. (From Kursh ED. No-incision endoscopic urethropexy. Cont Urol 1991;3:50.)*

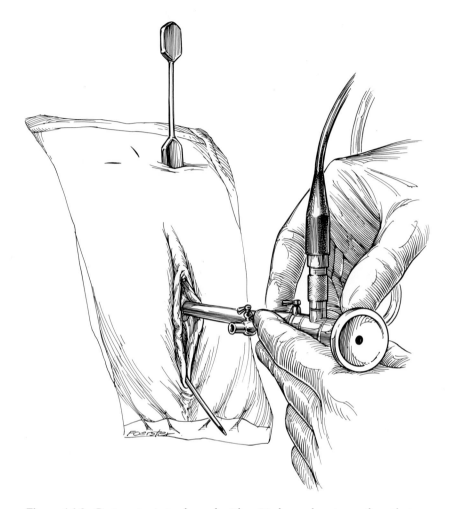

Figure 16-3. *Cystoscopy is performed with a 70-degree lens to confirm that the needle has not penetrated the bladder and that the needle is properly positioned adjacent to the bladder neck. (From Kursh ED. No-incision endoscopic urethropexy. Cont Urol 1991;3:50.)*

30-degree lens. An open bladder neck, especially if it is opened by posterior rotation of the distal tip of the cystoscope, should be discernible (Fig. 16-6). Elevation of the previously placed supporting sutures in the suprapubic area produces excellent closure of the bladder neck, and often a typical "smile" configuration is assumed at its corners (Fig. 16-7). Physiologic testing can also be performed. After bladder filling, the fluid

flows freely from the urethral meatus, especially when the bladder neck is rotated downward into an open position with the tip of the cystoscope. Elevation of either one or both of the suprapubic sutures should readily interrupt the flow of fluid (Fig. 16-8).

After maximal bladder filling, a punch suprapubic cystostomy tube, generally a 12 French size, is placed using cystoscopic guidance (Fig.

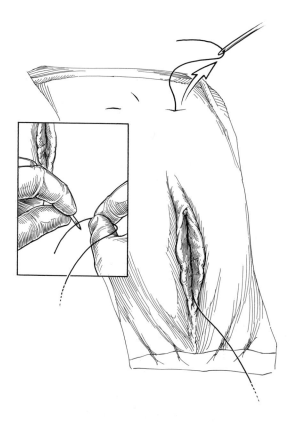

Figure 16-4. The eye of the Stamey needle is threaded with a no. 2 polypropylene suture. When the needle is withdrawn, one end of the suture is delivered from the vaginal area to the suprapubic area. (From Kursh ED. No-incision endoscopic urethropexy. Cont Urol 1991;3:50.)

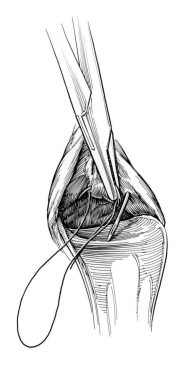

Figure 16-5. After the second pass of the Stamey needle, the vaginal end of the suture is threaded onto a Mayo needle. Several deep bites of vaginal mucosa are taken before threading the free end of the suture into the eye of the Stamey needle and delivering it to the suprapubic area. (From Kursh ED. No-incision endoscopic urethropexy. Cont Urol 1991;3:50.)

16-9). The patient is rotated to a Trendelenburg position to help bring the small bowel out of the pelvis and reduce the risk of small bowel injury. I prefer to use a Stamey type Malecot punch cystostomy tube because of its ease of placement and removal. Through the previously placed midline stab incision, the tube is advanced straight down, or its tip is angled slightly superiorly, which in fact represents tube passage approximately 20 degrees superiorly owing to the Trendelenburg position. Proper positioning is confirmed cystoscopically, and the tube is su-

tured in place with two 2–0 Prolene sutures. An indwelling urethral catheter is not employed.

The previously placed urethropexy supporting sutures are tied in the suprapubic stab sites with multiple knots. I prefer to tie the sutures snugly to achieve good urethral support and provide the greatest likelihood of a successful outcome, but it is emphasized that the sutures do not have to be tied overly tight. The suprapubic stab wounds are closed with one subcuticular stitch of 4–0 undyed Vicryl. Steri-Strips are also placed. At times, the stab sites are so small that it is impossible to place the subcuticular stitch, and Steri-Strips are used alone. If the surgeon so chooses, urethral length can be remeasured to

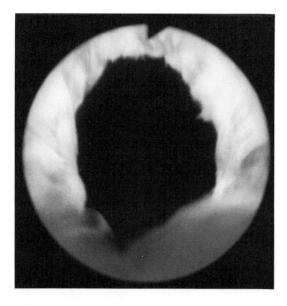

Figure 16-6. *An open bladder neck is visible on inspecting the urethra with a 30-degree lens.*

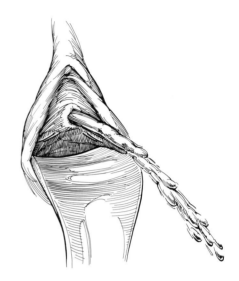

Figure 16-8. *With the bladder neck rotated downward into an open position and the bladder full, the fluid flows freely from the urethral meatus. Elevation of either one or both of the suprapubic sutures interrupts the flow. (From Kursh ED. No-incision endoscopic urethropexy. Cont Urol 1991;3:50.)*

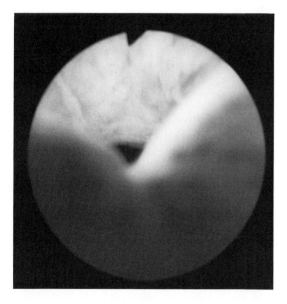

Figure 16-7. *Elevation of the supporting sutures in the suprapubic area closes the bladder neck; a typical "smile" configuration is often assumed.*

quantify the change in urethral length after placement of the urethropexy sutures.

The no-incision technique can be used in association with concomitant gynecologic surgery, such as a vaginal hysterectomy or vaginal repair of one form or another. If the anterior vaginal wall is not dissected during the gynecologic portion of the operation, it is unnecessary to extend the vaginal incision to perform a Raz or Stamey procedure, and the no-incision technique can be used instead in appropriately selected cases. The no-incision urethropexy was performed in association with concomitant gynecologic surgery in 25% of the patients operated on in my series.[4] Approximately one half of these women underwent vaginal hysterectomy and anterior or posterior vaginal repair, and the other half underwent a vaginal repair of one form or another.

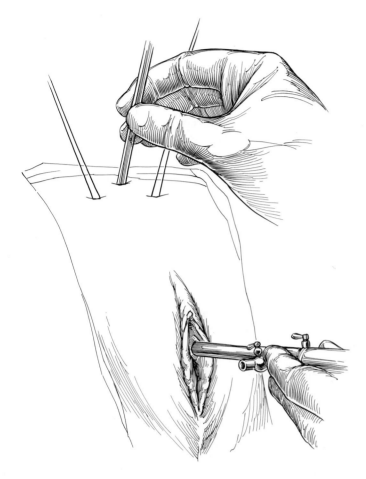

Figure 16-9. After maximal bladder filling, a punch supra-pubic cystostomy tube is advanced through the previously placed midline stab incision using endoscopic guidance. (From Kursh ED. No-incision endoscopic urethropexy. Cont Urol 1991;3:50.)

Postoperative Management

Prophylactic parenteral antibiotics are continued for 24 hours followed by oral therapy for approximately another week. I prefer both parenteral and oral cephalosporins. Early ambulation is encouraged beginning on the day of surgery.

The patient is instructed in the management of the suprapubic catheter on the first postoperative day. In patients who undergo concomitant gynecologic surgery, the training may be delayed for another day. The collection bag and tubing are disconnected from the end of the suprapubic catheter to facilitate ambulation and getting in and out of bed. The patient is taught to turn off the stop-cock on the suprapubic catheter. If she voids spontaneously, the stop-cock is opened to drain any residual urine from the bladder for measurement. If she is unable to void in the early postoperative period, which is normal for most patients, she is instructed to drain her bladder through the tube. When the patient is voiding reasonably well and residuals are consistently less than 100 ml, the suprapubic cystostomy tube is removed.

A variable period of urinary retention is expected after the no-incision technique.[3,4,7] Only 19% of my patients had the cystotomy tube removed in the hospital before discharge. The cystotomy tube remained in place a mean of 22 days and a median of 16 days with a range of 5 to as many as 90 days.[4] Despite prolonged urinary retention, more than 45 days in a small number of patients, all but one recent patient eventually voided satisfactorily. This patient required suture removal on one side before normal voiding ensued.

The median hospital stay in my series was 3 days, and the mean stay was 3.6 days. The mean hospital stay in the 27 patients who underwent concomitant gynecologic surgery was 5 days, which contributed to the increased stay noted for the entire group.[4] Today most patients who do not undergo concomitant surgery are discharged on the second postoperative day. The procedure has not been performed on an ambulatory basis, as some have suggested, because the patients experience modest postoperative pain and require instruction to manage the suprapubic catheter confidently.

After discharge, ambulation, including walking stairs, is not only allowed, but also encouraged. Patients are allowed to shower. They are also permitted to drive as soon as they feel capable of doing so. Strenuous physical activity is avoided for 6 weeks until a satisfactory scar is formed underneath the suture, which creates the so-called autologous pledget to help preserve a permanent support mechanism. As soon as satisfactory voiding is achieved with postvoid residuals consistently less than 100 ml, the patients return to the office for removal of the suprapubic cystostomy tube. Even if they are not voiding adequately, the patients are seen in the office 2 to 3 weeks after discharge to monitor their progress and to be certain that they do not have a urinary tract infection secondary to the cystostomy tube. At this time, it is surprising to note that the vaginal sutures are no longer visible or palpable in most

instances. Excellent urethral support is generally readily palpable on pelvic examination.

Results

In their initial report, Gittes and Loughlin noted an 87% success rate, but the follow-up period was relatively short.[3] In 1990, Loughlin and associates noted a success rate for the no-incision technique of 75% when no vaginal bites were taken to form the so-called autologous pledget and 86% in those patients who had a vaginal bite taken.[7] They also reported that analysis of the 25 failures revealed that many of them occurred in high-risk patients. Three of the 25 failures occurred in patients with neurogenic bladders, 2 had previous pelvic radiation, and 5 had failed a prior incontinence operation.[7]

I reported a cure rate of 81.5% using the relatively rigid criterion of a failure being considered any degree of incontinence after a minimum of 1 year follow-up.[4] These results are not as good as we initially reported in a small group of patients who underwent a no-incision urethropexy with a 94% cure rate.[8] The technique was particularly successful in women with grade 1 stress urinary incontinence (cure rate 97%) but was not effective in women with high-grade incontinence (45% in women with grade 3 stress urinary incontinence). These data demonstrate a significant correlation between the success rate and grade of incontinence ($P < 0.001$), suggesting that it is preferable to consider other surgical techniques for correction of patients with high-grade incontinence.[4]

It is noteworthy that there were no failures in the 36 premenopausal women in this review. The cure rate of 72% in the postmenopausal group represented a significant reduction ($P < 0.001$). These data suggest that the success of the repair is dependent on the strength and integrity of the vaginal mucosa. In the postmenopausal women who were taking hormones, the cure rate was only marginally better than those patients who were not taking exogenous hormones, being 75% in women who were taking hormones and 70% in women who were not.[4] It is possible that the failure rate noted in the postmenopausal patients who were taking hormones is dose dependent. As already mentioned, the excellent results noted in the premenopausal women has led to the current practice of administering estrogen vaginal cream preoperatively and postoperatively to postmenopausal patients.

This study also showed that the no-incision technique is effective in most properly selected patients who have failed previous anti-incontinence procedures, as evidenced by a cure rate of 82% in 22 patients in that group. Successful repair was achieved in some difficult incontinence patients, including one woman with three prior failures in 6 years, one woman with a failed Raz repair 6 months earlier, one woman with two failed Stamey procedures within the last year, one woman with two failed Marshall-Marchetti-Krantz operations, and one woman who failed a recent Stamey procedure 2 months postoperatively. Interestingly four of these five patients were premenopausal, and the other was only 51 years old but had undergone a prior total abdominal hysterectomy and oophorectomy.[4]

Another interesting observation in my series is that all but three of the failures occurred within 7 months of surgery, with the other failures occurring at 13 and 20 months and an unclear onset of incontinence in the last patient.[4] Because a large majority of failures occur early, it appears that if the procedure is successful in relieving incontinence for more than 6 to 8 months, long-term success can probably be anticipated in the overwhelming number of patients.

Complications

Because urinary retention is anticipated in most instances following the no-incision technique, it is not considered a complication. Prolonged urinary retention (longer than 45 days) was noted in 7% of my patients.[4] With rare exception, all patients eventually void if patience can be exercised by both the patient and physician.

Displacement of the suprapubic cystostomy tube has been observed in a small number of patients. The incidence of this complication should be low if the tube is properly positioned in the bladder using endoscopic control during surgery and is sutured well at the skin level.

Loughlin and associates reported one incidence of a bowel perforation secondary to placement of the percutaneous suprapubic cystostomy tube.[7] I have not experienced this problem in any of my patients, but others have informed me about the occurrence of intraperitoneal perforation or bowel perforation following a punch suprapubic cystostomy. To minimize the possibility of this complication, it is advisable to rotate the patient to a Trendelenburg position to bring the small bowel out of the pelvis. Additionally, the bladder should be maximally filled before placement of the punch cystostomy tube, and the tube should be placed using endoscopic guidance.

Other than prolonged urinary retention, complications were few in my review of 108 women. In addition to premature displacement of the cystostomy tube, there were three incidences of cellulitis around the suprapubic catheter, and one patient experienced severe suprapubic pain until the tube was removed. The only other complications were one instance of unexplained severe suprapubic pain for 10 days postoperatively and the development of a yeast infection in the suprapubic area in an obese woman.[4]

There is one group of patients that deserves particular mention. In an attempt to reduce the risk of the sutures migrating through the rectus fascia, 29 of 108 patients in my series had the supporting sutures tied over 2-mm-thick Gortex bolsters placed in the suprapubic stab sites. Five of the 29 patients developed infections in one of the stab sites, and 5 additional women had temporary tender nodules. One of the women with an infection eventually had the suture and bolster removed in the office owing to persistent drainage despite treatment, but fortunately she remained continent with only one supporting suture in place. These infections occurred despite the fact that copious amounts of antibiotic solution were used to irrigate the suprapubic incision throughout the operation.[5] This high complication rate in this group led to the abandonment of this modification for the no-incision endoscopic technique. It is postulated that bacteria in the vagina have the opportunity to migrate along the suture to reach the foreign body Gortex bolster until the vaginal stitch becomes buried. Until recently, infections have not been noted in my patients when foreign body material was not used or when it was employed in association with other techniques, but a woman developed an infected bolster requiring removal on one side following a Raz endoscopic urethropexy. Suture abscesses that required removal of one of the suspension sutures have been reported by others.[7]

Another complication that has also been noted is genitofemoral nerve entrapment resulting in discomfort in the groin and upper thigh.[9] I have not observed this complication, probably related to the fact that the stab incisions are made more medially than others have described.

Summary

It is concluded that the success of the no-incision endoscopic urethropexy is dependent on the strength of the vaginal mucosa. This technique appears to be particularly effective in premenopausal women even if they have complex cases of incontinence. The procedure is not as effective in postmenopausal patients or in women with severe high-grade incontinence. If the patient is noted to have poor-quality vaginal mucosa, it is preferable to employ another surgical technique, and the same can probably be said for women with high-grade stress urinary incontinence unless they are premenopausal. It is speculative whether or not the preoperative and postoperative administration of adequate doses of estrogens in postmenopausal women increases the success rate.

Use of an appropriate surgical technique is instrumental in enhancing the outcome of any type of urethropexy. To a major extent, this depends on the availability of strong supporting fascia or strong vaginal mucosa. The surgeon must keep this in mind when selecting a specific surgical approach for correction of stress incontinence.

References

1. Stamey TA. Endoscopic suspension of the vesical neck for urinary incontinence. Surg Gynecol Obstet 1973;136:547.
2. Raz S. Modified bladder neck suspension for female stress incontinence. Urology 1981;17:82.
3. Gittes RF, Loughlin KR. No incision pubovaginal suspension for stress incontinence. J Urol 1987; 138:568.
4. Kursh ED. Factors influencing the outcome of a no-incision endoscopic urethropexy. Surg Gynecol Obstet 1992;175:254.
5. Stamey TA. Endoscopic suspension of the vesical neck for urinary incontinence in females: Report on 203 consecutive patients. Ann Surg 1980; 192:465.
6. Tapp A, Versi E, Cardozo I. Is urethral pressure profilometry useful in the diagnosis of genuine stress incontinence? Proceedings of the International Continence Society, London, 1985:263.
7. Loughlin KR, Whitmore WF III, Gittes RF, Richie JP: Review of an eight-year experience with modifications of endoscopic suspension of the bladder neck for female stress urinary incontinence. J Urol 1990;143:44.
8. Kursh ED, Angell AH, Resnick MI. Evolution of endoscopic urethropexy: Seven-year experience with various techniques. Urology 1991;37:428.
9. Summers JL, Myers G. Complication of Gittes procedure. Presented at North Central Section Meeting AUA, Chicago, 1989.

17

Pubovaginal Sling

Jerry G. Blaivas

The use of a pubovaginal sling for the treatment of sphincteric incontinence has a long and variegated history. Von Giordano is credited with first describing a sling technique in 1907.[1] He fashioned a pedicle graft of gracilis muscle that was passed around the urethra. In 1910, Goebell used a pedicle flap of pyramidalis muscle that was passed through the retropubic space on either side of the vesical neck and sutured in the midline beneath the urethra.[2] Although he reported a successful outcome in two children—one with spina bifida and one with epispadias—no meaningful data were presented. Moreover, because the muscle was left attached to its insertion on the pubis, there was no way to adjust the tension, particularly if the muscle was too short. To obviate this problem, Frangenheim modified the procedure by incorporating an adjacent portion of rectus fascia to the pyramidalis muscle.[3] This technique provided sufficient length for the sling to pass around the urethra of a man who developed urinary incontinence after a perineal injury. In 1917, Stoeckel modified the procedure further. He plicated the vesical neck and raised bilateral rectangular flaps of rectus fascia and pyramidalis muscle. The flaps were passed through the retropubic space and around the plicated urethra and sutured in the midline.[4] Further modifications of these techniques became known as the *Goebell-Stoeckel-Frangen-*

heim operation.[5,6] These procedures were associated with a high complication rate, particularly urinary infection, hemorrhage, and obstruction, and were performed only infrequently for the better part of 30 years.

In 1931, Miller described a technique of passing a pedicle graft of pyramidalis or rectus muscle superficial to the pubis and around the urethra.[5] He believed that this obviated the need for an extensive dissection of the vesical neck from above and thereby lessened the likelihood of bleeding or injury to the bladder or urethra. Aldridge presented a meticulously detailed description of his slightly modified surgical technique in a single case report in 1942.[7] He raised bilateral rectus fascial strips that were detached laterally, passed through the rectus muscle, and sutured together in the midline beneath the urethra (Fig. 17-1). Further modifications were reported by a number of authors, but the procedure again fell into disfavor because of complications.[8–16]

The modern era of pubovaginal fascial sling surgery was introduced and popularized by the work of McGuire. In 1976, McGuire and colleagues introduced the concept of two generic types of sphincteric incontinence: urethral hypermobility and intrinsic sphincter deficiency.[36] They modified the Green classification by adding a new category, type III stress incontinence. Type

239

Female Urology, edited by Elroy D. Kursh and Edward McGuire. J. B. Lippincott, Philadelphia, © 1994.

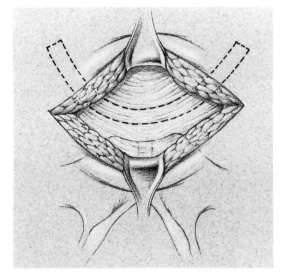

Figure 17-1. *A 2 to 3 cm wide graft is outlined keeping the incision parallel to the direction of the fascial fibers. The incision is extended laterally to the point where the rectus fascia divides and passes to the internal and external oblique muscles. (Modified from Blaivas JG. Pubovaginal sling procedure. In: Whitehead ED, ed. Current operative urology 1990. Philadelphia: JB Lippincott, 1990:93–101.)*

III stress incontinence was defined by an absence of urethral hypermobility, a low (proximal) urethral pressure, and an open vesical neck at rest. As the concept of type III stress incontinence continued to evolve, it became known as intrinsic sphincter deficiency. In 1978, McGuire and Lytton reported an 80% success rate in patients with type III stress incontinence after construction of a pubovaginal sling.[17] They stated that:

> Most patients with stress incontinence can be treated successfully, either with anterior colporrhaphy or with an anterior urethropexy. These procedures have resulted in the correction of the hypermobility of the posterior urethra and maintenance of its correct anatomical location above the pelvic diaphragm, so that sudden changes in intra-abdominal pressure are transmitted equally to the bladder and proximal urethra. The choice

of procedure depends upon the degree of mobility of the posterior urethra and the resultant anatomic deformity. . . . However, there remains a small group of patients in whom stress incontinence persists despite adequate anatomical correction of the position of the urethra and hypermobility, and most of these patients have a low urethral closing pressure exerted over a short distance. Many have undergone a previous operation for stress incontinence so that mobilization, elevation and fixation of the urethra may be difficult because of scarring and rigidity of the periurethral tissues. Insertion of a pubovaginal sling in these cases has usually been successful.

In their technique, a combined abdominal and vaginal approach was used. A 1 × 12 cm strip of rectus fascia and external oblique was left attached about 2 cm from the midline. The vesical neck was exposed through the retropubic space. A midline anterior vaginal wall incision was made and a tunnel created on either side of the vesicourethral junction. The free end of the sling was passed through the rectus muscle, around the vesical neck, and back through the rectus muscle on the contralateral side. Tension in the sling was adjusted by measuring urethral pressure; the intention was to raise urethral pressure by about 10 cm H_2O. The bladder was opened to ensure that there was no injury, and the sling was secured to the rectus fascia. The bladder was drained by suprapubic cystotomy.

A subsequent series by McGuire and others documented a success rate of 82% in 80 women with type III stress incontinence.[18,19] In this series, six women had concomitant urinary fistulas, and 28% had associated detrusor abnormalities. Most of the patients had failed previous attempts at surgical correction. Of the original 15 postoperative failures, 8 were due to detrusor instability or low compliance and 7 were due to persistent type III stress incontinence. Reoperation, including augmentation cystoplasty, repeat pubovaginal sling, and continent vesicostomy, resulted in an overall cure rate of 95%. Five patients (6%) had prolonged detrusor instability, and 18% required intermittent catheterization. Twelve of the patients on intermittent catheterization had neurologic conditions (mostly myelodysplasia).

Types of Graft Used

Blaivas and others, using the surgical technique described subsequently, reported a 91% success rate of operation in 67 women with complicated type III stress incontinence who were followed for a mean of 3.5 years (range 1 to 9 years).[20–22] In their technique, a free graft of rectus fascia is passed around the vesical neck without any dissection through the retropubic space; the entire dissection is performed through a vaginal incision. The sling is sutured to the rectus fascia on either side with no tension at all. The operation was performed as a single procedure in 39 patients and was combined with an operation for pelvic floor prolapse in 10. In 18 women, it was combined with a urethral reconstruction procedure. Sixty-two patients (93%) had failed 1 to 19 previous operations for stress incontinence, with a median of 3 previous surgeries. Overall, 55 women (82%) were dry under all circumstances and did not have symptoms of detrusor instability. Six (9%) had mild episodes of urinary incontinence, which occurred less often than once per week, and six were failures. The main cause of failure was urge incontinence; only two patients had persistent stress incontinence. Forty-two patients (63%) were unable to void satisfactorily on discharge on the seventh postoperative day and were sent home with a suprapubic catheter. Another voiding trial was undertaken 4 weeks postoperatively, and 36 were able to void satisfactorily. The remaining six patients were treated with permanent intermittent self-catheterization. Four of these had neurogenic bladders preoperatively, and urinary retention was an expected outcome. In the remaining two patients, postoperative videourodynamics revealed urethral obstruction at the site of the sling.

In 1933, Price first reported the successful use of a free graft of fascia lata as a sling in a young girl with sphincteric incontinence owing to sacral agenesis.[6] Others have used this technique, and the results compare favorably with the series that use rectus fascia.[1, 12, 23–25] Beck and colleagues reported a 92% success rate in 170 women, all of whom underwent the procedure after they had failed previous operations.[24] Only 3 of the 12 failures occurred because of recurrent stress incontinence; the remainder had persistent urge incontinence. For an excellent description of the surgical technique, the interested reader is referred to the work of Beck and Ridley[1, 26] (Fig. 17-2).

In our experience, it has always been possible to obtain a satisfactory strip of rectus fascia for use as a sling, even in patients who have had more than a dozen retropubic operations. Nevertheless, some concern has been voiced about the advisability of using fascia for the sling, particularly in patients who have undergone multiple previous abdominal or retropubic operations. A number of surgeons have used synthetic material instead of fascia for construction of the

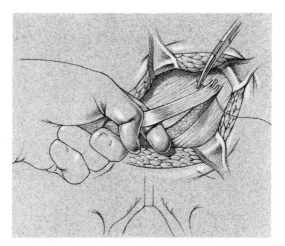

Figure 17-2. *A no. 2–0 nonabsorbable running horizontal mattress suture is placed across the lateralmost portion of the graft, and the ends are left long. (Modified from Blaivas JG. Pubovaginal sling procedure. In: Whitehead ED, ed. Current operative urology 1990. Philadelphia: JB Lippincott, 1990:93–101.)*

sling. Ox fascia, dura, collagen, and Silastic have been tried with limited success.[27-29] Synthetic polyester Dacron (Mersilene) has been used for almost four decades, but problems with erosion, infection, fistula, and sinus formation greatly limit its use.[10,11,15,16,30-34] In 1962, Williams and TeLinde described their technique using synthetic Dacron.[16] In this initial report, they cited an 83% cure rate in 12 patients. In one patient, the Dacron eroded into the urethra and was removed; a second patient developed a persistent sinus tract, but both of these patients were reportedly cured. Before this, these authors tried using a strip of nylon for the sling in two patients, both of whom ultimately developed abscess formation requiring complete removal. According to Ridley, the authors subsequently abandoned the use of synthetic material in favor of fascia lata because of the complication rate. Subsequently Moir reported an 83% "cure or substantial improvement" in 71 women with a Dacron sling.[10]

The most extensive experience with Dacron slings is that of Morgan and others.[32-34] They reported an 81% to 90% success rate in a cumulative series of more than 300 women followed as long as 15 years. In one report, 283 women with recurrent stress incontinence and 9 with primary stress incontinence underwent a Marlex sling operation through a two-team retropubic and vaginal approach. The authors stressed two important aspects of surgical technique, which they believe is critical to their success: (1) the necessity of completely mobilizing the vesical neck and proximal urethra "from a bed of scar, followed by repositioning of the bladder neck in an intra-abdominal retropubic position," and (2) placing the sling around the vesical neck with no tension at all—they do not even sew the sling in place. With a minimum follow-up of 5 years (range, 5 to 12 years), the success rate was 81%.[32,33] A subsequent series of 82 patients had a 93% cure rate with a 1- to 4-year follow-up.[34] In 16 patients with a *sloughed urethra*, the sling was used in conjunction with construction of a vaginal flap neourethra. Ten of these procedures resulted in ero-

sion and stone formation. Only two of the slings eroded in the rest of the 274 patients. Two patients underwent urinary diversion because of *end-stage contracted bladder*, 12 patients had persistent bladder outlet obstruction, and 2 are on routine intermittent catheterization. Overall, 5% of their patients had persistent urinary frequency and urgency.

Morgan has replaced Marlex with Dexon mesh. Although the mesh is absorbable, a rapid ingrowth of scar occurs within days of implantation resulting in a strong fibrous sling. Initial results with this procedure are superior to those of the Marlex slings.*

Despite the long-term success rate cited, pubovaginal sling never achieved widespread popularity.[8-12,15-25,26-30,32-34,35-38] This is primarily due to the perception that the procedure is technically more demanding than the standard urethropexy, and the complication rate, particularly in the hands of the inexperienced surgeon, is reportedly higher. The most common and troublesome complications are injury to the bladder or urethra, urinary retention, and detrusor instability. Urinary retention is largely preventable by insuring that the sling is passed beneath the vesical neck and sutured to the rectus fascia with no tension at all. In our experience, the major risk factor for developing postoperative detrusor instability is the presence of this symptom preoperatively. It may also be caused, however, if the sling is placed under too much tension, causing urethral obstruction. In our judgment, intraoperative injury to the bladder or urethra is no more likely during pubovaginal sling than any of the modified Peyrera operations. With either procedure, injury is entirely preventable by adhering to the surgical principles outlined by Aldridge in 1942:[7]

> [I]t requires a painstaking technique which should not be undertaken by a surgeon who has not acquired a modern conception of the anatomic structures in the anterior vaginal wall about the urethra and bladder. Dissection in this

* Morgan JE. Personal communication, 1992.

region is safe and nearly bloodless if carried out in the planes of cleavage described above. If these tissue planes are not followed, blood loss may be excessive and the bladder and urethra may be subjected to serious damage.

Despite these concerns, we believe that, for the experienced pelvic surgeon, pubovaginal sling offers the best chance for long-term cure of stress urinary incontinence, not only owing to complicated problems of intrinsic sphincter deficiency, but also owing to commonplace urethral hypermobility.

Indications

Historically the sling technique has been limited to patients who have failed previous surgery and those with intrinsic sphincter deficiency (type III stress incontinence). In a generic sense, intrinsic sphincter deficiency refers to malfunction of the intrinsic sphincteric properties of the vesical neck and proximal urethra. In the older literature, type III stress incontinence was recognized clinically by noting overt stress incontinence unaccompanied by appreciable descent of the vesical neck. With the advent of sophisticated multichannel videourodynamics, intrinsic sphincter deficiency is diagnosed primarily by observing radiographic contrast material in the vesical neck and urethra in the absence of a detrusor contraction (an open vesical neck).[20–22, 36, 37, 39] Intrinsic sphincter deficiency is most commonly due to recurrent stress incontinence after failed previous surgery, but it is also seen in neurologic disorders affecting urethral sphincter function.[20, 21, 36, 37] In some instances, intrinsic sphincter deficiency and urethral hypermobility coexist. Current diagnostic methodology does not clearly distinguish the two entities. Studies by McGuire, however, suggest that measurement of the *leak point pressure* is an important variable that can distinguish the two.* A complete list of the causes of type III stress incontinence is as follows:

* McGuire EM. Personal communication, 1992.

Previous incontinence surgery
Myelodysplasia
Lumbosacral spinal cord injury
Anterior spinal artery syndrome
Radical hysterectomy
Abdominoperineal resection of the rectum

Operative Technique

The procedure is performed in the dorsal lithotomy position. A Foley catheter is inserted into the urethra and the balloon inflated with enough saline to facilitate palpation of the vesical neck. To minimize blood loss, the abdominal portion of the procedure is completed first. The fascial strip to be used for the sling is harvested and stored in sterile saline while the vaginal portion of the operation is completed.

A Pfannenstiel incision is made and carried down to the rectus fascia. The surface of the rectus fascia is dissected free of subcutaneous tissue, and a suitable site is selected for excision of the fascial strip. If the patient has had previous surgery, there may be considerable scarring. It is not necessary to find "scar-free" fascia. Even the most scarred tissue, not even recognizable as fascia, may be used. In more than 150 cases, we have always been able to find a suitable strip to harvest.

Two parallel horizontal incisions, 2 to 3 cm apart, are made near the midline in the rectus fascia. The incisions are extended superolaterally for the entire width of the wound, following the direction of the fascial fibers (see Fig. 17-1). If a longer strip is necessary, the incisions may be extended superiorly in a vertical direction at the lateralmost aspect of the wound. The undersurface of the fascia is freed from muscle and scar. Before excising the strip, each end of the fascia is secured with a long no. 2–0 nonabsorbable suture using a running horizontal mattress suture that is placed at right angles to the direction of the fascial fibers (Figs. 17-2 and 17-3). No attempt is made to enter the retropubic space. It is not necessary to mobilize or expose the bladder or vesical neck from above

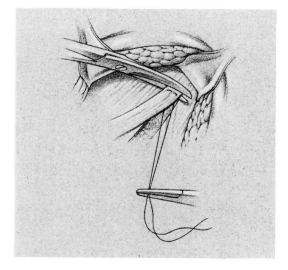

Figure 17-3. *Each end of the fascial graft is transected approximately 1 cm lateral to the mattress suture. (Modified from Blaivas JG. Pubovaginal sling procedure. In: Whitehead ED, ed. Current operative urology 1990. Philadelphia: JB Lippincott, 1990:93–101.)*

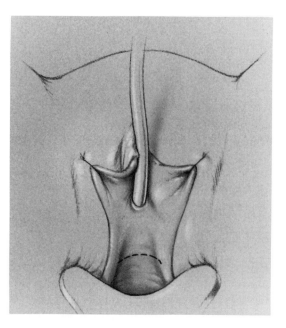

Figure 17-4. *Vaginal incision. A slightly curved horizontal incision is made at the vesical neck. (Modified from Blaivas JG. Pubovaginal sling procedure. In: Whitehead ED, ed. Current operative urology 1990. Philadelphia: JB Lippincott, 1990:93–101.)*

because this is accomplished through the vaginal dissection. The fascial defect is closed and the wound is temporarily packed with saline-soaked sponges, as attention is turned to the vagina.

The vesical neck is identified by placing gentle traction on the Foley catheter and palpating the balloon. In most patients, the actual position of the vesical neck is about 2 cm proximal to the palpable distal edge of the balloon. A gently curved horizontal incision is made in the anterior vaginal wall with the apex of the curve over the vesical neck (Fig. 17-4). It is important that this incision be made in the proper plane—just beneath the vaginal epithelium and superficial to the endopelvic fascia. The proper plane is identified by noting the characteristic shiny white appearance of the undersurface of the anterior vaginal wall. Although the plane is usually described as being bloodless, this is not always the case, but it usually provides the least blood loss.

Even more importantly, this plane insures that the dissection will proceed lateral to the bladder and urethra. If the initial vaginal incision is even a few millimeters too deep, injury to these structures may occur.

A small posterior vaginal flap is made for a distance of about 2 cm, just wide enough to accept the sling but narrow enough to prevent the sling from moving after it is passed around the urethra. The lateral edges of the wound are grasped with Allis clamps and retracted laterally. The dissection continues just beneath the vaginal epithelium with a Metzenbaum scissors pointed in the direction of the patient's ipsilateral shoulder until the periosteum of the pubis or ischium is palpated with the tip of the scissors (Fig. 17-5). During this part of the dissection, it is important

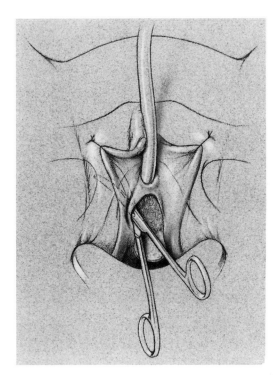

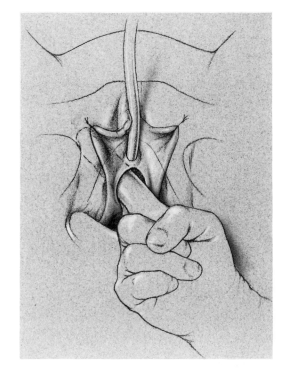

Figure 17-5. *Dissection beneath the vaginal epithelium with a Metzenbaum scissors to create a tunnel for passage of the sling. The tips of the scissors are directed toward the patient's ipsilateral shoulder. (Modified from Blaivas JG. Pubovaginal sling procedure. In: Whitehead ED, ed. Current operative urology 1990. Philadelphia: JB Lippincott, 1990:93–101.)*

Figure 17-6. *The endopelvic fascia is perforated with the index finger, and the retropubic space is entered. (Modified from Blaivas JG. Pubovaginal sling procedure. In: Whitehead ED, ed. Current operative urology 1990. Philadelphia: JB Lippincott, 1990:93–101.)*

to stay as far lateral as possible. This is best accomplished by dissecting with the concavity of the scissors pointing laterally and by exerting constant lateral pressure with the tips of the scissors against the undersurface of the vaginal epithelium.

Once the periosteum is reached, the endopelvic fascia is perforated and the retropubic space entered. In most instances, this is easily accomplished with blunt dissection by the surgeon's index finger (Fig. 17-6). The tip of the finger, opposite the nail, palpates the periosteum. With the back edge of the fingertip, the bladder and urethra are mobilized medially as the finger advances and perforates the fascia. This completely mobilizes the vesical neck and proximal urethra, freeing these structures from their vaginal attachments. If the dissection does not proceed easily, it may be necessary to complete it sharply with a Metzenbaum scissors. The scissors is introduced into the proper plane until the undersurface of the pubis is palpated. The tip of the scissors is pressed firmly against the bone and spread until it opens for a distance of 2 to 3 cm. This exposes the proper plane, and the index finger is reinserted to complete the dissection. Sometimes this maneuver has to be repeated several times before the vesical neck and proximal urethra are sufficiently mobilized. If the initial

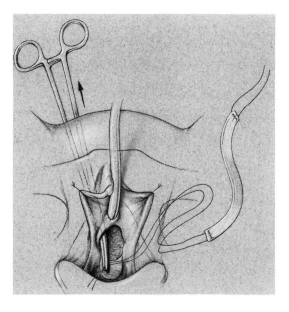

Figure 17-8. *The fascial graft is passed around the urethra and brought to the abdominal wound on either side. (Modified from Blaivas JG. Pubovaginal sling procedure. In: Whitehead ED, ed. Current operative urology 1990. Philadelphia: JB Lippincott, 1990:93–101.)*

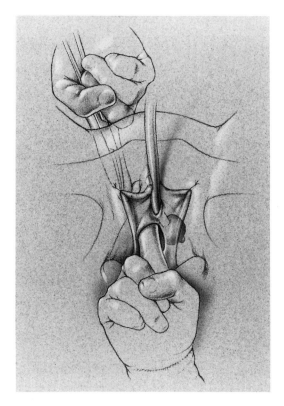

Figure 17-7. *A long DeBakey clamp is passed from the abdominal to the vaginal wound lateral to the urethra. (Modified from Blaivas JG. Pubovaginal sling procedure. In: Whitehead ED, ed. Current operative urology 1990. Philadelphia: JB Lippincott, 1990:93–101.)*

vaginal incision was made too deeply (beneath the endopelvic fascia), however, this part of the dissection will be dangerously close to the bladder and urethra, and inadvertent injury to either structure may occur.

The surgeon's left index finger is reinserted into the vaginal wound retracting the vesical neck and bladder medially. The tip of the finger indents the undersurface of the rectus fascia and is palpated by the index finger of the right hand in the abdominal wound. A 1-cm incision is made in the rectus fascia at the site where the left index finger was palpated.

This is usually just above the pubis and lat-

eral to the midline on either side. A long, sharp, curved clamp (DeBakey) is inserted into the incision and directed to the undersurface of the pubis. The tip of the clamp is pressed against the periosteum and directed toward the index finger, which is retracting the vesical neck and bladder medially (Fig. 17-7). In this fashion, the clamp is guided into the vaginal wound. When the tip of the clamp is visible, one end of the long suture, which is attached to the fascial graft, is grasped and pulled into the abdominal wound (Fig. 17-8). The procedure is repeated on the other side. The fascial sling is now positioned from the abdominal wall on one side around the undersurface of the vesical neck and back to the abdominal wall on the other side.

Cystoscopy is performed to ensure that there has been no damage to the urethra, vesical neck, bladder, or ureters. A trocar 12 French

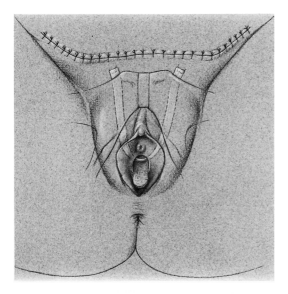

Figure 17-9. The sling is secured to the abdominal fascia on either side. (Modified from Blaivas JG. Pubovaginal sling procedure. In: Whitehead ED, ed. Current operative urology 1990. Philadelphia: JB Lippincott, 1990:93–101.)

suprapubic tube is inserted percutaneously into the bladder, and its position is visually inspected to be sure that it is well away from the trigone. The vaginal incision is closed with interrupted figure-of-eight sutures of no. 2–0 chromic catgut before securing the sling in place.

The sling is secured to the rectus fascia on either side using the long sutures attached to the ends of the fascial graft. In the majority of patients, great care is taken to ensure that the sling is sutured in place without any tension at all (Fig. 17-9). The only exception to this is when the goal of surgery is to create urinary retention and maintain the patient on intermittent catheterization. We have found no precise techniques for estimating the tension to be exerted on the fascial strip but through experience have decided that it is far better to err on the side of too little tension. At the present time, we use the following method to ensure that excessive tension is not applied: After securing one side of the strip to the rectus fascia, the other side is pulled up through the contralateral fascial incision until there is no slack in the strip. The suture is then dropped and the strip sutured in place without added tension. If the strip is too short to reach the fascia, it is sutured in place with a whatever gap is necessary to prevent tension. If the surgeon is unsure of whether or not there is excessive tension, cystoscopy is performed. With the end of the cystoscope in the bladder, the suture on the free end of the fascial strip is grasped and pulled upward, while downward pressure is applied to the cystoscope. This depresses the vesical neck and puts the sling on stretch. While maintaining the pressure on the cystoscope, the suture is released, removing the excess tension from the sling. The cystoscope is removed and the sling secured with no additional tension. A vaginal pack soaked in sterile lubricating jelly is left in place.

Postoperative Care

The vaginal pack is removed the day after surgery. Voiding trials are begun as soon as the patient is ambulating comfortably, usually 3 to 7 days after surgery. If the patient is able to void well, the suprapubic tube is removed. If she is unable to void, she is discharged with the suprapubic tube to gravity drainage. One day before her return visit, she again has a voiding trial at home. The suprapubic tube is removed, and if she is still unable to void well, she is begun on intermittent self-catheterization.

Complications

The most important complications of autologous fascial slings are (1) bladder or urethral injury, (2) urethral obstruction, and (3) symptomatic detrusor instability. Urethral obstruction and symptomatic detrusor instability occur in approximately 5% and 10% of patients. We have never encountered a bladder or urethral injury, and there is no modern literature reporting the incidence of such injuries. There has been a substantial number of such reported injuries, however, during modified Peyrera procedures, and we believe that there is a similar incidence with pubovaginal sling. When synthetic slings are used, the incidence of erosion and fistula formation is as high as 20%.

Conclusion

We believe that the success of the pubovaginal sling is primarily related to improvements in surgical technique. The most important aspects of surgical technique include (1) thorough familiarity of vaginal and retropubic anatomy; (2) confining the vaginal dissection to the "glistening white surface" just beneath the vaginal epithelium; (3) mobilization of the vesical neck from the vaginal approach, freeing it from tethering to the vagina; (4) use of a gently curved inverted U incision over the vesical neck to ensure that the sling cannot slip too far proximal or distal; (5) the use of free grafts of fascia for the sling instead of pedicle grafts; and (6) positioning the graft beneath the vesical neck without tension.

References

1. Ridley JH. The Goebel-Stoeckel sling operation. In: Mattingly RF, Thompson JD, eds. TeLinde's operative gynecology. Philadelphia: JB Lippincott, 1985:623–636.
2. Goebell R. Zur operativen beseitigung der angebornen incontinentia vesicae. Z Gynakol 1910;2:187–191.
3. Frangenheim P. Su operativen behandlung der inkontinenz der mannlichen harnohre. Verh Dtsch Ges Chir 1914;43:149–154.
4. Stoeckel W. Uber die verwendung der musculi pyramidalis bei der operativen behandlung der incontinentia urinae. Zentralbl Gynaekol 1917;41:11–19.
5. Miller NF. Surgical treatment of urinary incontinence in the female. JAMA 1932;98:628.
6. Price PB. Plastic operations for incontinence of urine and of feces. Arch Surg 1933;26:1043.
7. Aldridge AH. Transplantation of fascia for relief of urinary stress incontinence. Am J Obstet Gynecol 1942;44:398.
8. Jeffcoate TN. The results of the Aldridge sling operation for stress incontinence. J Obstet Gynaecol 1956;63:36–39.
9. McLaren HC. Late results of sling operation. Br J Obstet Gynaecol 1968;75:10–13.
10. Moir JC. The Guaze-Hammock operation. Br J Obstet Gynaecol 1968;75:1.
11. Narik B, Palmrich A. A simplified sling operation suitable for routine use. Am J Obstet Gynecol 1962;84:400–405.
12. Ridley JH. Surgical treatment of stress incontinence in women. J Med Assoc Ga 1955;44:135.
13. Studdiford WE. Transplantation of abdominal fascia for relief of urinary stress incontinence. Am J Obstet Gynecol 1944;47:764–775.
14. TeLinde RW. The modified Goebell-Stoeckel operation for urinary incontinence. South Med J 1934;27:193.
15. Wharton LR Jr, TeLinde RW. An evaluation of fascial sling operations for urinary incontinence in female patients. J Urol 1959;82:76.
16. Williams TJ, TeLinde RW. The sling operation for urinary incontinence using mersilene ribbon. Obstet Gynecol 1962;19:241.
17. McGuire EM, Lytton B. The pubovaginal sling in stress urinary incontinence. J Urol 1978;119:82.
18. McGuire EM, Wang C, Usitalo H, Savastano J. Modified pubovaginal sling in girls with myelodysplasia. J Urol 1986;135:94.
19. McGuire EM, Bennett CJ, Konnak JA, et al. Experience with pubovaginal slings for urinary incontinence at University of Michigan. J Urol 1987;138:525.
20. Blaivas JG, Salinas J. Type III stress urinary incontinence: The importance of proper diagnosis and treatment. Surg Forum 1984;35:472.
21. Blaivas JG, Olsson CA. Stress incontinence: Classification and surgical approach. J Urol 1988;139:727.
22. Blaivas JG, Jacobs BZ. Pubovaginal sling in the treatment of complicated stress incontinence. J Urol 1991;145:1214–1218.
23. Beck RP, Grove D, Arnusch D, et al. Recurrent stress incontinence treated by the fascial sling procedure. Am J Obstet Gynecol 1974;120:613.
24. Beck RP, McCormick, Nordstrom L. The fascia lata sling procedure for the treatment of recurrent genuine stress incontinence of urine. Obstet Gynecol 1988;72:699–703.
25. Parker RT, Ridley JH. Fascia lata urethrovesical suspension for stress urinary incontinence. Perspect Surg 1978;1:4.
26. Beck RP. The sling operation. In: Buchsbaum HJ, Schmidt JD, eds. Gynecological and obstetrical urology. 2nd ed. Philadelphia: WB Saunders, 1982:285–305.
27. Faber P, Beck L, Heidenreich J. Treatment of uri-

nary stress incontinence with the lyodura sling. Urol Int 1978;33:117.

28. Iosif CS. Porcine corium sling in the treatment of urinary stress incontinence. Arch Gynecol 1987; 240:131.

29. Stanton SL, Brindley GS, Holmes DM. Silastic sling for urethral sphincter incompetence in women. Br J Obstet Gynaecol 1985;92:747.

30. Hilton P, Stanton SL. Clinical and urodynamic evaluation of the polypropylene (Marlex) sling for genuine stress incontinence. Neurourol Urodynam 1983;2:145–153.

31. Irving M, Lee R. Delayed transection of urethra by mersilene tape. Urology 1976;8:580.

32. Morgan JE. A sling operation using Marlex polypropylene mesh for treatment of recurrent stress incontinence. Am J Obstet Gynecol 1970;106:369.

33. Morgan JE, Farrow GA. Recurrent stress urinary incontinence in the female. Br J Urol 1970;49:37.

34. Morgan JE, Farrow GA, Stewart FE. The Marlex sling operation for the treatment of recurrent stress urinary incontinence. Am J Obstet Gynecol 1985;151:224.

35. Hohenfellner T, Petri E. Sling procedures. In: Stanton SL, Tanagho EA, eds. Surgery of female incontinence. Berlin: Springer-Verlag, 1980.

36. McGuire EM, Lytton B, Kohorn EI, Pepe V. Stress urinary incontinence. Obstet Gynecol 1976; 47:255.

37. McGuire EM. Urodynamic findings in patients after failure of stress incontinence operations. In: Zinner NR, Sterling AM, eds. Female incontinence. New York: Alan R. Liss, 1980:351–360.

38. Sloan WR, Barwin BN. Stress incontinence of urine: A retrospective study of the complications and late results of simple suprapubic suburethral fascial slings. J Urol 1973;110:533.

39. Blaivas JG. Pubovaginal sling procedure. In: Whitehead ED, ed. Current operative urology. Philadelphia: JB Lippincott, 1990:93–101.

18

Injection Therapy for Urethral Incontinence

Rodney A. Appell

The choice of a proper therapeutic approach for treating urinary incontinence depends to a large degree on the underlying cause of the problem. The failure to store urine may be simplified by considering the problem to be located either at the level of the bladder or at the level of the urethra, and treatment modalities are directed accordingly. A knowledge of the physiology of the lower urinary tract (Chap. 3) and the functional anatomy of the female pelvis (Chap. 1) is essential in the understanding of both the causes and the treatments of urinary incontinence as well as patient selection for the latter.

When the incontinence is due to urethral dysfunction, it is important to distinguish whether the problem is a disorder of urethral support (Chap. 11) or urethral function (Chap. 12). Injectable therapy for urethral incontinence has its primary place in those patients with urethral functional incompetence, and just as a sling or artificial sphincter increases outflow resistance, so too are injectables designed to restore urinary control based on the principle of enhancing urethral resistance to the flow of urine by augmentation of intraurethral pressure.

Patient Selection

Candidates for periurethral injections are those with a primary incompetent proximal urethra (*e.g.*, myelodysplastic females) or those in whom the disorder of sphincteric function is secondary to sympathetic neural injury from trauma (*e.g.*, pelvic fracture) or pelvic surgery (*e.g.*, type III stress urinary incontinence). Therefore patient evaluation and selection as well as the diagnosis of bladder outlet incompetence are no different for the group of females considering periurethral injections than those for pubovaginal slings or artificial sphincters. Good candidates for these procedures are females with low urethral closing pressure in the most proximal portion of the urethra. Obviously urodynamic evaluation to ascertain the cause of incontinence is mandatory to demonstrate poor or absent urethral function. In this case, the bladder neck and proximal urethra are open at rest in the absence of a detrusor contraction. If the proximal portion of the urethra fails to close, the patient is a suitable candidate. The simplest manner in which to classify this disproportion between bladder and urethral pressures is to determine the leak point and the detrusor pressure at this point in time when urine leaks through the continence mechanism. This leak point pressure (LPP), from a practical point of view, corresponds to the urethral opening pressure, and the extent of urethral dysfunction resulting in incontinence may be obtained. Urethral failure is evidenced by a low or absent LPP, usually below 20 cm H_2O.

Female Urology, edited by Elroy D. Kursh and Edward McGuire. J. B. Lippincott, Philadelphia, © 1994.

Continence is attained by increasing this LPP with a sling, artificial sphincter, or suburothelial injection of a bulk-enhancing agent, such as polytetrafluoroethylene (Urethrin, Mentor Corporation, Goleta, California) or glutaraldehyde cross-linked collagen (Contigen, C. R. Bard, Covington, Georgia).

Historical Perspective

The treatment of urinary incontinence by the use of injectables has been considered and attempted with many different types of agents. The first such report using a sclerosing agent appeared in 1938 by Murless.[1] Sporadic studies using both sclerosing agents and bulk-enhancing agents have been conducted over the years, but complications and unsatisfactory patient selection have delayed the acceptance of this technique.[2,3] Despite a plethora of positive reports obtained using the bulk-enhancing agent Urethrin over the last two decades, this material has failed to gain universal acceptance.[4–9] A discussion of the probable reasons for the reluctance to use this compound as well as current investigative experience using Contigen in these patients follows.

Urethrin: Technique

Urethrin, Polytef, and Teflon are proprietary names for a paste consisting of a sterile mixture of polytetrafluoroethylene micropolymer particles (ranging in size from 4 to 100 μm), glycerin, and polysorbate. In theory, once injected, the particles are encapsulated by a fibrous reaction enabling a permanent bolstering effect. It has been found, however, that the particles migrate to other areas and organ systems and establish a granulomatous reaction, thus establishing concerns for its safety, which are discussed later.[10] Devices are available for both endoscopic (transurethral) and periurethral injection to allow the thick paste to be injected under pressure (Fig. 18-1).

TRANSURETHRAL INJECTION

Preoperatively the patients receive a prophylactic dose of a cephalosporin chosen for a spectrum to include anaerobic coverage and a povidone-iodine (Betadine) douche. Following general or regional anesthesia (local anesthesia may be used in selected patients using periurethral injectable 1% lidocaine and transurethral 2% lidocaine jelly with intravenous analgesic and amnesic agents—however, the pressure of the injection may be discomforting) and with the patient prepared and draped in the lithotomy position, this technique allows for direct visualization and therefore accurate placement of the 16-gauge needle just below the bladder neck at the 3, 6, or 9 o'clock positions to produce suburothelial cushions (Fig. 18-2).

PERIURETHRAL INJECTION

Although the transurethral technique may appear to be more accurate for needle placement, I believe the periurethral method is more advantageous for the surgeon and safer for the patient. Transurethrally it is difficult to prevent some paste from oozing out of the puncture site and into the bladder and urethra, where it tends to stick to the mucosa and is difficult to evacuate from the lower urinary tract. Additionally, there is the concern that violating the mucosal barrier in this manner may result in bleeding, urinary extravasation, or periurethral infection.

The patient is prepared and positioned as for the transurethral approach. Cystoscopic guidance is performed to check the position of the periurethral needle and subsequent injection of the material and to exclude bladder puncture and egress of Urethrin. In this manner, the bulk effect on urethral closure may be observed endoscopically. I use Bruning's injection device used by colleagues in otolaryngology, who have a great deal of experience with injections of Polytef for a variety of vocal cord problems for which the substance has long since had U.S. Food and Drug Administration (FDA) approval. This injection device resembles a caulking gun with a 16-gauge,

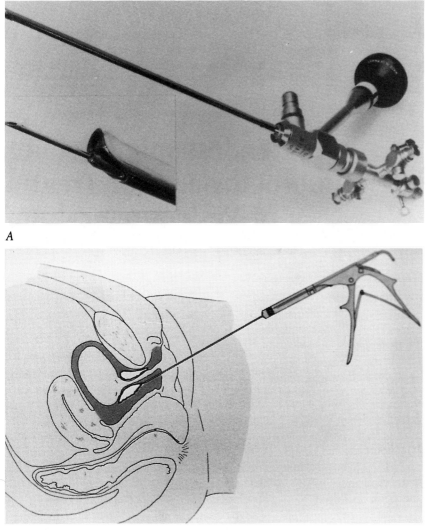

A

B

Figure 18-1. *Injection devices for Urethrin: (A) Transurethral; (B) periurethral. (From Appell RA. Commentary: Periurethral polytetrafluoroethylene (Polytef) injection. In: Whitehead ED, ed. Current Operative Urology 1990. Philadelphia: JB Lippincott, 1990.)*

9-cm length needle (see Fig. 18-1B). This technique requires an assistant to "pull the trigger" on the device because the surgeon must hold the cystoscope in one hand to observe the layering of the material and stabilize the needle periurethrally with the other hand.

Contigen: Technique

Clinical trials have been taking place since 1987 using this injectable glutaraldehyde cross-linked bovine collagen. Contigen is a sterile, non-pyrogenic material composed of highly purified

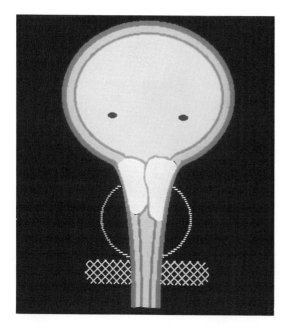

Figure 18-2. Schematic representation of cushions of Urethrin or Contigen just below the bladder neck.

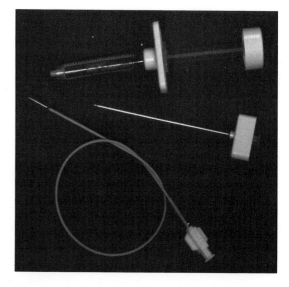

Figure 18-3. Injection delivery systems for Contigen.

bovine dermal collagen that is cross-linked with glutaraldehyde and dispersed in phosphate buffered physiologic saline. As a substance injected into humans, Contigen has the additional positive attribute of not eliciting a foreign body reaction. A minimal inflammatory response results from this noncytotoxic material, and there has been no evidence of particle migration.

The technique is (as with Urethrin) to attempt the injection either suburothelially through a needle placed directly through the cystoscope or periurethrally with a spinal needle through the tissues adjacent to the urethra. Obviously the cause of the defect, tissue condition at the injection site, and plane of placement of the injectable affect the degree of correction. For this reason, it may require repeated treatments to attain full continence regardless of the compound chosen. It has been my preference to inject males transurethrally and females periurethrally for the reasons discussed earlier in the section on Urethrin. Either way, the procedure is

under direct vision by way of the cystoscope. All women have been injected under local anesthesia in an outpatient setting. In my hands, I find the injection of females with Contigen much simpler than with Urethrin.

Preparation of the patient is identical to that discussed for Urethrin. The introitus and urethra are covered with 2% plain lidocaine jelly and left 10 minutes before cystoscopy begins. The transurethral delivery system consists of a beveled 20-gauge 1.5-cm needle attached to a 5 French thermoplastic catheter easily accommodated by a 21 French cystoscope sheath. I primarily use a 30-degree lens but often find a 0-degree lens to be helpful in selected individuals. The Contigen itself is provided in a 3-ml Luer-Lok syringe that easily attaches to the long needle (Fig. 18-3). Each syringe contains 2.5 ml of Contigen. In this manner, under direct vision, the bulking of the urethral mucosa may be observed with injection continuing until the urethra appears to close in the midline (Fig. 18-4).

Again the possible complications of bleeding and extrusion of the injectable substance are eliminated by using a periurethral rather than a

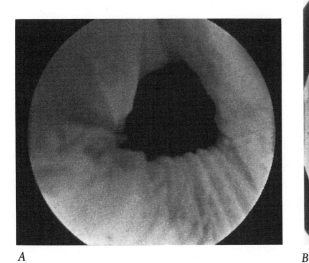
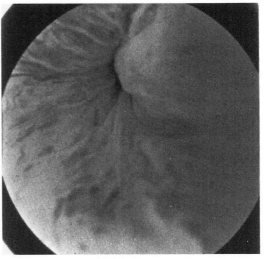

A   B

Figure 18-4. Endoscopic appearance of bladder neck before (A) and after (B) injection with Contigen. (From Appell RA. Periurethral collagen injection for female incontinence. Probl Urol 1991;5:134.)

transurethral approach (Fig. 18-5). Periurethrally at the 5 and 7 o'clock positions, 1% plain lidocaine is injected for a total of approximately 2 ml on either side of the urethra. Again, I usually use a 30-degree lens. A 22-gauge spinal needle is placed periurethrally at approximately 4 o'clock with the bevel of the needle directed medially (*i.e.*, toward the lumen), and it is slowly advanced while gazing through the cystoscope to notice the bulging of the tip of the needle against the lining of the urethra, so proper position of the needle can be ascertained before actual injection of the Contigen. When this point is reached, the 3-ml syringe of Contigen is attached to the spinal needle, and with one hand stabilizing the cystoscope for direct vision, the second hand injects the Contigen. One can actually see the material layering up outside the lining of the urethra gradually pressing the lumen closed (Fig. 18-4). At approximately the halfway point, the needle is removed and placed at the 8 o'clock position on the opposite side, and material is injected. Ultimately the appearance of the posterior urethra cystoscopically from the midurethra

reveals what appears to be two lateral lobes of a prostate "kissing" in the midline (Fig. 18-4). At this point, thinking that the procedure has been completed, one of the great advantages to local anesthesia is to have the patient stand and perform a few provocative maneuvers in an attempt to cause urinary leakage. When both the patient and the surgeon are satisfied, the procedure is officially terminated.

An important technical point is that repeated injections may be necessary to accomplish total continence. This is due to the difficulty in determining the quantity of material needed for each patient. Injections may be safely repeated every 7 days to achieve total continence.

Postoperative Management

An indwelling catheter is *not* used to prevent "molding" of the urethra around it. Difficulty in voiding, if present, is handled by intermittent catheterization using nothing larger than a 14 French catheter. This is an outpatient proce-

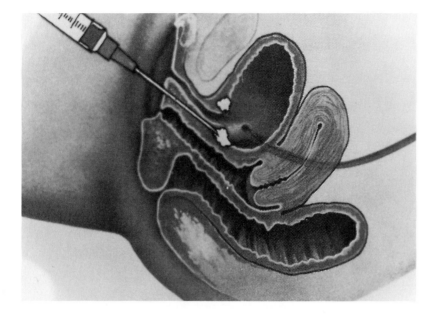

Figure 18-5. Periurethral Contigen injection procedure. (From Appell RA. Periurethral collagen injection for female incontinence. Probl Urol 1991;5:134.)

dure, and the patient is discharged on oral antibiotics and returns in 24 hours for evaluation, which includes determination of postvoid residual urine. Reinjection, if necessary, is then scheduled.

Efficacy and Safety of Urethrin and Contigen

The purpose of the procedure is to remedy the urinary incontinence problem, and the only truly acceptable result is complete dryness, even if this can be attained only after repeated injections. This demonstrates one of the major drawbacks to the procedure, that is, the inability to determine the quantity of injected material (Urethrin, Contigen, or whatever) needed for any individual patient. Although the statement concerning dryness is appropriate for the purist, most women (and therefore investigators) accept a certain amount of urinary leakage—so-called social continence, meaning urinary loss handled

by tissues or a minipad at most. If one also includes as "cured" those dry individuals who must empty their bladders by self-catheterization, results may appear astounding for slings, artificial sphincters, and injectables. Using these criteria, successful sling surgery occurs in 81% to 98%; successful sphincter surgery in more than 90% regardless of whether the abdominal or transvaginal approach is used; successful Urethrin injection in 70% to 95%; and successful Contigen injection in 64% to 95% of women.[11-14]

Because the results are comparable, why have injectables (easier for the patient and surgeon alike) not been universally accepted and performed? There are two glaringly objectionable aspects to injectable usage: (1) the inability to determine the quantity of material needed for an individual patient and (2) the safety of the material injected.

With respect to the first problem regarding quantity of material needed for a patient, I have no answers, and one does not improve at judging the quantity with experience. In the 149 women injected with Contigen between 10/87 and 1/91, 34 required less than 10 ml and 30 required more than 30 ml of material. The actual range to achieve continence in the females has been 2.5 to 85.0 ml. The simplicity of the procedure and the use of local anesthesia on an outpatient basis should make this of little import as long as the patient is aware of this fact preoperatively. Females have required an average of 2.2 injections and 19.2 ml of Contigen to attain continence.[14]

The second issue of safety explains the delay in approval of Urethrin and Contigen by the FDA. At the time of this writing, Urethrin has been approved only for men with postprostatectomy incontinence (thus relegating its usage to elderly men), and Contigen is still considered investigational. The concerns over the safety of Urethrin relate to particle migration and granuloma formation.[10,15] Of course, granuloma formation signifies a chronic foreign body reaction resulting long-term in fibrosis and possibly carcinogenesis, made more significant by the fact that related polymers of polytetrafluoroethylene have been shown to be carcinogenic in rats.[16] Despite this information, however, in the two decades of usage of Polytef in otolaryngology and certain centers for urinary incontinence in the United States and Europe, untoward sequelae have not been reported in humans, and the material may certainly be recommended for those women past the age of 60 years, especially since it has been approved for men in the same age group.

The concerns with the safety of Contigen are quite different than those enumerated with Urethrin. The fact that Contigen is biodegradable is both its strong point and its weak point. There is no concern over migration and granuloma formation as there is with Urethrin because this material begins to degrade in 12 weeks and is completely degraded in 9 to 19 months.[17] This brings to question the later need for repeated reinjections in patients rendered continent when the material degrades. Life-table analysis reveals that once continence has been attained with

Contigen, more than 80% of patients will not regress.[18] Contigen does elicit a minimal inflammatory response without granuloma formation that enables replacement of the degraded bovine collagen with the patient's own collagen because there is transformation of the injected collagen into living connective tissue.[19,20] The primary safety concern with Contigen is with respect to immunogenicity because there have been claims by patients who had collagen injections for soft tissue augmentation of signs and symptoms of collagen vascular disorders, such as dermatomyositis, which have resulted in litigation.

Despite these claims, there has been no evidence to link injection of bovine collagen with any disorder, as the injected patient population has thus far actually had a lower incidence of such disorders than would be expected in the general population. The multicenter investigative incontinence study includes skin testing to exclude any patients who may have an immunologic response. Only 5 of the first 333 patients have had a positive skin test result and were not injected for this reason. In addition, all patients have been evaluated by enzyme-linked immunosorbent assay (ELISA) for humoral antibodies, and no significant anticollagen antibody responses have been found following implantation of Contigen. In fact, there appears to be a significantly reduced potential to produce local immune-type reactions after collagen has been cross-linked with glutaraldehyde, and no patients in the multicenter trials have had an adverse event relating to immunogenicity.[21] The only adverse events have been transient urinary retention in 5 patients and urinary tract infection in 12 patients. Seventeen women have withdrawn from the study, but only 5 of these were due to lack of improvement. Thus far, Contigen appears safe as well as efficacious.

Conclusions

The goal of treatment of females with bladder outflow incompetence due to an intrinsic defect in the continence mechanism is to compress the proximal urethra, allowing coaptation without obstruction. In theory, this goal is best attained by the artificial urinary sphincter, but the difficulty in the surgery in females who have had multiple failed operations has caused surgeons to search for alternative forms of management. Periurethral injections have the potential to accomplish this need.

The best results with periurethral injections are in those patients who do not have detrusor problems, who have adequate bladder capacity, and who have no anatomic abnormality. Of the alternative treatments available to patients with severe urinary incontinence due to outlet incompetence, periurethral injections must be compared with the implantation of the artificial urinary sphincter and sling procedures. Many of the patients for whom these procedures are indicated are unsuitable surgical candidates owing to concomitant medical problems. Because therapy with injectables is less invasive than open surgery, a significant number of these patients can benefit from periurethral injection therapy, as their therapeutic options are extremely limited. With respect to materials currently available, the injection procedure using Contigen has been easy to perform under local anesthesia and thus far appears free of significant complications. This procedure should be restricted to those patients with clear-cut bladder outflow incompetence caused by a defect in the intrinsic continence mechanism because it is not helpful in detrusor instability or urethral hypermobility (genuine stress urinary incontinence).

References

1. Murless BC. The injection treatment of stress incontinence. Br J Obstet Gynaecol 1938;45:67.
2. Sachse H. Treatment of urinary incontinence with sclerosing solutions, indications, results, complications. Urol Int 1963;15:225.
3. Quackels R. Deux incontinences apres adenonectomic queries par injection de paraffine dans de perinee. Acta Urol Belg 1955;23:259.
4. Appell RA. Commentary: Periurethral polytetrafluoroethylene (Polytef) injections. In: Whitehead ED, ed. Current operative urology 1990. Philadelphia: JB Lippincott, 1990:63.
5. Berg S. Polytef augmentation urethroplasty: Correction of surgically incurable incontinence by injection technique. Arch Surg 1973;107:379.
6. Deane AM, English P, Hehir M, et al. Teflon injection in stress incontinence. Br J Urol 1985;57:78.
7. Lim KB, Ball AJ, Feneley RCL. Periurethral teflon injection: A simple treatment for urinary incontinence. Br J Urol 1983;55:208.
8. Politano VA. Periurethral teflon injection for urinary incontinence. Urol Clin North Am 1978;5:415.
9. Shulman CC, Simon J, Wespes E, Germeau F. Endoscopic injection of teflon for female urinary incontinence. Eur Urol 1983;9:246.
10. Malizia AA Jr, Reiman HM, Myers RP, et al. Migration and granulomatous reaction after periurethral injection of polytef (teflon). JAMA 1984;251:3277.
11. Blaivas JG. Treatment of female incontinence secondary to urethral damage or loss. Urol Clin North Am 1991;18:355.
12. Light JK, Scott FB. Management of urinary incontinence in women with the artificial urinary sphincter. J Urol 1985;134:476.
13. Appell RA. Techniques and results in the implantation of the artificial urinary sphincter in women with type III stress urinary incontinence by a vaginal approach. Neurourol Urodynam 1988;7:613.
14. Appell RA. Injectables for urethral incompetence. World J Urol 1990;8:208.
15. Mittleman RE, Marracini JV. Pulmonary teflon granulomas following periurethral teflon injection for urinary incontinence. Arch Pathol Lab Med 1983;107:611.
16. Oppenheimer BS, Oppenheimer ET, Stout AP. The latent period in carcinogenesis by plastic in rats and its relation to the presa-comatous stage. Cancer 1958;11:204.
17. Leonard MP, Canning DA, Epstein JI, et al. Local tissue reaction to the subureteric injection of glutaraldehyde cross-linked bovine collagen in humans. J Urol 1990;143:1209.
18. Bard CR. PMAA submission to US Food and Drug Administration for IDE #G850010, 1990.
19. Ford CN, Martin DW, Warren TF. Injectable collagen in laryngeal rehabilitation. Laryngoscope 1984;95:513.
20. Remacle M, Marbaix E. Collagen implants in the human larynx. Arch Otorhinolaryngol 1988;245:203.
21. Griffiths R, Shakespeare P. Human dermal collagen allografts: A three year histological study. Br J Plast Surg 1982;35:519.

Artificial Sphincter

Friedhelm Schreiter

Friedhelm Noll

In 1973, the artificial sphincter was introduced by Timm, Scott, and Bradley.[4,5] The currently available AS 800 (Fig. 19-1) is the result of an evolutionary process, which started with the first model AS 721. Every change in the design of the device (four different generations) produced better results in terms of postoperative continence and the number of necessary revisions. Wrong patient selection as well as a faulty surgical technique are now the most common causes of device failure. The AS 800 has a low failure rate. It can be easily handled by most of the patients and does not cause significant inconvenience in terms of limitations of daily activities.

Patient Selection

The artificial urinary sphincter (AUS) is able only to substitute a malfunctioning or absent sphincteric mechanism. The device is not intended to control detrusor hyperreflexia resulting in incontinence.[3] Detrusor function affects the clinical success of AUS implantation and should therefore be carefully tested preoperatively. The preoperative evaluation includes assessment of the following factors.

URODYNAMIC STATUS OF BLADDER

Urodynamics are necessary to evaluate the filling and storage phase of the bladder and exclude the presence of detrusor hyperreflexia. A normal bladder or detrusor areflexia with unaltered compliance is consistently associated with a high degree of success approaching 90%. Alternatively, augmentation cystoplasty may be necessary to create a low-pressure reservoir. Urodynamic testing is necessary in most cases of altered compliance to decide whether pharmacologic manipulation alone can achieve a low-pressure reservoir or whether augmentation cystoplasty is required.

BLADDER OUTFLOW RESISTANCE
AND RESIDUAL URINE

The presence or absence of significant outflow resistance is important if the bladder is to be emptied per urethra. Patients selected for sphincter implantation should have no residual urine. In patients with neuropathic lesions, surgery is usually required to decrease outflow resistance and residual urine. Women are best treated with augmentation of the urethra by a bladder flap

Female Urology, edited by Elroy D. Kursh and Edward McGuire. J. B. Lippincott, Philadelphia, © 1994.

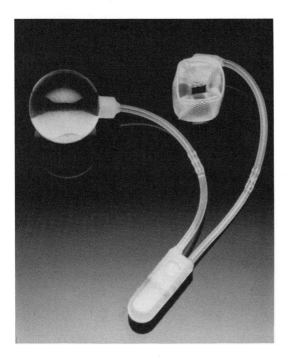

Figure 19-1. *The AS 800 is the currently available model of the artificial urinary sphincter.*

urethroplasty or an extensive Y-V-plasty. The level of outflow obstruction is in most cases at the external sphincter. The sphincter fails to relax, especially in neurogenic lesions. The decision to ablate any bladder outflow resistance rests with the implanting surgeon and the patient. If the desire to void per urethra is important for the patient, the additional risk of any procedure at the bladder neck is worth considering. If the patient is willing to apply intermittent catheterization postoperatively, however, procedures reducing the outflow resistance are not necessary.

OTHER DRAWBACKS

Perfusion of the tissue underneath the cuff is important because this is critical in avoiding cuff erosion. Any circumstances that significantly reduce the blood supply of this tissue increase the

risk of erosion occurring. Examples of this are irradiation, previous surgery at the bladder neck, and trauma. If the manual dexterity is altered, patients are usually not eligible for sphincter implantation. This is also true if there is any doubt regarding mental ability because the correct handling of the device and the micturition itself demand some understanding of what has been done to the bladder and its sphincter mechanism.

Operative Procedure

PREOPERATIVE PREPARATION

The following items are essential for sphincter implantation:

1. Sterile urine must be present. Any bacteriuria must be treated before surgery.
2. Intravenous antibiotics are routinely administered 12 hours before surgery.
3. The skin of the patient is washed for 15 minutes immediately before surgery with providone-iodine (Betadine) soap.
4. The final skin preparation uses an alcoholic betadine solution.

During the surgical procedure, the clinician should

1. Use vascular forceps whenever handling the device.
2. Use silicon-shod hemostats for cross clamping the tubing.
3. Avoid the entrance of blood or serum into the tubing. Irrigation is therefore performed during connections and whenever open tubing is handled. Gloves should be changed more often than usual.

SURGICAL PROCEDURE

The AUS in women must be placed around the bladder neck. The patients are placed in lithotomy position with thighs nearly parallel to the floor to allow access to the vagina during the surgical procedure. A vaginal pack is inserted to expand the vagina and allow easier identification of the dissection layer for cuff placement.

A low Pfannenstiel skin incision is made. The dissection proceeds thereafter to gain access to the retropubic space. Exposure of the bladder neck and the endopelvic fascia is a simple procedure in patients who have not undergone any previous retropubic surgery. Palpation of the balloon of a transurethral catheter allows easy identification of the bladder neck. At this point, the tissue posterior to the balloon of the indwelling catheter is grasped between the thumb and the index finger. The structure lying posteriorly is the vagina. In the absence of any previous anterior vaginal wall surgery, the plane between bladder neck and vagina is created relatively easily with a right-angled scissors.

Vaginal examination should be performed to ensure that the correct plane is dissected. If the vagina is perforated, the perforation should be repaired immediately. If previous surgery has obliterated this plane, an opening of the bladder is recommended. Palpating from below and above allows correct identification of the scarred plane and enables dissection without vaginal or bladder perforation. A right-angled clamp is then used to pull the cuff sizer through the previously dissected tunnel. After the catheter is withdrawn, the bladder neck diameter is measured and thus the correct cuff size determined. Bleeding from the tunnel usually ceases after insertion of the cuff. Estimation of cuff size may be a problem because it should neither be too large nor too small. The average size in women is 6 to 7 cm. The appropriately sized cuff is then pulled through with a right-angled clamp (Fig. 19-2). This is easily passed underneath the still present cuff sizer by slightly pulling it up. Care should be taken that the cuff does not twist during this maneuver. The cuff is snapped in position.

The balloon is inserted inside the perivesical space, which can be easily accessed. The hysteresis curve of the pressure-regulating balloon indicates that a fairly constant pressure is present with filling volumes of 18 to 22 ml. Therefore the

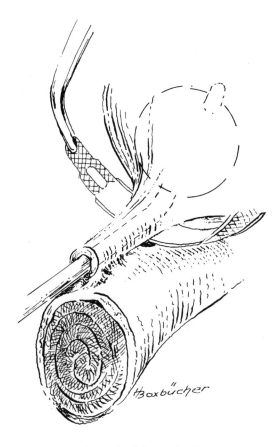

Figure 19-2. *The cuff of the artificial urinary sphincter is placed around the bladder neck.*

complicated method described by the manufacturer of the AS 800 is not necessary, and a simple filling with 22 ml of an isotonic mixture of sterile water and radiopaque medium provides the same device pressure. The cuff is maintained empty. To register the correct balloon pressure, each balloon is tested before implantation. It is filled with 20 ml of sterile water, and the exact balloon pressure is measured by way of a simple open tubing procedure. The fascia is then closed, and the rectus muscle is readapted using interrupted sutures of a monofilament absorbable suture. Inadvertent puncturing during closure must be avoided. Hemostasis is exceedingly important because preferably no drains should be used.

The tubing from the cuff and balloon are

then brought out separately using a passing tool. The tubing should exit through the full layer of muscles to enter the subcutaneous area. With the aid of a large clamp, a space is dissected in the subdartos area of the appropriate labia majora. The pump is inserted into this area and should be placed in a position where it will be easily accessible to the patient. The tubing is then cut to the appropriate length and connections made with quick connectors. The subcutaneous tissue is closed in layers followed by the skin. Final manipulation of the device confirms normal function before deactivation is performed by pressure on the poppet valve. A small 12 French Foley catheter is left indwelling for urinary drainage.

POSTOPERATIVE TREATMENT

Intravenous antibiotics are applied for 3 days postoperatively. The device is usually deactivated. The duration of deactivation depends on the clinical situation. When the patient is able to pump without any pain, the sphincter is activated routinely. Only when intraoperatively bad tissue had been recognized or other circumstances are present that demanded a longer healing period, activation was delayed for 6 to 8 weeks. At this time, the collateral circulation should be re-established. The duration of catheter drainage also depends on the clinical circumstances. The catheter is routinely removed in the first 48 hours. If the bladder has been opened intraoperatively, however, or an augmentation cystoplasty performed, catheter drainage is maintained for 7 to 10 days. One advantage of the AS 800 series is the ability to activate and deactivate at will. This allows the surgeon to decide when activation of the device should be performed.

Patients

From 1983 to 1992, we implanted an AS 800 artificial sphincter in 123 female patients. Of these, 80 remained in our continuous follow-up and are now followed for at least 2 years, with a

Table 19-1. *Etiology of Incontinence*

ETIOLOGY	NO.	NO.
Afunctional/hypotonic urethra	40	40
Neurogenic bladder		
Meningomyelocele	17	
Paraplegia	5	
Others	8	30
Extrophy/epispadia	4	
Stress	0	
Others (pelvic trauma)	6	10
Total	80	80

mean of 4.8 years. Forty of these female patients had afunctional urethras secondary to failed previous anti–stress incontinence procedures. Thirty suffered from neurogenic incontinence with sphincteric involvement, and 10 had congenital sphincter anomalies or traumatic sphincter weakness (Table 19-1). Those patients with an afunctional urethra had undergone multiple previous operations. Thirty-seven had urethral suspensions such as MMK, needle, or sling procedures; nine had bladder neck surgery. In 26 patients, gynecologic procedures had been performed. Twenty had paraurethral Teflon injec-

Table 19-2. *Previous Operations in Patients with an Afunctional Urethra*

OPERATION	NO.
Hysterectomy, abdominal	5
Hysterectomy, vaginal	8
Bladder neck	
TUR bladder neck	5
Bladder flap	1
Tanagho's neourethra	2
Urethral suspensions	
MMK	8
Burch	1
Alloplastic sling	7
Lyodura	6
Fascial sling	5
Stamey	10
Colporaphy	13
Teflon	20
Others	9
Total	100

Table 19-3. *Previous Operations in Patients with Neurogenic Bladder, Congenital Anomalies of the Urethra, or Incontinence after Pelvic Trauma*

OPERATION	NO.
Bladder neck	
TUR bladder neck	2
Bladder neck reconstruction	2
Bladder flap	11
Bladder	
Reimplantation of ureters	11
Augmentation	6
Urethral suspension	
MMK	3
Others	6
Total	41

Table 19-5. *Additional Operations*

ADDITIONAL OPERATIONS	NEUROGENIC BLADDER	AFUNCTIONAL URETHRA (NO.)
Ureteral reimplantation	4	1
Bladder flap	5	1
Augmentation	12	1
Total	21	3

another three were augmented. These three patients all developed upper tract dilatation soon after AUS implantation (Table 19-5).

tions, and 14 had radiation or extended pelvic surgery. All these previous operations add up to a remarkable number of 100 procedures in 40 patients (Table 19-2).

In the neurogenic group, 11 operations at the bladder neck, such as transurethral resection (TUR), Y-V plasties, or Tanagho's neourethra; 12 for bladder failures; and 7 for urethral suspensions had been performed before AS 800 implantation (Table 19-3).

The youngest patient was 16 years old, and the oldest was 74 years old. The most frequently used cuffs are 6 and 7 cm long, and nearly all patients had a 61 to 70 cm H_2O pressure-regulating balloon implanted (Table 19-4).

With AS 800 implantation, 21 additional procedures were performed, including 4 antireflux operations, 5 bladder flap procedures, and 12 augmentations. During follow-up, four patients had to be diverted into a Kock-Pouch, and

Results

Of the patients, 86.3% are completely continent, not needing a pad. A total of 3.8% are improved and use one or two pads a day, not requiring a reoperation. Four patients remained incontinent, and one is scheduled for a reimplantation. Four patients had been diverted into a continent Kock-Pouch. Thus, by AUS implantation alone, 90.1% of the patients became continent.

In regards to emptying, 81.3% are able to empty their bladder without residuals after opening of the sphincter; 8 have to apply additional clean intermittent self-catheterization (CIC) one to two times a day. Seven empty by CIC alone; the Kock-Pouch patients are listed among these.

In 38 of 80 patients, a total of 62 revisions were performed. Twenty-five had one, eight had two, and five had three or more operations (Table 19-6). Infection and erosion were the most

Table 19-4. *Pressure Regulating Balloon*

BALLOON PRESSURE (CM H_2O)	NO.
51–60	4
61–70	72
71–80	4
Total	80

Table 19-6. *Number of Revisions*

NO. REVISIONS	NO. PATIENTS	NO. OPERATIONS
1	25	25
2	8	16
≥3	5	21
Total	38	62

Table 19-7. *Reasons for Reoperations*

REASONS	NO.
Erosion	19
Tissue atrophy	13
Infections	10
Leakage	13
Wrong cuff sizing	2
Air in the system	2
Pump malfunction	3
Total	62

Table 19-9. *Previous Operations in Patients with Erosion*

OPERATION	NO.	PERCENTAGE
Bladder neck	21	
TUR bladder neck	2	28.5
Bladder flap	4	40
Tanagho's neourethra	2	100
Urethral suspensions	7	15
Teflon injections	6	30
Bladder	8	
Augmentation	6	31.5
Bladder reduction plasty (Zödler)	2	100
Ureteral reimplantation	0	
Others	1	
Radiation	1	20
Total	30	

common reasons for revision, constituting 48.2% of all revisions. The third most common reason was tissue atrophy underneath the cuff. Twenty-five percent of the revisions were due to device failures, most commonly cuff leakage (Table 19-7). This could be avoided by design changes of the cuff. Producing the cuff on a curved rather than a flat template offers one single curved cushion instead of a fourfold one. This eliminates the creases and thus avoids leakage, which always occurs at those sharp bends of the compressive cushion.

The most often performed revisionary operation was resizing of the cuff, which added up to 30% of all reoperations. Interestingly, 82% of the revisions are done in the first 21 months after AUS implantation. Thereafter the sphincter remained relatively stable. The most often cause for a late revision was cuff leakage (Table 19-8).

Fifty percent of the patients had undergone a previous operation at the bladder neck site, but

Table 19-10. *Number of Previous Operations in Patients with Erosion*

NUMBER PREVIOUS OPERATIONS	NO. PATIENTS
0	3
1	3
2	0
3	4
4	1
≥4	7

in the erosion group, operations at the bladder neck summed up to 79%, indicating the high risk in this group (Tables 19-9 and 19-10).

For tissue atrophy or infection, no special risk factor could be detected. Because of the high risk for erosion, AUS implantation should never be done with any bladder neck procedure in a one-stage setting.

Table 19-8. *Type of Revisionary Operation*

OPERATION	NO.
Explantation of AS 800	17
Change of AS 800	7
Cuff explantation	12
Change of cuff	18
Change of balloon	3
Change of pump	2
Others	3
Total	62

Discussion

The current AS 800 AUS is a reliable means of achieving urinary continence.[4,5] Strict adherence to basic prosthetic surgical principles is necessary, however, to achieve optimum results.

1. Continence can be achieved with an implantation of an AS 800 in more than 90% of female patients.
2. Most patients empty their bladder after opening the sphincter without residual urine.
3. Fifty percent of patients needed a reoperation; previous bladder neck procedures increase the risk for a revision. The enormous number of procedures before sphincter implantation contribute to the high reoperation rate. Most of the reoperations, however, are minor, could easily be performed, and were easily tolerated by the patients.
4. Patient acceptance is encouraging. Every woman who once had the experience of continence after AS 800 implantation wants to have this re-established as soon as possible when the sphincter fails. The ease of bladder emptying is an important factor for many women who choose to undergo sphincter implantation rather than another procedure, which may re-establish continence but demands intermittent catheterization.
5. AS 800 is truly an alternative to urinary diversion. In our opinion, there is no technique better than AUS for the properly selected patient.

References

1. Scott FB, Bradley WE, Timm GW. Treatment of urinary incontinence by an implantable prosthetic sphincter. Urology 1973;1:252.
2. Scott FB, Bradley WE, Timm GW. Treatment of incontinence by an implantable prosthetic urinary sphincter. J Urol 1974;112:75.
3. Mundy AR, Stephenson TP. Selection of patients for implantation of the Brantley Scott artificial urinary sphincter. Br J Urol 1984;56:717.
4. Khoury AE, Churchill BM. The artificial urinary sphincter. Pediatr Clin North Am 1987;34:1175.
5. Mundy AR. Artificial sphincters. Br J Urol 1991; 67:225.

20

Management of Complications Resulting from Stress Incontinence Surgery

Ernest M. Sussman

Shlomo Raz

As with any type of surgery, a fundamental anatomic and physiologic knowledge of the female vesicourethral unit is mandatory before the practicing urologist should embark on performing surgery for stress urinary incontinence (SUI). Obviously the best form of management for surgical complications is prevention. The "prepared mind" allows the operating urologist to recognize and deal with complications resulting during and after surgery for SUI.

Other chapters in this text elaborate on many of the intraoperative and postoperative complications to be mentioned in this chapter (bladder instability, detrusor incontinence, injuries to the urogenital organs, and management of genital and pelvic prolapse). First, intraoperative complications are discussed followed by postoperative sequelae that can be encountered. The later part of the chapter with regard to postoperative problems is further subdivided as to the urodynamic consequences of SUI surgery (recurrent SUI, instability, and retention) and general complications with respect to surgery in the retropubic region. Because our female urology patients have the majority of their procedures performed transvaginally, a certain bias may be introduced with respect to the gamut of complications presented on this subject.

Much of the urologic experience in the man-

agement of these complications can be traced back to the gynecologic literature covering injury to the urinary tract or intestine. The reported incidence during these gynecologic operations is about 5% to 8%.[1,2]

Intraoperative Complications

Intraoperative complications include bleeding, bladder and urethral perforations, ureteral injuries, and intestinal violations.

BLEEDING

The prevention of intraoperative bleeding begins before surgery. A thorough history detailing the patient's prior operations and responses to trauma must be documented. Appropriate preoperative screening with a platelet count, prothrombin time, and partial thromboplastin time provides a good estimate of clotting abnormalities. Patients are reminded to stop aspirin and other anti-inflammatory medications 7 to 10 days before surgery. Bleeding times are reserved for those patients in whom a positive history is obtained in the face of a negative routine hematologic workup.

Intraoperative bleeding can be venous or arterial in origin. Ignoring immediate hemostasis during surgery is dangerous even with the knowl-

Female Urology, edited by Elroy D. Kursh and Edward McGuire. J. B. Lippincott, Philadelphia, © 1994.

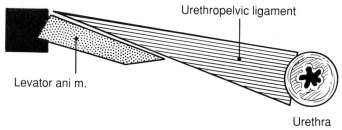

Tendinous arc

Urethropelvic ligament

Levator ani m.

Urethra

Figure 20-1. *Anatomic depiction of the anterolateral relationship of levator complex with respect to the urethropelvic ligament.*

edge that venous bleeding can be controlled by extrinsic pressure. Retropubic procedures usually provide better exposure of the bleeding source, and appropriate hemostasis (coagulation or ligatures) can be instituted.

Transvaginal approaches require a somewhat different philosophy. The most common source of bleeding during a transvaginal needle bladder neck suspension (BNS) is with violation of the periurethral fascia during dissection with either the Stamey or the modified Pereyra-Raz (MPR) BNS. If significant bleeding occurs, we advocate suture ligation with 3–0 braided absorbable suture for hemostasis. Another potential source of bleeding with either the MPR BNS or anterior colporrhaphy is entrance into the levator musculature, which occurs if dissection is carried too lateral when one is trying to dissect under the vaginal wall along the periurethral fascia toward its insertion into the tendinous arc (Fig. 20-1).

When attempting to ensure hemostasis, only vigorous venous and all arterial bleeding should be controlled. When performing the MPR BNS, a gauze sponge may be inserted into the retropubic space temporarily, while dissection proceeds on the contralateral side. This frequently provides a satisfactory tamponading effect. One should be cautious when coagulating directly on the urethra or bladder surface. This may lead to coagulation injury with subsequent necrosis and fistula formation. If coagulation becomes necessary, we prefer the bipolar electrocauterization forceps.

We routinely insert an antibiotic-soaked (mafenide [Sulfamylon] or povidone-iodine [Betadine]) vaginal pack following our transvaginal anti-incontinence procedures (AIPs), which provides a mild tamponading effect for cases with minimal oozing. When circumstances arise that call for more control in dangerous bleeding situations, the so-called umbrella pack of Mikulicz may be a lifesaving procedure.[3] Another option is the intravaginal insertion of a 30-ml balloon Foley catheter (instillation of 60 to 90 ml is usually required) as described by Katske[4] (Fig. 20-2). If bleeding occurs despite these measures, significant uncontrolled bleeding is evident.

PERFORATION

Bladder

Injuries to the bladder are more likely to occur in patients with a history of a prior AIP or pelvic surgery or in previously radiated patients. Parnell and colleagues reported 8 *urinary perforations* among 114 women undergoing the Marshall-Marchetti-Krantz (MMK) retropubic BNS after prior failed AIPs.[5] Conversely, Leach and Raz reported 54 reoperative patients undergoing the MPR BNS for recurrent SUI.[6] There were no instances of bladder or urethral perforation in this series.

Injuries to the bladder during transvaginal AIPs occur mainly at the base; however, anterolateral wall perforation may also occur and is

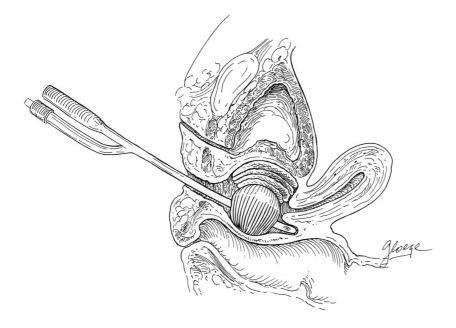

Figure 20-2. Intravaginal Foley catheter placed for tamponading effect. (Note: Vaginal packing lies between the anterior vaginal wall and Foley catheter.)

the direct result of the suprapubic Stamey needle passage. Bladder emptying before needle passage may reduce the chances of this event. Uniform use of a Foley catheter is invaluable in periodically assessing the bladder neck throughout these procedures. Also, by plugging the catheter during the course of the procedure, the collected urine can be assessed for hematuria, a sure sign of injury to the urinary tract. If the site of perforation is still unclear, intravesical instillation of any of the available vital dyes (indigo carmine or methylene blue) usually reveals the site of vesical disruption.

Obviously any iatrogenic bladder perforation should be promptly recognized and repaired appropriately. This involves a standard two-layer braided absorbable suture closure, with the first layer incorporating the full bladder wall thickness and the outer layer bringing together the seromuscular tissues in an interrupted fashion. If the insult occurs during the course of a transvaginal BNS, the suspension may be completed after repair of the unintentional cystotomy. Hadley and Myers presented 10 patients in whom a bladder perforation during the course of a transvaginal BNS was primarily repaired and the BNS completed with no instances of late sequelae, specifically no retropubic space infection nor fistula formation.

With either the retropubic or transvaginal approach, retropubic drainage is mandatory with a bladder perforation as with any violation of the urinary tract. This does not present a problem during the retropubic approach; however, draining a bladder perforation created during a transvaginal procedure requires a different plan. Having gained access into the retropubic space during the MPR BNS, a Kelly clamp is inserted transvaginally to tent up the abdominal wall just lateral to the bladder. A stab incision is made over the clamp, and a Penrose drain is guided down into the retropubic space. In no instance should the drain be allowed to exit from the vaginal side of the wound.

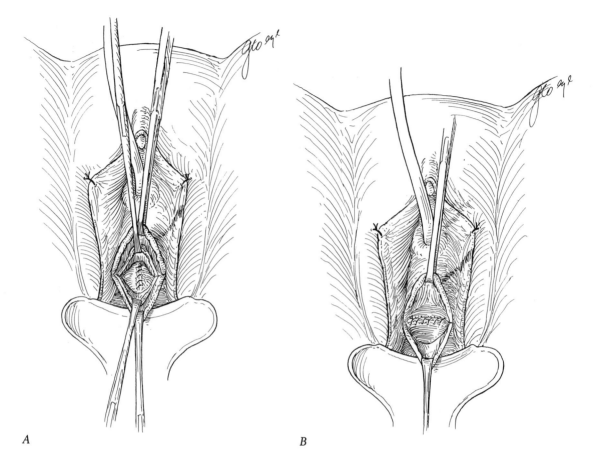

A   *B*

Figure 20-3. *(A) First layer of urethral reconstruction closes the full urethral wall thickness. (B) The periurethral fascia is closed transversely as the second layer of closure.*

Urethral

Inadvertent injury to the urethra is more likely to occur during transvaginal AIPs. This is because the female urethra lies just underneath the anterior vaginal wall and is separated from it by a thin periurethral and vaginal sheath. Once recognized, repair must be instituted to prevent postoperative sequelae, such as a diverticulum or fistula.[8]

A running suture of fine braided absorbable suture usually suffices in closure of these superficial defects. If the urethral lumen has been violated, a two-layer closure similar to that carried out for the repair of a urethral diverticulum should also be done (Fig. 20-3). After a full-thickness running suture of the urethral wall is done, reapproximation of the periurethral fascia ('the glistening surface') in a noncrossing fashion using braided absorbable suture completes the repair. Crushed or fulgurated tissue must be meticulously excised to prepare the urethral tissue before repair.

If the defect after excision is large and closure without narrowing the urethral lumen is impossible, a more extensive repair as performed in a neourethral formation is required.[9] A Martius fibrofatty graft of the labia then usually is required to complete the repair.[10,11]

BOWEL INJURY

Retropubic

The patient with prior surgery or radiation deserves special attention because inadvertent bowel injury is more likely in this subgroup of patients undergoing an AIP. Careful dissection and recognition of the injury are the best tenets to avoid violating the intestinal contents. Small perforations may be closed using usual general surgical principles, and the BNS may be completed because the absorbable sutures used in a retropubic BNS should not present a postoperative infectious problem.

Injury to the Bowel During Transvaginal Surgery

Again repair of iatrogenic injuries of the colon or small bowel during transvaginal surgery follows established criteria of general surgery. If inadvertent incision of the small bowel has occurred (with concomitant vaginal hysterectomy or enterocele repair), a two-layer closure may be obtained with the suture lines at right angles to each other.[12]

Special circumstances deserve attention within this discussion. Patients with prior abdominal surgery (anterior-posterior resection or hysterectomy) are at a much higher risk for perforation during a transvaginal BNS from the (1) suprapubic needle passage, (2) insertion of the suprapubic tube, or (3) entrance into the retropubic space during the MPR BNS. Maneuvers to avoid these complications include suprapubic cystostomy close to the symphysis pubis or, alternatively, omission of a cystostomy tube altogether with the institution of clean intermittent catheterization postoperatively to handle any prolonged retentive problems. As such, the urologist may opt to perform a retropubic BNS for more control in an effort to obviate these potentially serious post-BNS sequelae.

Although not a true complication, no major problems arise when the peritoneum has been opened during more involved transvaginal surgery for SUI (as in formal cystocele repair with BNS), provided that no bowel has been injured.[13]

With enough distance to the bowel, absorbable 2–0 pursestring sutures close the defect. If the opening is large (as exemplified after an enterocele repair or vaginal hysterectomy), a more formal closure has to be undertaken to prevent evisceration. This essentially involves the same principles used in an enterocele repair. Two sets of 1–0 pursestring sutures should incorporate the perivesical fasciae anteriorly: the broad, sacrouterine and cardinal ligaments laterally and the prerectal fascia posteriorly.

URETERAL INJURIES

Various authors report the incidence of ureteral involvement after gynecologic surgery to be from 0.3% to 3%.[14] Because AIPs are frequently done in combination with abdominal hysterectomies, the incidence of ureteral injuries can be expected to increase during these combined procedures. Ureteral injuries are, however, a rare complication of a routine BNS. The incidence of ureteral damage during BNS surgery in patients who have undergone prior abdominal surgery is significantly higher. Should there be extensive fibrosis and adhesions after previous surgery, preoperative insertion of ureteral stents may help facilitate intraoperative orientation.

During a retropubic BNS, the ureter may inadvertently become captured with one of the paravaginal sutures (more likely with a Burch or obturator shelf suspension) than with the periurethral sutures that are placed during a MMK procedure.[15-17] If the suture is removed immediately, surgical repair is usually not required. Prophylactic double-J stenting is, however, advisable. During our MPR BNS, we routinely perform cystoscopy at the end of the procedure after a previous intravenous injection of indigo carmine to assess for ureteral integrity by the observation of blue efflux. If no efflux is seen and suspicion is high for ureteral involvement, retrograde ureterography is required.

If there was some delay in the recognition of ureteral involvement during the procedure, intraoperative observation is in order. If there appears to be poor coloration of the ureter or if ischemic damage is strongly suspected, resection of the involved segment with either a ureteroureterostomy or reimplantation is required depending on the level of insult.

Postoperative Complications

For this portion of the chapter, problems that arise after surgery are divided into voiding dysfunction (recurrent SUI, retention, and urgency incontinence [UI]) and those general postoperative complications that may occur with surgery in the retropubic area.

CAUSE OF RECURRENT INCONTINENCE

An important point to remember is that the condition of SUI is the loss of urine per urethra coincident with an increase in intra-abdominal pressure in the absence of any involuntary detrusor activity. SUI may be due to malposition of the normal sphincteric unit (anatomic incontinence [AI]) or due to incompetence of the sphincteric unit itself (intrinsic sphincteric dysfunction [ISD]).

Aside from SUI, other sources for loss of urine from the urethral meatus include UI and urethral diverticula (Table 20-1). Watery discharge per vagina after an AIP is not always from the urethral meatus, and other causes for the extraurethral drainage (leakage) must be ruled out during the process of performing a detailed workup for recurrent SUI.

NONSTRESS INCONTINENCE

Urgency Incontinence

UI is an abnormal loss of urine per urethra caused by involuntary detrusor contractions and exists in between 15% and 30% of patients undergoing SUI surgery. Reportedly between 60% and 85% of these patients should have resolution or a vast improvement of UI after an AIP. *De novo* UI after surgery for SUI has been reported in between 5% and 15% of most reported series.

Table 20-1. *Differential Diagnoses for Fluid Leak from Vagina*

PER URETHRAL MEATUS

Stress urinary incontinence
    Anatomic incontinence
    Intrinsic urethral dysfunction
    Mixed anatomic incontinence and intrinsic sphincteric dysfunction
Urgency incontinence
Urethral diverticula
Congenital (ureteral ectopia)

EXTRAURETHRAL

Fistulas
    Vesicovaginal
    Urethrovaginal
    Ureterovaginal
Hydrops tubae profluens
Congenital (ureteral ectopia)
Vaginal cysts (Gartner's)

Careful history taking along with a properly performed urodynamic assessment should identify these patients both preoperatively and postoperatively.

Anticholinergic medications (oxybutynin, hyoscyamine sulfate, or propantheline bromide) with or without the addition of imipramine hydrochloride or estrogens have been helpful in this subgroup of patients in controlling UI. Urinary tract infections, occult carcinoma *in situ*, iatrogenic intravesical suture placement, and neurologic lesions must be ruled out before assigning a patient into this subgroup of idiopathic bladder instability.

Diverticula

Urethral diverticula as a cause of urinary incontinence are extremely rare. Patients with a urethral diverticulum frequently complain of lower tract irritative voiding symptoms along with postvoid dribbling. An anterior vaginal wall mass may be palpated, which after milking of the urethra can cause urine from the diverticular sac to be expressed at the external meatus.

As a cause of vaginal leakage after SUI surgery, either the patient had a preexisting diverticulum in addition to SUI or it developed secondary to the transvaginal procedure as a result of unsuspected injury to the urethral wall. With regard to the former scenario, if the diverticulum is recognized before BNS surgery, the transvaginal approach can be used to correct both problems simultaneously. Bass and Leach reported successful (no or minimal incontinence) combined management in 77% of 31 patients with a mean follow-up of 42 months.[18]

Fistulas

A urethrovaginal, ureterovaginal, or vesicovaginal fistula (VVF) should be highly suspected as a cause of extraurethral urinary leakage especially after a hysterectomy or complicated AIP. Patients with recurrent SUI may also have a VVF, which may actually mask their SUI component. The diagnosis of a VVF is made either with a cystogram or with the intravesical administration of any of the available vital dyes and a vaginally placed tampon.

Urethrovaginal fistulas may be more difficult to diagnose; however, a high index of suspicion should suggest this entity. Patients usually complain of alterations in their urinary stream and have leakage per vagina after urination. Physical examination, voiding cystography, cystoscopy, and vaginoscopy can help confirm the diagnosis.

Ureterovaginal fistulas can occur alone or in combination with a VVF. Ureteral genitourinary fistula can also be diagnosed using the pad-tampon test after either an oral urine colorizing agent (phenazopyridine) or intravenous agent (indigo carmine) is administered. A positive test result here in the face of a negative pad-tampon test after intravesical dye administration, thus ruling out a VVF, is almost confirmatory. Intravenous urography may demonstrate complete or partial obstruction and establish the diagnosis; however, retrograde studies are frequently necessary to delineate this abnormal communication fully.

Hydrops Tubae Profluens

Another rare form of vaginal drainage is hydrosalpinx, which is an abnormal fallopian tubova-

ginal leakage into the vaginal cuff after an abdominal hysterectomy. Leach and colleagues described two of these cases, one of which was found in coexistence with SUI.[19] Diagnosis may be aided by the demonstration of a negative oral phenazopyridine test ruling out urine as the source of leakage. Vaginoscopy and a vaginogram can then be used to locate the abnormal communication. Treatment consists of a transperitoneal repair with Burch colposuspension if coexisting SUI is present.

Congenital Abnormalities

Congenital abnormalities, including ureteral ectopia, should rarely persist into the SUI population without escaping detection. Depending on the degree of ectopy, urinary leakage may be periurethral or extraurethral. Young adolescents or even teenage girls with presumed SUI should be carefully evaluated for these rare forms of incontinence. Antegrade contrast studies along with voiding cystography can aid in the detection of these abnormalities.

RECURRENT STRESS URINARY INCONTINENCE

As with SUI, the pathophysiology of recurrent SUI must be considered in the context of either of two types: (1) AI due to displacement or hypermobility of the sphincteric unit or (2) ISD due to malfunction of the normal sphincteric unit as a result of radiation, multiple surgery, trauma, or neurologic disease (myelodysplasia). To help differentiate between AI and ISD, we advocate comprehensive evaluations to include a history, physical examination, cystourethroscopy, and urodynamic and radiologic study (videourodynamics).

AI is characteristically associated with mild to moderate subjective degrees of SUI, a well-coapted bladder neck endoscopically, and bladder neck hypermobility during straining cystourethrography (Fig. 20-4). Patients with ISD characteristically have more severe SUI produced with even the slightest of exertional movements, an atrophic or so-called pipestem urethra endoscopically, and a fixed or well-supported bladder

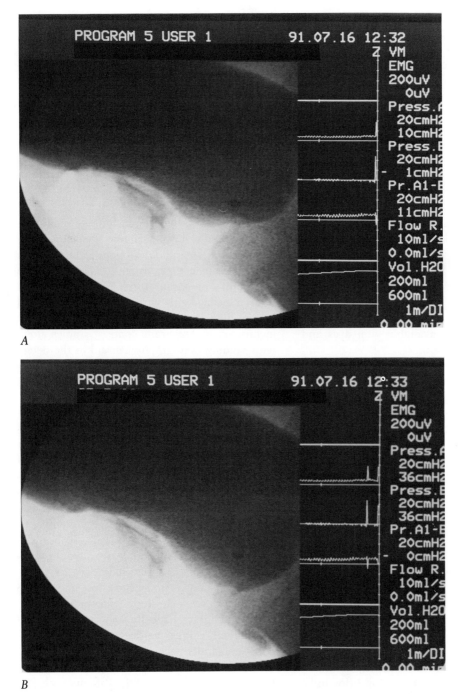

Figure 20-4. (A) Resting oblique cystogram in a patient with anatomic incontinence. (Note: Bladder neck is above the inferior border of the symphysis pubis.) (B) Straining phase in the same patient demonstrating both "funneling" and descent of the bladder neck below the symphysis.

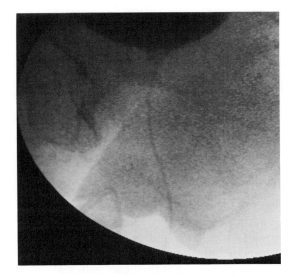

Figure 20-5. *Anteroposterior projection of an "open" bladder neck at rest in a patient with stress urinary incontinence caused by intrinsic sphincteric dysfunction.*

neck on straining maneuvers. In addition, ISD characteristically reveals "beaking" (urine in the proximal urethra) during the resting phase of cystourethrography (Fig. 20-5). If videourodynamics are performed, these patients characteristically demonstrate SUI with low Valsalva (*leak-point*) pressures.

The best chance of surgical cure for the SUI patient is that derived from the first operation. The choice as to which approach to use initially should be based on the particular expertise of the surgeon along with consideration as to the need for concomitant procedures. Many cases of recurrent SUI are usually complicated by periurethral fibrosis and fixation of various parts of the bladder and urethra to the retropubic area. In deciding which repair to perform, several factors should be taken into consideration before the most appropriate procedure is chosen. These factors include (1) severity of incontinence, (2) factors leading to ISD (numerous failed repairs, radiation, pelvic trauma, and congenital factors), (3) presence of associated vaginal pathol-

ogy (cystocele, enterocele, uterine prolapse, or rectocele), and (4) presence of obstruction.

Of the above-mentioned factors, the most important is deciding whether recurrent SUI is the result of recurrent bladder neck hypermobility producing AI, a poorly coapting urethra producing ISD, or both. Procedures for correcting the former aim to restore the bladder neck to its original retropubic position. The presence and degree of cystocele also have an impact on the type of reoperative approach that should be planned.

Pathophysiology of Recurrent Anatomic Incontinence

When the patient with recurrent SUI presents after having had a BNS for AI and the patient was well selected, the key factor in determining the pathophysiology of these operative failures is whether or not the bladder neck is adequately supported and whether the operation helped at all. Along with the history and physical examination, this can best be determined by combining voiding cystourethrography with urodynamics (videourodynamics). Within this context, recurrent SUI signifies that the BNS was initially curative, whereas persistent SUI indicates that the SUI was never helped. Three clinical scenarios are possible: (1) recurrent SUI with good support, (2) recurrent SUI with recurrent hypermobility, and (3) persistent SUI with or without hypermobility (the operation never helped).

If a patient has good support of the bladder neck after a BNS and has persistent or recurrent incontinence, the following diagnoses must be entertained in the pathophysiologic differential diagnoses of this abnormal urethral incontinence: (1) UI, (2) intrinsic pathology including foreign bodies or suture material, and, most importantly, (3) underlying ISD.

If the patient develops recurrent SUI after a prolonged period of clinical cure and has a bladder neck that is hypermobile, failure from either suture breakage or erosion from the paraurethral tissues is the most common cause. Factors that may predispose to recurrent SUI in these scenarios include (1) type of suture material (absorbable material has a higher tendency to fail), (2) quality of the tissues that are incorporated in the suspension, and (3) unusual physical stresses (chronic coughing or obesity).

If the patient with poor support has persistent SUI, that is, never having gained benefit from the BNS, most probably the sutures were never properly placed in the paraurethral tissues surrounding the bladder neck. Rarely inadequate suture tension may also contribute to this scenario. We have referred to these paraurethral tissues as the so-called good stuff that support the bladder neck and proximal urethra. These tissues represent the urethropelvic ligaments, which reside lateral to the bladder neck. Anatomically the urethropelvic ligament is a condensation of the periurethral and endopelvic fasciae and provides support of the above-mentioned structures to the tendinous arc on the lateral pelvic sidewall.

Reoperation for Anatomic Incontinence

Retropubic operations for recurrent SUI are quite common and again are used depending on the experience of the individual surgeon and the need for additional procedures. All of these procedures aim to increase urethral resistance effectively by tightening the musculofascial planes supporting the proximal urethra into a higher retropubic position. The MMK, paravaginal repair, and Burch suspension procedures are the most common.

The initial work of Peyrera signaled the advent of transvaginal needle BNSs for SUI. Since that time, modifications in this basic principle have led to a host of needle BNSs for the correction of SUI owing to AI, including the Cobb-Ragde, Stamey, Raz, and Gittes procedures.[20–23] At University of California, Los Angeles (UCLA), we perform the MPR procedure for all of our reoperative cases unless concomitant abdominal procedures are required, such as augmentation cystoplasty or ureteral reimplantation necessitating an abdominal or retropubic approach.

We reported our results of the MPR BNS in 206 patients.[24] With a mean follow-up of 16 months, 171 (83%) of the patients were cured

(no SUI), with an additional 16 (8%) patients significantly improved (rare SUI), giving successful results in 91% of this study population. Sixty percent of these patients had previous SUI surgery; interestingly, there was no statistical difference in the outcome within this reoperative group.

Pathophysiology of Recurrent Intrinsic Sphincteric Dysfunction

In patients with failure after a urethral sling or artificial urinary sphincter for ISD, the above-mentioned factors for recurrent SUI in a patient with good bladder neck support following a BNS for AI can be included. Failure to compress the urethra adequately during the initial operative procedure, however, is usually the source of the recurrent SUI in these patients with ISD.

Reoperation for Intrinsic Sphincteric Dysfunction

If a patient has been determined to have recurrent SUI based on ISD, therapy should be chosen accordingly to provide the necessary coaptation for this defect. The available modalities for the management of this type of recurrent SUI include (1) periurethral injection of an inert substance (collagen, Teflon, Fat, or silicon microspheres), (2) artificial urinary sphincter, (3) sling procedures, and (4) bladder neck reconstruction.

URINARY RETENTION

All approaches for the correction of SUI, whether done retropubically or transvaginally, have the potential to produce obstructive voiding symptoms. Complete urinary retention or obstructive voiding with overflow incontinence is rare in the routine BNS procedure. Whether a suprapubic tube is left indwelling or intermittent catheterization is instituted immediately postoperatively, most patients void with insignificant postvoid residuals (less than 60 ml) within 1 to 2 weeks. Patients may require longer intervals before voiding to completion, especially after sling procedures. Although not optimal, retention in sling patients is an acceptable alternative to this patient population with severe disabling SUI. Also, the patient's medications should be thoroughly reviewed along with a carefully performed neurologic evaluation.

Retention has not been a problem in our patient population, and the majority of patients with this condition could have been predicted preoperatively on a neurologic basis. Only 5 of our 206 patients presented earlier had prolonged retention, with only 1 of these (patient with a history of anterior-posterior resection for rectal carcinoma) requiring permanent intermittent catheterization.[24] Prolonged retention was noted in 10.7% of the group having a MMK operation.[5]

If retention is indeed due to the BNS, three causes for this iatrogenic obstruction need to be considered: (1) Sutures are too close to the urethra, (2) sutures are tied too tight, and (3) midurethral placement of the sutures has occurred. Re-evaluation is mandatory for both medicolegal and urodynamic concerns in an attempt to document either urethral obstruction (high pressure/low flow) or detrusor hypotonicity or atonicity (unfortunately, no classic pattern on cystometrogram).

Reoperation for Retention
After Bladder Neck Suspension

Regardless of which needle BNS is performed by way of the transvaginal approach, suture malposition is usually the etiologic agent for postoperative retention. This can be corrected suprapubically by initially taking down one set of sutures; if this is still not curative, the other set must be taken down. After 3 months postoperatively, cutting one of the sutures rarely causes recurrent SUI; however, if both require takedown, recurrent SUI can be expected at least 50% of the time, and patients should be informed of this risk.

If the patient is still obstructed, had a retropubic BNS, or is found to have recurrent SUI associated with the obstructed state, urethrolysis with a takedown of the previous suspension sutures and repeat BNS is required.[25] Only the retropubic and MPR BNSs afford the necessary exposure to accomplish this task.

Using the MPR BNS in these reoperative cases, the dissection of the anterior vaginal wall should proceed in the normal fashion. After the retropubic space is entered, blunt and sharp dissection between the anterior aspect of the urethra and the pubic symphysis (urethrolysis) is carried out. The old suspending sutures should be cut and removed at this time, although suture clearance is not mandatory if technically unfeasible. After these maneuvers, the surgeon's finger should be able to pass anteriorly around the urethra and bladder neck region, ensuring their total freedom from adhesions. The operation then proceeds with a resuspension in the normal fashion.

Nitti et al. reported on 41 patients who underwent transvaginal urethrolysis and resuspension of the bladder neck by the Raz technique for bladder outlet obstruction.[41] All patients voided normally prior to their original anti-incontinence procedure that produced the obstruction. With a mean follow-up of 21 months, 29 patients (71%) voided normally without significant residuals. Only preoperative post-void residual determination (values <100 ml) was predictive of successful voiding. Of these 41 patients, 19 had both recurrent SUI and obstructive voiding. Fifteen (79%) of this subgroup were cured of their SUI (totally dry), and 3 (16%) were significantly improved, with rare SUI not requiring protection.

If the transvaginal approach fails or indications exist for an open operation (augmentation enterocystoplasty or ureteral reimplantation), we then perform a retropubic urethrolysis. Several technical points deserve emphasis here. Careful dissection between the anterior urethra and undersurface of the pubic bone is mandatory to obtain total freedom of the urethra in the retropubic space. In Lee and associates' series of 322 patients from the Mayo Clinic undergoing a MMK BNS as their reoperative procedure, an intentional cystotomy was found useful to obviate inadvertent bladder or urethral perforation.[26] When performing a retropubic reoperation in these obstructed patients, if the lateral support of the bladder neck region is found to be intact in a continent patient, only urethrolysis with interposition of a pedicle-based omental flap is carried out. If, however, recurrent SUI is also present or poor support of the bladder neck is demonstrated, resuspension is indicated.

GENERAL POST–ANTI-INCONTINENCE PROCEDURE COMPLICATIONS

Unrecognized Bladder Perforation

Perivesical urinary extravasation from an unrecognized bladder perforation can cause prolonged hematuria, pain, ileus, or severe irritative voiding symptoms (frequency, urgency). If the cystogram is not diagnostic for a leak, the extravasation may be confirmed by other imaging techniques (computed tomography, ultrasonography). This condition usually resolves with conservative measures; however, signs of infection demand more aggressive management with either a retropubic or transvaginal drainage of this fluid collection.

Osteitis Pubis

Osteitis pubis, a culture-negative inflammatory condition affecting the pubic bone, has an incidence of being associated with patients undergoing retropubic BNSs ranging from 0.9% to 10%.[5, 26–28] Pain characteristically occurs over the pubis. Plain x-ray films reveal increased density or a mottled rarefaction; however, x-ray films are confirmatory in only up to 75% of the suspected cases.[5] Radionuclide bone scanning increases the diagnostic sensitivity by demonstrating increased uptake. Although this syndrome may initially be disabling, the disease is usually self-limited. Supportive therapy in the form of analgesics and anti-inflammatory agents is all that is usually needed, but in rare instances wedge resection of the pubic bone is required.

Ureteral Obstruction

Inadvertent ureteral injury may not always be picked up during the course of the AIP. Although extravasation may be possible, the most feared complication with BNS procedures is obstruction by one of the suspending sutures. Signs of

obstruction, including flank pain or costovertebral angle tenderness, should become obvious. Intravenous urography usually delineates the level and degree of obstruction; however, retrograde ureterography may become necessary. The late finding of a nonfunctioning hydronephrotic kidney is the most severe sequela.

Two approaches toward the management of this problem should be entertained. If only partial obstruction is demonstrated, attempts should be made to overcome the obstruction with double-J stenting either indirectly or with the aid of a ureteroscope. If total obstruction is evident or if the defect is unable to be negotiated with stenting, percutaneous nephrostomy is required.

With either maneuver, the length of therapy is mandated by the type of suture material used in the AIP. If chromic catgut was used, up to 3 weeks are necessary to allow the obstruction to subside. If, however, a braided absorbable suture was used, a minimum of 4 to 6 weeks of urinary diversion is required. Open surgery may still be required if either nonabsorbable suture material was used or if the obstruction fails to resolve despite these conservative measures instituted.

Neurologic Complications

Careful preoperative positioning generally avoids the postoperative peroneal or femoral neurapraxias that have been reported in patients placed in the lithotomy position for vaginal surgery.[14, 29] Most of these injuries are compressive in nature and if mild (neurapraxia) should resolve in 1 to 6 weeks. If the procedure was more involved with greater compression, these second-degree injuries (axonotmesis) may take up to 6 months to clear up.

Suprapubic Pain

Another problem directly related to transvaginal BNSs is suprapubic pain. This is thought to be related to nerve entrapment of either the ilioinguinal or genitofemoral sensory nerve branches when the suspending sutures are tied down over the anterior rectus fascia. Patients may complain of pain or a pulling sensation, with occasional radiation down the medial aspect of the inner thigh. Various series report an 8% to 16% rate of this complication in patients undergoing the different transvaginal BNSs.[30, 31] However empiric, we believe that the suprapubic incisions with any of the transvaginal BNSs should go down to the fascia to avoid entrapment of the more superficially located sensory nerves.

To avert this and other postoperative pain syndromes, Leach advocates performing the MPR suspension using a bone-fixation technique with the polypropylene suspension sutures being placed through the pubic tubercles with the aid of a Mayo trocar needle.[32] At UCLA, we continue to place the sutures routinely through the rectus fascia as close to the superior border of the symphysis pubis as possible, where there is minimal suture mobility. In Raz and associates' series mentioned earlier, a 2% suprapubic pain rate was reported.[24]

Prolapse

Secondary pelvic prolapse in the form of a cystocele, enterocele, or uterine prolapse may complicate AIPs. With the more common BNS procedures, repositioning the bladder neck to a higher retropubic position changes the axis of the vagina so potential spaces may develop allowing for either bladder, intestinal contents, or uterus to descend into the vaginal vault.

A cystocele is a prolapse of the bladder through the anterior vaginal wall (see Section IV). Cystocele formation after a BNS procedure presents as a vaginal mass, and a straining cystogram is confirmatory (equivalent to the physical examination in the standing position). In most cases of good bladder neck support with a posterior cystocele, an anterior repair (Kelly plication) suffices by reapproximating the lax pubocervical fasciae. If there is associated descent of the bladder neck in addition to the posteriorly based cystocele created by the bladder base, resuspension with cystocele repair in the form of either a Burch or a Tanagho retropubic BNS or our four-corner bladder neck and base suspension corrects this defect.[16, 17, 33] If full prolapse in the form of a grade IV cystocele complicates an AIP,

a formal cystocele repair with repeat BNS is in order.[13]

Enterocele formation following a BNS can be understood if one imagines that moving the bladder or uterus forward allows the potential space in the posterior cul-de-sac to develop between the uterosacral ligaments (Fig. 20-6). In our series, a 3% rate of enterocele formation was encountered.[24] This compares favorably with results reported for enterocele formation following the retropubic approaches with percentages as high as 16%.[16, 34] Langer and colleagues performed a prospective study looking at the effect of simultaneous hysterectomy on the cure for SUI when performing a Burch colposuspension; with regard to enterocele formation, no enteroceles were found in the hysterectomy group in which the Moschowitz procedure was routinely used to close the posterior cul-de-sac.[35, 36] Fourteen percent of their 22 patients in whom only the Burch was done without the Moschowitz procedure developed an enterocele.

Uterine prolapse can certainly occur by the same mechanisms already mentioned and requires vaginal hysterectomy in the majority of cases. In selected cases or if pre-existing medical conditions warrant, uterine suspension may be in order. The literature is mixed on the beneficial effects of routine hysterectomy in patients undergoing a BNS for SUI. Langer and associates' series failed to reveal any significant difference, although their study group was small.[35] Others, however, found that simultaneous hysterectomy did improve the cure rate for SUI.[37, 38]

Vaginal Pain, Shortening, and Stenosis

Although more common with the transvaginal BNSs, vaginal pain should fortunately be a rare complication. The best explanation to account for this is inadvertent inclusion of the levator complex with one of the suspending sutures, which in extreme cases requires a takedown with repeat BNS.

When a BNS is combined with either an enterocele repair or grade IV cystocele, care must be taken during the excision of redundant vaginal epithelium. Conscientious usage of Haney or

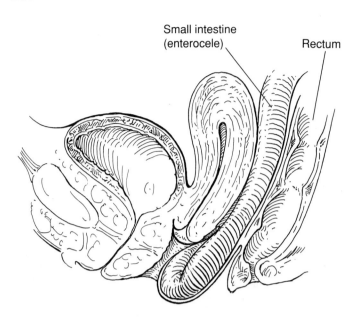

Small intestine
(enterocele)

Rectum

Figure 20-6. *Enterocele formation through the potential space created in the posterior cul-de-sac.*

other vaginal retractors throughout these procedures to ensure adequate vault capacity can prove invaluable.

Likewise, concomitant rectocele or perineal repair can cause undo stenosis of the vaginal introitus. Relaxing incisions in the lateral walls are sufficient for correction of moderate vaginal stenosis.[39] Sometimes after these incisions have been undermined for the purpose of increasing relaxation, the extension of these defects may require covering. Vaginal wall or free skin grafts can be used; however, with the latter case, an expandable intravaginal conformer should routinely be used until graft healing has occurred.[40]

Summary

Despite the various procedures for repositioning the bladder neck in an attempt to cure the condition of SUI, the anatomy and physiologic considerations have not changed much. A thorough understanding of retropubic and vaginal anatomy allows the urologist to have a better handle on how to manage the varied complications encountered. Another advancement in our understanding of SUI is the differentiation of incontinence owing to anatomic deficiencies of pelvic support (bladder neck hypermobility) versus those owing to intrinsic urethral dysfunction (poorly coapting proximal urethra).

With regard to either recurrent incontinence (stress or urgency) or urinary obstruction following these forms of reconstructive operations, a working knowledge of urodynamics becomes invaluable in the diagnosis and management of these complicated cases. A differential diagnostic list of the various forms of urethral and extraurethral incontinence also becomes invaluable in guiding therapy. As the field of female urology continues to expand, we can expect that fewer complications will occur as our expertise in gynecologic urology becomes more proficient.

References

1. Everett HS, Williams TI. Urology in the female. In: Campbell MF, Harrison JH, eds. Urology, Vol 3. Philadelphia: WB Saunders, 1970:1957–2014.
2. Nichols DH. Preface. In: Nichols DH, ed. Clinical problems, injuries and complications of gynecologic surgery. Baltimore: Williams & Wilkins, 1983.
3. Burchell C. The umbrella pack to control pelvic hemorrhage. Conn Med 1968;32:734.
4. Katske FA, Raz S. Use of Foley catheter to obtain transvaginal tamponade. Urol Urotech 1987; May:18.
5. Parnell JP, Marshall VF, Vaughan ED. Management of recurrent urinary stress incontinence by the Marshall-Marchetti-Krantz vesicourethropexy. J Urol 1984;132:912.
6. Leach GE, Raz S. Modified Pereyra bladder neck suspension after previously failed anti-incontinence surgery. Urology 1984;23:359.
7. Hadley RH, Myers RC. Complications of vaginal surgery: Does unintentional cystotomy result in vesicovaginal fistula? In: Proceedings of the Western Section, American Urological Association, Scottsdale, 1989:32.
8. Zimmern PE, Schmidbauer CP, Leach GE, et al. Vesicovaginal and urethrovaginal fistulae. Semin Urol 1986;4:84.
9. Blaivas JG. Treatment of female incontinence secondary to urethral damage or loss. Urol Clin North Am 1991;18:355.
10. Leach GE. Urethrovaginal fistula repair with Martius Labial fat pad graft. Urol Clin North Am 1991;18:409.
11. Martius H. Die operative Wiedersherstellung der vollkemmen fehlenden Harnrohre und des Schliessmuskels derselben. Zentralbl Gunak 1928;52:480.
12. Goodwin WE, Turner RD, Winter, CC. Rectourinary fistula: Principles of management and a technique of surgical closure. J Urol 1958;80:246.
13. Raz S, Little NA, Juma S, Sussman EM. Repair of severe anterior vaginal wall prolapse (grade IV cystourethrocele). J Urol 1991;146:988.
14. Benson RC, Hinman F Jr. Urinary tract injuries in obstetrics and gynecology. Am J Obstet 1955; 70:467.
15. Politano VA, Leadbetter WF. An operative technique for the correction of vesicoureteral reflux. J Urol 1958;79:932.
16. Cordonnier TT, Bowels WT. Surgery of the ureter and urinary conduits. In: Campbell MF, Harrison JH, eds. Urology. Philadelphia: WB Saunders, 1970:2289–2337.
17. Richardson AC, Edmonds PB, Williams NL. Treatment of stress urinary incontinence due to paravaginal fascial defect. Obstet Gynecol 1981; 57:357.
18. Bass JS, Leach GE. Surgical treatment of concomitant urethral diverticulum and stress incontinence. Urol Clin North Am 1991;18:365.
19. Leach GE, Yip CM, Donovan BJ, Raz S. Tubovaginal leakage: An unusual cause of incontinence. J Urol 1987;137:287.
20. Cobb OE, Ragde H. Simplified correction of female stress incontinence. J Urol 1978;120:418.
21. Stamey TA. Endoscopic suspension of the vesical neck for incontinence. Surg Gynecol Obstet 1973; 136:547.
22. Raz S. Modified bladder neck suspension for female stress incontinence. Urology 1981;17:82.
23. Gittes RF, Loughlin KR. No-incision pubovaginal suspension for stress incontinence. J Urol 1987;138:568.
24. Raz S, Sussman EM, Erickson DR, Bregg KJ, Nitti VW. The Raz bladder neck suspension: Results in 206 patients. J Urol 1992;148:845.
25. Zimmern PE, Hadley HR, Leach GE, et al. Female urethral obstruction after Marshall-Marchetti-Krantz operation. J Urol 1987;138:517.
26. Lee RA, Symmonds RE, Goldstein RA. Surgical complications and results of modified Marshall-Marchetti-Krantz procedure for urinary incontinence. Obstet Gynecol 1979;53:447.
27. McDuffie RW, Litin RB, Blundun KE. Urethrovesical suspension (Marshall-Marchetti-Krantz). Am J Surg 1981;141:297.
28. Peters WA, Thornton WN. Selection of the primary operative procedure for stress urinary incontinence. Am J Obstet Gynecol 1980;137:923.
29. Hawkins J, Hudson CN. Shaw's textbook of operative gynecology. Edinburgh: Churchill Livingstone, 1983.
30. Diaz DL, Fox BM, Walzak MP, et al. Endoscopic vesicourethropexy. Urology 1984;24:321.
31. Kelly MJ, Nielsen K, Roskamp D, et al. Long-term follow-up of the modified Pereyra bladder neck suspension for the correction of female stress urinary incontinence. Urology 1991;37:213.
32. Leach GE. Bone fixation technique for transvaginal needle suspension. Urology 1988;31:388.
33. Raz S, Klutke CG, Golomb J. Four-corner bladder and urethral suspension for moderate cystocele. J Urol 1989;142:712.
34. Stanton SL, Williams JE, Ritchie B. The colposuspension operation for urinary incontinence. Br J Obstet Gynaecol 1976;83:890.
35. Langer R, Ron-El R, Neuman M, et al. The value of simultaneous hysterectomy during Burch col-

posuspension for urinary stress incontinence. Obstet Gynecol 1988;72:866.

36. Moschowitz AV. The pathogenesis, anatomy and cure of prolapse of the rectum. Surg Gynecol Obstet 1942;15:7.

37. Green TH Jr. Urinary stress incontinence: Differential diagnosis. Pathophysiology and management. Am J Obstet Gynecol 1975;122:368.

38. Green TH Jr. Urinary stress incontinence: Pathophysiology, diagnosis and classification. In: Buchsbaum HS, Schmidt SB, eds. Gynecologic and obstetric urology. Philadelphia: WB Saunders, 1978:162–188.

39. Nichols DH. Complications and sequelae of vaginal surgery. In: Nichols DH, Randall CL, eds. Vaginal surgery. Baltimore: Williams & Wilkins, 1983.

40. Lesavoy MA. Vaginal reconstruction. Clin Obstet Gynecol 1985;12:515.

41. Nitti VW, Bregg KJ, Sussman EM, Raz S. Transvaginal urethrolysis for the treatment of obstruction following anti-incontinence procedures. J Urol 1993;149:401A.

IV

*Management
of Genital
and Pelvic Prolapse*

21

Relationship of Prolapse Syndromes to Symptoms

John O. L. DeLancey

Genital prolapse has plagued women since the beginnings of recorded history. It is described in the earliest Egyptian medical papyri 4 millennia before the time of Christ. At the end of the 19th century, gynecologic surgeons began to help women with this condition by devising surgical procedures intended to correct or ameliorate the prolapse and its symptoms. Since that time, many techniques have been tried to cure this condition with differing degrees of success. This surgery remains even today a reconstructive technique whose success depends on the surgeon's ability to understand the anatomy and pathophysiology of the pelvic supports and to correct the abnormalities present. This chapter is intended to address the cause of these conditions, their diagnosis, decisions concerning the appropriateness of surgery, and their relation to their symptoms, especially the problem of stress urinary incontinence.

Etiology of Prolapse

Prolapse develops because the force of intra-abdominal pressure pushes the vagina and uterus outside the body. Normally the levator ani muscles close the pelvic floor so the fasciae and ligaments that support the genital organs have little force applied to them.[1] Increases in abdominal pressure, failure of the muscles to keep the pelvic floor closed, and damage to the ligaments and fasciae all contribute to the development of prolapse.

The eversion of the vagina associated with prolapse has been likened to the eversion of the in-turned finger of a surgical glove that can be caused to turn out by closing the cuff of the glove and compressing the air trapped within it until the finger pops out.[2] Because the lateral aspects of the vagina are attached to the pelvic walls, prolapse usually involves protrusion of the anterior or posterior vaginal wall or the cervix. We therefore divide our consideration of this subject along these lines. Although prolapse is not caused by abnormalities in the bladder or rectum, anterior vaginal wall prolapse is usually referred to as a cystocele and posterior vaginal wall prolapse as a rectocele or enterocele depending on the organs that the vaginal wall fails to hold in place.

The protrusion of the uterus and vaginal wall that results in a uterine prolapse, cystocele, enterocele, or rectocele, occurs when some part of the normal supporting apparatus of the uterus and vagina no longer holds these organs in place. The supports may fail either from their inherent weakness or because such excessive loads have

Female Urology, edited by Elroy D. Kursh and Edward McGuire. J. B. Lippincott, Philadelphia, © 1994.

been placed on the pelvic floor that support structures possessing normal strength have broken. The idea that stretching of the pelvic fasciae was the mechanism by which prolapse developed has never had data to support it,[3] and newer observations[4] indicate that these structures break in the same way a mechanical structure such as a suspension bridge breaks rather than failing by stretching of mechanical elements.

The anatomy of the supportive mechanism has been covered in an earlier chapter. These supporting structures are made up of two different types of tissue. First, there are fibrous connective tissues that attach the vagina and uterus to the pelvic walls (cardinal and uterosacral ligaments; pubocervical and rectovaginal fasciae). Second, the levator ani muscles close the pelvic floor so the pelvic organs can rest on the muscular shelf they create. When these muscles effectively close the pelvic floor, there is no stress on the fasciae and ligaments. Damage to the muscles opens the pelvic floor. Once this has happened, the ligaments must support the vagina and uterus without assistance of the pelvic muscles. Breaks in the fasciae allow the wall of the vagina or cervix to prolapse downward. When this happens, the bladder or rectum prolapses as well. This is the nature of prolapse.

What Factors Contribute to Prolapse?

There are several factors that cause prolapse. It is easiest to understand them by using the structural analogy of a suspension bridge. The structural integrity of the bridge depends on the strength of its cables and piers. It can fail because these elements were too weak to begin with, because they have been damaged (*e.g.*, rust), because they are put under too much stress, or because the balance of parts in the design is defective. Table 21-1 summarizes these factors.

Each woman is born with an inherent strength for both the connective tissue and muscle. These can each be damaged by parturition or other factors. The degree to which this damage can be healed influences the likelihood that pro-

Table 21-1. *Factors Involved in Prolapse*

Inborn strength of connective tissue
Loss of connective tissue strength
    Damage at childbirth
    Deterioration with age
    Poor collagen repair
    Poor nutrition
Inborn strength of the levator ani muscles
Loss of levator strength
    Neuromuscular damage during childbirth
    Neural damage with chronic straining
    Metabolic diseases that affect muscle function
Increased loads on the supportive system
    Prolonged lifting
    Chronic coughing from chronic pulmonary disease
Disturbance of the balance of the structural parts
    Alteration of vaginal axis by urethral suspension
    Failure to reattach the cardinal ligaments at
      hysterectomy

lapse will develop. Given the strength of an individual woman's support structures, if she is involved in heavy lifting or has chronically increased intra-abdominal pressure, as can happen with persistent coughing, she is more likely to develop prolapse. Finally, the supportive mechanism of the pelvis is a balance of several factors, and simply disturbing this balance can precipitate prolapse. The prime example of this occurs when the anterior vaginal wall is pulled toward the top of the pubic bone, as it is during some urethral suspension procedures. The development of a postoperative enterocele in this instance is a well-recognized complication and occurs because of a disturbance of the balance of pelvic support rather than because of damage to the muscles or fasciae or a change in loads that the pelvic floor must withstand.[5]

Diagnosis

HOW TO EXAMINE PATIENTS
WITH PROLAPSE

The diagnosis of genital prolapse is made on physical examination. There are two important points to consider.

1. Examination must be made with the patient straining forcefully enough that the prolapse is at its largest.
2. The examiner must examine each different element of support independently.

If the patient is not able to strain sufficiently in the lithotomy position so that the prolapse is at its largest, examination in the standing position may be necessary. This is a critical point because it is only when the prolapse can be seen in its fullest extent that all of its various elements can be assessed. If the entire extent of the prolapse is not observed, some element may be overlooked. For example, a large cystocele may be seen initially when the patient strains, but the enterocele and apical prolapse may be recognized only with continued straining. To make sure all aspects of the prolapse can be evaluated, ask the patient how large her prolapse is at its largest and persist in the examination until that size is achieved. Once the prolapse is visible, the elements of the vagina and pelvic organs that have prolapsed can be evaluated. The examination then focuses on the specific defects that are present in support, how severe the prolapse is, and some evaluation of the cause of the prolapse.

EVALUATE THE SUPPORT OF EACH ASPECT OF THE VAGINA INDIVIDUALLY

Once the prolapse is maximally developed, begin by identifying how much the anterior wall, cervix, and posterior wall have prolapsed downward. The anterior and posterior walls should each be examined separately by retracting the opposite wall with the posterior half of a vaginal speculum (Fig. 21-1). This is important because a large cystocele, for example, may hold a potential rectocele in place and therefore hide it. If this is not recognized preoperatively, the rectocele may not be repaired and will become symptomatic postoperatively.

Examination of the *anterior wall* should establish the status of urethral support as well as that of the bladder. In addition, it should determine whether the cystocele is caused by a defect in the pubocervical fascia through which the bladder has herniated or a separation of the pubocervical fascia from its normal attachments to the pelvic wall at the white line and the cervix.

The urethra and vaginal wall are fused,[6] and the status of urethral support can be determined by careful attention to the location of the lower one third of the anterior vaginal wall below the urethrovaginal crease (Fig. 21-2). The vaginal wall in this area should be above the hymenal ring during straining. Flattening of this crease during straining often occurs in patients with stress urinary incontinence owing to loss of urethral support and corresponds with the loss of the posterior urethrovesical angle on radiographic studies. The lower anterior vaginal wall is mobile in all women and may move significantly in the continent multipara. Therefore motion of this region does not establish that the patient has stress incontinence but rather indicates the degree to which the support of the urethra has failed. Descent below the hymenal ring is definitely abnormal and indicates the presence of a cystourethrocele whether or not stress incontinence is present.

The anterior wall above the urethrovesical crease usually lies in a flat plane at about a 45-degree angle from the horizontal (Fig. 21-2). Descent below the level of the hymenal ring is significant. This descent can be caused by one of three things: (1) separation of the paravaginal attachment of the pubocervical fascia from the white line, (2) loss of the vagina's attachment to the cervix, or (3) tearing in the pubocervical fascia that results in herniation of the bladder through this layer.

The pubocervical fascia is normally attached laterally to the pelvic wall at the white line. This can be recognized vaginally as the area where the superior lateral sulcus of the vagina meets the vaginal sidewall (Fig. 21-3). In the event that this attachment breaks, this crease falls down to lie below its normal line of attachment to the pelvic side wall (a line that runs between the inferior edge of the pubic symphysis and the ischial spine). The anterior vaginal wall

(*continued on page 290*)

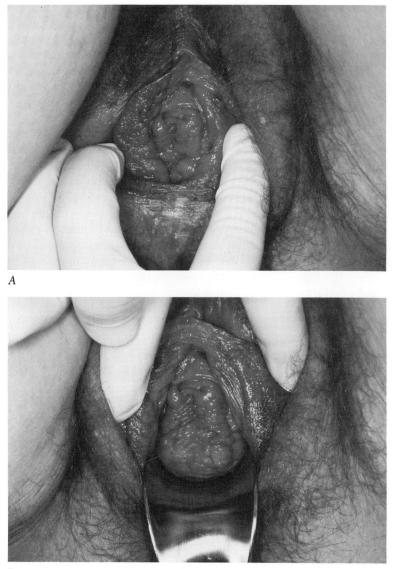

A

B

Figure 21-1. *Examination of the anterior and posterior vaginal walls separately using a half speculum to retract the posterior and anterior walls separately. (A) Displacement cystourethrocele. (B) Full extent of cystourethrocele demonstrated by placement of the speculum.*

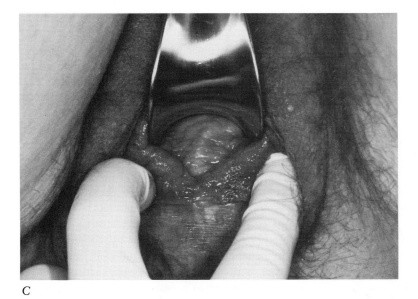

C

Figure 21-1. (continued) (C) *Small rectocele, not evident when the cystocele is present, revealed by placing a speculum anteriorly. (Copyright John O. L. DeLancey, 1992.)*

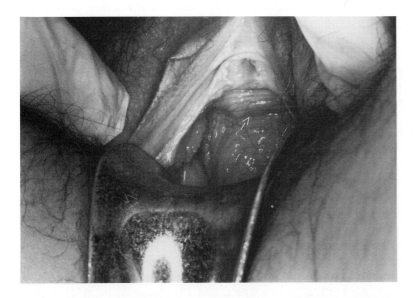

Figure 21-2. *Urethrovesical crease* (arrow) *in the anterior vaginal wall indicating the location of the junction between the urethra and bladder. (Copyright John O. L. DeLancey, 1992.)*

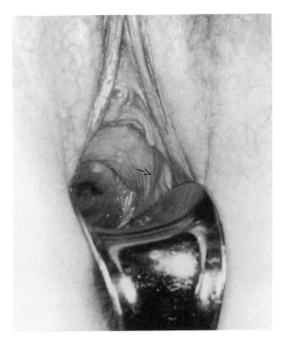

Figure 21-3. Superior lateral vaginal sulcus (arrow) *where the relatively flat anterior vaginal wall is attached to the lateral vaginal wall at a point where the anterior wall attaches to the arcus tendineus fasciae pelvis. (Copyright John O. L. DeLancey, 1992.)*

in these patients retains its rugal folds and is not stretched as it is in other patients. It is referred to as a *displacement cystourethrocele* (Fig. 21-4). Many of these individuals also have an avulsion of the pubocervical fascia from the uterine cervix, and this can be recognized by loss of the anterior fornix between the cervix and vagina.

These defects have clinical importance. For example, traditional anterior colporrhaphy works best for a distention cystourethrocele (Fig. 21-5) that arises from a central defect in the fascia rather than its detachment from the pelvic side wall. In the case of paravaginal detachment of the pubocervical fascia, anterior colporrhaphy only gathers the pubocervical fascia in the midline but does not elevate it. Elevation of the lateral borders of the pubocervical fascia is necessary in these individuals. Similarly, in the event

that the pubocervical fascia has detached from the cervix, it should be retrieved at the time of vaginal hysterectomy and included in the closure of the vagina to elevate the anterior wall better by connecting the upper edge of the pubocervical fascia to the cardinal and uterosacral ligaments that can elevate it to a more normal position.

The location of the cervix is used to gauge the severity of uterine prolapse (Fig. 21-6). Its position relative to the hymenal ring should be noted while the prolapse is at its largest. If the cervix is not visible because of the presence of a cystocele or rectocele, its location may be palpated while having the patient strain. When the cervix descends to within a centimeter of the hymenal ring, there is a significant loss of support. In planning surgery for stress incontinence where the uterus is not necessarily going to be removed, the normality of uterine support should be further tested before assuming that the uterus is well supported. This can be done by grasping the cervix with a tenaculum or ring forceps and applying traction until it stops descending.[7] Occult prolapse in which the cervix comes below the hymenal ring can be detected in this way and addressed at the time of surgery.

In addition to seeing how far the cervix descends, its length should be determined. Cervical elongation is frequent in individuals with prolapse, and the uterine corpus may often lie at a normal location. In instances of cervical elongation, knowing this fact preoperatively allows the surgeon to proceed expeditiously with the hysterectomy, rather than hoping with every pedicle that the uterine arteries will soon appear. In addition, it is important to recognize that the upper portions of the cardinal ligaments in patients with cervical elongation are in a normal location. They can be attached to the vaginal apex at the completion of the hysterectomy to resuspend the vagina. In instances in which the cervix is not elongated, the strength of the entire cardinal/uterosacral ligament complex should be suspect, and efforts should be made to perform a modified McCall cul de plasty in such a way that it elevates the vaginal apex. In patients who have previously undergone hysterectomy,

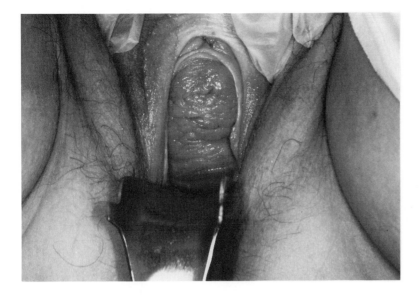

Figure 21-4. *Displacement cystourethrocele with descent of the anterior vaginal wall but preservation of the rugal folds. (Copyright John O. L. DeLancey, 1992.)*

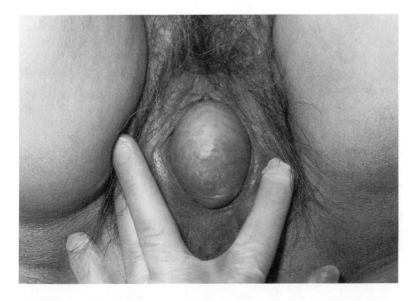

Figure 21-5. *Distention cystourethrocele with absence of rugal folds. (Copyright John O. L. DeLancey, 1992.)*

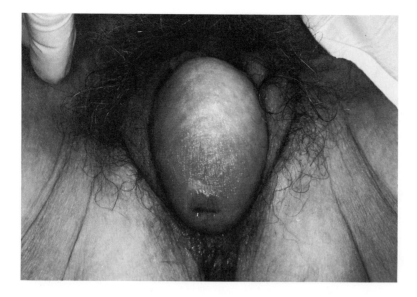

Figure 21-6. *Uterine prolapse with a cystocele. (Copyright John O. L. DeLancey, 1992.)*

special care is needed to identify the location of the vaginal apex because the uterine cervix, which is an indicator of support of the top of the vagina, is missing. This is given special consideration later in this chapter.

Evaluation and correction of posterior vaginal wall support challenge even the most experienced gynecologic surgeon, and this is probably the pelvic support defect that is least understood. The problem of distinguishing a high rectocele from an enterocele is difficult for even the experienced examiner. Because dyspareunia can follow repair, correction of asymptomatic posterior wall defects is not without risk.[8] Having a rectocele or enterocele develop after vaginal hysterectomy and anterior colporrhaphy, on the other hand, is an equally undesirable outcome, and careful consideration of posterior vaginal wall support is important.

There are three questions that should be asked when examining the posterior wall:

1. Is it normally supported?

2. Is it a true rectocele or a pseudorectocele?
3. Is there an enterocele present?

When the posterior vaginal wall descends below the hymenal ring, there is significant prolapse. This can be caused by a rectocele, an enterocele, or both. There are also occasions in which the posterior wall appears to bulge into the vagina not because the rectal wall is poorly supported but because a deficiency exists in the perineal body. This has been referred to by Nichols as a pseudorectocele and can be easily differentiated from a true rectocele because the anterior rectal wall contour is normal on rectal examination[9] (Fig. 21-7).

The hallmark of a typical rectocele is the formation of a pocket below the anal sphincter. When performing a rectal examination with the prolapse fully developed, a rectocele exists if there is an extension of the rectal lumen below the hymen (Fig. 21-7). This provides not only the diagnosis, but also illustrates the mechanism by which rectoceles create their symptoms. As long

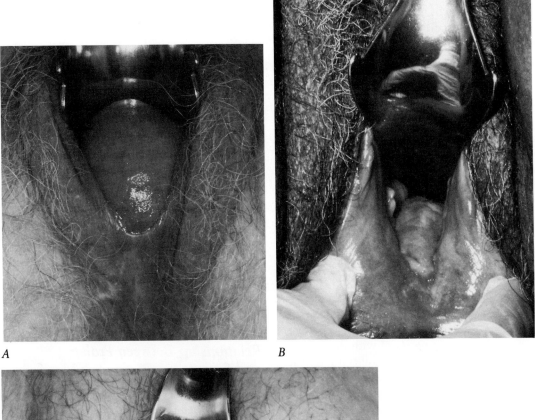

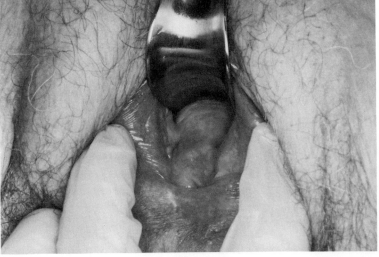

Figure 21-7. (A) Rectocele—note posterior vaginal wall extends below hymen. (B) Pseudorectocele—perineal body is separated, creating the illusion of a bulge, but the posterior vaginal wall does not extend below the plane of the hymenal ring, and the pseudobulge is simply a reflection of the absence of the perineal body. (C) Enterocele in upper portion of posterior vaginal wall overriding a rectocele. (Copyright John O. L. DeLancey, 1992.)

as the anterior rectal wall has a smooth contour, even though it may be more mobile than normal, stool passes through the anus easily. When a pocket develops as an individual strains, however, stool becomes trapped, and difficulty with evacuation can occur.

A protrusion of the upper part of the posterior vaginal wall can be caused by either an enterocele or a high rectocele. The distinction between these two conditions is made on rectovaginal examination performed in the standing position. With the index finger in the rectum and the thumb in the vagina, the examiner determines whether small bowel can be palpated between these two viscera. If so, an enterocele is present. If the bulge is created by a sacculation of the rectal wall, a high rectocele is present. This distinction is critical because an undetected enterocele may persist postoperatively and create a surgical failure. This determination must be carried out on the awake patient because the bowel in the enterocele is present only when the patient strains. In the operating room with the patient anesthetized and supine, this ability to see the enterocele develop and palpate the bowel in its sac is lost, and therefore it is imperative to determine whether or not an enterocele is present before the patient is anesthetized.

Prolapse Subsequent to Hysterectomy

Special consideration should be given to patients who have prolapse after hysterectomy to assess whether prolapse of the vaginal apex is present. When the uterus is *in situ*, the cervix calls attention to the fact that the cervix and upper vagina are poorly supported. In instances of posthysterectomy vaginal prolapse, descent of the vaginal apex is more easily missed. When prolapse of the vaginal apex is overlooked and an anterior and posterior colporrhaphy are not accompanied by suspension of the vaginal apex, the colporrhaphies fail to cure the prolapse, and the problem is not corrected.

Examination of the patient who has previously had a hysterectomy should include a spe-cific effort to determine the location of the vaginal apex when the prolapse is at its largest. The apex is identified by the scar that exists where the cervix was removed (Fig. 21-8). Vaginal prolapse is present when the vaginal apex lies below the level of the hymenal ring.[10] If the apex descends to within the lower one-third of the vagina with straining, this is significant, and the vagina should be resuspended during repair. Another technique to evaluate the degree to which descent of the apex is responsible for prolapse is to place the posterior half of a vaginal speculum into the vagina to its full extent. Because a speculum is the length of a normal vagina, inserting it to its full extent elevates the apex to a normal position. If this eliminates the bulge both when the half speculum is placed posteriorly *and* anteriorly, it is the elevation of the apex that has corrected the problem rather than support of the anterior or posterior wall.

Relationship Between Prolapse and Symptoms

There are several symptoms that all types of prolapse have in common. Once the vagina prolapses below the introitus, it is the structural layer that lies between intra-abdominal pressure and atmospheric pressure. The downward force this pressure differential creates puts tension on the fasciae and ligaments that support the ligaments and vagina. This results in a dragging feeling where the tissues connect to the pelvic wall (usually identified by the patient as occurring in the groin) and sacral backache caused by traction on the uterosacral ligaments. This type of discomfort resolves when the patient lies down, and the downward pressure is reduced. In addition, exposure of the moist vaginal walls leads not only to sensation of perineal wetness, which may be confused with urinary incontinence, but also can give rise to ulceration of the vaginal wall. Most patients also have an underlying sense of insecurity that is difficult for them to describe and often is expressed as a feeling that "something is just not right." Although this is

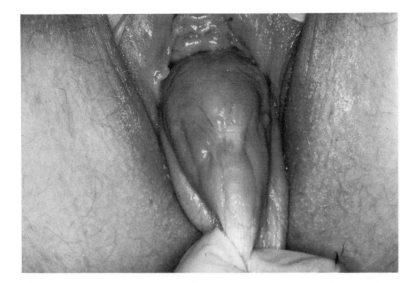

Figure 21-8. *The puckered scar that indicates the location previously occupied by the cervix is below the hymen indicating the presence of vaginal prolapse. (Copyright John O. L. DeLancey, 1992.)*

difficult for patients to put into words, it is a constant finding and one that should not be ignored.

SYMPTOMS OF ANTERIOR WALL PROLAPSE

The symptoms of cystourethrocele are varied, and the two primary ones are paradoxical.[11] On the one hand, loss of urethral support and support of the lower vaginal wall and urethra are associated with stress urinary incontinence. On the other hand, loss of support of the upper anterior vaginal wall and bladder base can cause difficulty in emptying the bladder. This inability to empty the bladder completely is probably related to those women who void by Valsalva. If there is a detrusor contraction, there should be no reason why a woman with a cystocele does not empty her bladder completely, and many women with significant cystocele have a normal postvoid residual urine volume. When a woman strains to void, however, the cystocele simply gets bigger, and no impulse is provided for urine to flow through the urethra.

In addition to these functional symptoms, many patients with a cystourethrocele complain of urinary urgency and frequency. This probably comes from the stretching of the bladder base that accompanies its prolapse through the vaginal introitus and is often less pronounced at night when the patients are supine.

Patients have a varying combination of support loss under the urethra or bladder, and symptoms vary along the spectrum from incontinence to urinary retention. As is true for other forms of prolapse, it is important to correlate the patient's symptoms with the physical findings to address these problems.

SYMPTOMS ASSOCIATED WITH PROLAPSE OF THE UTERUS, VAGINAL APEX, OR ENTEROCELE

There are few specific symptoms related to prolapse of the uterus or vaginal apex or to formation of an enterocele. These patients usually complain of the generalized symptoms of prolapse mentioned earlier. Some have urgency and frequency, probably related to the pressure of the prolapse on the bladder base, but this is variable. In addition, occasional patients with large thin enteroceles have a sense of impending rupture. Although this is an uncommon problem, it should not be ignored.

SYMPTOMS OF RECTOCELE

The cardinal symptom of a rectocele is difficulty in emptying the rectum.[8] As a woman bears down to evacuate the rectum, stool is pushed into the rectocele, and the harder she strains, the bigger the rectocele becomes. Because constipation is common in older women, it is important to differentiate between infrequent bowel movements owing to poor motility or inadequate dietary fiber and difficulty owing to a rectocele. Many women have found that if they press between the vagina and rectum to elevate the rectocele, this maneuver helps with defecation. This finding supports the fact that the rectocele is the source of the problem.

Who Should Be Treated Surgically

A decision about when an operation for prolapse should be performed is based on each individual woman's situation. It depends on the size of the prolapse, the presence or absence of symptoms, and whether or not physiologic complications have arisen because of the presence of the prolapse.

When the prolapse extends only to the level of the hymenal ring, surgery should be performed only if definite symptoms are present and can be reliably attributed to the prolapse. An example of this is the patient with a cystourethrocele at the hymen who has significant stress incontinence or a woman with the cervix in the lower third of the vagina whose symptoms are relieved by placement of a supportive pessary. A patient with a small rectocele in whom a definite pocket can be detected on rectal examination and in whom elevation of the perineum relieved problems with defecation is another example.

It is unusual for a woman in whom the uterus has not yet descended to the level of the hymenal ring to have symptoms caused by descent of the uterus. Symptoms of pressure, back pain, or feelings that something is coming out should be studied to confirm that they are related to the prolapse and not to other factors before deciding to operate. If the symptoms go away when a pessary is placed or if the patient notices prompt relief when she lies down, this helps to confirm the fact that the prolapse is the source of the symptoms. A woman with low back pain, whose discomfort persists after she is supine, is more likely to have musculoskeletal pain than pain on the basis of uterine prolapse, and the results of surgery are likely to be a disappointment for her.

There is no justification for operating simply because a woman's prolapse might get worse. Patients can be examined over a period of time to see if this is beginning to occur and a repair performed once the prolapse has demonstrated its progressive nature. With frequent examination, the prolapse will not become so large that it is more difficult to repair. Problems such as dyspareunia, iatrogenic stress incontinence, or postoperative pain are uncommon but unacceptable complications for the woman who had no significant symptoms before the surgery.

In patients whose prolapse descends several centimeters below the hymenal ring, symptoms are usually present, and surgery relieves these patients of this distress. Some women with a large prolapse deny any symptoms because they do not wish to undergo surgery or because they simply are not troubled by the presence of the prolapse. Their wishes should be respected, but potential problems from the prolapse should be considered and discussed frankly so possible complications from the prolapse are taken into account.

Specific problems that would indicate that prolapse should be repaired despite its lack of symptoms include the presence of recurrent urinary tract infections associated with an increased postvoid residual urine volume. Ureteral dilatation, which may cause an impairment of renal function, occurs in some patients with large prolapses and should be considered an indication for repair. An intravenous pyelogram and renal function testing can detect these abnormalities and indicate the need for treatment. The intravenous pyelogram should include films made with the patient *standing* and the prolapse present because the supine position may mask the presence of significant dilatation.

Rupture of the vagina caused by prolapse is an extremely rare, although serious complication.[12] It occurs primarily in the elderly patient with an enterocele and extremely thin atrophic vaginal wall. Ulceration of the vagina that occurs over the bladder is unlikely to rupture but when it occurs over an enterocele it is potentially dangerous.

Advanced age alone is not a contraindication to surgery, and a patient should not be denied relief from the discomfort of the prolapse because she is elderly. Situations occasionally arise when the patient's medical condition contraindicates surgery. In this situation, a pessary is usually the best treatment. With the improvements in anesthesia and postoperative care, however, this is becoming an increasingly uncommon necessity. Colpocleisis can be performed under local anesthesia and provides excellent relief of symptoms.

The *timing* of a patient's surgery is usually not critical. Because this is not an emergent problem, the patient should be in optimal medical condition before surgery and any pulmonary or cardiac problems carefully evaluated before surgery. If an ulcer is present on the prolapse, making sure that it is not infected is important. Treatment of the vaginal mucosa with topical estrogens helps improve the pliability of the tissue in the operating room and may help with treating ulcerations, but it is rarely possible to eradicate an ulcer completely. Any suspicious ulcer should be biopsied.

Management of Patients with Both Stress Incontinence and Prolapse

The management of stress incontinence and genital prolapse should give equal emphasis to both of these conditions. Care must be exercised not to overlook either the incontinence that may be present with prolapse or the prolapse that may be present with incontinence. There is not a good correlation between urethral support and stress incontinence, and so all patients should be carefully examined with a full bladder to see if they are incontinent during cough or Valsalva.

Urethropexy should be performed when stress incontinence exists with prolapse or when it occurs with the prolapse reduced. It is imperative to examine patients for stress incontinence with the prolapse present and to reduce the prolapse to see if incontinence becomes evident when the prolapse is replaced. In replacing the prolapse to see if stress incontinence will be present after the operation, it is necessary to avoid overcorrecting the prolapse. In normal continent women, if the anterior vaginal wall is stretched too much, stress incontinence can be artificially induced. The goal of the preoperative examination for stress incontinence is to try to reproduce, as exactly as possible, the degree of correction that is anticipated from the surgery.[13] It has been suggested that a pessary be placed to see if this causes incontinence, but it would be naive to think that having a large object in the vagina was a good reproduction of what will occur with surgery.

When stress incontinence is present on examination either spontaneously or with the prolapse reduced, equal attention to curing the stress incontinence should be given to these patients as to those who have stress incontinence alone. In addition, the possibility that this may be caused by type III incontinence should also be kept in mind, especially in patients who have previously had an operation for prolapse where the vesical neck may have been damaged.

When Should Surgery for Prolapse Accompany Urethropexy

Postoperative enteroceles can occur in as many as 15% of patients who have had a urethropexy, and other forms of prolapse may occur in an additional 10%.[14] When a patient has stress incontinence, she should be examined as outlined earlier to see if prolapse is present that the patient has not mentioned.

Prolonged and forceful straining is sometimes needed to cause the prolapse to come down, and traction on the cervix or vaginal apex should be employed if any question about the adequacy of these supports exists. If the uterus is well supported and traction on the cervix does not cause it to descend into the lower third of the vagina, it may be left in place if there are no other gynecologic indications for its removal. If there is concern about the support of the uterus and the woman does not wish to retain the ability to bear children, a hysterectomy with suspension of the vaginal apex using the uterosacral and cardinal ligaments should be performed. It is not rare for a woman to develop uterine prolapse after a urethropexy, and therefore erring on the side of addressing this possibility at the time of the first surgery is justified with the patient's consent.

Separate examination of the anterior and posterior walls with a half speculum is mandatory to uncover a rectocele that is being masked by the presence of a larger cystourethrocele. Postoperative dyspareunia may follow a posterior colporrhaphy. This operation should therefore not be performed as a routine. Nevertheless, the possibility that eliminating a cystocele may leave the rectum unsupported and therefore precipitate the enlargement of a rectocele must be kept in mind and given careful consideration. It is not possible to make exact rules about when these lesions should or should not be repaired. The strength of the supports present on examination, whether the patient plans to be sexually active, and degree to which activity will stress these supports should all be assessed in making this decision. If the urogenital hiatus in the pelvic floor is unusually enlarged, a perineorrhaphy to narrow this is in order.

References

1. Paramore RH. The supports-in-chief of the female pelvic viscera. J Obstet Gynaecol Br Emp 1908;13:391.
2. Bonney V. The principles that should underlie all operations for prolapse. Br J Obstet Gynaecol Br Emp 1934;41:669.
3. Goff BH. The surgical anatomy of cystocele and urethrocele with special reference to the pubocervical fascia. Surg Gynecol Obstet 1948;87:725.
4. Richardson AC, Lyons JB, Williams NL. A new look at pelvic relaxation. Am J Obstet Gynecol 1976;126:568.
5. Burch JC. Cooper's ligament urethrovesical suspension for stress incontinence. Nine years' experience—results, complications, technique. Am J Obstet Gynecol 1968;100:764.
6. Krantz KE. The anatomy of the urethra and anterior vaginal wall. Am J Obstet Gynecol 1951; 62:374.
7. Bartscht KD, DeLancey JOL. A technique to study cervical descent. Obstet Gynecol 1988; 72:940.
8. Arnold MW, Stewart WR, Aguillar PS. Rectocele repair. Four years' experience. Dis Colon Rectum 1990;33:684.
9. Nichols DH, Randall CL. Vaginal surgery. 2nd ed., Baltimore: Williams & Wilkins, 1983.
10. Morley GW, DeLancey JOL. Sacrospinous ligament fixation for eversion of the vagina. Am J Obstet Gynecol 1988;158:872.
11. Gardy M, Kosminski M, DeLancey JOL, et al. Stress incontinence and cystoceles. J Urol 1991;145:1211–3.
12. Friedel W, Kaiser IH. Vaginal evisceration. Obstet Gynecol 1975;45:315.
13. Bump RC, Fantl JA, Hurt WG. The mechanism of urinary continence in women with severe uterovaginal prolapse: Results of barrier studies. Obstet Gynecol 1988;72:291.
14. Wiskind AK, Creighton SM, Stanton S. The incidence of genital prolapse following the Burch colposuspension operation. Neurourol Urodynam 1991;10:453.

22

Surgical Treatment of Cystocele and Rectocele

Mark D. Walters

Defects of anterior and posterior vaginal wall support are common problems in women and may coexist with disorders of micturition and defecation. Mild cystoceles and rectoceles frequently occur in parous women but usually present few problems for the patient. As pelvic support defects progress and symptoms develop and worsen, treatment may be indicated. This chapter reviews the anatomy and pathology of cystocele and rectocele and describes methods of their surgical repair.

Anatomy and Pathology

CYSTOCELE

Cystocele is defined as pathologic descent of the anterior vaginal wall and overlying bladder base. According to Nichols and Randall, cystoceles are classified as distention cystoceles or as displacement cystoceles.[1] *Distention cystocele* is a result of overstretching and attenuation of the anterior vaginal wall. It is mainly due to overdistention of the vagina associated with vaginal delivery or to atrophic changes associated with aging and menopause. Rugal folds of the anterior vaginal epithelium are usually diminished or absent owing to thinning or loss of midline vaginal fascia. *Displacement cystocele* results from

pathologic detachment or elongation of the anterolateral vaginal supports to the pelvic diaphragm. These may occur unilaterally or bilaterally and frequently coexist with some degree of distention cystocele and with descent of the proximal urethra.[2] Although a true cystocele is usually associated only with symptoms of pelvic prolapse, descent of the proximal urethra and bladder base may be associated with stress urinary incontinence.

RECTOCELE

Rectocele may be defined as herniation or bulging of the posterior vaginal wall and underlying rectum anteriorly into the vaginal lumen. Rectocele is fundamentally a defect of the vagina and its support, not of the rectum.[3] It is predominantly due to stretching and dehiscence of the rectovaginal septum and the adjacent vaginal fascial envelope during childbirth.[3–5] Within the rectovaginal septum, there is a thin membrane-like connective tissue called the *fascia of Denonvilliers* that is fused to the underside of the posterior vaginal wall.[3,6] This tissue extends downward from the bottom of the cul-de-sac of Douglas to its attachment to the upper margin of the perineal body. When this caudal attachment is avulsed, as during childbirth, the perineum is

Female Urology, edited by Elroy D. Kursh and Edward McGuire. J. B. Lippincott, Philadelphia, © 1994.

destabilized. Such weakness is one cause of rectocele and perineal descent.[3]

Failure of peritoneal fusion of the obliterated extension of the pelvic cavity in the rectovaginal septum can result in congenital deepness of the cul-de-sac and congenital weakness of the posterior vaginal wall in adults. This accounts in part for the frequent coexistence of high rectocele with enterocele.[3] So frequent is this association that when one condition is found, the other must be routinely sought and repaired at the same time.

Rectocele and enterocele appear to be disorders confined to parous women. One or both were seen in 39% of asymptomatic women who underwent laparoscopy for other indications.[4] Parturition is associated with a significant increase in the length of the dorsal vaginal wall. This increase in dorsal vaginal length was ascribed to the increase in length of the rectovaginal septum alone, as there was no change in the depth of the cul-de-sac between parous and nulliparous women.[4]

Evaluation

HISTORY

When evaluating women with urogenital prolapse or stress incontinence, attention should be paid to all potential pelvic support defects. These include the anterior vaginal wall and overlying urethra and bladder base; the uterus (if present) and vaginal apex; and the posterior vaginal wall, rectum, and perineum. Careful assessment should be made of the rectovaginal space to detect enterocele, which frequently coexists with, and mimics, rectocele. It is the responsibility of the reconstructive surgeon to determine the specific sites and causes of damage for each patient, with the ultimate goal to restore both anatomy and function.[3]

Patients with vaginal prolapse complain either of symptoms related directly to the herniated tissue in the vagina or of associated symptoms, such as urinary incontinence or voiding difficulty. Symptoms directly related to genital prolapse include the sensation of a mass or bulge in the vagina, pelvic pressure and pain, low back pain, and sexual difficulty.[7] Urinary incontinence and voiding difficulty may be related to anterior vaginal wall prolapse. Postevacuation rectal discomfort or the inability to empty the bowel completely, requiring manual vaginal or perineal expression to evacuate, sometimes are related to rectocele. Constipation *per se* is not a symptom of rectocele, although they may coexist.[3]

PHYSICAL EXAMINATION

The physical examination should be conducted with the patient in lithotomy position as for a routine pelvic examination. The examination is first done in the supine position, then if symptoms do not correspond to physical findings, the woman is re-examined in the standing position. The standing rectovaginal examination is the most reliable position to examine for enterocele.

The genitalia are inspected, and if no displacement is apparent, the labia are gently spread to expose the vestibule and introitus. The integrity of the perineal body is evaluated, and the approximate size of all prolapsed parts is assessed. After the resting examination, the patient is instructed to strain down forcefully or to cough vigorously. During this maneuver, the order of the descent of the pelvic organs is noted, as is the relationship of the pelvic organs at the peak of straining.[8,9] Anterior vaginal wall descent usually represents a cystocele with or without rotational descent of the urethra. Less commonly, an anterior enterocele can mimic a cystocele on physical examination. Posterior vaginal wall prolapse represents a rectocele or an enterocele or both (Fig. 22-1). A rectovaginal examination is done to differentiate between these conditions. The rectal finger is elevated into the vagina to assess for anterior displacement of the rectal wall (rectocele) and for the integrity and thickness of the perineal body. An enterocele is diagnosed on rectovaginal examination by noting a sac of tissue, which may or may not contain

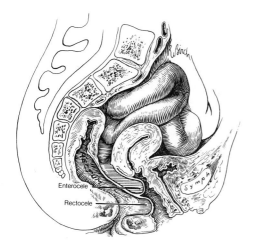

Figure 22-1. Sagittal section of pelvis, showing relative position of rectocele and enterocele. (From Mattingly RF, Thompson JD. TeLinde's Operative gynecology. 6th ed. Philadelphia: JB Lippincott, 1985:574.)

small bowel, in the rectovaginal space. When a standing rectovaginal examination is done, small bowel can frequently be felt to herniate into this space between the fingers.

With the patient supine at rest and straining, the position of the cervix and uterus or, if absent, the vaginal apex should be assessed. Descent of the cervix or vaginal apex to or past the midvagina represents abnormal uterovaginal support. Digital depression of the perineal body while the patient strains produces an artificial enlargement of the genital hiatus, which leads to the protrusion of the cervix and anterior vaginal wall in some parous women. Although this maneuver may be helpful to visualize the anatomy, it may overestimate the amount of pelvic relaxation at rest.

DIAGNOSTIC TESTS

After careful history and physical examination, few diagnostic tests are needed to evaluate patients with genital prolapse. A urinalysis should be done to rule out urinary infection if incontinence or dysuria are noted. If the patient's estro-gen status is unclear, vaginal cytologic smears can be obtained to assess maturation index. For severe uterovaginal prolapse, a pyelogram or renal ultrasound should be done to evaluate for ureteral patency and hydronephrosis, which frequently result.[10,11]

If coexistent urinary incontinence is present, further diagnostic testing may be indicated to differentiate detrusor incontinence from urethral incontinence. Urodynamic, endoscopic, or radiologic assessments of filling and voiding function are probably necessary only when symptoms of incontinence or voiding dysfunction are present. Even if no urologic symptoms are noted, some assessment of voiding function should be done to evaluate for completeness of bladder emptying. This usually involves only a timed, measured micturition or electronic uroflowmetry, followed by urethral catheterization to measure residual urine volume.

Although mild to moderate prolapse is often associated with stress urinary incontinence, patients with severe genitourinary prolapse and cystocele extending beyond the vaginal introitus often do not have urinary incontinence. Further, stress incontinence may occur after prolapse surgery, and severe genital prolapse is a risk factor for recurrence of stress incontinence after surgery.[12-14] The mechanism underlying this observation may be that severe uterovaginal prolapse results in urethral kinking, which generates increased urethral resistance.[13] It may also be that direct compression on the urethra occurs by descending parts of the genital tract. Urethrovesical angulation or extrinsic compression could explain the high pressure transmission ratios that are observed when urethral pressure profiles are done in women with uterovaginal prolapse.[15]

It is important to check urethral function after the prolapse is repositioned in women with severe uterovaginal prolapse and large cystoceles. A pessary can be used to reduce the prolapse before clinical or electronic urodynamic testing.[13,16] If urinary leaking occurs with stress or the urethral closure pressure profile becomes positive after reduction of the prolapse, the urethral sphincter is probably incompetent, even if the patient is normally continent. Using this maneuver, the surgeon can choose an anti-incontinence procedure or, if sphincteric incompetence is not present, an anterior colporrhaphy.

Surgical Repair Techniques

CYSTOCELE

Anterior Colporrhaphy with Vesical Neck Plication

The patient is supine, with the legs elevated and abducted and the buttocks placed just past the edge of the operating table. The vagina and perineum are sterilely prepared and draped, and a 16 French Foley catheter with a 5 to 10 ml balloon is inserted sterilely into the bladder. One to three perioperative intravenous doses of an appropriate antibiotic should be given as prophylaxis against infection. If a suprapubic catheter is to be placed into the bladder, it may be done at this time.

A weighted speculum is placed into the vagina. Hemostatic solutions or saline may be injected submucosally, along the midline of the anterior vaginal wall, to decrease bleeding and to aid in dissection of the vesicovaginal space. The labia minora may be sutured to the adjacent skin of the thigh if desired. If a vaginal hysterectomy is to be done, it should be completed before the anterior colporrhaphy.

If a vaginal hysterectomy has been done, the incised apex of the anterior vaginal wall is grasped transversely with two Allis clamps and elevated. A third Allis clamp is placed about 1 cm below the posterior margin of the urethral meatus and pulled up. The points of a pair of curved Mayo scissors are inserted between the vaginal epithelium and the bladder wall and gently forced upward while partially opening and closing the scissors. Countertraction during the maneuver is important to minimize the likelihood of perforation of the bladder lumen.[17] After development of the vesicovaginal space, the vaginal epithelium is incised in the midline. When the entire vaginal wall has been cut, the edges are grasped

with Allis clamps or T-clamps and drawn laterally for further mobilization. Dissection of the vaginal flaps and mobilization of the cystocele are then accomplished by turning the clamps back across the forefinger and incising the vaginal fascia with a scalpel, while constant traction on the bladder is maintained superiorly and medially by the assistant. This procedure is done bilaterally until the entire bladder base has been dissected free. The spaces lateral to the urethrovesical junction are sharply and bluntly dissected toward the urogenital diaphragm, as with a Pereyra procedure.

When the vaginal flaps have been developed and the cystocele delineated, the urethrovesical junction can be identified visually or by pulling the Foley catheter downward until the bulb obstructs the vesical neck. Repair should begin at the urethrovesical junction. In most cases, regardless of whether the patient suffers from urinary incontinence, plicating sutures at the urethrovesical junction should be placed to preserve posterior urethral support and to ensure that stress incontinence, if not present at the time of operation, does not develop postoperatively.[18, 19]

The vesical neck and cystocele are repaired by turning in the remains of the submucosal fascia and bladder adventitia with vertically placed Lembert sutures, using no. 0 delayed absorbable suture. The first plicating suture is placed into the periurethral endopelvic fascia at the urethrovesical junction (Fig. 22-2). After the urethrovesical junction is supported with two or three sutures, the remaining cystocele is repaired with several additional plication sutures, so each successive stitch incorporates some of the previous stitch. Depending on the size of the cystocele, one or two rows of plication sutures may be necessary. After the entire cystocele has been repaired, vaginal epithelium is trimmed bilaterally, and the anterior vaginal wall is closed with a running no. 3–0 subcuticular suture.

Needle urethropexy procedures effectively treat small cystoceles associated with descent of the urethra and bladder base. Larger cystoceles usually involve bulging of the posterior bladder wall above the interureteric ridge and cannot be

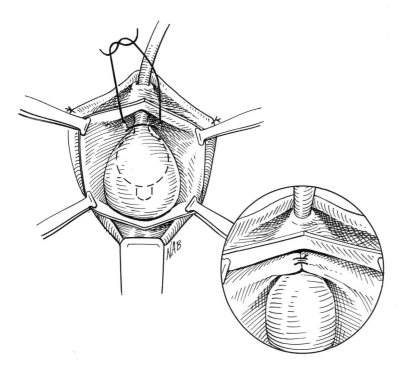

Figure 22-2. *Vesical neck plication for repair of urethral descent associated with cystocele.*

treated adequately with needle urethropexies. In these cases, a cystocele repair should be accomplished using the procedure of anterior colporrhaphy described earlier. If the cystocele is large, a purse-string suture may be placed to reduce the cystocele partially. This is followed by standard plication sutures of the bladder muscularis, trimming of the anterior vaginal wall, and closure. If this is combined with a needle urethropexy, it is probably easier to repair the cystocele before the urethropexy sutures are tied.

The main indication for anterior colporrhaphy with vesical neck plication is for repair of cystocele. This procedure is also effective for treatment of mild stress incontinence associated with urethral hypermobility. Several studies have described continence rates as high as 90% after 1 year, although recurrences frequently occur with longer follow-up times.[20,21] One prospective randomized study showed that conti-

nence rates after 1 year were similar between anterior colporrhaphy and needle urethropexy in women with urethral incontinence and pelvic relaxation.[22]

Abdominal Cystocele Repair

Retropubic surgical procedures are effective for treating small cystoceles, although they are generally not used for that purpose. Both the Burch colposuspension and the vaginal obturator shelf and paravaginal repairs suspend the anterior vaginal wall for the treatment of genuine stress incontinence. These operations effectively treat displacement cystoceles, although the Burch colposuspension may leave a distention cystocele located above the trigone.

Abdominal repair of a posterior distention cystocele can be accomplished after abdominal hysterectomy.[23] After the cervix has been amputated from the vagina, the bladder is dissected off the anterior vaginal wall, nearly to the level of the ureters. A full-thickness midline wedge of anterior vaginal wall is excised, and the vagina is closed with running delayed absorbable suture. The vaginal cuff is then repaired as per the surgeon's preference. This procedure has no effect on bladder neck or urethral support, and care should be exercised that latent urethral incontinence is not unmasked by treatment of a high cystocele without simultaneous urethral suspension.[18]

PERINEAL RELAXATION AND RECTOCELE

The repair of a relaxed perineum and of a rectocele are two distinct operative procedures, although they are usually performed together. Before beginning the repair, the surgeon should estimate the severity of the rectocele and perineal defect as well as the desired postoperative caliber of the vagina and introitus.[24] The ultimate size of the vaginal orifice is determined by placing Allis clamps on the inner aspect of the labia minora bilaterally and approximating them in the midline. The final vaginal opening should admit three fingers easily, taking into account that the levator ani and perineal muscles are completely relaxed from the general anesthesia and that the vagina may further constrict postoperatively.

To begin the posterior colporrhaphy, Allis clamps are placed bilaterally on the posterior perineum. A triangular-shaped incision is made in the perineal body, and the overlying perineal skin is removed. A subepithelial tunnel is made in the rectovaginal space using Mayo scissors and extending the dissection to the apex of the vagina. The posterior vaginal wall is incised in the midline along its entire length. In a manner similar to the anterior colporrhaphy, lateral traction is placed on each vaginal flap, and the underlying rectum is dissected bluntly and sharply (Fig. 22-3A,B). The dissection should be extended laterally as far as possible to mobilize perirectal fascia and to expose the medial margins of the puborectalis muscles. The terminal ends of the bulbocavernosus and transverse peri-

neal muscles are also freed from the adherent mucosa in the lower vagina.

Vertical mattress sutures of no. 0 delayed absorbable suture are used to plicate the pararectal fascia over the rectal wall. Repair of this fascia may be sufficient to treat small rectoceles. If the rectocele and levator hiatus are large, however, additional no. 0 delayed absorbable sutures are placed deeply into the medial portions of the puborectalis muscles, and the muscles are brought together in the rectovaginal space (Fig. 22-3C,D).[24] Although levator plication effectively treats rectocele, it also tends to decrease the caliber of the vaginal lumen and to create a transverse ridge in the posterior vaginal wall, both of which may lead to dyspareunia. After the pararectal fascia and levator muscles are plicated, as appropriate, redundant vaginal epithelium is trimmed bilaterally, and the posterior vaginal wall and epithelium are closed with no. 3–0 delayed absorbable running suture (Fig. 22-3E). The perineal body is then repaired by placing deep sutures into the perineal muscles and fascia to build up the perineal body. The overlying vulvar skin is closed with no. 3–0 running subcuticular suture.

For anterior and posterior colporrhaphy, a vaginal pack is placed and removed the first postoperative day. Ambulation and diet are advanced rapidly as tolerated by the patient. The bladder is routinely drained after anterior colporrhaphy for 2 or 3 days, after which trials of voiding are begun.

Results

Few studies have addressed the long-term success of vaginal plastic procedures for treating cystocele and rectocele. Recurrences of vaginal prolapse occur with increasing age, but their actual frequency are unknown. Early recurrences of vaginal prolapse are usually due to failure to identify and repair individually all support defects, including the anterior vaginal wall, vaginal apex, rectovaginal septum, poste-

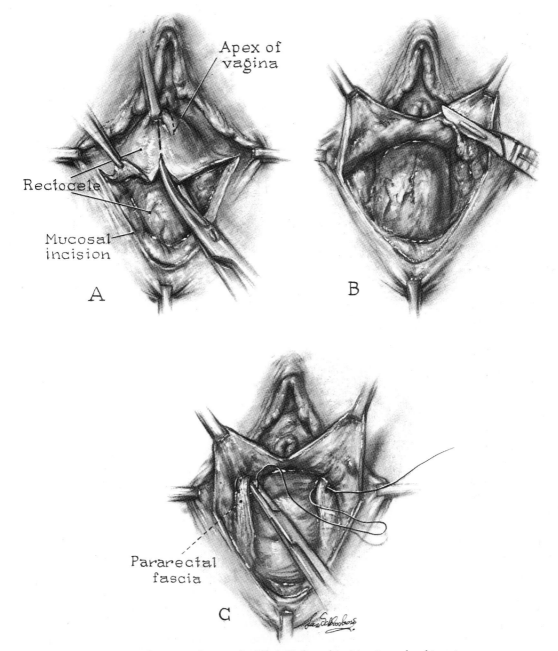

Figure 22-3. *Repair of moderate-sized rectocele. (A) A V-shaped incision is made of introitus over perineal body; midline vertical incision extends to apex of vagina. (B) Pararectal fascia is separated from mucosa by sharp dissection and (C) plicated over anterior wall of rectum.*

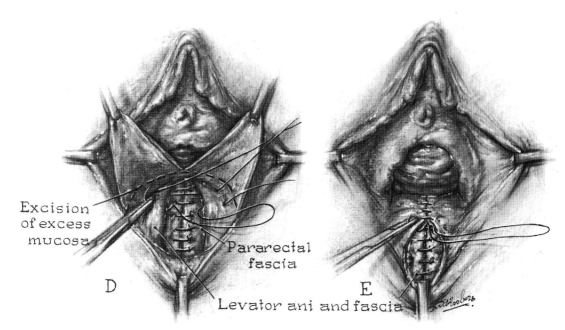

Excision of excess mucosa

Pararectal fascia

D   E

Levator ani and fascia

Figure 22-3. *(continued) (D) Levator ani muscles are approximated in the midline with deep sutures of no. 0 or 1 delayed absorbable material. The excess vaginal mucosa is excised, and the margins are closed (E) with either an interrupted or continuous suture. (From Mattingly RF, Thompson JD. TeLinde's Operative gynecology. 6th ed. Philadelphia: JB Lippincott, 1985:578.)*

rior vaginal wall, and perineum. Late recurrences are probably due to weakening of the patient's own supporting tissue, which occurs with advancing age and after menopause. Other characteristics that may increase chances of recurrence are pregnancy, heavy lifting, chronic pulmonary disease, smoking, obesity, absence of estrogen replacement after menopause, and genetic predisposition.

Complications

The intraoperative complications of anterior and posterior colporrhaphy include blood loss re-

quiring a blood transfusion and damage to the lumina of the bladder and rectum. Accidental cystotomy or proctotomy should be repaired in layers at the time of the injury. After repair of cystotomy, the bladder is generally drained for about 7 days to allow for adequate healing. After repair of proctotomy, oral feedings should not begin postoperatively until after approximately 48 hours, during which time intravenous fluid replacement is maintained and bowel function is gradually restored. Patients can then advance to clear liquids and to a soft, low-residue diet for an additional 48 hours. A regular diet may be started after patients pass flatus or following the first soft bowel movement. The use of laxatives should be avoided for 4 or 5 days to keep the terminal rectum and anal canal free of fecal material for as long as possible postoperatively, until the mucosal suture line is healing adequately.[24] Failure of healing can result in formation of rectovaginal fistula.

Voiding difficulty can occur after anterior colporrhaphy. This occurs primarily in women with subclinical preoperative voiding dysfunction, especially those with low micturition flow rates and absent detrusor contractions with voiding.[25] Treatment is bladder drainage or intermittent self-catheterization until spontaneous voiding resumes, usually within 6 weeks. Other rare complications include ureteral damage, intravesical or urethral suture placement (and associated urologic problems), and fistula, either urethrovaginal or vesicovaginal. These complications occur rarely; their actual incidences are unknown.

Sexual function may be positively or negatively affected by the vaginal operations for genital prolapse and urinary incontinence. Francis and Jeffcoate found that about one half of sexually active women had some sexual problems after anterior and posterior colpoperineorrhaphy with or without hysterectomy.[26] Fifty-five percent of these patients reported loss of sexual desire or impotence (male or female), which frequently predated the vaginal surgery. The remaining women had shortened or stenotic vaginas, dyspareunia, or fear of injury as the cause of their sexual difficulties.

Haase and Skibsted studied 55 sexually active women who underwent a variety of operations for stress incontinence or genital prolapse.[27] Postoperatively 24% of the patients experienced improvement in their sexual satisfaction, 67% experienced no change, and 9% experienced a deterioration. Improvement often resulted from cessation of urinary incontinence. Deterioration was always due to dyspareunia following posterior colporrhaphy. These authors concluded that the prognosis for an improved sexual life is good after surgery for stress incontinence, but that posterior colpoperineorrhaphy causes dyspareunia in some patients.[27]

References

1. Nichols DH, Randall CL. Vaginal surgery. 3rd ed. Baltimore: Williams & Wilkins, 1989:239.
2. Richardson AC, Lyon JB, Williams NL. A new look at pelvic relaxation. Am J Obstet Gynecol 1976;126:568.
3. Nichols DH. Posterior colporrhaphy and perineorrhaphy: Separate and distinct operations. Am J Obstet Gynecol 1991;164:714.
4. Kuhn RJP, Hollyock MD. Observations on the anatomy of the rectovaginal pouch and septum. Obstet Gynecol 1982;59:445.
5. Harrison JE, McDonagh JE. Hernia of Douglas' pouch and high rectocele. Am J Obstet Gynecol 1950;60:83.
6. Milley PS, Nichols DH. A correlative investigation of the human rectovaginal septum. Anat Rec 1969;163:443.
7. Addison WA, Livengood CH, Parker RT. Posthysterectomy vaginal vault prolapse with emphasis on management by transabdominal sacral colpopexy. Postgrad Obstet Gynecol 1988;8:1.
8. Porges RF. A practical system of diagnosis and classification of pelvic relaxations. Surg Gynecol Obstet 1963;117:769.
9. Beecham CT. Classification of vaginal relaxation. Am J Obstet Gynecol 1980;136:957.
10. Stabler J. Uterine prolapse and urinary tract obstruction. Br J Radiol 1977;50:493.
11. Hadar H, Meiraz D. Total uterine prolapse causing hydroureteronephrosis. Surg Gynecol Obstet 1980;150:711.
12. deGregorio G, Hillemanns HG. Urethral closure function in women with prolapse. Int Urogynecol J 1990;1:143.
13. Richardson DA, Bent AE, Ostergard DR. The effect of uterovaginal prolapse on urethrovesical pressure dynamics. Am J Obstet Gynecol 1983;146:901.
14. Arnold EP, Webster JR, Loose H, et al. Urodynamics of female incontinence: Factors influencing the results of surgery. Am J Obstet Gynecol 1973;117:805.
15. Bump RC, Fantl JA, Hurt WG. The mechanism of urinary continence in women with severe uterovaginal prolapse: Results of barrier studies. Obstet Gynecol 1988;72:291.
16. Bhatia N, Bergman A. Pessary test in women with urinary incontinence. Obstet Gynecol 1985;65:220.
17. Mitchell GW. Vaginal hysterectomy: Anterior and posterior colporrhaphy; repair of enterocele; and prolapse of vaginal vault. In: Ridley JH, ed. Gynecologic surgery: Errors, safeguards, salvage. 2nd ed. Baltimore: Williams & Wilkins, 1981:49.

18. Symmonds RE, Jordan LT. Iatrogenic stress incontinence of urine. Am J Obstet Gynecol 1961; 82:1231.

19. Pelusi G, Bacchi P, Demaria F, Rinaldi AM. The use of Kelly plication for the prevention and treatment of genuine stress urinary incontinence in patients undergoing surgery for genital prolapse. Int Urogynecol J 1990;1:196.

20. Beck RP, McCormick S. Treatment of urinary stress incontinence with anterior colporrhaphy. Obstet Gynecol 1982;59:269.

21. Stanton SL, Norton C, Cardozo L. Clinical and urodynamic effects of anterior colporrhaphy and vaginal hysterectomy for prolapse with and without incontinence. Br J Obstet Gynaecol 1982; 89:459.

22. Bergman A, Koonings PP, Ballard CA. Primary stress urinary incontinence and pelvic relaxation: Prospective randomized comparison of three different operations. Am J Obstet Gynecol 1989; 161:97.

23. Macer GA. Transabdominal repair of cystocele, a 20 year experience, compared with the traditional vaginal approach. Am J Obstet Gynecol 1978; 131:203.

24. Mattingly RF, Thompson JD. TeLinde's Operative gynecology. 6th ed. Philadelphia: JB Lippincott, 1985:569.

25. Bhatia NN, Bergman A. Use of preoperative uroflowmetry and simultaneous urethrocystometry for predicting risk of prolonged postoperative bladder drainage. Urology 1986;28:440.

26. Francis WJA, Jeffcoate TNA. Dyspareunia following vaginal operations. Br J Obstet Gynaecol 1961;68:1.

27. Haase P, Skibsted L. Influence of operations for stress incontinence and/or genital descensus on sexual life. Acta Obstet Gynecol Scand 1988; 67:659.

23

Surgical Repair of Uterine Prolapse and Enterocele

John O. L. DeLancey

Early in the evolution of surgery for genital prolapse, the vaginal approach to hysterectomy arose as a logical solution to the removal of the protruding ulcerated uterus in women with procidentia. Because vaginal surgery avoided the peritonitis and shock involved in abdominal exploration, it was the method of choice for hysterectomy before the advent of antibiotics, anesthesia, blood transfusion, and intravenous fluid supplementation. Its lower morbidity, absence of postoperative ileus, and lack of complications resulting from an abdominal incision continue to make it an excellent choice when compared with abdominal hysterectomy.[1,2]

The vagina is fused with the uterine cervix, so prolapse of the uterus cannot occur without some degree of prolapse of the vagina. When we speak of vaginal hysterectomy for the treatment of prolapse, we are therefore speaking of a reconstructive rather than an extirpative procedure, one portion of which includes removal of the uterus to gain access to the supportive ligaments, but the critical element of this procedure has to do with shortening the cardinal and uterosacral ligaments and reattaching them to the vagina. Although these operations are thought of in strictly mechanical terms, they have important implications for the function of the pelvic organs

as well and remain the mainstay of operative therapy.[3]

The relationship between vaginal hysterectomy and the treatment of stress urinary incontinence is an important one. Patients may have stress urinary incontinence without uterine prolapse and vice versa, although the two frequently coexist. If obvious prolapse is present, vaginal hysterectomy is clearly indicated. Whether a hysterectomy improves the outcome of surgery for stress incontinence has been debated, and there is no compelling physiologic or clinical information that it does.[4] Prolapse of the uterus and stress incontinence so frequently occur together that combined treatment should be the rule rather than the exception. It is also logical that a woman whose urethral supports are weak and who develops urethral prolapse may also have weak uterine supports and develop uterine prolapse later in life. It is therefore prudent to evaluate the need for hysterectomy at the time of surgery for stress incontinence and not simply to reserve it for patients with clinically obvious prolapse. These considerations raise the following question: In patients in whom prolapse is not a presenting complaint, when should a vaginal hysterectomy be performed in conjunction with surgery for stress incontinence?

Female Urology, edited by Elroy D. Kursh and Edward McGuire. J. B. Lippincott, Philadelphia, © 1994.

Vaginal Hysterectomy

INDICATIONS

Women with stress incontinence and normal uterine support should be evaluated for concomitant gynecologic problems that may necessitate surgery. A detailed discussion of this subject would obviously be a summary of indications for hysterectomy and is beyond the scope of this book. Most commonly, uncontrolled hypermenorrhea or refractory dysmenorrhea that is not satisfactorily alleviated with medication should be evaluated to see if problems such as endometriosis, uterine leiomyomas, or adenomyosis are present. A Papanicolaoce smear must be obtained and any history of previously abnormal cytologies evaluated. The woman's future reproductive plans should be explored with her not only to discuss with her the possibility that a future pregnancy might disrupt a successful repair, but also to raise the issue of whether a tubal ligation should be considered if she wants no more children and if the uterus is to be retained.

There is no unanimity of opinion concerning the issue of *prophylactic* hysterectomy at the time of stress incontinence surgery in the absence of specific gynecologic disease to eliminate menses and prevent the subsequent development of gynecologic malignancy, which occurs in more than 1 in 50 women. In the case of ovarian malignancy, which has a hereditary tendency in certain families, women with a strong family history of ovarian cancer should have the option of having their ovaries removed. Because hysterectomy in these situations is elective, the patient must know the risks of hysterectomy and fully understand the possibility that complications may arise from the surgery.

Beyond the obvious need for hysterectomy in patients with overt prolapse, there is a need to consider patients with lesser degrees of pelvic relaxation. The surgeon must critically evaluate the likelihood that the supportive ligaments of the uterus are weak and that prolapse may become manifest soon after a repair for stress incontinence. This determination is best performed during the patient's initial examination.

Simple inspection of the status of support in the lithotomy position with the patient at rest is inadequate. The support of the uterus and vaginal walls should be tested with the patient straining forcefully. In addition, both the anterior and the posterior vaginal wall must be inspected separately by inserting the fixed half of a vaginal speculum first anteriorly then posteriorly when the patient is straining. If there is any doubt about the presence of uterine prolapse, a tenaculum or ring forceps should be placed on the cervix and traction applied. If the lateral border of the cervix descends below the level of the hymenal ring, the uterine supports are inadequate, and consideration should be given to performing a hysterectomy at the time of surgery for stress incontinence.

CONTRAINDICATIONS

During a vaginal hysterectomy, the surgeon's ability to visualize the pelvic contents is limited, and it is difficult to extend the scope of the operation if unexpected disease is present. Careful preoperative assessment is the key to avoiding operative compromise. Contraindications to vaginal surgery are usually listed as individual items (Table 23-1). Common sense and the operator's skill must be used to individualize these rigid guidelines. The colpotomy performed at the beginning of the operation is an ideal time to re-evaluate the pelvis for unexpected findings and switch to an abdominal approach if unfavorable factors are discovered. In a few selected cases, a preoperative laparoscopy may be useful, providing reassurance that previous salpingo-oophoritis or endometriosis has not so distorted pelvic anatomy that a vaginal hysterectomy would not be feasible. The safety of the surgery often depends on numerous factors, and several small negatives may be enough to warrant abdominal hysterectomy, whereas a single problem may often be accommodated in a vaginal approach.

In patients with malignant disease of the genital tract, vaginal hysterectomy is limited to the occasional patient with microinvasion of the

Table 23-1. *Contraindications to Vaginal Hysterectomy*

ABSOLUTE

Malignancy of the genital tract
Ovarian tumor
Large uterus with inadequate access for morcellation
History of endometriosis whose extent is unknown
Desire for future childbearing

RELATIVE

Inadequate room or mobility
Fixed uterus
Large uterus
Cervical myoma
Small pelvis
Narrow subpubic arch
Stenotic vagina
Adherent cul-de-sac
Extensive pelvic adhesions

NOT CONTRAINDICATIONS IN THE HANDS OF AN EXPERIENCED SURGEON

Previous adnexal surgery or adhesions
Previous cesarean section
Large uterus
Previous abdominal surgery

cervix meeting specific stringent criteria and well-differentiated stage I adenocarcinoma of the endometrium in experienced hands, among women in whom the risk of abdominal exploration carries some unusual risk, as it does in the massively obese individual.[5] Although it is possible to remove large uteri vaginally when adequate mobility and access are available, it is unwise to plan this approach if exposure is compromised, the uterine arteries are not accessible before morcellation as is true with cervical myomas, or if the operator is not experienced in techniques of morcellation. If endometriosis has been previously diagnosed, it may obliterate the cul-de-sac and increase the likelihood of rectal injury. Information from the operative report or a laparoscopy may be of help in determining if the cul-de-sac is free of disease. Finally, a hysterectomy should not be performed against a pa-

tient's wishes without considerable discussion or if she desires to have more children.

Several factors do not preclude vaginal hysterectomy but may make it more difficult and must be considered in choosing this approach. The size of the uterus, its mobility, and the adequacy of the pelvic and vaginal canals are all such factors. Any one of these factors can usually be managed by an experienced surgeon, but multiple factors probably make abdominal hysterectomy a better approach. A fixed uterus, one that does not move with traction, especially in the face of a narrow subpubic arch, poses significant problems. In addition, the presence of a cervical myoma below the uterine arteries can be removed only with considerable blood loss. A cul-de-sac that is nodular and that is not supple may indicate that the rectum has become adherent to the posterior uterus from endometriosis and might be entered inadvertently. Finally, previous pelvic inflammatory disease may create enough adhesions that hysterectomy may be difficult.

Several factors that have often been listed as contraindications deserve special mention. Previous adnexal or abdominal surgery and previous cesarean section both may cause adhesions between the intestines and the uterus or the bladder and cervix. Once the posterior colpotomy is made, the extent of adhesions can be assessed, and rarely do they preclude vaginal hysterectomy. In the instance of previous cesarean section, in which the bladder may be adherent to the anterior cervix, this needs to be addressed whether the surgery is done abdominally or vaginally and must be performed skillfully in either approach. Vaginal hysterectomy should not be excluded in this situation unless the previous operative report describes particular difficulty.

PREOPERATIVE PREPARATION

In addition to the usual thorough history and physical examination and other medical measures necessary before any major operation, preoperative preparation for vaginal hysterectomy should include a pelvic examination, Papanicolaou smear, and urinalysis. Special care should be taken, as previously mentioned, to determine the degree of prolapse present and detect any potential ovarian malignancy. A Fleet enema the night before surgery empties the rectum in the event that a rectal examination is required during surgery and provides more room posteriorly, improving exposure. Patients should receive prophylactic antibiotics to minimize the risk of postoperative infections (500 mg cephazolin intramuscularly or intravenously on call to the operating room is appropriate).[6] If abnormal uterine bleeding has been present, the endometrium should have been sampled preoperatively. Finally, special consideration should be given to assessing whether or not concomitant cystocele, stress incontinence, enterocele, or rectocele is present, as outlined in Chapter 21.

TECHNIQUE OF VAGINAL HYSTERECTOMY

Before beginning the hysterectomy, the bladder is drained and a sterile preparation performed.

An indwelling catheter is usually not placed at this point, so the bladder can accumulate enough urine so an inadvertent cystotomy may easily be recognized. Care should be taken in positioning and draping the patient to avoid nerve compression and yet to gain adequate access to the operative site. An examination should be performed under anesthesia to assess once again whether or not it is wise to proceed with a vaginal hysterectomy or to switch to an abdominal approach.

The elements of vaginal hysterectomy in the United States are derived from the operation by Heaney.[7,8] It is begun by making a circumscribing incision through the vaginal wall at the cervicovaginal junction (Fig. 23-1). Anteriorly it is placed at the lower edge of the bladder to allow for entry into the vesicocervical space. The lower edge of the bladder can be palpated against the cervix to determine where this incision should be made. In addition, the junction of the vaginal rugae and the smooth mucosa of the cervix can be used as a landmark to identify the proper site

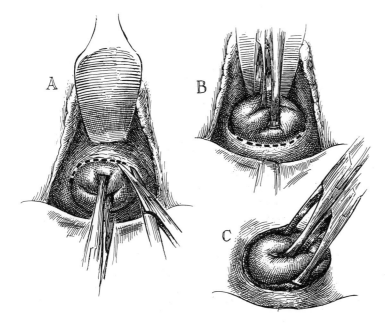

Figure 23-1. *Circumscribing the cervix. This should be done at the cervicovaginal junction and may be accomplished by the use of scissors or a knife. (From Nichols DH, Randall CL. Vaginal surgery. 3rd ed. Baltimore: Williams & Wilkins, 1989.)*

of incision. Care should be taken when the anterior fornix is absent. In this instance, the bladder has prolapsed over the cervix into a position where it can easily be damaged. In this situation, or in those in which the cervix is greatly hypertrophied from long-standing prolapse, a vertical incision on the anterior vaginal wall as is done with an anterior colporrhaphy allows the bladder to be mobilized off of the cervix. The circumscribing incision can then be made with exact knowledge of the bladder's position. Some operators inject saline into the tissues around the cervix to facilitate dissection, but this should not contain a vasoconstrictor because these increase the incidence of postoperative pelvic infection.[9]

The incision should be made through the full thickness of the vaginal wall. This can be determined by placing a retractor anteriorly while pulling forcefully on the cervix so the vaginal wall is placed under tension. Once it has been transected, it separates, exposing the underlying cleavage plane. On the posterior aspect of the cervix, this exposes the area of the cul-de-sac. Blunt dissection here frees the peritoneum, which can then be grasped and entered (Fig. 23-2). Care should be exercised so as not to

dissect the peritoneum off of the uterus because that makes entry more difficult. Once the cul-de-sac incision has been extended laterally as far as the medial margins of the uterosacral ligaments, it can be sutured to the posterior vaginal cuff to minimize bleeding. At this point, it is appropriate to palpate the adnexal structures through the colpotomy to detect unsuspected tumors and also to make a final decision concerning the feasibility of the vaginal approach if any doubt had existed. This is an easy time to acquire this valuable information, and if unsuspected disease is found, an abdominal approach can be taken.

Next a long-bladed posterior weighted retractor is placed into the cul-de-sac and attention turned to entering the anterior cul-de-sac. Dissection along the vesicocervical plane is best performed by lifting the fascia anteriorly while cutting with Mayo scissors placed tip down on the cervix (Fig. 23-3). This avoids the problems with dissecting into the cervix that sometimes happens when a knife is used because the scissors held in this orientation do not cut into the cervical stroma. Once the cleavage plane of the vesicocervical space is reached, gentle dissection with a gloved finger is all that is needed to elevate

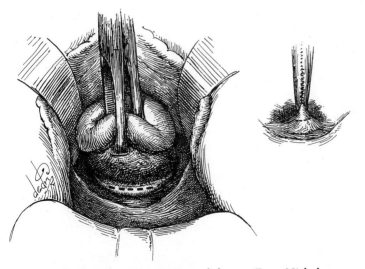

Figure 23-2. Entering the posterior cul-de-sac. (From Nichols DH, Randall CL. Vaginal surgery. 3rd ed. Baltimore: Williams & Wilkins, 1989.)

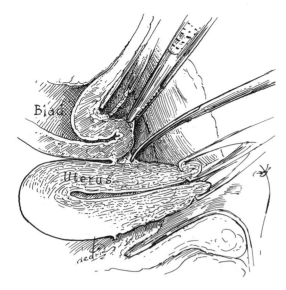

Figure 23-3. *Dissecting the bladder off of the anterior surface of the uterus before entering the anterior cul-de-sac. (From Nichols DH, Randall CL. Vaginal surgery. 3rd ed. Baltimore: Williams & Wilkins, 1989.)*

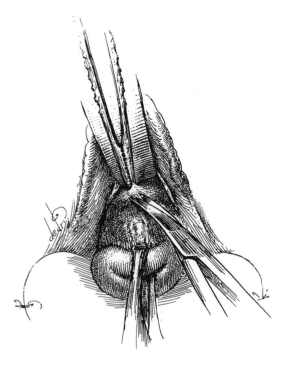

Figure 23-4. *Incising the peritoneum of the anterior cul-de-sac. (From Nichols DH, Randall CL. Vaginal surgery. 3rd ed. Baltimore: Williams & Wilkins, 1989.)*

the bladder off of the cervix. If the bladder pillars are prominent, they can be clamped next to the cervix, transected, and ligated to provide more lateral exposure. The peritoneum is palpated by sliding a finger back and forth and feeling the way in which the two slippery mesothelial surfaces slide on one another. It can then be lifted up, transilluminated, and incised (Fig. 23-4). After extending the incision laterally, a suture can be placed in its vesical edge and held with a hemostat to facilitate its later identification at the time of reperitonealization.

If difficulty is encountered in entering the anterior cul-de-sac, it may be easier after the uterosacral and cardinal ligaments have been transected, provided that the bladder and ureters have been adequately mobilized off of the cervix. The additional downward descent that is achieved by severing the suspensory ligaments frequently brings the peritoneum into closer proximity to the operator and facilitates its identification. If this still does not provide access, the

first two fingers of the right hand can be inserted through the posterior cul-de-sac incision, brought over top of the broad ligament and down between the bladder and uterus, carrying the peritoneum with them. It can then easily be cut.

Once the cul-de-sacs have been entered, the ureter should be palpated to determine its position before shortening and transecting the cardinal ligaments. This is a critical step because it is only if the ligaments are shortened that the vagina is held at a higher level than the prolapsed cervix was. Place a retractor in the lateral fornix of the vagina and a finger in the anterior cul-de-sac. Because the ureter must pass under the uterine artery and reach the bladder that is anterior to the finger, it can be palpated against the retractor blade. The characteristic snap of the ureter permits its identification and can be followed

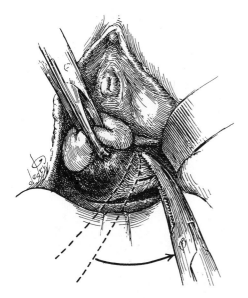

Figure 23-5. *Shortening the uterosacral ligaments before their transection to enhance vaginal support when the uterosacral ligaments are attached to the vagina at the completion of the operation. (From Nichols DH, Randall CL. Vaginal surgery. 3rd ed. Baltimore: Williams & Wilkins, 1989.)*

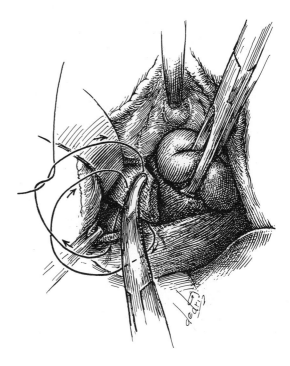

Figure 23-6. *Suture ligation of the shortened uterosacral ligament and transfixing it to the vagina to help elevate the vagina. (From Nichols DH, Randall CL. Vaginal surgery. 3rd ed. Baltimore: Williams & Wilkins, 1989.)*

for some distance by moving the retractor and examining finger.

Having identified the location of the ureter, the uterosacral and cardinal ligaments are then shortened by clamping them at a safe distance from the ureter but somewhat lateral to the cervix (Fig. 23-5). After cutting and suture ligating the ligaments (Figs. 23-6 and 23-7), the sutures are left long and marked for use in resuspending the vagina at the end of the procedure. The uterine arteries are similarly clamped, transected, and suture ligated but not tagged for suspension purposes.

At this point, the corpus of the uterus is usually brought through the posterior colpotomy by pulling on it with a tenaculum to expose the connections between the adnexal structures and the uterus. When this is not possible because of a small vagina or large uterus, the uterus can be divided along its sagittal plane and one half pushed up into the peritoneal cavity, while leav-

ing a long tenaculum attached to allow for its later retrieval while the contralateral adnexal pedicles are dealt with. Whatever technique has been used to expose the adnexa, clamps are then placed across the adnexal structures, exercising care not to include bowel or adjacent structures, and the pedicles are transected. If there is little tissue in this area, one clamp may suffice, but commonly one can be brought in from either side of the uterus and overlapped, minimizing the size of each pedicle (Fig. 23-8). Next the uterus is removed to improve exposure, and the pedicles are ligated (Fig. 23-9). Consideration should then be given to removal of the ovaries.[10] If the ovaries are to be removed, this is accomplished at this time by clamping the mesovarium or infundibulopelvic ligament; removing the ovary, with or without the fallopian tube; and

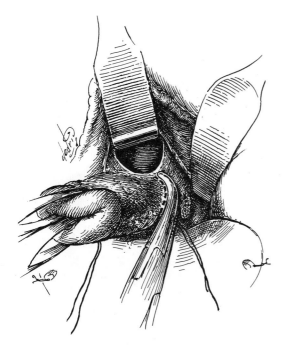

Figure 23-7. Clamping the cardinal ligament. (From Nichols DH, Randall CL. Vaginal surgery. 3rd ed. Baltimore: Williams & Wilkins, 1989.)

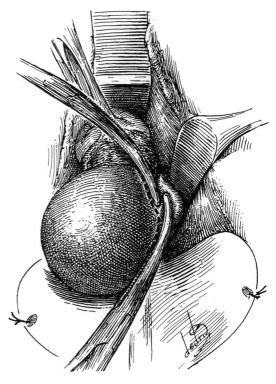

Figure 23-8. Clamping the cornual structures before removing the uterus. (From Nichols DH, Randall CL. Vaginal surgery. 3rd ed. Baltimore: Williams & Wilkins, 1989.)

suture ligating the remaining pedicle (Fig. 23-10). In premenopausal women, after hemostasis has been assured, the sutures are cut to allow the ovaries to retract upward away from the vaginal apex because attaching them to the vagina carries the risk of subsequent dyspareunia. In postmenopausal women, in whom the ovaries seem to be less sensitive, these pedicles can be used to provide additional support at the time of vaginal closure if significant prolapse is present.

MANAGEMENT OF THE CUL-DE-SAC AND SUSPENSION OF THE APEX

Once the uterus has been removed and the ligaments prepared by shortening them, the reconstructive phase of the operation begins. Its goals are to close the peritoneum and suspend the vaginal apex and to correct any enlargement of the cul-de-sac that exists. The peritoneum of the cul-de-sac attaches to the uterus, and so whenever the uterus prolapses, it pulls the cul-de-sac peritoneum with it. If this extension is not distended with bowel, it is referred to as a traction enterocele. When the cul-de-sac is not only elongated, but also filled with bowel and distended during increases in abdominal pressure, it is referred to as a pulsion enterocele, a true enterocele.

When little prolapse has been present (the cervix does not extend below the hymenal ring), simple closure of the cul-de-sac and attachment of the ligaments suffice. A Foley catheter is usually placed at this time to drain the bladder. This brings the anterior peritoneum closer to the surgeon and thereby facilitates its closure. The peritoneum is closed with a pursestring suture of

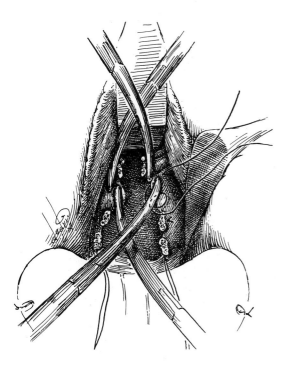

Figure 23-9. *Suture ligating the cornual structures when the ovaries are to be retained. (From Nichols DH, Randall CL. Vaginal surgery. 3rd ed. Baltimore: Williams & Wilkins, 1989.)*

0 silk placed at the highest level possible beginning on the vesical peritoneum, continuing laterally to the position of the pedicles, skipping the vascular structures, and continuing across the posterior cul-de-sac from one uterosacral ligament to the other and then anteriorly again (Fig. 23-11). A finger is placed in the peritoneum while this suture is tied to avoid trapping intraabdominal contents and removed as the suture is snugged down.

If there is a pulsion enterocele present or if severe uterine prolapse exists where the ligaments are particularly elongated, a modified McCall culdoplasty can be used to elevate the posterior vagina and to close the cul-de-sac.[11] This is done by placing a suture through the vaginal wall in its upper posterior extent, placing it through the uterosacral ligament as high as possible, and then similarly including the uter-

osacral ligament and vaginal wall on the other side. The uterosacral ligament is identified by placing an Allis clamp on its severed end and putting it on tension so it becomes tight and therefore palpable. This pulls the vagina higher and posteriorly in the pelvis as well as obliterating the cul-de-sac (Fig. 23-12). When a particularly large pulsion enterocele is present, the excess peritoneum and stretched vaginal wall must be removed. This may be done by removing a V-shaped wedge of vaginal wall and peritoneum. Sutures placed in the uterosacral ligaments may be used to close this defect, not only approximating the edges of the vaginal incision, but also suspending it. If a cystocele is present, it is repaired at this time.

To complete the suspension of the vagina, one of several techniques can be used to connect the shortened cardinal and uterosacral ligaments. The angle sutures described by Heaney can be used, wherein a suture is placed through the anterior lateral vaginal wall, cardinal ligaments, uterosacral ligaments, and then the posterior vaginal wall, so when the suture is tied, it reattaches the vaginal apex to the suspensory ligaments. Alternatively, the ends of the sutures attached to the ligaments can be sewn directly into the vaginal wall using a threadable needle and thereby closing the cuff. The cardinal ligaments are placed laterally and the uterosacral ligaments medially. This avoids having to place a needle through a potentially vascular pedicle and also minimizes the amount of suture in the wound, while at the same time closing the vaginal apex.

ROLE OF ANCILLARY REPAIR

At this point, an anterior or posterior colporrhaphy is performed. Enteroceles are discussed later in this chapter.

Enterocele After Hysterectomy

The previous description concerns the technique of vaginal hysterectomy as it is usually performed and discusses the management of an enterocele

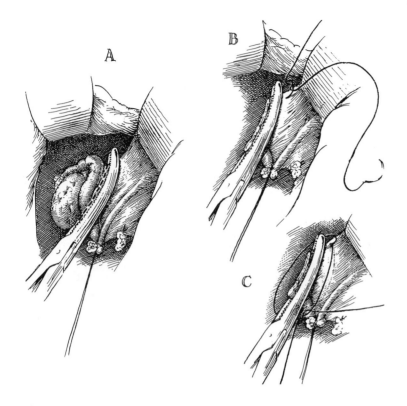

Figure 23-10. *Removal of the tube and ovary. (From Nichols DH, Randall CL. Vaginal surgery. 3rd ed. Baltimore: Williams & Wilkins, 1989.)*

encountered with the uterus *in situ*. Because the problem of enterocele after hysterectomy is a significant complication, it is considered separately here. There are two reasons why discussion of enterocele is especially important in patients with stress urinary incontinence. First, some techniques of urethropexy (e.g., Burch procedure), by pulling the vagina into an unnaturally anterior position high on the pubic bone, can pull the cul-de-sac open and precipitate the development of a new enterocele.[12] Second, if an enterocele is already present and not detected and repaired at the time of surgery, it may become larger postoperatively and present as a recurrent prolapse despite the correction of other aspects of pelvic support.

There is always a cul-de-sac between the upper vagina and the rectum. This allows a culdocentesis to be performed and permits a colpotomy to be made through the posterior vaginal wall at the beginning of a vaginal hysterectomy. This peritoneal pouch extends 3 to 4 cm beyond the junction of the vagina and cervix.[13] An enterocele is absent in normal women, therefore, because the cul-de-sac is closed, not because a peritoneal space does not exist. In normal women, the vagina lies above (cephalad) the rectum, so an increase in abdominal pressure forces the vagina against the rectum and closes the cul-de-sac. The position of the vagina is determined by the upward and posterior traction on the vagina by the cardinal and uterosacral ligaments of the vagina. The relatively horizontal position of the rectum on which the vagina rests is determined by the action of the levator ani muscles. These factors explain two clinical observations.

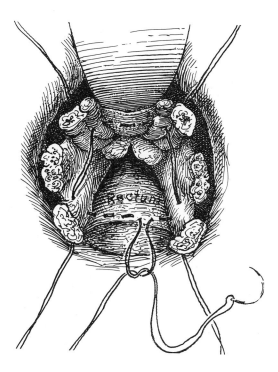

Figure 23-11. Pursestring closure of the perito-neum, including the uterosacral ligaments to bring them together in the midline. (From Nichols DH, Randall CL. Vaginal surgery. 3rd ed. Baltimore: Williams & Wilkins, 1989.)

First, as previously mentioned, anterior traction on the vagina as occurs during high urethral suspension may cause an enterocele by pulling the cul-de-sac open. Second, it explains the association between poor function of the levator ani muscles and genital prolapse.[14] Therefore the factors that close the cul-de-sac are equally important to its depth. In fact, the enlarged cul-de-sac present in an enterocele *reflects* the dilation of this peritoneal pouch caused by factors that open it and subject it to dilation.

As mentioned in the earlier section dealing with enterocele associated with uterine prolapse, there are two types of enteroceles: pulsion and traction. A pulsion enterocele exists when the cul-de-sac is distended and presents as a bulging mass that is inflated by increases in abdominal

pressure. This may occur with the vaginal apex or uterus well suspended, in which case the cervix or vaginal apex is at a normal level, and the enterocele dissects between the vagina and the rectum. When an enterocele is also associated with prolapse of the uterus or vaginal apex, the prolapse and enterocele occur together.

A traction enterocele represents a situation in which prolapse of the uterus pulls the cul-de-sac peritoneum with it. In this instance, there is no bulging or distention of the cul-de-sac when abdominal pressure rises. This situation is usually found at the time of vaginal hysterectomy when the cervix has prolapsed. It represents a potential enterocele rather than an actual enterocele because there is no bulging mass separate from the uterus. The enterocele should be carefully repaired because once the uterus is removed, it may develop into a clinically symptomatic pulsion enterocele.

PREOPERATIVE CONSIDERATIONS

In contrast to uterine prolapse, which is obvious on examination, an enterocele may be difficult to distinguish from a large cystocele or rectocele. Therefore the key to detecting an enterocele lies in actively looking for it whenever a patient who has prolapse is examined. Detection of an enterocele is best performed in the awake straining patient and may not be suspected in a supine individual at rest. Anatomically an enterocele extends from the apex of the vagina downward, whereas a rectocele typically begins in the lower portion of the vagina. It is sometimes evident as a bulge that overrides the more caudal rectocele. Careful inspection of the posterior vaginal wall with a speculum retracting the anterior wall can suggest this diagnosis. Although an enterocele may be evident in the supine position, there may not be sufficient force on the pelvic floor to cause it to distend with the patient lying down. The most sensitive examination to detect this is to have the patient stand and to place the index finger in the rectum and the thumb in the vagina. Then with the patient straining, the rectovaginal space may be palpated to detect the bulge of the

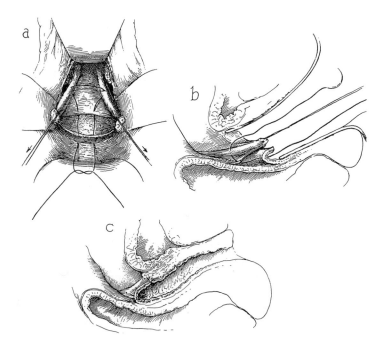

Figure 23-12. *Modified McCall culdoplasty. (From Nichols DH,*
Randall CL. Vaginal surgery. 3rd ed. Baltimore: Williams &
Wilkins, 1989.)

enterocele and the presence of small bowel, omentum, or large bowel in this region. In addition to looking for the enterocele during clinical examination, its presence should also be sought in the operating room and the cul-de-sac evaluated once the peritoneum has been opened.

REPAIR OF THE ENTEROCELE

Repair of an enterocele should not only obliterate the cul-de-sac, but also should pull the vagina over the rectum by shortening the ligamentous suspension of the vagina. In addition, if the vaginal wall has been stretched because of its protrusion below the pelvic floor, the excess vaginal wall must be excised. Although transabdominal enterocele repairs (Moschcowitz or Halban) are useful as prophylaxis at the time of abdominal repair, an enterocele that presents after hysterectomy can almost always be repaired vaginally, and this is the preferred method because it avoids the morbidity of an abdominal incision and is much easier to perform.

The vaginal wall is opened over the enterocele sac. If a concomitant rectocele is present, this may be done by extending the incision made for the posterior repair up to the apex of the vagina. If a pure enterocele is present, the incision may be made directly over the enterocele. In instances in which the prolapsed vaginal wall has become stretched, a diamond-shaped incision may be made to excise the excess vaginal skin. These incisions should be made through the vaginal mucosa and the fascia. The proper depth has been reached when firm traction and countertraction cause the vaginal wall to separate and the loose areolar tissue of the subperitoneal space is encountered. It is easiest to reach this plane 2 to 3 cm from the scar where the cervix had previously been present.

When the enterocele is large, identification of the peritoneal sac is usually easy. In instances

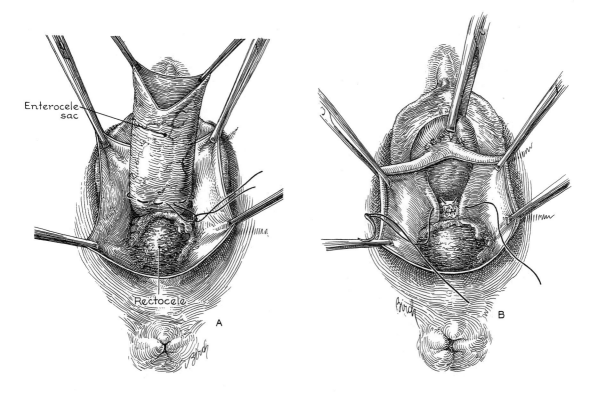

Figure 23-13. *Transvaginal closure of an enterocele. (A) Pursestring closure of the entero-cele after it has been dissected free of the vaginal wall. (B) Plication of the uterosacral ligaments under the peritoneal closure. Although shown with the cervix in situ, this is usu-ally encountered after hysterectomy, where the position of the cervix is replaced by the vaginal apex. (From Mattingly RJ, Thompson JD, eds. TeLinde's operative gynecology. 6th ed. Philadelphia: JB Lippincott, 1985.)*

in which prolapse is associated primarily with a large cystourethrocele but in which a definite enterocele sac is present, identification of the sac may be more difficult. In these situations, make sure that the incision is made posterior to the scar in the vaginal apex to avoid injury to the bladder. If the peritoneum is still difficult to find, it may be brought closer to the operator by using its attachment to the anterior rectal wall. Placing a finger in the rectum and pulling the rectum anteriorly through the vaginal incision into the operative field usually draws the peritoneum into view.

Once identified, the peritoneum is separated from the vagina. The peritoneum may be sepa-rated from the surrounding vaginal wall, but is attached to the vaginal cuff and to the rectum. These form the limits to which the peritoneum may be dissected free. Once the peritoneum has been mobilized to this level, a pursestring perma-nent suture is placed at a high level to obliterate the peritoneum (Fig. 23-13A). Once this has been done, the excess peritoneum is excised.

Next the remnants of the uterosacral liga-ments are brought together under the perito-neum and attached to the vaginal apex to im-prove its support (Fig. 23-13B). They may be identified by pulling forcefully in an anterior direction to put them on stretch. This makes them palpable and allows their substance to be appreciated. Several sutures may be used to plicate them under the peritoneum to reinforce the peritoneal closure. At that point, any excess vaginal wall is trimmed, a posterior repair performed if needed, and the vaginal incision closed.

Most enterocele repairs should be accompanied by a posterior colpoperineorrhaphy. A lack of pelvic floor closure below the uterus and vagina is critically important to the development of prolapse and its recurrence. Inadequate closure is manifested by the gaping introitus and diastasis of the levator ani muscles. This does not occur because of a deficient perineal body or separation of the bulbocavernosus muscles as often thought but rather because of damage to the levator ani muscles. In women with uterine prolapse or enterocele, it is important to consider the status of the pelvic floor, and if it is gaping, a careful posterior colporrhaphy should be performed in an attempt to narrow the enlarged opening and therefore lessen the strain on the fascial and ligamentous tissues that have been used in the repair.

References

1. White SC, Wartel LJ, Wade ME. Comparison of abdominal and vaginal hysterectomies. Obstet Gynecol 1971;37:530.
2. Porges RF. Changing indications for vaginal hysterectomy. Am J Obstet Gynecol 1980;136:153.
3. TeLinde RW. Prolapse of the uterus and allied conditions. Am J Obstet Gynecol 1966;94:444.
4. Langer R, Ron-El R, Neuman M, et al. The value of simultaneous hysterectomy during Burch colposuspension for urinary stress incontinence. Obstet Gynecol 1988;72:866.
5. Peters WA, Andersen WA, Thornton WN, Morley GW. Selective use of vaginal hysterectomy in the management of adenocarcinoma of the endometrium. Am J Obstet Gynecol 1983;146:285.
6. Hemsell DL, Johnson ER, Hemsell PG, et al. Cefazolin for hysterectomy prophylaxis. Obstet Gynecol 1990;76:603.
7. Heaney NS. Report of 565 vaginal hysterectomies performed for benign pelvic disease. Am J Obstet Gynecol 134;28:751.
8. Heaney NS. Vaginal hysterectomy: Its indications and technique. Am J Surg 1940;48:284.
9. England GT, Randall HW, Graves WL. Impairment of tissue defenses by vasoconstrictors in vaginal hysterectomies. Obstet Gynecol 1983; 61:271.
10. Sheth SS. The place of oophorectomy at vaginal hysterectomy. Br J Obstet Gynaecol 1991;98:662.
11. McCall ML. Posterior culdeplasty: Surgical correction of enterocele during vaginal hysterectomy. A preliminary report. Obstet Gynecol 1957;10:595.
12. Burch JC. Cooper's ligament urethrovesical suspension for stress incontinence Am J Obstet Gynecol 1968;100:764.
13. Kuhn RJP, Hollyock VE. Observations on the anatomy of the rectovaginal pouch and septum. Obstet Gynecol 1982;59:445.
14. Smith ARB, Hosker GL, Warrell DW. The role of partial denervation of the pelvic floor in the aetiology of genitourinary prolapse and stress incontinence of urine: A neurophysiological study. Br J Obstet Gynaecol 1989;96:24.

V

Injuries to the Urogenital Organs

24

Ureteral Injuries

Elroy D. Kursh

The ureter is predisposed to injury during surgical procedures in the female pelvis owing to its close embryologic development to the female genital tract. The incidence of ureteral injury has been variably reported to be between 0.20% and 0.56%. Two prospective studies reported more than 30 years ago indicated that the incidence of ureteral injury may be as high as 2.4% to 2.5%.[1,2] In 1988, Daly and Higgins noted an incidence of 1.5% in 1093 women who underwent pelvic procedures.[3] It is clear, therefore, that the incidence of ureteral injury is substantial. All surgeons operating within the pelvis must be familiar with the techniques to prevent ureteral injury and, if necessary, to manage this complication correctly.

Anatomy of the Ureter

The adult ureter is approximately 25 cm long and divided into two roughly equal parts, the abdominal and pelvic portions. The ureters enter the pelvis by passing over the pelvic brim, where they cross the division of the common iliac artery into the internal and external iliac arteries. The pelvic ureter courses along the posterior lateral pelvic wall anterior to the internal iliac artery until it is deep in the pelvis. In this area, it lies just medial to branches of the internal iliac artery,

where it attaches to the medial leaf of the broad ligament. Next the ureter courses beneath the uterine artery, where it is only approximately 1.5 cm lateral to the cervix. As the ureter approaches the bladder, it passes medially over the anterior fornix of the vagina to enter the bladder wall.

The blood supply of the ureter comes from multiple sources, including the renal artery, the gonadal artery, the aorta, the internal iliac artery, the superior vesicle arteries, and the inferior vesicle arteries. The number of vessels supplying the ureter varies from three to nine arteries, with an average of five per ureter. The ureteral blood supply varies from that of the bowel in that it does not branch into arcades away from its lumen. Instead its blood supply lies in close relation to the ureter, being positioned between its muscular wall and its adventitial sheath. In a majority of cases, a single artery runs the length of the ureter within its sheath, but in approximately 20% of dissections, multiple nonanastomosing vessels are found to supply the ureter. It is important to note that the blood supply of the abdominal ureter comes from medial sources, whereas below the pelvic brim, it comes from lateral sources. This knowledge may help the pelvic surgeon avoid injury to the blood supply when dissecting near the ureter.[4]

Ureters are usually single and bilateral, but it

Female Urology, edited by Elroy D. Kursh and Edward McGuire. J. B. Lippincott, Philadelphia, © 1994.

must be remembered that they may be partially or completely duplicated and may cross the midline when the kidney is ectopic. Therefore the pelvic surgeon must be aware that ureteral injury may occur to anomalous ureters.

Etiology and Pathogenesis

Approximately two thirds of all iatrogenic ureteral injuries occur during gynecologic surgery, the common procedures being abdominal hysterectomy or excision of adnexal mass.[5,6] The hysterectomy is frequently described as being straightforward and uncomplicated.[7] A variety of pelvic inflammations and masses may displace the ureter and contribute to its injury, such as pelvic inflammatory disease, endometriosis, uterine tumors, and ovarian tumors. Interestingly, a preoperative intravenous pyelogram (IVP) or computed tomography (CT) scan does not appear to prevent ureteral damage.[8] Angulation and obstruction of the ureter has also been known to occur rarely following suprapubic urethropexy.[9]

Nongynecologic surgery may also be responsible for ureteral injury. Abdominoperineal resection or anterior resection of the rectosigmoid colon may be injurious. During colon resection, it has been noted that the ureters are at risk near the site where the inferior mesenteric artery is ligated.[10,11] Vascular surgery also accounts for a number of ureteral injuries.[12] Radiation injury to the ureter is uncommon, but it does occur even today with the more sophisticated methods of delivering treatment.[13] It is also important to note that the more complicated operative procedures, particularly those associated with pelvic cancer, have a higher incidence of associated ureteral injury. Not only may the ureter be invaded by the cancer, but also more frequently the tumor is stuck to its sheath. Therefore the ureter may become devascularized while it is being dissected off of the malignancy.

Ureteral injury most often occurs while hemostasis is being obtained. Therefore the most common sites of injury are close to where the ureter converges with major pelvic vessels: (1) the location where the uterine artery crosses ventral to the ureter and (2) the region of the infundibulopelvic ligament where the ureter closely approximates the ovarian vessels. Another common sight of injury during pelvic dissection is between the cardinal and ureterosacral ligaments, where the ureter emerges from Waldeyer's sheath and the bladder wall.

Other risk factors that have been identified in association with ureteral injury are (1) previous operation in the pelvis, (2) operation at the pelvic brim, (3) distorted anatomy at the pelvic side wall and pelvic brim, (4) removal of the remaining adnexa after hysterectomy, (5) removal of ovarian neoplasm, and (6) repair of injuries to the bladder.[3]

Most injuries of the ureter are a result of crushing the ureter with a clamp, ureteral ligation, avulsion, or transection. Ureteral devascularization, or obstruction of the ureter from angulation by adjacent sutures, is not usually recognized until the postoperative period, when the patient develops a urinoma, fistula, or evidence of ureteral obstruction.

The advent of ureteral instrumentation is making urologic causes of iatrogenic ureteral injury a much more common occurrence. Lytton and associates reported a 9% incidence of minor ureteral perforations and a 3% incidence of major ureteral injury, including avascular necrosis and stenosis.[14] Major perioperative complications with urinary extravasation or hemorrhage is reported by others to be about 4%.[15,16] Fortunately, most of these ureteral injuries are perforations, which are generally managed relatively easily with ureteral stent placement. Avulsion, requiring immediate surgical repair, occurs in approximately 0.5% of cases.[15,17] Ureteral strictures, which are not an infrequent complication of ureteroscopy, may require subsequent balloon dilatation or possible open surgical repair.

Clinical Presentation

Most ureteral injuries occur during uncomplicated pelvic surgery when trauma to the ureter is not a concern or consideration.[7] Unfortunately, fewer than a third of the injuries are recognized intraoperatively.

Injury to the ureter may be suspected during surgery if an unusual collection of fluid is noted in the pelvis secondary to extravasation of urine. It should also be suspected if dissection in the vicinity of the ureter is tedious or difficult.

Unfortunately, a disturbingly high incidence of surgical ureteral injuries is not recognized until the postoperative period, when the patient develops unexplained abdominal pain, a mass, fever, or a paralytic ileus. It is emphasized that postoperative symptoms may be subtle, and a conscientious surgeon should entertain the possibility of ureteral injury when the patient experiences any of these symptoms. Another possible presentation postoperatively is extensive prolonged drainage from operative drain sites, which may represent urine leakage.

Diagnosis

The opportune time to recognize an operative ureteral injury is during surgery. Immediate repair of the injury is usually straightforward and generally associated with a good outcome.[5, 11] When the surgeon suspects injury to the ureter, the intravenous administration of furosemide (Lasix) increases the amount of draining urine. Additionally, the intravenous administration of a vital dye, such as methylene blue or indigo carmine, stains the extravasated urine to help identify the drainage as urine.

If ureteral injury is suspected during a difficult pelvic procedure, it is wise to dissect and identify the ureters. The ureters are usually recognized by the relatively glistening appearance of its sheath, its characteristic peristalsis, and its particular feel to palpation.

If the surgeon is concerned about possible ureteral occlusion, patency can be established by opening the bladder through a longitudinal cystotomy and observing the escape of the urine from the ureteral orifices.[18] As already mentioned, a brisk diuresis can be established with intravenous furosemide, and visualization from the orifices can be enhanced by the administration of a vital dye. If uncertainty persists, the suspected ureter should be catheterized with a 5 French ureteral catheter.[18] Another method that has been suggested for demonstrating ureteral patency intraoperatively employs the placement of a cystoscope through a stab incision at the dome of the bladder at the center of a pursestring suture. Ureteral orifices can be observed for patency as described earlier. In one instance, ureteral catheters were passed bilaterally from this approach in a patient in whom no efflux of dye solution was visualized from either ureteral orifice.[19]

In the postoperative period, excess drainage from the incision, drain sites, or vagina may represent urine leakage secondary to ureteral injury. Unfortunately, it is not uncommon for the surgeon to interpret the drainage to represent serum, often leading to a delay in establishing a correct diagnosis. Analysis of the drainage for urea nitrogen and creatinine confirms the diagnosis of urine leakage by observing a concentration substantially greater than that of serum (usually 10 to 20 times).

If the patient experiences postoperative signs and symptoms suggestive of possible ureteral injury, an intravenous urogram should be performed. This study is most helpful in defining the presence and site of ureteral injury. Extravasation of contrast media from the ureter helps identify urine leakage or a fistula. Various degrees of occlusion of the ureter may be recognized by nonvisualization or reduced visualization of the kidney and collecting system or varying degrees of hydroureteronephrosis. Filling of the vagina with contrast media indicates the presence of a ureterovaginal fistula, particularly if it is associated with a degree of hydroureteronephrosis, which is common for a ureterovaginal fistula.

Ultrasonography may provide useful information but is not as diagnostic as the IVP. Ultrasonography reveals the presence of hematoma or urinoma and also demonstrates an obstructed segment, but the study is not as accurate as an IVP in defining the site of injury. Therefore I reserve ultrasonography for patients with an elevated creatinine level. A CT scan of the abdomen is valuable in demonstrating the extent of the fluid collection, which may represent a urinoma or hematoma. If the collecting system is not well visualized on an IVP or the site of injury is not defined, retrograde urography is usually diagnostic.

If the patient experiences leakage of fluid from the vagina that possibly represents urine, the visualization of dye in the vagina after the intravenous administration of indigo carmine or methylene blue confirms the diagnosis of an ureterovaginal fistula if a vesicovaginal fistula has been ruled out.

Prevention

The best means of avoiding ureteral injury is to define the ureter by means of careful retroperineal dissection.[7,18] This is particularly true for difficult pelvic dissections in which the pelvic pathology may distort the pathway of the ureter. To expose the ureter, the posterior peritoneum is incised at the level of the pelvic brim over the bifurcation of the common iliac artery, where the ureter is readily visible. The pelvic ureter is dissected on its anterior medial surface to avoid its blood supply, which comes from a lateral direction. Dissection proceeds outside its adventitial sheath, and it is sufficient and advisable to avoid extensive mobilization to prevent ureteral devascularization. Mobilization and visualization of the pelvic ureter, as it advances through the vesicouterine ligament into the bladder, can usually be accomplished in a few minutes with minimal bleeding.

The value of preoperative placement of catheters to help prevent ureteral injury has been subjected to debate. Numerous authors have shown that the preoperative placement of catheters has not necessarily avoided ureteral injury.[7,20] Possibly the greatest value in having ureteral catheters in place is that the appearance of the catheter may identify an injured or transected ureter. Simmonds has stressed that careful identification and dissection of the ureter are the most important means of avoiding injury.[7] Three cases of reflux anuria were reported in 59 patients undergoing colorectal surgery, who had prophylactic ureteral catheters placed.[21] It is unclear whether the so-called reflux anuria is caused by edema of the ureteral orifices or results from neurogenic factors initiated by ureteral manipulation resulting in vasoconstriction in the renal cortex.[22] Therefore, although the prophylactic placement of ureteral catheters during any pelvic dissection may help identify the course of the ureter, it is not an innocuous procedure.[21,23]

Management of Ureteral Injuries Discovered During Surgery

It is not advisable simply to ligate a ureter if it is found to be injured or transected during the course of an operation unless the patient has a life-threatening problem, such as cardiac arrest or a massive pulmonary embolus. If the patient's condition stabilizes after undergoing ligation of the ureter, a postoperative percutaneous nephrostomy should be performed. Otherwise, simple ligation of the ureter in a normal functioning unit results in pyelonephritis, pyelonephrosis, or hydronephrotic atrophy of the kidney, which produces symptoms necessitating surgical removal in approximately 20% of cases.[4] I have not hesitated to ligate a nonfunctioning or minimally functioning renal unit with low urine output during a variety of ureteral reconstructive procedures following transplantation. These patients, with a minimally or nonfunctioning renal unit, do not experience problems related to ureteral ligation, and use of their native ureters, which requires ligation above the utilized segment, provides a valuable option for repairing posttransplant urine leaks.

In life-threatening situations, an option that is almost as rapid as ureteral ligation is to cannulate the ureter with an 8 or 10 French feeding tube, tie the distal end of the ureter to the tube, and lead the tube and ureter to the skin. Not only does this maneuver afford drainage of the kidney, but also it allows measurement of the urine output and easy localization of the ureter when reoperating to repair the injury.

A formal operative nephrostomy is never necessary today in the expanding era of percutaneous techniques. If nephrostomy is needed, a percutaneous nephrostomy can be performed in the postoperative period. Additionally, operative nephrostomy is not a rational adjunct for management of lower ureteral injuries because it is time-consuming and requires extension of the surgical incision.

Clamping or ligating the ureter may be of little significance if recognized intraoperatively because these injuries usually include adjacent tissue in the clamp or ligature to help protect the ureter. Release of the clamp or suture with catheterization of the ureter for a week or possibly longer with a double J ureteral stent is usually sufficient therapy. If the ureter is not protected by adjacent tissue, there may be significant vascular impairment of a small portion of ureter. Unfortunately, there is a regrettable tendency to underestimate such injuries. If there is any concern about the viability of any segment of ureter, it is preferable to excise the segment and perform a primary repair. Evidence of vascular impairment of the ureter includes discoloration, lack of peristalsis, and absence of bleeding from the end of the ureter if it is transected. When vascular injury is suspected, the ureter should be debrided until it bleeds readily before performing repair.

Ureteroneocystostomy

Ureteral injuries that occur during hysterectomy often occur deep in the pelvis, in which case ureteroneocystostomy is the procedure of choice. It is controversial whether the ureteral vesical anastomosis should be nonrefluxing or a fish-mouth end-to-side anastomosis. I prefer to perform an end-to-side ureteroneocystostomy. Ureteral reflux is rarely a problem in the adult, and I have never observed upper tract changes or evidence of pyelonephritis in an adult who underwent an end-to-side anastomosis of a normal diameter ureter. An antirefluxing anastomosis has a higher risk of exhibiting varying degrees of obstruction.

The anastomosis must be tension free, and the surgeon should ensure the viability of the distal ureter. Mobilization of the bladder helps achieve a tension-free anastomosis. Another advantage of an end-to-side anastomosis is that it is more likely to be tension free. Ureteral mobilization is done well outside its adventitia but should be limited to as little as possible to avoid ureteral devascularization.

The distal ureter is brought through a convenient site in the bladder. The ureter is spatulated superiorly, and the ureterovesical anastomosis is performed using fine absorbable suture material (4–0 chromic or Vicryl). After taking a bite of the ureter with the suture, a substantial bite of both muscularis and mucosa is taken in the bladder wall with the inferior and two lateral sutures to achieve good fixation of the ureter. Between these initial sutures, the ureter is sutured to the bladder, taking smaller bites of the bladder mucosa with interrupted sutures to complete the anastomosis (Fig. 24-1).

If there is any doubt that the anastomosis is not tension free, a psoas hitch should accompany the ureteroneocystostomy. Mobilization of the bladder is the initial step in performing a psoas hitch. Tension on the anterior surface of the bladder establishes a horn on the side of the ureterovesical anastomosis, which is sutured to the iliopsoas muscle with interrupted absorbable suture. The site of the psoas muscle chosen is usually lateral and above the external iliac artery, and care should be taken to avoid injuring the genitofemoral nerve (Fig. 24-2).

Antirefluxing techniques should be employed in children and is a reasonable alternative in young women. I generally use a double J ureteral stent, which can be easily removed in the

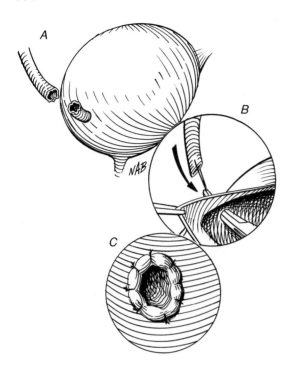

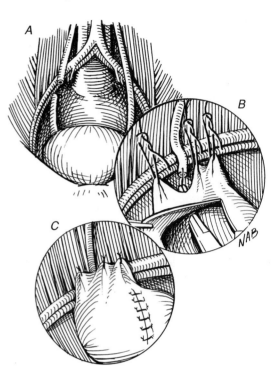

Figure 24-1. *Ureteroneocystostomy. (A) Injury to the ureter deep in the pelvis. (B) Distal ureter is brought through a convenient site in the bladder and spatulated superiorly. (C) Tension-free end-to-side anastomosis is completed using fine absorbable suture.*

Figure 24-2. *Psoas hitch. (A) Injury to the ureter deep in the pelvis. (B) After adequate bladder mobilization, a horn is established on the side of the ureterovesical anastomosis by suturing the bladder to the psoas muscle lateral to the external iliac vessels using O chromic or Vicryl sutures. (C) Completed psoas hitch reduces tension on the ureterovesical anastomosis. Not only does the procedure provide a few centimeters of extra length, but also it offers fixation of the anastomosis, which is an advantage if an antirefluxing technique is used by preventing angulation at the hiatus.*

office under topical anesthesia. A Jackson-Pratt drain is placed in the retroperineum close to the anastomotic site.

Ureteroureterostomy

Ureteroureterostomy is a relatively uncomplicated method of repair that restores ureteral continuity and preserves the vesicoureteral junction. Years ago, the technique was discouraged because of the high incidence of ureteral stenosis. Modern techniques of minimizing ureteral leakage at the anastomotic site have reduced the fibrotic response and associated renal atrophy.

To reduce ureteral leakage, the anastomosis is made watertight if at all possible. If there is any

concern about the integrity of the anastomosis, it can be wrapped with adjacent fat or, if necessary, omentum. It is also important to provide adequate drainage with closed suction drainage, such as with a Jackson-Pratt drain. Another controversial issue is whether or not to stent the anastomosis. I prefer to use an indwelling double J ureteral catheter because it is inert, retains its position well, and minimizes leakage at the anastomosis. It is emphasized that the double J stent

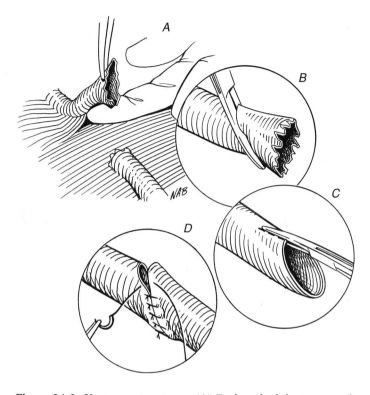

Figure 24-3. *Ureteroureterostomy. (A) Each end of the transected injured ureter is identified. (B) After mobilizing a sufficient length of each end of the ureter to ensure a tension-free anastomosis, the respective ends of the ureter are debrided of any possible nonviable tissue by transecting diagonally. (C) Each end of the ureter is spatulated on opposing ends to enlarge the circumference of the anastomosis. (D) A watertight anastomosis is performed using 4–0 absorbable suture.*

is not completely diverting because urine can reflux up the stent if the patient has a full bladder. Therefore when a double J stent is employed, it is advisable to keep the bladder empty with an indwelling urethral catheter for approximately 7 days to avoid a possible leak at the ureteroureterostomy site. It is also wise to keep the closed suction drain in place near the ureteroureterostomy until the Foley catheter is removed to be certain that leakage does not occur at the anastomotic area.

When performing ureteroureterostomy, each end of the ureter is debrided to ensure via-bility of the respective ends. The ureter is mobilized proximally and distally for a sufficient length to prevent tension on the anastomosis. An oblique anastomosis is achieved by transecting the ureter diagonally and also spatulating the ureter on the opposing ends to enlarge the circumference of the anastomosis. A watertight anastomosis is performed using interrupted 4–0 absorbable suture material through the full thickness of the ureteral wall (Fig. 24-3).

For ureteral injuries above the pelvic brim, additional ureteral length can be obtained by mobilizing the kidney. The kidney can be displaced downward by performing a nephropexy resulting in additional ureteral length of 2.5 cm to up to 5 cm.

Boari Bladder Flap

A Boari bladder flap can be employed when a larger section of a distal ureter is missing or has been devascularized. When a patient has a normal bladder, as much as 15 cm of the ureter can be replaced using this technique. I prefer to regard the creation of a bladder flap as the establishment of a large bladder diverticulum rather than a narrow thin tube of ureteral replacement. Conceptionally this is more likely to provide a well-vascularized bladder flap, which is much less prone to scarring and stricture formation.

The bladder flap is constructed by making two roughly parallel but converging incisions diagonally across the anterior bladder wall with the base of the flap posteriorly. A trapezoid pedicle should be mapped out with the base of the flap being at least 4 to 5 cm wide and the apex being approximately 3 cm wide. It is frequently helpful to distend the bladder with normal saline before planning and marking the flap with stay sutures. The mobilized bladder flap is swung superiorly, and the ureter is anastomosed 1 to 2 cm from the distal end of the flap using interrupted 4–0 absorbable sutures. The ureter may be reimplanted into the bladder flap using a submucosal tunnel to establish an antirefluxing anastomosis or, as I prefer, in a fishmouth end-to-side fashion. A ureteral stent is generally employed. The bladder flap is closed with interrupted sutures of 2–0 absorbable suture material to complete the procedure (Fig. 24-4).

Transureteroureterostomy

Another alternative for managing extensive ureteral loss is the performance of a transureteroureterostomy. Generally it is advisable to use other methods of establishing ureteral continuity if at all possible, especially in the acute set-

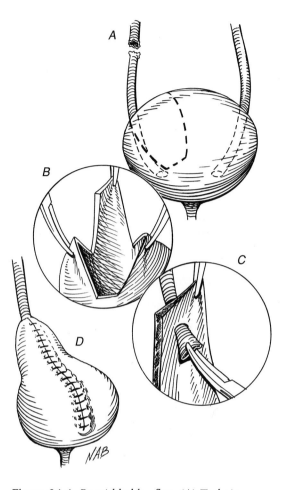

Figure 24-4. Boari bladder flap. (A) Technique used for high pelvic ureteral injury when a large section of distal ureter is missing or has been devascularized. Bladder flap is outlined by mapping out two roughly parallel but converging incisions diagonally across the anterior bladder wall with the flap based posteriorly. (B) Bladder flap is created and swung superiorly. (C) The ureter is brought through a hiatus 1 to 2 cm from the distal end of the bladder flap, and an end-to-side anastomosis is performed. (D) Bladder flap is completed by closing the anterior bladder and tubularizing the flap using 2–0 absorbable suture.

ting. One should not hesitate to employ this technique if inflammation or cancer is present at the site of injury or the defect cannot be bridged in any other way. There are a number of contraindications to this procedure, including bilateral renal disease, urothelial cancer, tuberculosis, recurrent urinary calculi, and pelvic radiation.

When performing a transureteroureterostomy, the posterior peritoneum is incised for an adequate distance to expose the ureters, usually in the vicinity where the ureters cross the iliac arteries. The injured ureter to be transplanted is dissected from its bed well outside its adventitia for a sufficient length to allow a gentle sweep across the retroperitoneal space. The donor ureter is divided as low as possible in the proximity of the injury and ligated distally with 2–0 absorbable suture. A tunnel at the base of the mesosigmoid is established bluntly, preferably above the inferior mesenteric artery, although it can generally be sacrificed with impunity if the remainder of the left colon blood supply is intact. The donor ureter is drawn through the tunnel, transected obliquely, and spatulated on its medial edge. After identifying the recipient ureter, which is mobilized minimally or not at all, a longitudinal incision is made on its anterior medial surface for approximately 1.5 cm. The anastomosis between the oblique end of the donor ureter and the opening in the recipient ureter is accomplished using interrupted 4–0 or 5–0 absorbable suture material, usually with the aid of magnifying lenses. Stenting is optional, although I prefer to use a double J stent placed through the anastomosis down the recipient ureter to the bladder and up the donor ureter to the donor renal pelvis. The vicinity of the anastomosis is drained extraperitoneally through a separate stab wound with closed suction drainage (Fig. 24-5).

Other alternatives for ureteral replacement include an ileal ureter and renal autotransplantation. These alternatives are not advisable in an acute setting owing to the magnitude of performing them, especially in patients with unprepared bowel.

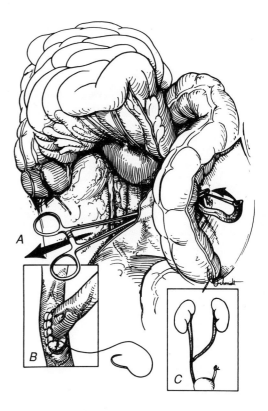

Figure 24-5. Transureteroureterostomy. (A) After adequate mobilization, the donor ureter is brought through a tunnel at the base of the mesosigmoid. (B) The donor ureter is spatulated on its medial edge and anastomosed to the recipient ureter using interrupted fine absorbable sutures. (C) Completed anastomosis. (From Guerriero WG. Ureteral trauma. In: Guerriero WG, ed. Urologic injuries. Norwalk, CT: Appleton-Century-Crofts, 1984.)

Repair of Ureteral Injuries Discovered Postoperatively

After the nature and extent of a ureteral injury discovered postoperatively are defined, initial consideration should be given to an attempt to manage the injury by endoscopic means. If the patient has a urinoma secondary to a small partial incision in the ureter, the surgeon should try to pass a guidewire followed by a double J stent. If the extravasation resolves, any degree of ob-

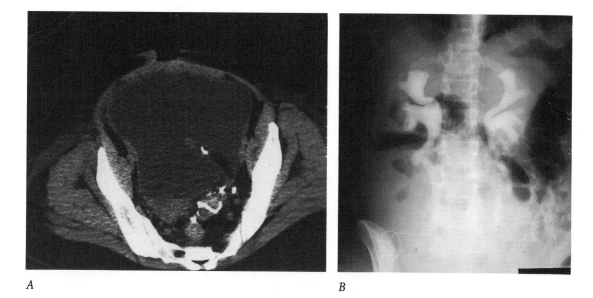

A   B

Figure 24-6. This 41-year-old woman with a right ureteral injury discovered following a difficult colon operation was managed by endoscopic means. (A) Computed tomography scan reveals huge fluid-filled mass (urinoma) in the abdomen, which extends into the pelvis. (B) Intravenous pyelogram shows bilateral hydronephrosis with right ureter dilated to level of transverse process of L-5 and a huge abdominal mass displacing the bowel. A catheter has been inserted into the fluid-filled mass percutaneously. The creatinine of the fluid was significantly elevated, proving that the contents of the mass represented urine.

struction is relieved, and there is adequate control of urinary infection, it is reasonable to observe the fistula while providing prolonged urinary stenting with the double J catheter (Fig. 24-6). Because ureteral stenosis may result, close observation with follow-up IVPs after stent removal is essential. Subsequent therapy, such as balloon dilatation of a stenotic ureter or possible open surgical intervention, may be required.

In the past, many authors recommended staging or delaying ureteral repair when it was discovered in the postoperative period. Today there is little evidence to support the tradition that there is an advantage in delaying repair.[24] Of course, if the patient is unstable, the patient is septic, or there is extensive hematoma or abscess formation at the site of ureteral injury, surgery should not be undertaken. In these instances, it is preferable to provide renal drainage with percutaneous nephrostomy and delay surgery until the problem is resolved. Alternatively, most ureteral injuries occur in healthy female patients with good cardiovascular systems who do not have chronic debilitating diseases. They are apt to tolerate the second surgical procedure well, and the psychological strain of facing a second surgical procedure at a later date can be avoided.

Surgical exploration of the injured ureter is performed if endoscopic management is not possible. If the ureter is obstructed or kinked from sutures in the vicinity of the ureter, it may be possible to relieve the obstruction by simple de-ligation or suture removal.[25] A ligature around the ureter may include sufficient adjacent tissue

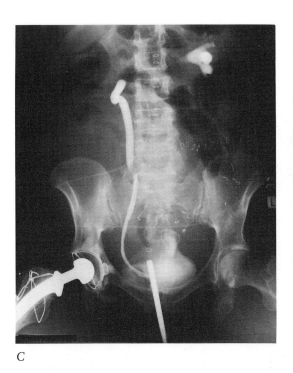

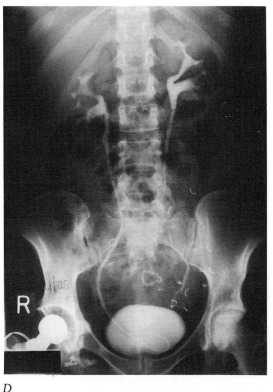

C

D

Figure 24-6. (continued) (C) Retrograde pyelogram demonstrates site of ureteral injury near transverse process of L-5. (D) A double J stent was inserted into the right kidney. Three months later, an intravenous pyelogram reveals normal upper tracts with the stent still in place. A follow-up intravenous pyelogram remained normal after stent removal.

to prevent ureteral necrosis and maintain blood supply. In this setting, ureteral deligation may again be all that is required,[25] but it is probably advisable to stent the injured ureter for a prolonged period with a double J catheter. In most instances, it is necessary to employ one of a variety of surgical techniques to correct ureteral obstruction, extravasation, or fistulas discovered postoperatively. These alternatives have been discussed thoroughly in the previous section on repair of ureteral injuries discovered during surgery. Other options that can be considered postoperatively include ileal ureter and renal auto-

transplantation, although it is preferable to select one of the simpler alternatives presented in this chapter if at all feasible.

Management of Ureterovaginal Fistula

Because fistulas become progressively stenotic as they heal, it has generally been concluded that open operative treatment is required. Hoch and associates did not observe spontaneous healing in any of their patients with ureterovaginal fistulas, all of whom required surgical correc-

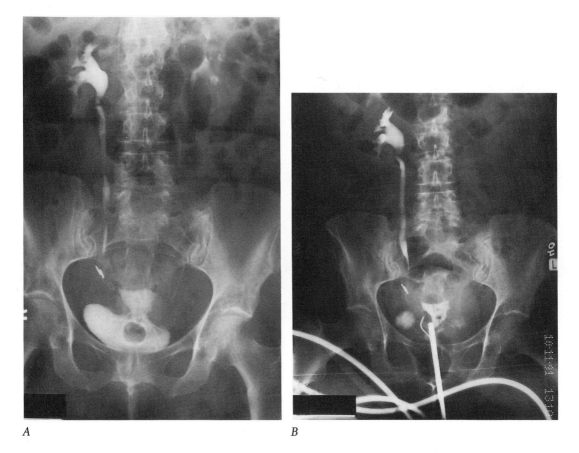

A   B

Figure 24-7. *This 68-year-old white woman, who developed a right ureterovaginal fistula following an upper vaginectomy for recurrent microinvisible cervical cancer, was managed endoscopically. (A) Intravenous pyelogram demonstrated a right ureterovaginal fistula with contrast media filling a cavity, which drained into the vagina posterior to the bladder. (B) A retrograde pyelogram confirmed the diagnosis of a ureterovaginal fistula.*

tion.[26] Therefore they encouraged early aggressive operative correction of most women with ureterovaginal fistulas.[26]

In the past, conservative management of a ureterovaginal fistula by passing a catheter up the ureter through the fistula site occasionally led to resolution of the fistula. Peterson and associates indicated that conservative management is a consideration if there is minimal or no obstruc-

tion of the injured ureter, mild periureteral extravasation, documentation of upper tract improvement on follow-up examinations, adequate control of urinary tract infection, and use of absorbable suture material in the initial operative procedure.[27]

We recently retrospectively reviewed 20 ureterovaginal fistulas in 19 patients managed in the last 20 years. Healing occurred in all seven

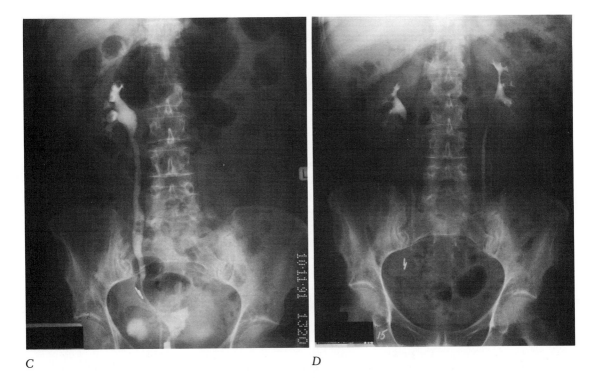

C   D

Figure 24-7. (continued) *(C) Insertion of a double J stent into the right renal pelvis for 3 months resulted in complete resolution of incontinence. (D) A follow-up intravenous pyelogram 3 months after stent removal shows healing of the fistula and normal upper urinary tracts without development of a ureteral stricture.*

patients who had a self-retaining ureteral stent placed in either a retrograde (five) or antegrade (two) manner for a minimum of 4 to 8 weeks. Endourologic management was not attempted in any women in the 1970s, was successful in 4 of 12 women in the 1980s, and has been successful in 3 of 4 women since 1990 (Fig. 24-7). This trend is based on the increased likelihood of passing an internal stent with evolving endourologic technology. Therefore, we conclude that modern endourologic management will result in resolution of a ureterovaginal fistula if it is feasible to pass a suitable internal stent, and every effort should be made to manage a ureterovaginal fistula endourologically rather than resort to immediate open surgery.

When open surgical repair of a ureterovaginal fistula is required, a ureteroneocystostomy is performed, frequently accompanied by a psoas hitch. The technique is the same as described for management of injuries sustained during surgery (Fig. 24-1).

Laparoscopic Ureteral Injury

With an increasing use of laparoscopy for tubal ligation, diagnosis, and as a therapeutic modality, an increasing number of ureteral injuries are being reported. In 1990, Grainger and associates summarized the eight previously reported cases of laparoscopic ureteral injury and presented five additional cases.[28] The indications for laparoscopy were sterilization (four), endometriosis (five), adhesions (two), diagnosis (one), and ureterosacral ligament transection (one).[28] Except for a trochar injury in the patient undergoing a diagnostic laparoscopy, electrocoagulation was used in each instance of ureteral injury.

The authors emphasize that the ureters are usually easy to identify in the upper pelvis but cannot be identified reliably in the vicinity of the ureterosacral ligaments, particularly in the presence of diseases such as endometriosis. Thickened nodular ureterosacral ligaments should alert the operator to potential distortions of normal anatomy of the ureter in this area. The proximity of the ureter to the cervix is also implicated because this is a difficult area to visualize.[28]

During sterilization, it is thought that the likely cause of ureteral injury is a result of the cautery forceps touching the pelvic side wall during application of the current. Therefore it is essential to grasp the tube in the bipolar forceps and move it away from the side wall before applying current. It is erroneous to assume that bipolar coagulation is safe because five of the reported ureteral injuries occurred using this method.[28]

The common presenting symptoms are abdominal pain with peritonitis, leukocytosis, and fever in the early postoperative period. As in other forms of ureteral injury, passage of a ureteral stent may lead to resolution of extravasation with ureteral healing, but any of the other options already discussed may be used. Unfortunately, nephrectomy was required in two of the reported cases owing to pyelonephritis and persistent obstruction after treatment.[28]

References

1. St. Martin EC, Trichel BE, Campbell JH, Locke CH. Ureteral injuries in gynecologic surgery. J Urol 1953;70:51.
2. Solomons E, Levin EJ, Bauman J, Baron J. A pyelographic study of ureteric injuries sustained during hysterectomy for benign conditions. Surg Gynecol Obstet 1960;111:41.
3. Daly JW, Higgins KA. Injury to the ureter during gynecologic surgical procedures. Surg Gynecol Obstet 1988;67:19.
4. Guerriero WG. Ureteral injury. Urol Clin North Am 1989;16:237.
5. Witters S, Cornellissen M, Vereecken R. Iatrogenic ureteral injury: Aggressive or conservative treatment. Am J Obstet Gynecol 1986;155:582.
6. Grace PA, Murphy DM, Butler MR. Surgical injury to the ureter: A report on 21 injuries in 19 patients. Irish Med J 1983;76:418.
7. Simmonds RE. Ureteral injuries associated with gynecologic surgery: Prevention and management. Clin Obstet Gynecol 1976;19:623.
8. Mann WJ, Arato M, Patsner B, Stone ML. Ureteral injuries in an obstetric and gynecology training program: Etiology and management. Obstet Gynecol 1988;72:82.
9. Kissinger DH, Beaugard EP, Affuso PS. Ureteral obstruction complicating urethropexy. J Med Soc NJ 1982;79:747.
10. Hughes ES, McDermott FT, Polglase AL, et al. Ureteric damage in surgery for cancer of the large bowel. Dis Colon Rectum 1984;27:293.
11. Fry DE, Milholen L, Harbrecht PJ. Iatrogenic ureteral injury. Options in management. Arch Surg 1983;118:454.
12. Spirnak JP, Hampel N, Resnick MI. Ureteral injuries complicating vascular surgery: Is repair indicated? J Urol 1989;141:13.
13. Sefert HJ, Gillenwater JY. The consequences of ureteral irradiation with special reference to subsequent ureteral injury. J Urol 1972;107:369.
14. Lytton B, Weiss RM, Greon DF. Complications of ureteral endoscopy. J Urol 1987;137:649.
15. Weinberg JJ, Ansoung K, Smith AD: Complications of ureteroscopy in relation to experience: Report of survey and author experience. J Urol 1987;137:384.
16. Flam TA, Malone MJ, Roth RA. Complications of ureteroscopy. Urol Clin North Am 1988;15:167.
17. Kahn RI. Endourological treatment of ureteral calculi. J Urol 1986;135:239.
18. Boyd NE. Care of the ureter in pelvic surgery. Can J Surg 1987;30:234.
19. Timmons MC, Addison WA. Suprapubic teloscopy: Extraperitoneal intraoperative technique to demonstrate ureteral patency. Obstet Gynecol 1990;75:137.
20. Leff EI, Groff W, Rubin RJ, et al. Use of ureteral catheters in colonic and rectal surgery. Dis Colon Rectum 1982;25:457.

21. Sheikh FA, Khubchandani IT. Prophylactic ureteric catheters in colon surgery—how safe are they? Dis Col Rectum 1990;33:508.

22. Shearlock K, Howard SS. Postoperative anuria: A documented entity. J Urol 1976;115:212.

23. Songco A, Rattner W. Reflex anuria. Urology 1987;29:432.

24. Badenoch DF, Tiptaft RC, Thakar DR, et al. Early repair of accidental injury to the ureter or bladder following gynecological surgery. Br J Urol 1987;59:516.

25. Herman G, Guerrier K, Persky L. Delayed ureteral deligation. J Urol 1972;107:723.

26. Hoch WH, Kursh ED, Persky L. Early, aggressive management of intraoperative ureteral injuries. J Urol 1975;114:530.

27. Peterson DD, Lucey DT, Fried FA. Nonsurgical management of ureterovaginal fistula. Urology 1974;4:677.

28. Grainger DA, Soderston RM, Schiff SF, et al. Ureteral injuries at laparoscopy: Insights into diagnosis, management and prevention. Obstet Gynecol 1990;75:839.

25

Bladder and Urethral Injuries

J. Patrick Spirnak

Bladder injury may occur either as a result of external trauma (penetrating or blunt) or during the course of any pelvic surgical procedure (operative trauma). When diagnosed and effectively treated, bladder injury seldom leads to long-term complications. When these injuries are undiagnosed or mismanaged, however, complications such as urinary ascites, pelvic abscess, or fistula formation may occur (Fig. 25-1). To minimize the incidence of operative injuries, the pelvic surgeon must be familiar with the spatial relationship of the bladder to the surrounding pelvic organs. In those cases in which bladder injury is unavoidable, appropriate surgical management minimizes morbidity. Similarly, it is imperative that any physician involved in the evaluation and care of trauma victims be familiar with the indications for evaluation of the lower urinary tract, the proper way to perform the indicated studies, and the appropriate way to manage these injuries.

Anatomic Considerations

The urinary bladder is primarily an extraperitoneal organ, which functions as a storage reservoir for urine. In the adult, it is well protected by the rigid bony pelvis. In children, the bladder is an abdominal organ lying just beneath the anterior abdominal wall. Only after about the sixth year of life has the bony pelvis enlarged sufficiently to allow the bladder to assume its permanent pelvic position beneath the pubic symphysis.[1]

The bladder when empty has a tetrahedral shape. It consists of four surfaces: the superior, posterior, and two inferolateral surfaces.[1] The superior surface is directed upward, is triangular in shape, and is the only surface covered completely by peritoneum. It has a direct relationship with both the sigmoid colon and loops of small bowel. The uterus lies on and indents the superior surface. The bladder's posterior surface, better known as the base or fundus, is loosely attached to the upper part of the anterior vaginal wall, cervix, and uterus (Fig. 25-2). The two inferolateral surfaces are separated from the obturator internus muscle, the pelvic diaphragm, and back of the pubis by loose fatty areolar tissue. Loose connective tissue occupies the prevesical space (*i.e.*, space of Retzius). This space allows for both the easy mobilization of the bladder from adjacent viscera and the performance of extraperitoneal surgical repair.

The pubovesical ligaments attach the bladder directly to the pubic symphysis.[2] Inferiorly the pelvic floor provides the chief support. Posteriorly the bladder base is supported by the vagina and uterus. Anteriorly the medial and paired

341

Female Urology, edited by Elroy D. Kursh and Edward McGuire. J. B. Lippincott, Philadelphia, © 1994.

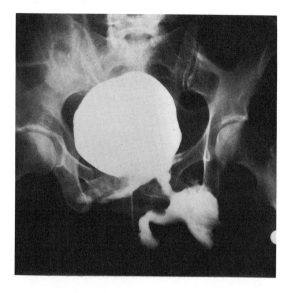

Figure 25-1. *Vesicocutaneous fistula in a patient with a pelvic fracture and a missed extraperitoneal bladder perforation.*

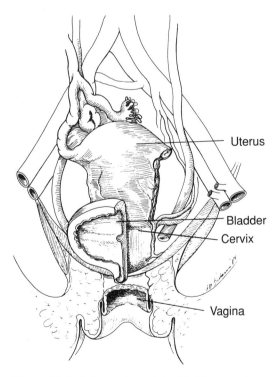

Figure 25-2. *Relationship of the bladder to other pelvic viscera.*

lateral umbilical ligaments provide support (Fig. 25-3). With the exception of the fixed bladder neck, the remainder of the bladder is free to move and expand in response to bladder filling, and it assumes a globular shape when distended.

The main blood supply to the bladder is derived from branches of the hypogastric or internal iliac artery. The superior vesical artery supplies the superior lateral bladder wall. Branches from the obturator, internal pudendal, and inferior gluteal arteries supply the anterior bladder wall. The middle hemorrhoidal artery provides a branch to supply the posterior bladder surface. Additional vascular supply is provided by branches from the uterine and vaginal arteries.[3] The venous drainage is primarily by way of the lateral vesical plexus, which lies in close proximity to the bladder neck and eventually drains into the internal iliac veins.

Operative Bladder Injuries

BLADDER INJURIES ASSOCIATED WITH OBSTETRIC-GYNECOLOGIC PROCEDURES

Bladder injury may occur during any pelvic gynecologic procedure. The majority occur during either abdominal or vaginal hysterectomy, usually as a result of a difficult pelvic dissection. The typical injury occurs either on the trigone between the ureteral orifices or on the posterior bladder wall just above the trigone. The injury usually occurs while attempting to mobilize the base of the bladder off of the cervix, upper vagina, or uterine fundus or while closing the vaginal cuff when the bladder has not been adequately mobilized. Often, unforeseen bleeding has occurred, making recognition of the surgical planes difficult and thus increasing the probability of bladder injury. Other gynecologic procedures that can result in intraoperative bladder injury include surgery for incontinence when performed either transvaginally or transabdominally, transvaginal cystocele repair, or excision of a suburethral diverticulum. Bladder injury is also a recognized potential complication of laparoscopy and suction curettage.[4–6] Obstetric

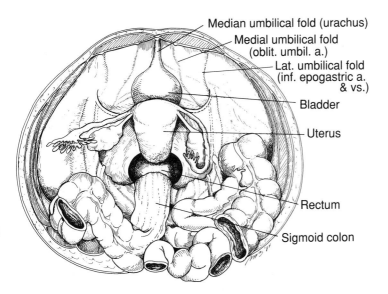

Median umbilical fold (urachus)
Medial umbilical fold (oblit. umbil. a.)
Lat. umbilical fold (inf. epogastric a. & vs.)
Bladder
Uterus
Rectum
Sigmoid colon

Figure 25-3. *The bladder is supported by the pelvic floor, vagina, and uterus.*

bladder injuries, although rare, may occur as a complication of cesarean section, prolonged labor, or forceps delivery.[7]

Graber and associates reviewed more than 800 hysterectomies and noted only 16 bladder injuries, an incidence of less that 2%.[8] Eleven were recognized at the time of surgery and repaired without further complications. All five patients with bladder injury, undiagnosed at the time of hysterectomy, developed postoperative vesicovaginal fistula. Other large series corroborate the low incidence of bladder injury associated with gynecologic procedures.[9-11] Wharton reviewed more than 16,000 major gynecologic procedures and noted only 83 bladder injuries, an incidence of about 0.5%.[12] In the 77 patients in whom the injury was noted and corrected at the time of surgery, complications related to the bladder injury did not occur. Postoperative vesicovaginal fistula occurred in all six patients with unrecognized bladder injury. In 15 patients, the bladder was injured during initial abdominal incision, and in 62, the injury occurred while attempting to dissect the bladder from the cervix or some other abdominal viscera. The majority

of bladder injuries occurred during surgery for benign disease (65%) and usually in the presence of adhesions owing to pelvic inflammatory disease or endometriosis. Morbidity associated with recognized bladder injury included prolonged hospital stay, urinary tract infection, and hematuria. No patient died as a direct result of the bladder injury or repair.[13]

To avoid operative bladder injury, one must be aware of the exact bladder location at all times. An empty bladder is less susceptible to bladder injury. A urethral catheter placed before making a lower abdominal incision decompresses the bladder and lessens the chance of bladder injury. During hysterectomy complicated by dense pelvic adhesions, prior urologic surgery, or severe pelvic bleeding, distention of the bladder with saline may help identify the bladder and may prevent bladder laceration. The use of saline colored with methylene blue or indigo carmine has been described as a useful adjunct not only in identifying the bladder, but also in recognizing small lacerations at the time they are made.[8] Palpation of the inflated Foley catheter balloon is also helpful in localizing the urinary bladder during difficult pelvic dissection. Other surgical techniques useful in avoiding bladder injury have been extensively described in the literature.[8, 10, 14–16]

Obstetric bladder injury is a well-recognized complication of cesarean section. Jones reviewed more than 2500 cases and found only four bladder injuries.[17] Kaskarelis and associates identified three injuries in more than 300 patients for an incidence of less than 1%.[18] With indications for cesarean section broadening, an increase in the number of bladder injuries may be expected. The usual cause of bladder injury is the inadequate reflection of the bladder from the lower uterine cervical segment. Other recognized causes include failure to empty the bladder before surgery and mistaking the vagina for the lower uterine segment. In pregnant women, the bladder is usually displaced out of the pelvis by the gravid uterus. Failure to empty the bladder before cesarean section may result in the bladder being lacerated at the time of the initial incision. An effaced dilated cervix may, on occasion, be mistaken for the lower cervical segment, and bladder injury may occur as a result of the incision being made into the vagina.[19]

In the past, prolonged difficult labor usually owing to cephalopelvic disproportion often resulted in bladder ischemia and necrosis as a result of the fetal head compressing the bladder against the pubis for prolonged periods of time.[2] Fortunately, these injuries are rare today except in undeveloped countries. Bladder injury resulting from difficult forceps delivery may also occur.

When unrecognized at the time of delivery, bladder injury usually results in either vesicovaginal or vesicouterine fistula. Youssef has also described the syndrome of menouria occurring without urinary incontinence in select patients with vesicocervical fistula.[20]

BLADDER INJURIES ASSOCIATED WITH GENERAL SURGICAL PROCEDURES

As a result of the bladder's intimate relationship with the sigmoid colon and rectum, abdominoperineal resection for rectal carcinoma and sigmoid resection for tumor or inflammatory bowel disease may threaten bladder integrity.[21] Ward and Nay reviewed 150 cases of abdominoperineal resections and noted a 2% incidence of bladder injury.[22] Lapides and Tank reviewed more than 2000 abdominoperineal resections and reported an incidence of bladder injury of less than 5%.[23] When noted at the time of surgery and adequately repaired, complications directly related to bladder injury seldom occur. When unrecognized, bladder laceration frequently results in vesicocutaneous or colovesical fistula.

Traumatic Bladder Injury

Traumatic bladder perforation may occur as a result of either penetrating or severe blunt abdominal trauma. Bladder rupture is classified as either intraperitoneal or extraperitoneal. Bladder trauma is frequently associated with other life-threatening abdominal or thoracic injuries, which may require immediate surgical exploration and preempt radiographic evaluation. Under such circumstances, the diagnosis of bladder injury is made at the time of exploration. In the clinically stable patient, properly performed radiographic studies are diagnostic. Bladder rupture occurs in about 4% to 15% of all pelvic fractures.[24–26] The perforation may be extraperitoneal (50% to 85%), intraperitoneal (15% to 45%), or rarely both (0 to 12%)[26] (Fig. 25-4).

Extraperitoneal bladder rupture associated with pelvic fracture usually involves the anterolateral aspect near the bladder neck.[27] Until recently, extraperitoneal perforation was believed to result exclusively from direct penetration of the bladder wall by a bony spicule or by disruption of the ligamentous attachments between the bladder and pelvis.[28–30] Carroll and McAninch, however, noted only 35% of the bladder injuries in their series to be on the same side as the pelvic fracture.[31] Cass and Luxenberg reported similar findings and proposed a second mechanism of injury.[32] With the bladder empty,

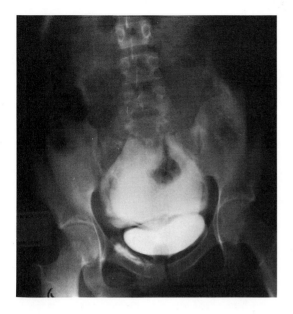

Figure 25-4. A cystogram showing both intra-peritoneal and extraperitoneal extravasation of contrast material.

severe lower abdominal trauma may cause a bursting or extraperitoneal perforation similar to that which occurs with the bladder full.[31-33] Thus the pelvic fracture associated with extra-peritoneal perforation may be coincidental rather than causative, as initially thought.

An intraperitoneal rupture usually consists of a large horizontal tear in the dome of the bladder (Fig. 25-5). It is believed to occur as a result of a blow delivered to the lower abdomen when the bladder is full. The intravesical pressure becomes acutely elevated, and the bladder perforates at its weakest point. Oliver and Ta-guchi have shown the bladder dome to be the least supported by adjacent structures and the area of the bladder wall where the muscle fibers are most widely separated, thus making the dome the weakest and most frequent site of intraperitoneal perforation.[34]

Evaluation of the Patient with Suspected Traumatic Bladder Injury

It has been recommended that all patients with pelvic fracture or pelvic fracture associated with

(*continued on page 348*)

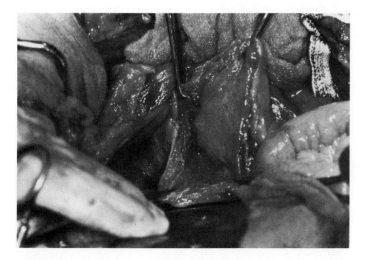

Figure 25-5. Typical appearance of large intraperitoneal perfora-tion involving the dome of the bladder.

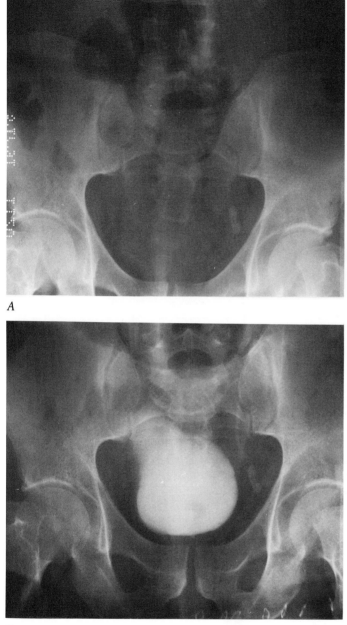

A

B

Figure 25-6. *Complete bladder evaluation requires four films.*
(A) Scout. (B) Anteroposterior film with the bladder distended.

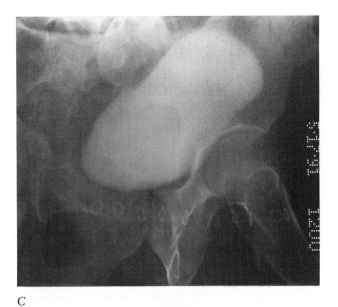

C

D

Figure 25-6. (continued) *(C) Oblique film with the bladder distended. (D) Drainage film.*

microscopic hematuria undergo radiographic evaluation of the lower urinary tract to rule out urologic injury.[30,35,36] Antoci and Schiff reviewed 234 patients with pelvic fracture and found 120 patients with microscopic hematuria.[37] All underwent lower tract evaluation, which failed to yield a single case of bladder or urethral perforation. Their review of the literature also failed to reveal a single case of a patient with a pelvic fracture and concomitant microscopic hematuria who had a significant lower urinary tract injury. Fallon and associates reviewed 200 patients with pelvic fracture and found significant urologic injury in 32 (16%).[38] Twenty-nine (91%) had gross hematuria, a urine sample was not obtained in two, and one patient had microscopic hematuria. It appears that the finding of microscopic hematuria in the absence of other urologic signs and symptoms is a poor predictor of the presence of a significant urologic injury in pelvic fracture patients.

All female patients with pelvic fracture undergo a careful visual examination of the urethra. Radiographic studies are indicated in patients with either gross hematuria or an inability to void.[39] Individuals who sustain severe blunt lower abdominal trauma who present with gross hematuria also require lower tract evaluation.

A properly performed cystogram is a highly accurate study and is rarely associated with a false-negative result.[40] In the adult, 300 to 500 ml of dilute water-soluble contrast material is administered under gravity. When contrast material no longer flows into the bladder, an additional 10 to 15 ml is injected under slight pressure to distend the bladder adequately. With the bladder distended, a radiograph is obtained in the anteroposterior projection. A complete bladder study requires oblique and lateral projections with the bladder full and a postdrainage film, but in the severely injured immobile patient, the oblique films are frequently omitted, adding more importance to the postdrainage film.[24] Small amounts of extravasation not seen behind a contrast-filled bladder are readily identified on the drainage film[41] (Fig. 25-6). Weyrauch and Peterfy demonstrated the importance of bladder distention when they showed in dogs that bladder lacerations as long as 2 cm could be missed by cystography if the bladder was not sufficiently distended[42] (Fig. 25-7).

The characteristic cystographic finding of an extraperitoneal bladder perforation is extravasation of contrast material confined to the pelvis (Fig. 25-8). The extravasated contrast material may appear as flamelike wisps or linear streaks or may assume a stellate or sunburst pattern. Extravasation may be more obvious on the postdrainage film (Fig. 25-9).

Radiographically intraperitoneal bladder perforation may produce diffuse extravasation of contrast material throughout the peritoneal cavity with no discernible pattern (Fig. 25-10). Extravasated contrast material may accumulate in the dependent portion of the pelvis, obscuring the superior aspect of the bladder and producing an hourglass configuration.[28] Contrast material may also accumulate in the paracolic gutters or beneath the diaphragm.

A normal cystogram in the presence of gross hematuria and in the absence of renal injury is diagnostic of a bladder contusion. Treatment consisting of catheter drainage is maintained until the urine is grossly clear. There is no need to perform a cystogram before removing the catheter.

Treatment of Bladder Rupture from External Trauma

INTRAPERITONEAL BLADDER PERFORATION

All intraperitoneal bladder perforations require surgical exploration and repair.[31,43-45] A vertical midline incision allows adequate exposure for abdominal exploration and repair of any coexistent abdominal organ injuries. The tear in the dome is usually large (5 cm or greater). It may be extended anteriorly if necessary to allow thorough examination of the bladder neck area. This is an important consideration in patients with pelvic fracture, who may have a concomitant extraperitoneal injury. Extraperitoneal tears are closed from within with running 2–0 or 3–0 chromic suture. In patients with pelvic fracture,

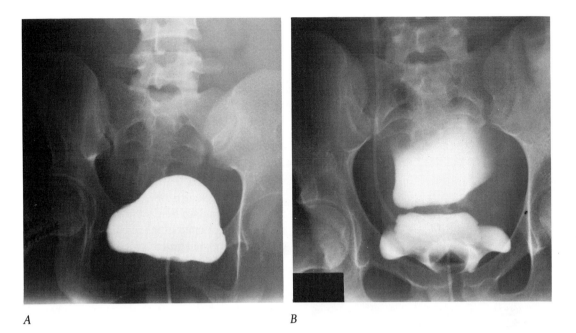

A   *B*

Figure 25-7. *(A) Bladder is inadequately distended with 180 ml of contrast material. The study was interpreted as being normal. (B) The same patient now with a ureteral stent in place. Intraperitoneal extravasation is now obvious after bladder distention with 450 ml of contrast material.*

care is taken not to disturb the pelvic hematoma. The bladder is closed in watertight fashion using a two-layered technique. The bladder mucosa is closed with a running locking 3–0 chromic suture. The muscle is closed as a separate layer using a 2–0 chromic Lembert type stitch (Fig. 25-11). The adequacy of the repair is tested by distending the bladder with saline. Small leaks are repaired with an interrupted figure-of-eight suture. A Penrose or closed suction type drain is placed in the space of Retzius unless there is a pelvic fracture with a large pelvic hematoma. In those cases in which the hematoma has not been disturbed, a drain is not routinely used. Suprapubic tubes are used when there is extensive bladder injury and a watertight closure is impossible to obtain. If the bladder closure has been watertight, a cystogram is not routinely obtained before removing the catheter (usually in 7 to 10 days).

EXTRAPERITONEAL BLADDER PERFORATION

Before the 1970s, it was believed that all traumatic bladder perforations required surgical exploration and repair.[46,47] Bacon, in 1943, reported that of 21 patients not operated on, 19 died, and similar results were reported by Culp.[46,47] It was not until 1969 that Waterhouse and Gross first proposed a nonoperative approach to the management of bladder rupture.[48] Mulkey and Witherington in 1974 reported the successful nonoperative management of a ruptured bladder in two patients with pelvic fracture.[49] McConnell and associates in 1982 and Cass and associates in 1983 recommended nonoperative management be reserved only for female patients with small extraperitoneal lacerations and no other indications for surgical exploration.[43,50] Because it is impossible to assess accurately the size of a bladder laceration solely with cystographic findings,

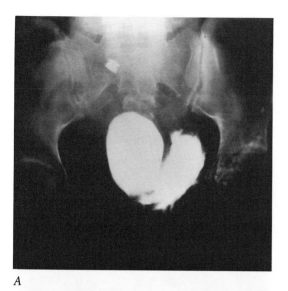

A

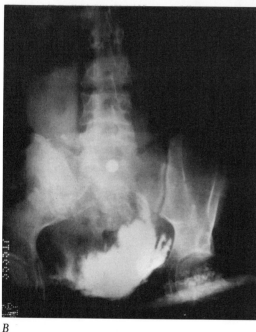

B

Figure 25-8. *Patient with a pelvic fracture and obvious extraperitoneal extravasation of contrast material. (A) Anteroposterior film with the bladder distended. (B) Drainage film with contrast material confined to the pelvis.*

surgical selection based only on the degree of extravasation does not seem reasonable.[44] More than 100 patients with extraperitoneal bladder perforation have been successfully managed using a nonoperative or conservative approach with minimal morbidity.[28,32,44,45,51] Corriere and Sandler treated 39 patients solely by bladder drainage without consideration given to the size of the bladder perforation; bladder repair was reserved for patients requiring exploration for other associated injuries.[44] Cystograms performed 10 days after the injury showed no extravasation in 34 patients (87%). Bladder drainage was maintained in the remaining five patients until the extravasation resolved. Antibiotics were not routinely used. Septic complications and hemorrhage did not occur.

Patients undergoing exploratory laparotomy for other abdominal injuries have all concomitant bladder lacerations repaired as previously described. All other patients with extraperitoneal bladder perforations are initially managed by catheter drainage alone, unless there is a suspected bony spicule perforating the bladder. In those rare cases, the bladder is repaired and the spicule removed.

Nonoperative management implies simple catheter drainage and close clinical observation. Broad-spectrum antibiotics are routinely given. A cystogram is obtained before catheter removal, usually after 7 to 10 days (Fig. 25-12). Severe bleeding with clots, sepsis, and persistent urinary extravasation are indications for surgical exploration.

Evaluation of Suspected Operative Bladder Injury

If during the course of a difficult pelvic or transvaginal surgical procedure the integrity of the bladder is questioned, the surgeon is obligated to rule out bladder injury. A catheter, if not already present, is sterilely placed and the bladder distended with sterile saline. Any leakage is diagnostic and mandates proper surgical repair. A dilute solution of indigo carmine or methylene blue to distend the bladder may prove helpful in

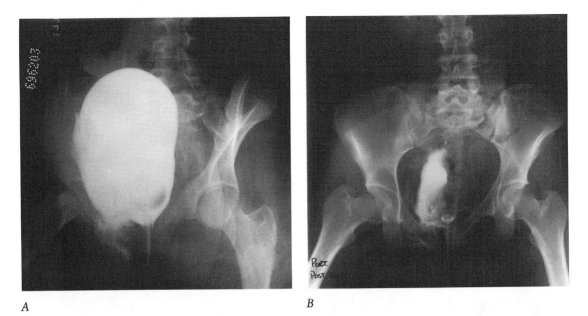

A   B

Figure 25-9. *Extraperitoneal bladder perforation with extravasation more obvious on the drainage film. (A) Anteroposterior film with bladder distended. (B) Extravasation readily apparent on the drainage film.*

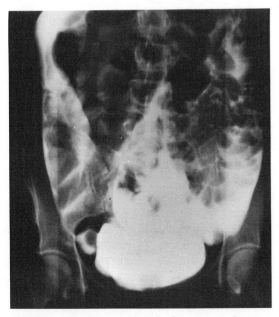

Figure 25-10. *Appearance of intraperitoneal extravasation of contrast material.*

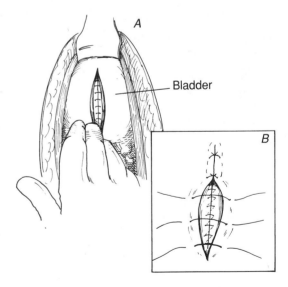

Figure 25-11. *Technique of two-layered bladder closure. (A) The mucosa is closed with a running chromic suture. (B) Lembert type stitches are used to close the seromuscular layer.*

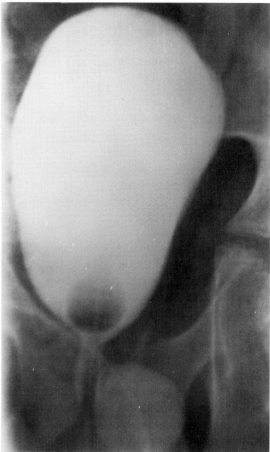

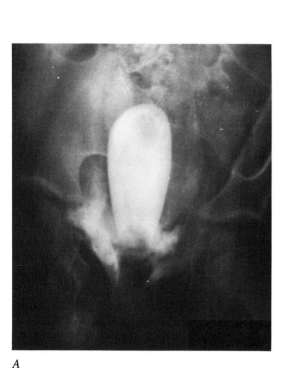

A   B

Figure 25-12. *(A) Cystogram showing extraperitoneal extravasation of contrast material. Patient was treated with catheter drainage. (B) Cystogram repeated 7 days later showing a normal bladder.*

identifying small bladder lacerations or a wayward stitch inadvertently placed through the bladder wall.[8] If bladder injury is suspected during a vaginal procedure, cystoscopy may be readily performed to evaluate the extent of the injury.

If the injury is to the posterior bladder wall or trigone, ureteral patency must be assessed before repairing the bladder. Several techniques may be used to document ureteral integrity. The

bladder may be opened anteriorly and ureteral catheters placed. If one is unable to pass the catheters into the renal pelvis, ureteral injury must be suspected. Alternatively, cystoscopy may be performed and ureteral catheters placed. If one is unable to identify the ureteral orifices, intravenously administered indigo carmine may prove helpful in assuring ureteral patency. Large posterior wall defects are closed from within. While repairing the trigone, ureteral catheters help avoid ureteral injury. Large injuries that occur during transvaginal procedures are repaired using a suprapubic approach.

In the absence of extensive bladder injury, radiation cystitis, or severe bleeding, a 20 to 24 French urethral catheter provides adequate urinary drainage. In the severely debilitated patient, however, in whom prolonged catheter drainage is anticipated or in the presence of one of the aforementioned conditions, a large suprapubic catheter is also placed. In those instances in which suprapubic drainage is desired, a 22–26 Pezzer, Malecot, or Foley catheter is brought out through a separate stab incision in the anterior bladder wall and sutured with chromic to the rectus fascia. Care is taken to position the catheter so it does not traverse the peritoneal cavity.

Before closing the incision, the perivesical space is drained with either a large Penrose drain or one of the closed suction-type drains. Postoperative bladder spasms are treated with anticholinergics. Antibiotic therapy, if not instituted preoperatively, is begun at the time of injury and continued until the catheter is removed.

In the uncomplicated situation in which a watertight bladder closure has been obtained, the catheter is removed after 5 to 7 days. In the presence of severe radiation cystitis or extensive bladder injury, a cystogram is obtained before removal of the suprapubic tube.

Complications occurring as a result of bladder injury seldom occur provided that the injury is readily identified and surgically repaired, and continuous unobstructed bladder drainage is obtained.

The late recognition of bladder injuries is not uncommon. Usually these patients present with a clear vaginal discharge. Cystography performed in conjunction with cystoscopy is diagnostic. When identified in the immediate (3 to 5 days) postoperative period, primary repair may be performed if the patient is clinically stable and there is no sign of concomitant infection.[52] Bladder injuries that become manifest later in the postoperative period (10 to 15 days) are usually associated with extensive inflammation and devitalized tissue. In these cases, delayed repair is

undertaken once the inflammatory response has resolved (usually in 3 to 4 months).

Urethral Injury

Traumatic urethral disruption is less common in women than men.[38] The relative mobility of the female urethra and its lack of attachments to the pubis are believed to be the primary reason for the rarity of this injury.[53] In female trauma victims with pelvic fracture and gross hematuria, a urethrogram is not routinely performed before bladder catheterization. Traumatic urethral lacerations are repaired primarily over a Foley catheter.

The female urethra is rarely injured during surgical procedures on adjacent organs. It may be lacerated, however during any anterior vaginal wall procedure. The diagnosis is usually obvious, and repair is performed over a urethral catheter, which is left in 7 to 10 days.

References

1. Basmajian JV. Grant's Method of Anatomy. Baltimore: Williams & Wilkins, 1971:287.
2. Moir JC. Injuries of the bladder. Am J Obstet Gynecol 1961;82:124.
3. Gray H. The urogenital system. The urinary bladder. In: Goss CM, ed. Anatomy of the human body. Malvern, PA: Lea & Febiger, 1973;17:1290.
4. Georgy FM, Fetterman HH, Chefetz MD. Complications of laparoscopy. Two cases of perforated urinary bladder. Am J Obstet Gynecol 1974; 120:1121.
5. Homburg R, Segal T. Perforation of the urinary bladder by the laparoscope. Am J Obstet Gynecol 1978;130:597.
6. Rous SN, Major F, Gordon M. Rupture of the bladder secondary to uterine vacuum currettage: A case report and review of the literature. J Urol 1971;106:685.
7. Guerriero WG. Gynecologic injuries to the ureter, bladder and urethra. In: Raz S, ed. Female urology. Philadelphia: WB Saunders, 1983:357.
8. Graber EA, O'Rourke JJ, McElrath T. Iatrogenic bladder injury during hysterectomy. Obstet Gynecol 1964;23:267.
9. Bown WC. Bladder fistulas and ureteral injuries. J Urol 1966;96:706.

10. Falk HC. Prevention of vesicovaginal fistula in total hysterectomy for benign disease. Obstet Gynecol 1966;29:865.

11. Ullery JC, Villalon R. Urinary tract infection in obstetrics and gynecology. West Virginia Med J 1968;64:127

12. Wharton LR. Methods of preventing injury to the ureters and bladder during gynecological operations. Ann Surg 1956;143:752.

13. Everett HS, Mattingly RF. Urinary tract injuries resulting from pelvic surgery. Am J Obstet Gynecol 1956;71:502.

14. Graber EA, Barber HRK, O'Rourke JJ. Bladder mobilization in hysterectomy. Obstet Gynecol 1967;30:591.

15. Knapp RC, Donahue VC, Friedman EA. Dissection of paravesical and pararectal spaces in pelvic operations. Surg Gynecol Obstet 1973;137:758.

16. Ridley JH. Prevention and management of operative injuries to the urinary tract. Clin Obstet Gynecol 1981;24:1267.

17. Jones OH. Cesarean section in present-day obstetrics. Presidential address. Am J Obstet Gynecol 1976;126:521.

18. Kaskarelis D, Sakkas J, Aravantinos D, et al. Urinary tract injuries in gynecological and obstetrical procedures. Int Surg 1975;60:40.

19. Faricy PO, Augspurger RR, Kaufman JM. Bladder injuries associated with cesarean section. J Urol 1978;120:762.

20. Youssef AF. "Menouria" following lower segment Cesarean section. A syndrome. Am J Obstet Gynecol 1957;73:759.

21. Daly JM, DeCosse JJ. Complications in surgery of the colon and rectum. Surg Clin North Am 1983;63:1215.

22. Ward JN, Nay HR. Immediate and delayed urologic complications associated with abdominoperineal resection. Am J Surg 1972;123:642.

23. Lapides JL, Tank ES. Urinary complications following abdominal perineal resection. Cancer 1971;28:230.

24. Carroll PR, McAnininch JW. Major bladder trauma: The accuracy of cystography. J Urol 1983;130:887.

25. Montie J. Bladder injuries. Urol Clin North Am 1977;4:59.

26. Wolk DJ, Sandler CM, Corriere JN Jr. Extraperitoneal bladder rupture without pelvic fracture. J Urol 1985;134:1199.

27. Corriere JN Jr. Current urologic therapy. Philadelphia: WB Saunders, 1986:253.

28. Brosman SA, Fay R. Diagnosis and management of bladder trauma. J Trauma 1973;13:929.

29. Morehouse DD, MacKinnon KJ. Urologic injuries associated with pelvic fractures. J Trauma 1969;9:479.

30. Pokorny M, Pontes JE, Pierce JM. Urologic injuries associated with pelvic trauma. J Urol 1979;121:455.

31. Carroll PR, McAninch JW. Major bladder trauma: Mechanisms of injury and a unified method of diagnosis and repair. J Urol 1984;132:254.

32. Cass AS, Luxenberg M. Features of 164 bladder ruptures. J Urol 1987;138:743.

33. Wolk DJ, Sandler CM, Corriere JN Jr. Extraperitoneal bladder rupture without pelvic fracture. J Urol 1985;134:1199.

34. Oliver JA, Taguchi Y. Rupture of the full bladder. Br J Urol 1964;36:524.

35. Moy HN. Lower urinary tract injuries. Br J Urol 1970;42:739.

36. Clark SS, Prudencio RF. Lower urinary tract injuries associated with pelvic fractures: Diagnosis and management. Surg Clin North Am 1972;52:183.

37. Antoci JP, Schiff M Jr. Bladder and urethral injuries in patients with pelvic fractures. J Urol 1982;128:25.

38. Fallon B, Wendt JC, Hawtrey CE. Urological injury and assessment in patients with fractured pelvis. J Urol 1984;131:712.

39. Spirnak JP. Pelvic fracture and injury to the lower urinary tract. Surg Clin North Am 1988;68:1057.

40. Carroll PR, Taylor SR, McAninch JW. Major bladder trauma. In: McAninch W, ed. Blaisdell and Trunky trauma management. New York: Thieme-Stratton, 1985:69.

41. Peters PC, Bright TC III: Management of trauma to the urinary tract. Adv Surg 1976;10:197.

42. Weyrauch HM Jr, Peterfy RA. Tests for leakage in the early diagnosis of the ruptured bladder. J Urol 1940;44:264.

43. McConnell JD, Wilkerson MD, Peters PC. Rupture of the bladder. Urol Clin North Am 1982;9:293.

44. Corriere JN Jr, Sandler CM. Management of the ruptured bladder: Seven years of experiences with 111 cases. J Trauma 1986;26:830.

45. Hayes EE, Sandler CM, Corriere JN Jr. Management of the ruptured bladder secondary to blunt abdominal trauma. J Urol 1983;129:946.

46. Bacon SK. Rupture of the urinary bladder: Clinical analysis of 147 cases in the past 10 years. J Urol 1943;49:432.

47. Culp OS. Treatment of ruptured bladder and urethra: Analysis of 86 cases of urinary extravasation. J Urol 1942;48:266.

48. Waterhouse K, Gross M. Trauma to the genitourinary tract: A 5 year experience with 251 cases. J Urol 1969;101:241.

49. Mulkey AP Jr, Witherington R. Conservative management of vesical rupture. Urology 1974; 4:426.

50. Cass AS, Johnson CF, Khan AU, et al: Nonoperative management of bladder rupture from external trauma. Urology 1983;22:27.

51. Palmer JK, Benson GS, Corriere JN. Diagnosis and initial management of urological injuries associated with 200 consecutive pelvic fractures. J Urol 1983;130:712.

52. Pierce JM, Riehle RA. Lower genitourinary tract trauma. Curr Trends Urol 1981;1:139.

53. Kaiser TF, Farrow FC. Injury of the bladder and prostatomembranous urethra associated with fracture of the bony pelvis. Surg Gynecol Obstet 1965;120:99.

VI   *Vesicovaginal Fistula*

26

Etiology, Evaluation, Preoperative Management, and Endoscopic Management of Vesicovaginal Fistula

Elroy D. Kursh

Historical and Social Perspective

Although vesicovaginal fistula (VVF) almost certainly occurred at the beginning of recorded time, little is mentioned about this problem in ancient literature. The finding of a large VVF in an Egyptian mummy dating back to the year 2000 B.C. verifies the ancient existence of VVF. Surprisingly, the insightful manuscripts of Hippocrates that covered so many phases of disease never mentioned this entity. The first known individual to record the occurrence of a VVF was a Perso-Arab physician, Avicenna (980–1037 A.D.). Interestingly, he recognized the relationship between this malady and a difficult labor.[1]

In 1852, the young American physician, Jay Marion Sims, published a monumental work describing the surgical technique to cure vaginal tears. For several years, he experimented in a small Montgomery, Alabama, slave hospital before successfully suturing a vaginal tear in a slave patient, Anarcha. Some of Sims' success was related to technical advances that he designed. Sims used a duck-billed speculum at the time when most physicians were loath to examine women's genitals. The *Sims' position* afforded improved visibility to increase the success of suturing the fistula. Sims' enthusiasm and outgoing personality enhanced the importance of the treatment of diseases of women in American medicine and eventually won him the title of "The Father of Gynecology."[2]

VVF remains a social calamity in some areas of the world. One report described 1443 patients who underwent operative treatment for VVF during a 12-year period in a city in Northern Nigeria.[3] In some areas in Northern Nigeria, 300 new cases come to the gynecology clinic each month, whereas in other areas, the waiting list is said to be 1000 patients, with only one surgeon doing a few surgical repairs a week.[4,5] At the Addis Ababba Fistula Hospital in Ethiopia, more than 7000 fistulas have been repaired.[6] This huge number of patients clearly illustrates the magnitude of the problem in some communities. Many or even a majority of uneducated women living in these backward areas customarily marry early and practice sexual intercourse even before menarche. The incomplete growth of the pelvis during their first pregnancy is responsible for the cephalopelvic disproportion causing difficult labor and excessive pressure on the bladder. The obstructed labor leads to bladder necrosis and the development of a VVF. Operations such as the gishiri cut, which is performed throughout Northern Nigeria, is also responsible for many fistulas. This tradition consists of cutting the anterior and rarely the posterior as-

Female Urology, edited by Elroy D. Kursh and Edward McGuire. J. B. Lippincott, Philadelphia, © 1994.

pect of the vagina with a razor blade to treat a variety of conditions, including obstructed labor, infertility, dyspareunia, amenorrhea, goiter, backache, dysuria, and other complaints. The gishiri cut may be superficial, but deeper cuts have resulted in VVF, hemorrhage, or sepsis. In Tahzib's study, 13% of all fistulas were directly related to this practice.[3]

The exact number of deaths attributable to obstructed labor is unknown, but there is considerable information about those unfortunate survivors who develop a VVF afterward. Their own society goes to great lengths to ostracize these young women. Not only does the offensive odor of urine make these girls a social outcast, but also the odor becomes confused with venereal disease, causing the affected family and patient to feel a deep sense of shame.[7]

Etiology

Advances in obstetrics have greatly reduced the incidence of obstetric VVF in developed nations. Far and away the most common cause of VVF in the developed areas of the world is iatrogenic damage to the bladder during surgery. Gynecologic surgery accounts for approximately 70% to 80%, with the majority occurring after an abdominal hysterectomy, but vaginal hysterectomy may also be responsible. Other causes of VVFs include gastrointestinal procedures, urologic operations (procedures such as surgery on the bladder neck and ureteral reimplantation) and surgery for management of pelvic trauma. In a review by Lee and associates, the following conditions and procedures were responsible for 190 VVFs: abdominal hysterectomy (132), vaginal hysterectomy (20), radical hysterectomy (4), vaginal repair (3), cesarean section (5), cesarean section with postpartum hysterectomy (6), forceps delivery (8), trauma (6), and radiation (6).[8] Unusual causes of VVF that have been reported include erosion into the bladder from a pessary or vaginal diaphragm, erosion induced by an intravesical foreign body, tuberculosis of the bladder, and fistular development postcoital 6 months following surgery for cervical cancer.[9–13]

VVFs may also develop following radiation therapy. These fistulas present a particularly vexing management problem. Although most complications of radiation therapy appear relatively soon after treatment is completed, usually within 6 to 12 months after cessation of therapy, there is evidence that urinary and rectosigmoid complications are increasing in incidence 5 years after treatment has been completed and may be noted even 30 years later.[14] Not only does the radiation therapy cause significant tissue injury, but also tissue necrosis may be enhanced by progressive arteriosclerotic vascular disease, which frequently occurs with aging.

Various theories have been proposed to explain the cause of VVF after hysterectomy. The most commonly stated explanations were that the fistula results from avascular necrosis of the base of the bladder or erosion from sutures placed between the bladder and vaginal cuff. It has also been implied that a fistula that develops shortly after an operation may result from an intraoperative bladder injury. Therefore in the past, the exact cause of VVF has been ambiguous.

We reported evidence that many or most VVFs develop from an unsuspected bladder injury that has generally not been considered to play a causative role. In an attempt to determine the cause of VVF, the records of 12 patients who had a fistula develop after total abdominal hysterectomy were compared with 12 consecutive patients who underwent total abdominal hysterectomy without fistula formation. Most of the patients who developed VVFs had excessive postoperative abdominal pain, distention, or paralytic ileus. Hematuria and symptoms of severe bladder irritability and reduced urine output either immediately postoperative or after the Foley catheter was removed were also noted in some of the patients in the fistula group, and prolonged postoperative fever and increased white blood count occurred more often. In contrast, the postoperative course was uncomplicated in the nonfistula group.[15]

The clinical course observed in many of the patients with VVFs suggests that the patients had an unrecognized bladder injury resulting in urinary extravasation. It is postulated that a VVF develops when the urinoma drains into the vaginal cuff, which is dependent and usually not closed.[15] Our study also confirmed the finding that there is an increased likelihood of developing a VVF when the hysterectomy is technically difficult to perform.[16] In fact, 3 of the 12 patients who developed VVFs had significant bleeding during the operation, requiring ligation of one or both hypogastric arteries.[15]

The results of this study suggest that the development of excessive abdominal pain, distention, or paralytic ileus after total abdominal hysterectomy signals the possibility of an unsuspected bladder perforation. Contamination of the peritoneal cavity with urine or the undrained urinoma extraperitoneal behind the bladder or both are responsible for these symptoms. The logical drainage site of urine leaking from the injured bladder is the vaginal cuff, which is dependent and usually not closed. A VVF develops when the tract between the bladder and vagina becomes epithelialized.[15] The fact that VVFs invariably involve the vaginal cuff supports this theory.[17]

The frequent practice of ignoring varying amounts of vaginal leakage in the hope that it represents vaginal discharge or seroma must be avoided if a bladder injury or a diagnosis of impending VVF is to be established early. The development of excessive abdominal pain, distention or paralytic ileus, hematuria, reduced urine output, symptoms of marked bladder irritability after the catheter is removed, and possibly even prolonged postoperative fever or increased white blood count should alert the surgeon to consider the possibility of an unsuspected bladder perforation, which might lead to the development of a VVF.

The early establishment of a correct diagnosis of a bladder perforation affords the physician the opportunity to provide adequate bladder drainage and possibly abort the development of a VVF. Therefore appropriate diagnostic studies should be expeditiously performed to rule out an unsuspected bladder perforation if

this diagnosis is considered. If a relatively small leak is noted extraperitoneally behind the bladder or directly into the vagina, a large Foley catheter should be placed in the urethra for an extended period (minimum 3 to 4 weeks) to provide maximum drainage. Before removing the catheter, the diagnostic studies are repeated to determine if the leak is still present and to assess the size of the perforation. If the perforation is present but smaller, it is worthwhile to provide an additional period of bladder drainage to attempt to have the perforation seal and avoid the epithelialization of a chronic fistulous tract. Once a sizable fistula is formed with epithelialization of the tract, it is extremely unlikely that the fistula will close despite adequate bladder drainage. Therefore, if the fistula remains unchanged, further drainage with the hope of spontaneous fistula closure is probably futile. Bladder perforations with extravasation of large amounts of urine intraperitoneally should be closed immediately on recognition.

Presenting Symptoms

Patients usually note the onset of a painless watery discharge of varying amounts from the vagina, most often occurring 7 to 14 days after surgery. The volume of leakage can vary substantially depending on the size and location of the fistula. Most VVFs are located in a dependent portion of the base of the bladder and large enough to result in leakage of most, if not all, of the urine from the vagina. A very small fistula may result in vaginal leakage of a small amount of urine intermittently. Leakage may occur only when the bladder is full and may even be misinterpreted as stress incontinence because it may be enhanced by the elevated pressure on the bladder during maneuvers such as coughing or sneezing. This problem of unrecognized small VVFs was emphasized in a report of three patients with persistent urinary incontinence after total abdominal hysterectomy, two of whom underwent unsuccessful Marshall-Marchetti-Krantz operations to attempt to resolve suspected stress urinary incontinence.[18]

Unfortunately, it is not uncommon to attribute small amounts of vaginal discharge as drainage of serous fluid, which may lead to considerable delay in establishing a correct diagnosis. As already emphasized, the onset of drainage is often preceded by excessive abdominal pain, distention, or paralytic ileus, hematuria, and symptoms of bladder irritability after the catheter is removed.

Radiation-related fistulas may develop several months or even many years after therapy. Whenever a radiation fistula develops, the patient should be considered to have recurrent cancer until proved otherwise. Surgical repair of the fistula should not be entertained until this possibility has been carefully evaluated.

Diagnosis

If a VVF is suspected, it is imperative to evaluate the patient for this possible diagnosis urgently if there is any hope of aborting the development of a chronic fistula with an epithelialized tract. Once urine leakage is suspected, it may be valuable to identify the discharge as urine by obtaining chemical analysis of the fluid for blood urea nitrogen and creatinine. If the blood urea nitrogen and creatinine values exceed that of serum (usually 20 times), urinary leakage is proved.

A cystogram may be valuable in establishing a diagnosis of bladder perforation or VVF. When performing this study, it is important to obtain a satisfactory x-ray film in the lateral position with a postevacuation film (Fig. 26-1).

Even if cystography reveals a VVF, cystoscopy is imperative to identify the number, size, and location of the fistulas and assess the degree of associated inflammation in the bladder. Traditionally it has been claimed that the cystoscopic examination should be performed under general anesthesia to assess both the bladder and the vaginal sides of the fistula and confirm the diagnosis with other tests. I have not found it necessary to employ general anesthesia to do these examinations in most instances and advise it only when there is a question of ureteral involvement and one intends to do retrograde urography or attempt insertion of a ureteral stent. Usually the fistula is easy to identify cystoscopically, but at times it may be masked by considerable associated inflammatory change. Findings may be quite subtle in a small fistula, and all that might be noted is a small dimple at the fistula site, or the fistula may be hidden by a band of scar tissue in the bladder. At times, it may be helpful to attempt to pass a small ureteral catheter through the suspected fistula site to determine if it enters the vagina. During the cystoscopic examination, a bladder filling test is done by instilling fluid into the bladder while observing the vagina with a speculum for leakage. Inspection of the vagina almost always reveals considerable inflammation of the vaginal cuff, which is the inevitable site of most VVFs.

If the diagnosis of a VVF is still in doubt, various dye studies can be performed either separately or at the time of performing cystoscopy. Methylene blue or indigo carmine solution is instilled into the bladder, with care taken to avoid leakage from the urethra. The suspected site of the fistula in the vagina is observed for possible leakage of the dye solution. Another technique is to insert a tampon into the vagina after the bladder is filled with the dye solution. Staining of the uppermost part of the tampon indicates a VVF, whereas staining of the outermost part of the tampon may represent urinary incontinence or a urethrovaginal fistula.

Because it is not uncommon for a ureterovaginal fistula to be associated with a VVF, it is extremely important to consider the possibility of this entity also.[19] If placement of a Foley catheter leads to complete resolution of the leakage, it is highly probable that a ureterovaginal fistula is not present. Ureterovaginal fistulas are almost always associated with varying degrees of ureteral obstruction, making intravenous or, at times, retrograde urography a valuable part of the workup. In addition to demonstrating ureteral obstruction, a ureterovaginal fistula may be directly visualized radiographically with the extravasation of contrast media from the ureter into the vagina on either of these studies. Finally, an intravenous dye test may be used to confirm

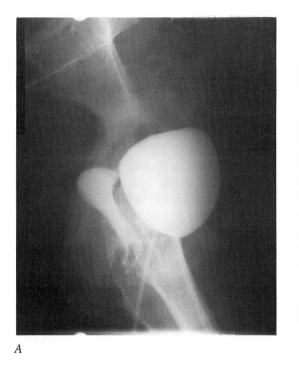

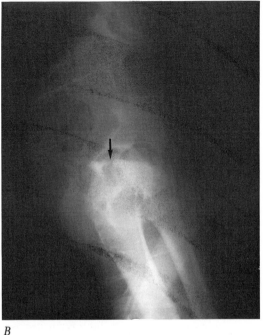

A   *B*

Figure 26-1. *Lateral cystogram. (A) A large vesicovaginal fistula is demonstrated. Vagina is filled with contrast media posterior to the bladder. (B)* Arrow *depicts fistula on post-evacuation film.*

the diagnosis of a ureterovaginal fistula. If a VVF is not confirmed with the standard techniques, indigo carmine or methylene blue may be administered intravenously. Staining of a vaginal tampon indicates the presence of a ureterovaginal fistula if a tampon did not similarly stain following bladder instillation of dye solution.

Although ultrasonography has been described to delineate a VVF,[20] it has little or no merit for the diagnosis of this entity because the studies already described provide reliable data and are easy to perform. The use of computed tomography (CT) has also been described and may be advantageous in some instances. CT has the ability to assess for a possible contiguous pelvic mass or the extent of extraluminal disease and may provide a clue about the underlying cause of a fistula that occurs following radiotherapy, such as recurrent cancer.[21]

Generally speaking, it is not necessary to perform all of these studies to establish a correct diagnosis. Cystoscopy with bladder filling and observation of the vagina are all that is usually required to confirm the presence of a VVF. The only other assessment that is essential is confirmation that a ureterovaginal fistula is not present before undertaking surgical correction.

Preoperative Management

A major problem for the patient is the management of urinary leakage while awaiting surgical repair. The continual wetness, odor, and discomfort present difficult social problems. A small fistula may be managed by frequent voiding and vaginal tampons, but this is rarely sufficient. Unfortunately, most of the fistulas are in the dependent portion of the bladder base and tend to cause considerable leakage. Usually incontinence underpants with various urine collection pads are necessary. Silica-impregnated pads are preferable because they trap the urine and help prevent extensive contact with the perineum. Today there are a variety of urine collection pads that are effective in trapping the urine and preventing excoriation of the genital area.

Use of the contraceptive diaphragm is another alternative to attempt to trap enough urine to reduce urinary leakage. The diaphragm must completely cover the fistula and should be well fitted to ensure good contact between its rim and the vaginal mucosa. Even a properly fitted diaphragm does not usually provide a watertight seal, making the addition of absorption collection devices necessary. A technique for construction of a vaginal prosthesis made of methylmethacrylate has also been described to help control urinary incontinence in a patient with a VVF secondary to recurrent cervical cancer following radiation therapy.[22] Although this prosthesis appears to be cumbersome, technology is likely to provide improved appliances to help collect vaginal leakage.

Although some patients may require an indwelling Foley catheter for hygienic and psychological reasons, they are best avoided because of the risk of infection and inflammation that is invariably associated with them. Even a large indwelling Foley catheter may not adequately vent all of the urine to prevent perineal soiling if the fistula is large and in a dependent position.

Early use of estrogen vaginal cream is strongly recommended in postmenopausal or postoophorectomy patients. Not only does estrogen replacement aid in the healing of the vagina, but also it provides improved vascular supply and turgor of the vaginal wall before surgery. Generally I prefer to use estrogen vaginal creams rather than oral estrogen replacement.

Timing of Surgery

Over the years, the standard management of a VVF was to delay surgery for a minimum of 3 months and for a period of usually 5 to 6 months to allow the edema and inflammation to resolve beforehand. A delay in repair usually provides a better healed operative site with less inflammation, making it easier to establish proper surgical planes and increasing the likelihood of a successful surgical outcome.

The social inconvenience and psychological impact imposed by delayed repair has led to attempts to repair VVFs shortly after they are diagnosed. Persky and associates reported six successful repairs in seven patients performed 7 to 10 weeks after the initial surgery.[23] The only failure in their series occurred in a patient with a combined cystoureterovaginal fistula. Fourie reported five successful repairs in six patients employing an early suprapubic surgical approach.[24] Cruikshank reported successful early repairs in all of nine patients, 13 to 19 days posthysterectomy, using a vaginal approach.[25] Badenoch and colleagues reported primary healing in all of 19 patients using an abdominal approach whether or not surgery was done in less than 6 weeks (7 women) or more than 6 weeks (12 women) posthysterectomy.[26] Finally, Wang and Hadley advocated early nondelayed repair of simple nonradiated VVFs using a transvaginal approach because they noted 100% success in patients repaired before a 3-month waiting period elapsed.[27]

My own preference is to time the repair on the basis of the amount of visible associated inflammation. Patients are examined every 4 weeks. The vaginal side of the fistula is examined first with a speculum. If the vagina appears uninflamed, well epithelialized, and free of granulation, cystoscopy is performed with topical or no anesthesia. If similar findings are noted in the bladder and pelvic examination reveals a pliable vagina without induration, surgery is scheduled. Several studies have supported this approach. Robertson noted a 97% surgical cure rate in 100 patients when endoscopic timing of the repair was employed.[28] Fearl and Keizur noted that endoscopic timing led to repair an average of 2.4 months earlier in 20 patients compared with an empiric delay with no decrease in the success rate.[29] Using this approach, I have scheduled surgery as early as several weeks after the primary procedure that led to the fistula and often before 6 to 12 weeks have elapsed. I believe, however, that a surgeon should not allow himself or herself to be pressured into scheduling surgery at a time when he or she does not think there is a high likelihood of achieving a successful outcome. If surgery is performed early and fails, the surgeon will undoubtedly be held accountable.

Radiation VVF represents a different problem. Most radiation fistulas appear relatively soon after cessation of therapy, occurring within 6 to 12 months after completion of radiation treatment. In this instance, it is critical to await resolution of the acute radiation injury, necessitating a delay of at least 6 to 12 months before undertaking surgery. During this time, it is imperative to investigate for possible recurrent cancer by obtaining biopsy specimens of the edge of the fistula. Repeat pelvic and speculum examinations of the vagina are performed to estimate the degree of necrosis and inflammation and to be certain that the inflammatory process has stabilized before considering surgery.

Rarely radiation VVFs may develop years after completion of radiation therapy. There is evidence that urinary and rectosigmoid complications are increasing in incidence 5 years after treatment has been completed and may be noted even 30 years later.[14] Fistulas that develop years after radiation insult are more rigid, indurated, and fixed in appearance and have less associated necrosis and acute inflammation. In this instance, it may be possible to avoid the long delay when timing the surgical procedure.

Percutaneous Management of Incurable Vesicovaginal Fistulas

At times, patients have incurable pelvic disease resulting in large VVFs and total urinary incontinence. Included in this category of incurable pelvic disease are women with preterminal recurrent pelvic cancer following radiotherapy and patients with extensive pelvic scarring from radiation therapy with associated severe bowel disease, making it impossible to employ any segment of bowel for urinary diversion.

The only alternative for making these unfortunate individuals dry is nephrostomy with ureteral occlusion. Today percutaneous techniques can usually be used to establish a nephrostomy, even in the undilated system. Various percutaneous techniques have also been attempted to occlude the ureters to prevent varying amounts of urine from reaching the fistula site. Reported alternatives for ureteral occlusion include embolization of the ureter with isobutylcyanoacrylate, percutaneously applied ureteral clips, and radiofrequency endoluminal electrocautery.[30–33] There is little doubt that as laparoscopic and endourologic techniques evolve, effective ureteral occlusion will be feasible to assist in the management of these vexing problems.

Endoscopic Management of Small Fistulas

In 1957, Falk and Orkin reported the use of cystoscopic electrocoagulation to treat VVFs. In their series, 8 of 10 patients were successfully managed using this technique, the only failures occurring when the fistula was greater than 3 mm in diameter.[34]

We recently reviewed our experience with endoscopic fulguration of vesicovaginal fistulas in 14 women.[35] In all instances fistula size was estimated to be 2–3 mm or less. A Bugbee electrode was inserted into the fistula either cystoscopically from the bladder or from the vagina (Fig. 26-2). Following the procedure the bladder was decompressed via a large indwelling catheter for 2 to 4 weeks. Ten of the 14 women (71%) had complete resolution of the fistula and one had only a minor degree of residual incontinence.

The theory behind the use of fulguration is that it destroys the epithelial lining of the fistula tract, allowing the bladder and vagina and their respective mucosal surfaces to heal from side to side. Experience has shown that the fistulous tract must be minute or very small and it is futile to attempt electrocoagulation of those larger

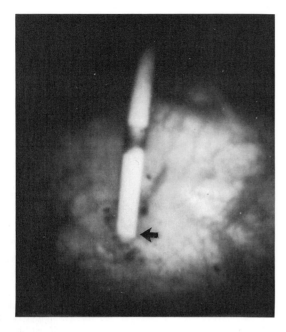

Figure 26-2. A 5 French ureteral catheter is inserted into the bladder from the vagina. The site of the fistula in the bladder is noted (arrow). The ureteral catheter was replaced with a Bugbee electrode, which was withdrawn into the fistula using endoscopic guidance as the fistula was fulgurated. This resulted in resolution of the fistula after 3 weeks of bladder decompression using a large Foley catheter.

than a few mm. It is recommended that a relatively low current be applied to attempt to confine the destruction to the epithelial lining of fistula and avoid injuring the surrounding tissues. A pediatric Bugbee electrode is often preferable to the larger adult size. It is also important to ensure sterilization of the urine both pre- and postoperatively.

The data indicate that fulguration is usually effective in managing small vesicovaginal fistulas a few mm in diameter. Therefore, it is concluded that this relatively simple technique should be attempted first in appropriately selected cases rather than resort to a formal vaginal or abdominal fistula repair.

References

1. Falk HC, Tancer ML. Vesicovaginal fistula: An historical survey. Obstet Gynecol 1954;3:337.
2. McGregor DK. Female disorders in nineteenth-century medicine: The case of vesicovaginal fistula. Caduceus 1987;3(1):1.
3. Tahzib F. Epidemiological determinants of vesicovaginal fistulas. Br J Obstet Gynaecol 1983; 90:387.
4. Harrison KA. Child bearing, health and social priorities: A survey of 22,774 consecutive hospital births in Zaria, Northern Nigeria. Br J Obstet Gynaecol 1985;92(suppl 5):1.
5. Tahzib F. An initiative on vesicovaginal fistula. Lancet 1989;1:1316.
6. Hebert DB. Vesicovaginal fistula: A therapeutic challenge. Infect Urol 1988;July/Aug:63.
7. Harrison KA. Commentary—obstetric fistula: one social calamity too many. Br J Obstet Gynaecol 1983;90:385.
8. Lee RA, Symmonds RE, Williams TJ. Current status of genital-urinary fistula. Obstet Gynecol 1988;72:313.
9. Goldstein I, Wyse GJ, Tancer ML. A vesicovaginal fistula and intravesical foreign body: A rare case of the neglected pessary. Am J Obstet Gynecol 1990;163:589.
10. Kwa DM, Malloy TR. Vesicovaginal fistula and its complications due to prolonged use of vaginal diaphragm. Aust NZ J Obstet Gynaecol 1984; 24:225.
11. Mhiri MN, Amous A, Mezghanni M, et al. Vesicovaginal fistula induced by an intravesical foreign body. Br J Urol 1988;62:271.
12. Singh A, Fazal R, Sinha SK, et al. Tuberculous vesicovaginal fistula in a child. Br J Urol 1988; 62:615.
13. Oumachigui A, Reddy NS, Rajaram P. Postcoital vesicovaginal fistula following surgery for cancer cervix. Int J Gynaecol Obstet 1989;28:77.
14. Zoubek J, McGuire EJ, Noll F, DeLancey JOL. The late occurrence of urinary tract damage in patients successfully treated by radiotherapy for cervical carcinoma. J Urol 1989;141:1347.
15. Kursh ED, Morse RM, Resnick MI, Persky, L. Prevention of the development of a vesicovaginal fistula. Surg Gynecol Obstet 1988;166:409.
16. Turner-Warwick R. Urinary fistulae in the female. In: Campbell's urology. Walsh PC, Gittes RF, Perlmutter AD, Stamey TA, eds. Philadelphia: WB Saunders, 1986;2718–2738.
17. Tancer ML. Post-total hysterectomy (vault) vesicovaginal fistula. J Urol 1980;123:839.
18. Drutz HP, Mainprize TC. Unrecognized small vesicovaginal fistula as a cause of persistent uri-

nary incontinence. Am J Obstet Gynecol 1988; 158:237.

19. Hoch WH, Kursh ED, Persky L. Early, aggressive management of intraoperative ureteral injuries. J Urol 1975;114:530.

20. Carrington BM, Johnson RJ. Vesicovaginal fistula: Ultrasound delineation and pathological correlation. J Clin Ultrasound 1990;18:674.

21. Kuhlman JE, Fishman EK. CT evaluation of enterovaginal and vesicovaginal fistula. J Comput Assist Tomogr 1990;14:390.

22. Green DE, Phillips GL Jr. Vaginal prosthesis for control of vesicovaginal fistula. Gynecologic Oncol 1986;23:119.

23. Persky L, Herman G, Guerrier K. Non-delay in vesicovaginal fistula repair. Urology 1979;13:273.

24. Fourie T. Early surgical repair of post-hysterectomy vesicovaginal fistulas. S Afr Med J 1983; 63:889.

25. Cruikshank SE. Early closure of post-hysterectomy vesicovaginal fistulas. South Med J 1988; 81:1525.

26. Badenoch DF, Tiptaft RC, Thakar DR, et al. Early repair of accidental injury to the ureter or bladder following gynaecological surgery. Br J Urol 1987;59:516.

27. Wang W, Hadley HR. Non-delayed transvaginal repair of high lying vesicovaginal fistula. J Urol 1990;144:34.

28. Robertson JR. Vesicovaginal fistulas. In: Slate WG, ed. Disorders of the female urethra and urinary incontinence. Baltimore: Williams & Wilkins, 1982:282–249.

29. Fearl CL, Keizur LWA. Optimum time interval from occurrence to repair of vesicovaginal fistula. Am J Obstet Gynecol 1969;104:205.

30. Hennessy OF, Gibson RN, Allison DJ. Therapeutic ureteric embolization. Br J Radiol 1984; 57:1151.

31. Stern JL, Maroney TP, Lacey CG. Management of incurable urinary fistulas by percutaneous ureteral occlusion. Obstet Gynecol 1987;70:958.

32. Darcy MD, Lund GB, Smith TP, et al. Percutaneously applied ureteral clips: Treatment of vesicovaginal fistula. Radiology 1987;163:819.

33. Kopecky KK, Sutton GP, Bihrle R, Becker GJ. Percutaneous transrenal endoureteral radiofrequency electrocautery for occlusion: Case report. Radiology 1989;170:1047.

34. Falk HC, Orkin L. Nonsurgical closure of vesicovaginal fistulas. J Obstet Gynecol 1957;9:538.

35. Kursh ED, Stovsky M, Ignatoff JM, Nanninga JB, O'Conor VJ. Use of fulguration in the treatment of vesicovaginal fistulas. 1993;149:292A.

27

Transvaginal Vesicovaginal Fistula Repair

Philippe Zimmern

Gary Leach

Despite much progress in preventing and surgically correcting vesicovaginal fistulas (VVFs), their exact pathophysiology remains unclear. This is particularly true because the human model for a VVF, also called *vaginal cystotomy*, was reported to have no adverse effects. Moir, in his review on the reconstruction of the urethra in 1964, stated:

> I have occasionally provided additional drainage by means of a vaginal cystotomy. A hooked glass tube is inserted through this artificially created fistula and kept in position for one week, after which the drainage is continued through the already-placed polythene urethral tube. The cystotomy has in my experience always closed spontaneously.[1]

For many surgeons at present, the mystery resides not so much in the pathophysiology of VVFs but more in how to comprehend and master the vaginal techniques, permitting in the words of Sims a "safe and perfect cure."[2]

This chapter therefore focuses on the preoperative, intraoperative, and postoperative steps involved in the vaginal repair of a nonradiated VVF.

Then associated vaginal pathologies requiring simultaneous correction are discussed. Alternative vaginal techniques such as the colpocleisis (Latzko operation) and the Martius labial fat pad graft are reviewed. Finally, a brief update on the management of radiated VVFs is presented.

Vaginal Repair of a Nonradiated Vaginal Vault Vesicovaginal Fistula

The focus of this first section is on the management of a *VVF*, that is, a fistula entering the vaginal cuff. The choice made of describing such a highly located fistula stems from the current trend of being involved more and more with such supratrigonal VVFs.

PREOPERATIVE MANAGEMENT

Knowledge of Fistula Characteristics

Because more than half of VVFs occur after simple abdominal hysterectomy, the most common anatomic location of VVF is currently seen at the vaginal apex or vault.[3] Objective documentation of fistula characteristics is best obtained from a voiding cystourethrogram with adequate oblique and lateral views[4] (Fig. 27-1). Preoperative cystoscopy, however, with bilateral bulb retrograde ureteropyelograms is essential to examine the site and size of the fistula precisely; to assess its distance from the ureteric orifices; to look for a

Female Urology, edited by Elroy D. Kursh and Edward McGuire. J. B. Lippincott, Philadelphia, © 1994.

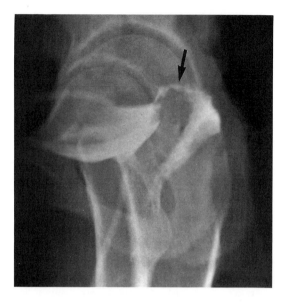

Figure 27-1. Lateral cystogram demonstrating a classic high vault vesicovaginal fistula (arrow) after abdominal hysterectomy. An anteroposterior view alone can easily miss the posteriorly located vesicovaginal fistula behind the outline of the bladder.

secondary fistula tract, which if missed could cause immediate failure; and to verify the integrity of both ureters. In large series, a ureterovaginal fistula has been found associated with a VVF in 10% to 25% of cases.[5,9] A normal appearing intravenous pyelogram does not exclude a small ureterovaginal fistula.

Timing of Repair

Classically it is recommended to wait 3 to 6 months before undertaking the repair of a VVF. This waiting period was thought to be essential for the inflammatory reaction at the fistula site to subside. A trend of nondelay in the last 30 years has gained wider acceptance for three reasons:[1,6-9]

1. The emotional and social consequences of a fistula are tremendous for the patient and her family.
2. There is no satisfactory management to con-

trol the severe urinary leakage resulting from a VVF.
3. A limited waiting period with repair of the fistula within a month from the initial injury (which is the average time it takes to recognize and diagnose its presence) offers the same chance of success in historical series as a longer waiting period has afforded in the past.

For all these reasons, a limited waiting period averaging 4 to 6 weeks has been adopted, during which the patient is prepared for the upcoming operation. In small size fistulas, an attempt at closure with an indwelling Foley catheter for 3 weeks can be considered but is rarely successful. Medications during this waiting period have a limited role, mostly hormonal replacement to enhance vaginal wall pliability and control of a urinary tract infection if present to achieve sterile urine at the time of the repair.[10]

Consent

Assuming that an isolated 1- to 2-cm VVF has been identified in the trigone, not involving the ureteric orifices and surrounded by healthy tissues permitting an immediate repair, the patient can be told that she has an 85% to 90% chance of being cured at the first repair (Table 27-1). The consent should include a discussion of possible complications, such as fistula recurrence, bleeding, and infection. Narrowing of the upper vagina and dyspareunia should be mentioned, although those complications have rarely been encountered in our practice. Also, when the fistula is close to the ureteric orifice (especially if the patient has a solitary kidney), the placement of a ureteral catheter is highly suggested.[5,10]

Finally, consent should be obtained for the intraoperative placement of a suprapubic tube catheter and for the possible use of a Martius labial fat pad graft or a peritoneal flap interposition if the repair appears tenuous or in case of prior failure.

Infection

Infection at the time of the repair must be avoided at all costs because it often precludes a

Table 27-1. *Summary of Series of Transvaginal Repair of Vesicovaginal Fistulas in the Last 20 Years*

AUTHOR	YEAR	NO.	SUCCESS, FIRST REPAIR (%)	FAILURE, NO. PATIENTS	SUCCESS, REOPERATION (%)*
Collins *et al*	1971	29	72.5	8	100
Lawson	1972	65	85	10	98
Steg *et al*	1977	40	70	10	92.5
Keetel *et al*	1978	157	—	9	94.3
Symmonds	1979	260	88	32	92.5
Kelly	1979	160	81	13	—
Goodwin and Scardino	1980	22	77	—	95
Leach and Raz	1983	20	100	—	—
Benchekroun *et al*	1987	276	98	—	—
Wang and Hadley	1990	16	94	1	—
Zimmern	1991	37	84	6	92
Total		1092	85.2		95.6

* Ultimate success after two or more repeated vaginal surgeries.

successful result. The patient should receive vaginal douching (povidone-iodine [Betadine]) the evening before and the morning of the operation. In addition, broad-spectrum antibiotic therapy (ampicillin/gentamicin [Garamycin] or ampicillin/sulbactam sodium) is initiated intravenously on the morning of the procedure. In patients presenting with an indwelling Foley catheter or documented urinary tract infection preoperatively, a course of oral antibiotics is recommended to sterilize the urine. The use of the Foley catheter preoperatively should be discouraged because the presence of the catheter maintains bladder wall inflammation.

OPERATIVE PROCEDURE

Indication for Vaginal Approach

The vaginal approach is preferred by surgeons familiar with vaginal surgery. It is agreed upon, however, and we insist on the fact that the surgeon's experience should dictate the choice of approach. Advantages of the vaginal approach include the avoidance of a laparotomy and a cystotomy, the possibility of simultaneous repair of other vaginal pathology (*i.e.*, bladder neck suspension), an easier recovery for the patient, and a shorter hospital stay.

Contraindication to Vaginal Approach

A narrow vagina, a high vault fistula, and the proximity of the ureteric orifice can constitute relative contraindications. A relaxing posterior vaginal wall incision to facilitate adequate exposure, as described later, and ureteral catheter placement can represent easy solutions to these problems. Lack of experience with vaginal surgery and an associated ureterovaginal fistula are definite contraindications to proceed vaginally.

Patient Position and Preparation

Sims' technique of using the knee-elbow position is rarely used.[2] Pneumatic compression devices are routinely used as a simple prophylaxis against deep venous thrombosis. Foam boots are wrapped around the foot and ankle for protection in stirrups. The patient is then placed in high exaggerated lithotomy position. Proper positioning is important not only for adequate vaginal exposure, but also for preventing nerve plexus injury (femoral neuropathy), which can result from prolonged overflexing and abducting of the thigh. Also, lateral peroneal nerve compression over poorly padded metal stirrups is avoided.

After the preparation is completed, a povidone-iodine–soaked gauze is inserted in the rectum to facilitate proper identification of the rectum. Then a sterile drape is placed across the field to separate the rectum from the vaginal area. Drapes are placed in a standard fashion, and their margin bordering the vaginal fourchette is secured to the perineal skin above the rectum with interrupted nonabsorbable sutures. The labia are retracted with the stay hooks of the Scott retractor.

Cystoscopy and Suprapubic Tube Placement

Careful inspection of the fistula tract is recommended at the start of the procedure to reassess its location and size and the quality of the adjacent bladder wall lining. A suprapubic tube is then inserted using either the direct punch technique if the bladder can be appropriately inflated or the curved Lowsley retractor.[11] Our experience with the latter technique has been excellent, allowing safe and rapid placement of a large size (20 to 24 French) suprapubic Foley catheter.

Techniques to Enhance Exposure to Vaginal Vault

Exposure of a VVF located at the vault can be greatly enhanced by the following four steps: (1) use of a self-retaining vaginal retractor, such as the Scott retractor; (2) placing the patient in Trendelenburg position; (3) wearing a headlight; and (4) catheterizing the fistula with a small Foley or Fogarty catheter, depending on its size, from the vagina into the bladder. This simple maneuver allows traction on the fistula tract and adequate dissection of the tissues surrounding the tract (Fig. 27-2). Occasionally the fistula tract is tortuous or small, and catheterization can be performed only from the bladder side. In such instances, a 0.038 floppy tip guidewire or a whistle tip ureteral catheter is inserted through the fistula and advanced into the vagina. A small, open-ended catheter is then passed over the wire, or a small Foley or Fogarty catheter can be attached to the ureteral catheter and guided back inside of the bladder.

Incision and Vaginal Wall Flap

The anterior vaginal wall incision is a key step of the procedure and should be planned with three

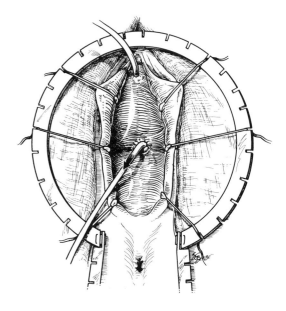

Figure 27-2. *Traction on a small Foley or Fogarty catheter inserted in the fistula tract per vagina facilitates exposure by bringing the fistula tract closer to the operative field.*

goals in mind:[12] First, the anterior vaginal wall flap created serves to cover the underlying fistula repair at the end of the procedure. Second, the base of the flap should be broad to maintain flap vascularity and also to accommodate the vaginal wall tendency to retract. In addition, the flap may have to cover additional interposed bulky tissue, such as a Martius labial fat pad as described later. Third, the flap should have a U-shaped form, with its base directed anteriorly for a high vault fistula and its tip at the fistula tract (Fig. 27-3).

The planned line of incision is infiltrated with normal saline to facilitate the dissection between the vagina and the underlying perivesical tissues. After completion of the incision and creation of a large broad-base anterior vaginal wall flap, the incision is extended to circumscribe the fistula with an approximately 5- to 10-mm margin of vaginal wall remaining around the edges of the fistula (Fig. 27-4).

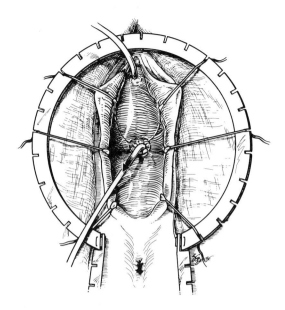

Figure 27-3. Anterior vaginal wall incision creating a large broad-based flap. The tip of the flap is adjacent to the incision, which circumscribes the fistula tract.

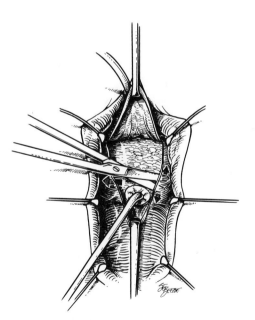

Figure 27-4. Dissection is performed beneath the vaginal wall, lateral to the fistula to achieve wide mobilization of the fistula tract.

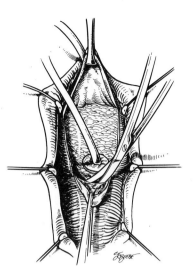

Figure 27-5. The posterior flap is dissected with care to avoid entry into the rectum or peritoneal cavity. Should a peritoneal opening be made, a peritoneal flap can be laid over the fistula repair.

Dissection of the Vesicovaginal Fistula

Using long curve Metzenbaum scissors and traction on the catheter placed through the fistula tract, vaginal wall flaps are dissected laterally between bladder and vagina as well as anteriorly and posteriorly (Fig. 27-4). This circular dissection around the fistula tract is needed to achieve sufficient mobilization to permit closure without tension. In this case of a high vault VVF, the posterior flap dissection is likely to result in a peritoneal opening (Fig. 27-5). This is of no consequence and sometimes even elected, so a peritoneal flap can be laid over the VVF repair as an interposition graft. Of more potentially serious consequence, a rectal injury could also occur during this posterior dissection. A povidone-iodine–soaked gauze placed in the rectum before the perineal draping has facilitated proper identification of the rectum in our practice.

Closure of the Vesicovaginal Fistula without Excision

The fistula tract is closed in two layers without excision of the tract[5, 12] (Figs. 27-6 through

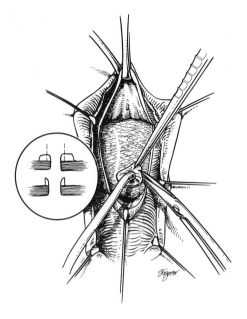

Figure 27-6. *The edges of the tract are trimmed without excision of the fistula tract.*

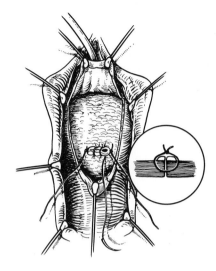

Figure 27-7. *First layer of fistula closure. Two corner sutures are placed. One of them is run transversely across the fistula with careful imbrication of the fistula edges.*

27-8). Excision of the fistula tract has been classically advocated, but we have found it unnecessary. Fistula excision is always accompanied by bleeding, enlargement of the defect, and possible risk of endangering a nearby ureteric orifice.

The fistula tract edges are neatly trimmed (Fig. 27-6). Hemostasis is carefully obtained to facilitate the repair and avoid secondary hematoma. Then absorbable sutures are placed at each corner of the fistula tract to serve as traction once the small Foley or Fogarty catheter is removed from the fistula tract. One of the corner sutures is run across the fistula opening transversely toward the opposite side with care taken to imbricate the edges of the fistula tract (Fig. 27-7).

A second layer of interrupted absorbable sutures is performed at right angle from the underlying suture line. This second layer incorporates the adjacent and widely mobilized perivesical tissues to cover over the fistula first line of closure (Fig. 27-8).

Diluted methylene blue dye is then dripped

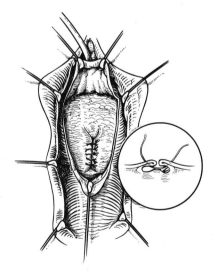

Figure 27-8. *Second layer of fistula closure at right angle to the first layer of closure. Interrupted absorbable sutures incorporate the adjacent, widely mobilized perivesical tissue.*

in the bladder under gravity through the suprapubic tube, while the site of fistula closure is carefully inspected for leakage. After the watertightness of the repair has been demonstrated, the suprapubic tube is placed on drainage, and a urethral Foley catheter is inserted (if not placed at the beginning of the procedure).

Techniques of Interposition and When to Use Them

When the repair appears tenuous, the tissues are of poor quality, or there has been a prior failed attempt at repair, interposition of a peritoneal flap or a labial fat pad (Martius technique) should be performed.[13] (See description to follow.)

The peritoneal cul-de-sac is often entered during the posterior vaginal wall flap dissection, and an adequate flap of peritoneum can be rotated and secured over the fistula repair. Otherwise, a long and broad-based labial fat pad can be harvested from the labia and tunneled beneath the vaginal side wall to cover the fistula repair site, as described subsequently.

Vaginal Flap Advancement

When the repair is completed, the initially raised anterior vaginal wall flap is advanced posteriorly. The apical edge of the flap is trimmed. Advancement of this vaginal wall flap provides excellent coverage of the underlying fistula tract closure without overlapping suture lines. Two running absorbable sutures are used from the apex to each side of the base of the flap (Fig. 27-9). A vaginal packing with antibiotic ointment is placed in the vagina for 24 to 48 hours. All urinary catheters are left indwelling.

POSTOPERATIVE CARE

Immediate Postoperative Care

Uninterrupted catheter drainage of both the urethral and the suprapubic catheters for 10 to 14 days is vital because clot retention or kinking of the catheter tubing can lead to excessive bladder distention, disruption of the suture lines, and immediate recurrence of the VVF. The patient as

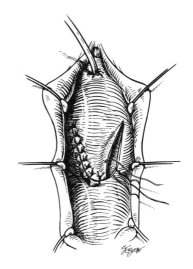

Figure 27-9. *Third layer of fistula closure. After the watertightness of the repair has been demonstrated, the anterior vaginal wall flap is advanced over the fistula site, avoiding overlapping of the suture lines.*

well as the nurses must be instructed regarding the importance of monitoring vigilantly the urinary drainage of both catheters.

The patient position with feet up and head down trying to minimize the exposure of the suture lines to urine is no longer judged important. Anticholinergic medications to avoid bladder spasms (including belladonna and opium suppositories) and antibiotics are maintained while the urinary catheters are in place.

Follow-Up Assessment

Approximately 2 weeks postoperatively, the urethral Foley catheter is removed, and a suprapubic tube cystogram is obtained to document the closure of the fistula. The suprapubic catheter is then clamped and removed after documentation of two postvoid residuals less than 100 ml. Regular clinic visits are scheduled until the vaginal healing is completed. Mild exercises and sexual activity can usually be resumed by 3 months postoperatively.

RESULT

For the first attempt at repair, most series report a success rate of 85% to 95%[14–18] (Table 27-1). It should be noted that there is a tremendous variability in all series in regard to the techniques employed and the duration and mode of follow-up. Failures by the transvaginal approach are usually dealt with by a repeat transvaginal approach or a suprapubic approach.

COMPLICATIONS

Intraoperative Complications

Loss of Fogarty Catheter. When the balloon of the Foley or Fogarty catheter ruptures during the procedure or is pulled out of the tract during the dissecting maneuvers, it can be sometimes extremely difficult to find the fistula tract again. For this reason, we tend to use a safety guidewire over which the catheter is advanced through the fistula tract.

Ureteral Injury. Without excision of the tract as recommended in the technique described here, the risk of injuring the ureter is virtually eliminated. Placement of a ureteral stent, however, is advisable if the fistula is close to one orifice, in case of a solitary kidney, or in a repeat operation in which the trigonal anatomy is abnormal after prior repair. Should ureteral damage occur, a laparotomy to repair the injury must be performed. Finally, it is emphasized once more that a VVF with a known associated ureterovaginal fistula is a strict contraindication to a vaginal approach.

Rectal Injury. Should a rectal injury occur and be recognized, a two-layer closure of the rectal wall with appropriate antibiotic coverage and hyperalimentation for a few days to leave the bowel at rest should result in a satisfactory outcome. Unrecognized, such an injury could lead to a rectovaginal fistula, pelvic abscess, or other complication.

Bleeding. Bleeding is rarely a significant problem during the repair of a VVF. Excision of the tract is avoided in part to minimize this risk.

Inadequate hemostasis can lead to a vaginal wall hematoma, which can become infected or result in a breakdown of the suture lines under tension. The insertion of the vaginal packing at the completion of the surgery is useful in facilitating hemostasis.

Postoperative Complications

Recurrence. Although uncommon, failures can result from errors, as follows: errors in diagnosis, especially when a second fistula tract is not recognized; errors in technique with uncontrolled preoperative urinary tract infection, inadequate identification of the tract, poor hemostasis, or overlapping of the suture lines; or errors in postoperative care with bladder overdistention from unrecognized catheter plugging. Depending on the surgeon's experience, a repeat vaginal procedure can be considered when a recurrent fistula develops (Table 27-1). In such an instance, the use of a Martius labial fat pad is highly recommended as a simple means of interposition.

Dyspareunia. Unless a Latzko procedure (partial colpocleisis, as described later) is performed, this is not a common long-term complication. Intercourse can be resumed safely once the vagina is healed, around 3 months postoperatively. The use of lubrication and of estrogen cream in the postmenopausal patient is advisable.

Small Bladder Capacity. An unused bladder can theoretically suffer irreversible wall damage, although even the initially small bladders have been seen to re-expand to normal capacity once the fistula was closed. A bladder augmentation is therefore not usually indicated primarily.

Stress Urinary Incontinence. A pre-existing history of stress urinary incontinence can sometimes be elicited. Moderate symptoms of stress urinary incontinence secondary to urethral hypermobility are not uncommon in postmenopausal patients, but the severity of the leakage associated with the VVF can mask its presence. Both conditions can be treated at the same time transvaginally.[12, 19] The bladder neck suspension is performed first (but the suspension sutures not tied), followed by the repair of the VVF.

Vesicovaginal Fistula and Rare Associated Pathologies

NARROW VAGINA

A narrow vagina is not an absolute contraindication to proceed with a vaginal approach. A posterolateral relaxing incision similar to an episiotomy can be easily done to enlarge the exposure. Such a difficult anatomy, however, can render the repair of a high vault VVF extremely hazardous, thereby forcing the decision for a safer abdominal approach or even a combined abdominovaginal approach.

VESICAL CALCULI

A report of five cases of vesical calculi and VVF with vaginal stone formed over a nonabsorbable suture suggested a two-step repair, with crushing of the stone initially and fistula repair 3 months later.[20] In one similar instance, the vesical stone was crushed endoscopically, the suture was removed vaginally, and the fistula was closed at the same setting with no problems.[19]

TRAUMATIC VESICOVAGINAL FISTULA

Extensive perineal tears from falls or impalement with involvement of the bladder, vagina, and occasionally rectum must be considered for immediate repair, if feasible, to prevent the development of a large VVF. Simple catheter drainage is not sufficient.[19]

Martius Operation

INDICATION

This simple technique should be considered when the idea comes to the mind of the repairing surgeon.[13] Other than this subjective indication, which derives from experience more so than from a rationale attitude, a tenuous repair with poor tissues, a repeat operation, or an associated

vaginal wall pathology are classic examples of when to perform this procedure.[21]

TECHNIQUE

A vertical incision is made over the labia majora from the level of the mons pubis to the posterior fourchette. Skin flaps are developed on each side of the incision to expose the fat and fibromuscular content of the labia. The labial fat pad is freed down to the underlying fascia (Fig. 27-10A). Because the vascular supply comes inferiorly from the external pudendal vessels, the superior aspect of the fatty pad is commonly divided as high as needed.

Then a large tunnel is created beneath the side wall of the vagina through which the labial fat pad is advanced toward the site of fistula tract closure, with care not to twist the pad at the base. The pad is secured in place at two or three sites over the first two layers of fistula repair (Fig. 27-10B). The initial broad-base vaginal flap is then advanced to cover the Martius labial fat pad. The labia is closed over a small Penrose drain. Ice packs are applied to limit the swelling.

Latzko Procedure

PRINCIPLE AND INDICATION

The Latzko operation results from a simple principle, which is that in a woman after hysterectomy the anterior vaginal wall lies over the posterior vaginal wall. So when the area surrounding the fistula is denuded, the corresponding raw surfaces of the two vaginal walls can be simply reapproximated without tension. In the case of a vault VVF, this technique of *high occlusion* of the vagina is technically easy to perform, leads to minimal vaginal shortening, and has a good success rate.[22]

TECHNIQUE

The fistula tract is circumscribed at a 1- to 2-cm distance. The whole vaginal epithelium of this circumscribed area to the edge of the fistula tract

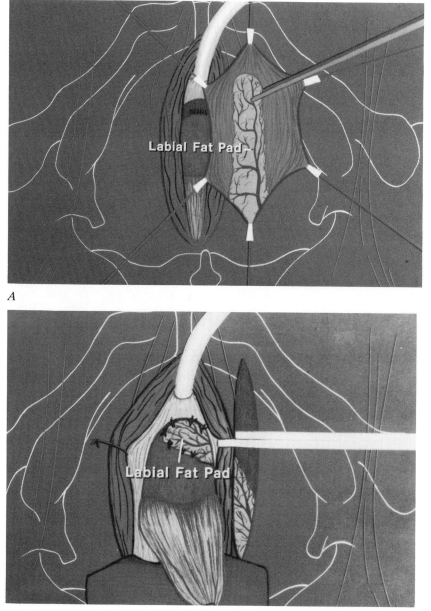

A

B

Figure 27-10. *Martius labial fat pad graft. (A) Through a generous vertical incision over the labia majora, the labial fat pad is mobilized with preservation of the posterior external pudendal vessel supply. (B) The Martius graft is tunneled beneath the side wall of the vagina and secured over the site of fistula repair. (From P. Zimmern, G. Leach. Vesicovaginal fistula repair. Prob Urol 1991;5: 171–182.)*

is excised but not the fistula tract itself. There is no dissection of the bladder wall and minimal risk of injuring the ureter.

The colpocleisis is performed with absorbable sutures in a vertical anteroposterior direction, followed by a transversal vaginal wall closure over the underlying fistula tract repair. Bladder drainage is mandatory for 7 to 10 days.

RESULT

This simple partial colpocleisis procedure is associated with minimal bleeding, limited vaginal shortening in case of a high vault fistula, and an excellent success rate (almost 100%).[23–25] When this operation fails, a repeat procedure can be easily performed with a good chance of success according to the author.[23] Total colpocleisis is rarely needed to treat a VVF and would be indicated only as a last resort in an elderly, nonsexually active patient.

Radiated Vesicovaginal Fistula

Radiated fistulas represent an extremely difficult challenge to the surgeon. This section reviews the pathophysiology, diagnosis, and surgical options available to treat these defects.

PATHOPHYSIOLOGY

Radiation VVFs are the most complex form of fistulas, incorporating tissue injured by the radiation, often large defects, and rigid and fibrotic tissue around the fistula tract. VVFs classically occur after radiation therapy for cervical carcinoma, with an incidence of 1% to 5%.[26,27] The fistula can develop from the necrosis of the tumor (during the radiation therapy) or directly from the high radiation dosage (after completion of the radiation therapy). VVFs have also been reported in radiated patients after electrofulguration to stop bleeding from radiation cystitis and after embolization of the hypogastric arteries for life-threatening vaginal bleeding.[28]

TIMING AND INDICATIONS FOR REPAIR

Part of the decision to intervene depends on the result of the biopsy specimens taken at the edges of the fistula tract to exclude recurrent or persistent cancer. Other factors to consider are the overall condition of the patient, the status of the bladder wall damage and of the upper tracts, and the degree of resolution of the radiation injury. Indeed most authors recommend to wait at least 1 year after the appearance of the VVF to contemplate a possible repair.[5,27,29,30] The acute radiation reaction should have subsided, and the fistula tract should be of stable size with a rigid and fibrotic perimeter on clinical examination and cystoscopic inspection.

Finally, should the radiated VVF be satisfactorily repaired, the surgeon may be faced with other effects of the radiation injury reducing the functional bladder capacity or damaging the urethral sphincteric mechanism (type III stress urinary incontinence).[5,27] A careful clinical evaluation should permit early detection of these adverse surgical factors.

SURGICAL ALTERNATIVES FOR REPAIR OF RADIATED VESICOVAGINAL FISTULAS

Standard fistula closure techniques are notoriously unsuccessful. Temporary or permanent urinary diversion, although viewed as a last resort, often concludes a series of frustrated attempts at a more simple means of eradicating the problem in an otherwise clinically cured patient.

Vaginal techniques used in the largest series reported (averaging 20 to 80 patients) include the Latzko partial colpocleisis, the Martius labial fat pad graft, and more extensive techniques of graft interposition with gracilis or rectus muscles.[26,27,29–31] Description of those techniques is beyond the scope of this chapter. Success rates range from 25% to 75% in experienced hands. In our experience, the technique of partial colpocleisis was found ideally suited for a high vault fistula because of its simplicity and minimal invasiveness. The Martius operation can be combined quite easily with the Latzko procedure either primarily or in case of failure. It has been suggested that this well-vascularized labial pad stabilizes or reverses the radiation-induced obliterative endarteritis, thereby enhancing the healing process.[32] A theoretical disadvantage of the use of the Martius flap or even the rectus muscle graft includes their potential initial involvement in the field of radiation. This concern has led to the development of the gracilis muscle interposition, which consists of mobilizing the gracilis muscle from the inner thigh on the proximal profunda femoris artery and transposing the muscle through a wide tunnel beneath the proximal thigh to the lateral vaginal wall to cover the area of fistula repair.[33,34]

References

1. Moir JC. Reconstruction of the urethra. J Obstet Gynecol 1964;71:349.
2. Sims MJ. On treatment of vesicovaginal fistula. Am J Med Sci 1852;23:59.
3. Symmonds RE. Prevention and management of genitourinary fistula. J Cont Educ Obstet Gynecol 1979;2:13.
4. Zimmern PE. The role of voiding cystourethrography in the evaluation of the female lower urinary tract. Probl Urol 1991;5:23.
5. Zimmern PE, Hadley HR, Staskin DR, Raz S. Genito-urinary fistulae: Vaginal approach for repair of vesicovaginal fistulae. Urol Clin North Am 1985;12:361.
6. Barnes R, Hadley H, Johnston O. Transvaginal repair of vesicovaginal fistulas. Urology 1977;10:258.
7. Benchekroun A, Lakrissa A, Essakali HN, et al. Vesicovaginal fistula. Review of 600 cases. J d'Urol 1987;3:151.
8. Couvelaire R. Les fistules vesicovaginales complexes. J d'Urol 1982;88:353.
9. Goodwin WE, Scardino PT. Vesicovaginal and ureterovaginal fistulae: A summary of 25 years of experience. J Urol 1980;123:370.
10. Keetel WC, Sehring FG, DeProsse CA, et al. Surgical management of urethrovaginal and vesicovaginal fistulas. Am J Obstet Gynecol 1978;131:425.
11. Zeidman E, Chiang H, Alarcon A, Raz S. Suprapubic cystostomy using Lowsley retractor. Urol 1989;33(suppl):11.
12. Leach GE, Raz S. Vaginal flap technique. A method of transvaginal vesicovaginal fistula repair. In: Raz S, ed. Female urology. Philadelphia: WB Saunders, 1983:372.
13. Martius H. Gynaecological operations and their topographic-anatomic fundamentals. Chicago: Canterbury Press, 1939:271–276.
14. Collins CG, Collins JH, Harrison BR. Early repair of vesicovaginal fistula. Am J Obstet Gynecol 1971;4:524.
15. Lawson J. Vesical fistulae into the vaginal vault. Br J Urol 1972;44:623.
16. Steg A, Vialatte P, Olier C. Treatment of vesicovaginal fistulas by Chassar-Moir technique. Report of 40 cases. Ann Urol 1977;2:103.
17. Kelly J. Vesicovaginal fistulae. Br J Urol 1979;51:208.
18. Wang Y, Hadley HR. Nondelayed transvaginal repair of high lying vesicovaginal fistula. J Urol 1990;144:34.
19. Zimmern PE, Leach GE. Vesicovaginal fistula repair. Probl Urol 1991;5:171.
20. Mahapatra TP, Rao MS, Rao K, et al. Vesical calculi associated with vesicovaginal fistulas. Management considerations. J Urol 1986;136:94.
21. Birkhoff JD, Weschler M, Romas NA. Urinary fistulas: Vaginal repair using a labial fat pad. J Urol 1983;130:1073.
22. Latzko W. Behandlung hochsitzender Blasen und Mastdarmscheidenfisteln nach Uterusextirpation mit hohem Scheidenverschluss. Zentrabl Gynak 1914;38:905.
23. Latzko W. Postoperative vesicovaginal fistulas. Am J Surg 1942;58:211.
24. Tancer ML. The post-total hysterectomy (vault) vesicovaginal fistula. J Urol 1980;123:839.
25. Kaser O. The Latzko operation for vesicovaginal fistula. Acta Obstet Gynaecol Scand 1977;56:427.
26. Kottmeier HL. Complications following radiation therapy in carcinoma of the cervix and their treatment. Am J Obstet Gynecol 1964;88:854.
27. Boronow RC. Repair of the radiation-induced vaginal fistula utilizing the Martius technique. World J Surg 1986;10:237.
28. Behnam K, Jarmolowski CR. Vesicovaginal fistula following hypogastric embolization for control of intractable pelvic hemorrhage. J Reprod Med 1982;27:304.
29. Bastiaanse MA, Van B. Bastiaanse's method for surgical closure of very large irradiation fistulae of the bladder and rectum. In: Youssef AF, ed. Gynecological urology. Springfield, IL: Charles C. Thomas, 1960;280–297.
30. Ingelman-Sundberg A. Pathogenesis and operative treatment of urinary fistulae in irradiated tissue. In: Youssef AF, ed. Gynecological urology. Springfield, IL: Charles C. Thomas, 1960:263–279.

31. Graham JB. Vaginal fistulas following radiotherapy. Surg Gynecol Obstet 1965;120:1019.
32. Svanberg L, Astedt B, Kullander S. On radiation decreased fibrinolytic activity of vessel walls. Acta Obstet Gynaecol Scand 1976;55:49.
33. Zinman L. Use of myocutaneous and muscle interposition flaps in management of radiation-induced vesicovaginal fistula. In: McDougal WS, ed. Difficult problems in urologic surgery. Chicago: Year Book Medical Publishers, 1989: 143–163.
34. Obrink A, Bunne G. Gracilis interposition in fistulas following radiotherapy for cervical cancer: A retrospective study. Urol Int 1978;33:370.

28

Transabdominal Vesicovaginal Fistula Repair

Elroy D. Kursh

Both vaginal and abdominal approaches have been employed for surgical correction of vesicovaginal fistulas (VVFs), and a variety of modifications of each technique have been described. Testimonials have been written regarding the value of an individual approach by various gynecologic and urologic surgeons. Whichever route a surgeon selects, the best operation for repair of a VVF is probably the first operation. In most instances, it is preferable for the surgeon to select an approach that he or she is most comfortable with, based on training and experience.

This chapter describes the use of an abdominal approach or a combined transabdominal and vaginal technique. Most urologists are more familiar with the abdominal exposure, whereas gynecologists usually prefer a vaginal repair.

The abdominal technique has several advantages for complex VVFs (*e.g.*, recurrent or multiple fistulas or those that occur following radiation therapy). It affords the opportunity to interpose a variety of pedicle materials between the bladder and vagina. VVFs that are located close to a ureteral orifice can be more readily repaired without risk of injury or obstruction of the ureter, or, if necessary, the ureter can be reimplanted into the bladder in a different location. Finally, a transabdominal technique allows for the possibility of bladder augmentation when

repairing radiation-induced fistulas, which are frequently associated with vesical contraction and poor compliance.

Preoperative Preparation

TIMING OF SURGICAL PROCEDURE

Over the years, the traditional management of a VVF was to delay surgery for 3 to 6 months to allow the edema and inflammation to resolve. The issue of the optimal time to undertake surgical correction is discussed in Chapter 26. My own preference is to time the repair on the basis of the apparent associated inflammation. Pelvic and vaginal speculum examination is repeated until the vagina appears uninflamed, well epithelialized, and free of granulation tissue. At this time, cystoscopy is performed to inspect the appearance of the fistula from the bladder side. If similar findings are observed and pelvic examination reveals a reasonably pliable vagina without induration, surgery is undertaken.

IMMEDIATE PREOPERATIVE PREPARATION

Preoperative preparation includes mechanical and antibiotic bowel preparation because it is frequently necessary to lyse a significant number

Female Urology, edited by Elroy D. Kursh and Edward McGuire. J. B. Lippincott, Philadelphia, © 1994.

of adhesions to gain access to the pelvis. If the bowel is inadvertently entered, it can be closed with little or no increased risk of infection.

It is important to ensure sterilization of the urine before undertaking surgery. Urine cultures are repeated shortly before the scheduled surgical date, and antibiotics are prescribed according to the culture data. Broad-spectrum parenteral antibiotic coverage is started preoperatively, usually a combination of an aminoglycoside and ampicillin or a cephalosporin. A povidone-iodine douche is also administered the night before surgery.

Surgical Technique

A variety of transabdominal approaches have been described, including transvesicle approaches, combined transvesical-vaginal approach, transvesical extraperitoneal approach, transvesical transperitoneal approach, and a bladder flap method.[1–6]

TRANSVESICAL APPROACH

The transvesical approach has been largely abandoned by most pelvic surgeons owing to the relatively restricted exposure, although even today we still see an occasional report using modifications of the basic technique because of its simplicity.[2] Transvesical dissection may include mobilization of the bladder off the vagina with a multilayer closure or merely dissection and closure of the mucosa off the closed fistula without excision of the fistulous tract.[2] A classic transvesical approach is depicted in Fig. 28-1 primarily for historical interest and not because it is recommended.

TRANSVESICAL EXTRAPERITONEAL APPROACH

O'Conor was instrumental in describing the suprapubic approach of bivalving the bladder to the level of the fistula.[4] The procedure is usually

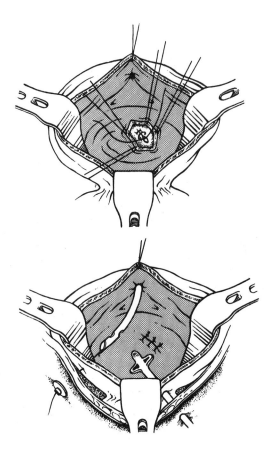

Figure 28-1. *Classic transvesical approach to vesicovaginal fistula repair. After the bladder is opened, the bladder component of the fistula is dissected off the vaginal component, and each is closed separately. (From Turner-Warwick R. Urinary fistulae in the female. In: Walsh PC, Gittes RF, Perlmutter AD, Stamey TA, eds. Campbell's urology. 5th ed. Philadelphia: WB Saunders, 1986:2724.)*

done extraperitoneally, although if exposure is difficult or if the surgeon contemplates using omentum, the peritoneum may be opened. The fistulous tract is excised on both the bladder and the vaginal sides. After the bladder is dissected well off the vagina, each is closed separately (Fig. 28-2).

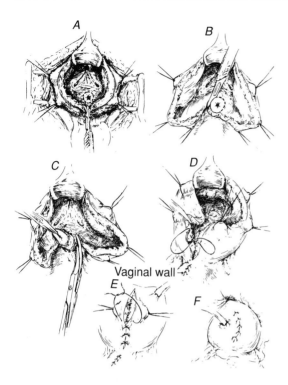

Figure 28-2. Transvesical extraperitoneal approach to vesicovaginal fistula repair. (A) The dome of the bladder is opened. (B) The incision is extended posteriorly, and the fistula tract is excised in a racquet fashion. (C) After excision of the fistula, the bladder is widely mobilized off the anterior vagina. (D) After the vaginal closure is completed, the bladder closure is started using absorbable sutures. (E) The initial bladder closure is reinforced with a second inverting layer. (F) Closure is completed, and a suprapubic cystostomy tube is placed. (From O'Conor VJ Jr. Review of experience with vesicovaginal fistula repair. J Urol 1980;123:367.)

TRANSVESICAL, TRANSPERITONEAL APPROACH

I prefer a transabdominal, transvesical, transperitoneal approach. This technique is particularly valuable for complicated fistulas because it allows for a multilayered closure and the interposition of a variety of pedicle materials between the bladder and vagina.

If the fistula is not particularly complex, such as a difficult recurrent fistula or one associated with radiation treatment, the patient is positioned in a standard supine position with the lower extremities spread slightly apart. Sequential compression devices are placed on the lower extremities. During preparation of the patient, the vagina is thoroughly prepared with povidone-iodine, and it is often helpful to pack the vagina with a packing soaked with povidone-iodine before preparing and draping the abdomen. This greatly assists in localization of the vagina intra-abdominally later in the procedure. Likewise, the abdomen is prepared with povidone-iodine, and the patient is draped in the standard manner for a lower abdominal midline incision. This incision is preferred to a transverse incision because it can be extended if it is decided to interpose an omental flap between the bladder and vagina later in the operation.

A lower abdominal midline incision is made. The rectus muscle is split in the midline, and the peritoneum is opened. Any adhesions holding the small bowel in place are transected, and the small bowel is delivered from the pelvis and packed out of the pelvic cavity.

The bladder is opened anteriorly between Allis clamps. Bivalving the bladder is avoided to prevent a large posterior bladder closure later in the procedure. Avoidance of bivalving the bladder may also help preserve a bladder that is compromised from radiation therapy and may facilitate maintenance of bladder capacity. Placement of a small Foley catheter, or even a Fogarty catheter, through the fistulous tract after the bladder is opened often aids in identification of the fistula as the plane is established between the bladder and vagina. Generally ureteral catheters are also passed to aid in locating the orifices and preventing ureteral injury (Fig. 28-3).

Dissection proceeds by establishing a plane between the vagina and bladder. The previously packed vagina facilitates intra-abdominal palpation of the vagina to locate the correct site of this plane. The peritoneum overlying this site is incised. Dissection between the bladder and vagina

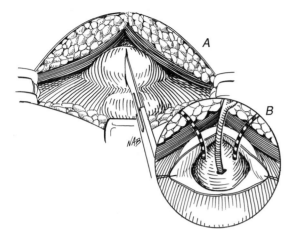

Figure 28-3. (A) The bladder is opened anteriorly. (B) A small Foley catheter is inserted through the fistula into the vagina. Ureteral catheters are usually inserted also.

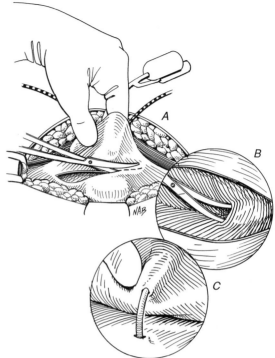

Figure 28-4. (A) The peritoneum overlying the plane between the posterior bladder wall and anterior vagina is incised. (B) Blunt and sharp dissection is used to dissect the vagina off the posterior bladder wall. (C) Dissection is completed behind the bladder and in front of the vagina well below the fistula, which is defined by the catheter previously placed through it.

proceeds both bluntly and sharply, but usually sharp dissection is required. Establishment of the correct plane is greatly facilitated by dissecting along the taut anterior vaginal wall, which is readily palpable owing to the previously placed vaginal pack. According to the judgment of the surgeon, it may be easier to begin this dissection before opening the bladder. The dissection behind the bladder and in the front of the vagina is done until the fistula is entirely defined and a plane of at least a centimeter or two caudal to the fistula is established (Fig. 28-4).

The traditional approach for repairing a VVF or any other fistula has usually included wide excision of the fistulous tract to freshen the margins and remove all of the inflammatory and granulation tissue. I prefer to debride any inflammatory tissue and epithelium at the rim of the fistula sharply, but no attempt is made to excise the entire vesicle or vaginal sides of the fistulous tract for a particular distance (Fig. 28-5A). It is amazing how excision of a small fistulous tract can result in large openings in the bladder and vagina. Therefore the major advantage of avoiding wide excision is diminishing the size of the defects in each component of the

fistula. Other advantages include minimizing excessive bleeding from the freshly excised margins and possibly avoiding the need for ureteral reimplantation. In my hands, this method of handling the fistula margin has not compromised the outcome.

After the vaginal pack is removed, the vagina is usually closed in a transverse direction using 2–0 chromic catgut or Vicryl. The seromuscular layer of the bladder is closed from the posterior surface of the bladder, usually in an opposite longitudinal fashion to avoid apposing suture lines using interrupted 2–0 chromic catgut or Vicryl sutures. If the fistula is not too large

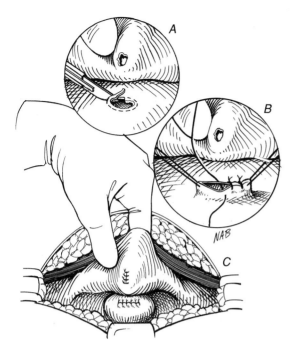

Figure 28-5. (A) Inflammatory, granulation, or indurated tissue at the rim of the fistula is sharply debrided for a short distance. (B) Vaginal component of the fistula is closed in a transverse direction. (C) Both components of the fistula are completely closed in opposite directions.

and the bladder is reasonably pliable, it is usually feasible to invert the initial bladder closure with a second layer of Lembert type sutures using 2–0 or 0 absorbable suture material. The mucosa of the bladder is closed from inside the bladder using a running 4–0 chromic catgut. It is by no means necessary always to close the bladder or vagina in a particular direction. Each component of the fistula is closed in a manner that the surgeon deems is easiest based on the size and location of the fistula or multiple fistulas, the proximity of the ureteral orifices, and the patient's individual anatomy (Fig. 28-5).

A peritoneal flap is usually established and interposed for a substantial distance over the vaginal closure. If there is any concern about the integrity of the closure or when dealing with

larger, more complex fistulas, an omental pedicle graft is used instead or in addition to the peritoneal flap (see Chap. 29). Another particularly valuable pedical material that can be used when repairing complex fistulas is the rectus abdominus muscle flap (Chap. 29).

Alternative Surgical Technique for Complex Vesicovaginal Fistulas

After anesthesia is induced, the patient is placed in the lithotomy position with the lower extremities strapped in adjustable foot restraints so the surgeon has access to both the abdomen and the vagina. I have found the Allen universal stirrups to be particularly valuable for maintaining the lithotomy position because of their ease in manipulation and the good support they provide to the lower extremities while still allowing access to each thigh if it is decided to use a gracilis muscle flap. It is also possible to use sequential compression devices when using the Allen stirrups, but only the knee-high devices are employed when contemplating using a gracilis flap. The vagina, perivaginal area, entire abdomen, and the upper portion of both lower extremities to below the knees are prepared with povidone-iodine, and the patient is draped to allow exposure of the suprapubic area, the vagina, and medial aspect of each thigh if it is decided to use a gracilis flap.

A lower abdominal midline incision is made. As described earlier, a transverse incision should be avoided because it may be necessary to extend this incision to gain adequate access to the upper abdomen to mobilize an omental flap. The procedure proceeds in an identical fashion as already described for the transvesical, transperitoneal approach, with some modifications depending on the choice of pedical material.

When establishing the plane between the vagina and the bladder, it is helpful for the surgeon to keep either the index and long fingers of the free hand or the hand of an assistant in the vagina to determine the exact location of the anterior vaginal wall. As already stated, a povidone-iodine–soaked pack inserted in the vagina can also be used to assist in identifying the anterior vaginal wall intraperitoneally. After an adequate plane is established between the vagina and bladder with the use of Metzenbaum scissors, the diseased necrotic tissue from the bladder and vaginal edges of the fistula is excised sharply, but for the reasons stated earlier, care is taken to avoid wide excision if at all possible. The one exception when adequate debridement of the diseased tissue at the edge of the fistula is imperative is during repair of a relatively acute radiation fistula, which is apt to be associated with poorly vascularized necrotic tissue.

Depending on the degree of inflammation or associated radiation-induced injury, the viability and strength of the tissue supporting the sutures, and the satisfaction of the repair that has already been completed, a decision is made regarding the type of pedicle material to interpose between the bladder and vagina. If there is any concern about the adequacy of repair or there is a high risk of recurrence as in radiation fistulas, a viable rectus abdominis or gracilis muscle flap is interposed between the bladder and vagina. The techniques for using the various muscle flaps are discussed in Chapter 29.

If a decision is made to interpose well-vascularized muscle between the bladder and vagina, my preference is to use a rectus abdominis flap if at all feasible (Fig. 28-6). When considering use of the rectus muscle for repair of a radiation-induced fistula, the surgeon should be confident that the rectus has not sustained associated radiation injury. Observation of the skin of the lower abdomen preoperatively might provide a clue about the vascular status of the rectus muscle. Advantages of employing a rectus flap instead of a gracilis flap include avoiding an incision and dissection in the thigh and the inferior dissection between the bladder and vagina, which may be difficult, particularly in radiation-induced fistulas. The rectus abdominis flap is particularly appealing if the fistula is not located inferior in the bladder base, making it difficult to fix the flap in place well below the fistula site in

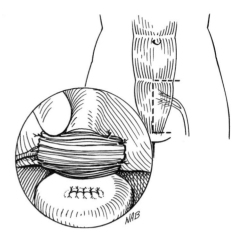

Figure 28-6. *Use of the rectus abdominis muscle flap to repair a vesicovaginal fistula. A segment of rectus muscle is mobilized on its blood supply from the inferior epigastric artery. The muscle flap is completely detached both superiorly and inferiorly at its attachment to the symphysis pubis to allow ample mobility to swing it into the pelvis. The muscle is delivered on its pedicle through a defect in the linea semilunaris. Inset shows muscle sutured in place to cover the repaired bladder component of the fistula.*

the bladder. Alternatively, it is relatively easy to suture a gracilis flap in place to cover an inferiorly positioned bladder defect.

Fleischmann and Picha described an abdominal approach for interposition of a gracilis muscle flap.[7] Dissection proceeds between the bladder and vagina caudal to the fistula under the contralateral ureter in the direction of the thigh of the donor gracilis muscle. Again it is helpful for the examiner to keep the examining fingers of the free hand in the vagina to define the anterior edge of the vagina. This dissection terminates near the bladder neck in a plane beneath the endopelvic fascia in the prevesicle space. The endopelvic fascia is incised anteriorly on the side of the donor thigh. This incision extends for several centimeters, which is large enough to admit the belly of the gracilis muscle. A plane is therefore established in the endopelvic fascia, which connects to the already established plane between the bladder and vagina where the gracilis muscle flap will sit (Fig. 28-7). After the gracilis muscle is mobilized, it is delivered through an opening in the urogenital diaphragm and passed through the opening in the endopelvic fascia to enter the space posterior to the bladder (Fig. 28-8). The muscle is properly positioned and affixed in place to the adjacent endopelvic fascia with a few interrupted 2–0 absorbable sutures. The distal end of the muscle is sutured in place on the bladder to cover the previously closed bladder side of the fistula completely[7] (Fig. 28-9). Both a gracilis muscle flap and omental flap may be interposed between the bladder and vagina, and it is even feasible to use two gracilis flaps from each thigh. Use of the omentum has the added advantage of helping absorb adjacent fluid collections that might accumulate in the pelvis.

After the repair of the fistula is completed, the ureteral stents are removed. A large Foley catheter is employed as a cystotomy tube, which is brought through a separate stab incision, and a urethral Foley catheter is also inserted. Generally a closed suction drain such as a Jackson-Pratt is placed in the space of Retzius and brought through a separate stab incision.

POSTOPERATIVE MANAGEMENT

Careful attention to fluid and electrolyte balance is maintained. Repair of more complex fistulas is often associated with a paralytic ileus. Nasogastric suction is usually employed until there is ample evidence of normal bowel activity. Parenteral antibiotics are continued for several days, and oral antibiotics are administered when the patient resumes a normal diet.

Sequential compression devices are used until the patient is ambulating well. For a standard uncomplicated VVF repair in which a gracilis flap is not employed, early ambulation is encouraged. If a gracilis flap is used, the lower extremity of the donor gracilis muscle is kept relatively adducted, and the bed is adjusted so the lower extremities are elevated with the hips flexed. The

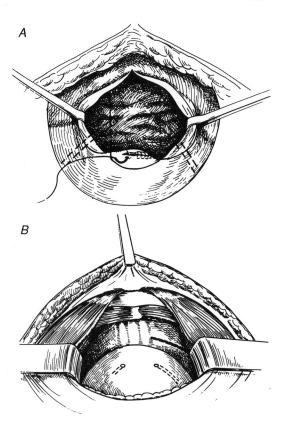

Figure 28-7. (A) After exposure of the fistula, the vaginal component of the fistula is closed. Dissection proceeds by creating a subvesical tunnel caudal to the fistula. (B) A tunnel is established between the bladder and vagina, which extends to the prevesical space through an incision in the endopelvic fascia. A parallel opening is also made in the urogenital diaphragm to admit delivery of the gracilis muscle into the pelvis. (From Fleischmann J, Picha G. Abdominal approach for gracilis muscle interposition and repair of recurrent vesicovaginal fistulas. J Urol 1987;140:552.)

patient is allowed to ambulate after a few days, but sitting in a chair is avoided to minimize the risk of venous stasis and subsequent venous thrombosis.

Drains are left in place until drainage is minimal. The urethral catheter is usually removed 5 to 7 days postoperatively. The patient is often

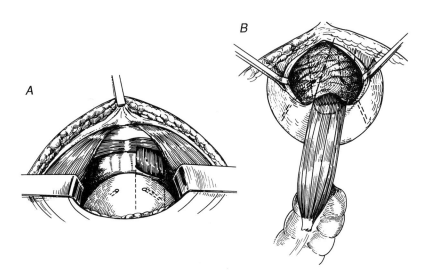

Figure 28-8. (A) The gracilis muscle is brought to a position behind the bladder by delivering it through the openings in the urogenital diaphragm and endopelvic fascia. (B) Gracilis muscle is in position behind the bladder interposed between the vaginal and bladder components of the fistula. (From Fleischmann J, Picha G. Abdominal approach of gracilis muscle interposition and repair of recurrent vesicovaginal fistulas. J Urol 1987;140:552.)

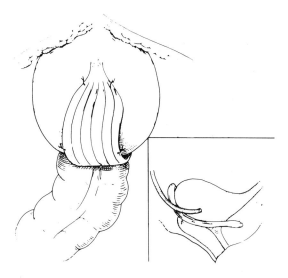

Figure 28-9. Gracilis muscle is sutured in place to bolster the vesicle closure. (From Fleischmann J, Picha G. Abdominal approach for gracilis muscle interposition and repair of recurrent vesicovaginal fistulas. J Urol 1987;140:552.)

discharged with the suprapubic cystostomy tube in place. For complex fistulas or following surgical correction of radiation-induced fistulas, the cystotomy tube is left in place for 2 to 3 weeks. Often a cystogram is obtained before removal of the cystostomy tube to verify the adequacy of repair.

RESULTS

Various results have been reported in the literature depending on the type of repair employed and the complexity of the VVF. Udeh reported an 86% success rate after the first operative attempt using a simple transvesical approach.[2] Using primarily a transvesical technique, Hedlund and Lindstedt reported 22 successful repairs in 24 patients who had no irradiation after the first operation, whereas a second operation was necessary in the two initial failures before the fistula was successfully closed.[8] Of the 14 patients treated by irradiation, 9 had primary healing after the first operation, and 2 required additional operations; there were 3 failures.[8]

In 1973, Persky and Rabin reported 100% success in 12 patients, using the basic transabdominal, transvesical, transperitoneal technique described in this chapter.[5] During the last 18 years at university hospitals of Cleveland and Case Western Reserve University, we have achieved 100% success rate in 20 patients who have undergone this approach that have not been associated with radiation therapy.

Gil-Vernet and associates reported 100% success in 42 consecutive patients using a transvesical approach with a posterior bladder wall flap covering the excised fistula.[6] The excellent results noted in this series suggests that greater use of this technique may be warranted. The technique presents a new procedure for vesical autoplasty that appears to be relatively uncomplicated. A flap is obtained from the posterior superior bladder wall that slides down to cover large lesions, even in low-capacity bladder reservoirs. Most of the patients in their series had complex VVFs that had been previously repaired unsuccessfully, and included were three patients with irradiation VVFs.[6]

In general, the overall cure rates using an abdominal approach are slightly lower than for vaginal repairs, but this is related to the fact that abdominal techniques are employed for more complicated, difficult fistulas and not because the procedure is less successful. Generally cure rates between 80% and 90% have been reported for the variously described abdominal techniques. The results are not nearly as good for radiation-induced VVFs, with the reported success being in the vicinity of 60%.

COMPLICATIONS

Stress urinary incontinence has been noted to develop following VVF repair owing to the development of hypermobility of the urethra. If a hypermobile urethra is observed during surgery or established during the surgical dissection, performing a urethropexy is a consideration. Other reported complications include a contracted bladder, bladder stones, ureteral injury, and prolonged paralytic ileus.

References

1. Landes RR. Simple transvesical repair of vesicovaginal fistula. J Urol 1979;122:604.
2. Udeh FN. Simple management of difficult vesicovaginal fistulae by the anterior transvesical approach. Int Urol Nephrol 1985;17:159.
3. Frang D, Jilling A. Techniques for surgical repair of vesicovaginal fistulae. Int Urol Nephrol 1983; 15:161.
4. O'Conor VJ. Review of experience with vesicovaginal fistula repair. J Urol 1980;123:367.
5. Persky L, Rabin R. Experience with vesicovaginal fistulas. Am J Surg 1973;125:763.
6. Gil-Vernet JM, Gil-Vernet A, Campos JA. New surgical approach for treatment of complex vesicovaginal fistula. J Urol 1989;141:513.
7. Fleischmann J, Picha G. Abdominal approach for gracilis muscle interposition and repair of recurrent vesicovaginal fistulas. J Urol 1988;140:552.
8. Hedlund H, Lindstedt E. Urovaginal fistulas: 20 years of experience with 45 cases. J Urol 1987; 137:926.

29

Use of Interposition Pedicle Material for Vesicovaginal Fistula Repair

Brian Windle

Elroy D. Kursh

Patients with complex, recurrent, or irradiation-induced vesicovaginal fistulas (VVFs) present particularly vexing surgical management problems. The persistence of incontinence after an attempted VVF repair leads to increasing anger and frustration for the patient as well as frustration for the physician. Large or multiple VVFs or fistulas associated with radiation therapy represent demanding surgical challenges with high failure rates. Therefore, when faced with any of these complicated fistulas, it is essential for the surgeon to employ a technique that maximizes the chance for a successful outcome, which invariably requires the interposition of fresh, well-vascularized tissue between the bladder and vagina after the fistula is closed.

A variety of tissues have been used to strengthen the repair and increase vascularity, including peritoneum, omentum, rectus abdominis muscle, gracilis muscle, and bulbocavernosus muscle and fat pad. Although other muscles have been used for interposition pedicle material, the aforementioned tissues are most accessible and employed most often. This chapter describes the use of these more commonly employed pedicle materials and the advantages and disadvantages of each.

Preoperative Preparation

Whatever approach the surgeon chooses, careful attention to preoperative preparation is essential. A mechanical and antibiotic bowel preparation is advisable, particularly when using an abdominal approach because it is often necessary to lyse a significant number of adhesions to gain adequate exposure of the pelvis. If the bowel is inadvertently entered, it can be closed with little or no increased risk of infection. Care is taken to ensure sterilization of the urine before entering the hospital. Additionally, broad-spectrum parenteral antibiotic coverage is started preoperatively. It is also advisable to administer a povidone-iodine douche the night before surgery.

PERITONEAL FLAPS

Peritoneal flaps are frequently employed when using the abdominal approach. Because the peritoneum is readily accessible, it is relatively easy to design a variety of flaps, based on a wide pedicle, that can be rotated between the bladder and vagina. Two peritoneal flaps can even be used by rotating separate flaps from each side of the abdomen.

393

Female Urology, edited by Elroy D. Kursh and Edward McGuire. J. B. Lippincott, Philadelphia, © 1994.

Peritoneal flaps provide tissue that can be placed between each component of the fistula, but they are not particularly vascular and add little to promote healing of a structure that may already have compromised vascularity.

Little and associates have also described the use of a peritoneal flap when using the vaginal approach for fistula closure.[1] The dissection of the posterior vaginal flap is extended to the peritoneal reflection, and the peritoneum is freed from adhesions to the posterior bladder wall. After completion of the two initial layers of fistula closure, the fistula and perivesical fascia, the peritoneum is advanced to cover the repair. After the peritoneal flap is sutured in place, the last layer to be closed is the vaginal wall flap, which covers the entire area.

MARTIUS FLAP

The use of the bulbocavernosus muscle and fat pad was described by Martius in the late 1920s, but this technique was not introduced into the United States until the American translation of Martius' work in 1957.[2] Not only has this flap been used extensively to repair VVFs, but also it has been used for rectovaginal fistulas, urethral vaginal fistulas, sloughed urethras, rectal strictures, and radiation-induced fistulas.[3–7]

Today most surgeons use the labial fat pad alone without going to the extent of dissecting out the bulbocavernosus muscle as initially described. Elkins and associates reported anatomic studies in a cadaver demonstrating that the standard Martius graft is composed of fibroadipose tissue from the labia majora and not from the bulbocavernosus muscle.[8]

Elkins and associates also demonstrated the anatomic dissection planes. The graft tissue itself represents an elongated band of adipose tissue. After the initial incision, the superficial fibrous layer is mobilized from the undersurface of the skin. The lateral border of the dissection is the labiocrural fold, where a sheet of fibrous tissue attaches the skin of the fold to the ischiopubic ramus and the fascia lata. The medial plane of the dissection separates the adipose layer from the fascia covering the inner aspect of the labia minora, bulbocavernosus muscle, and vestibular bulb. The deep portion of the dissection follows the deep fascia (Colles' fascia), over the urogenital diaphragm. Lying within the adipose layer are terminal fibers of the round ligament of the uterus, although these fibers are not prominent. The superficial fibrous layer, which is similar to the dartos layer of the scrotum, lends further strength to the graft.[8]

This precise anatomic dissection also included the injection of latex to help identify the arterial supply of the graft. The bulbocavernosus fat pad has a rich blood supply coming from several directions. Posteriorly and inferiorly the graft is supplied by the posterior labial branches of the internal pudendal artery and vein. Anteriorly and superiorly a branch of the external pudendal vessels proceeds medially from its origin at the femoral vessels to enter the anterior lateral aspect of the graft. Laterally branches of the obturator vessels, which are transected during mobilization, also supply the graft. Within the fibrofatty tissue is a rich capillary network that is contiguous with the capillary blood supply of the subcutaneous tissue of the mons pubis.[8] The dual blood supply of the fat pad from the external pudendal anteriorly and the internal pudendal posteriorly allows the surgeon the prerogative of basing the graft either anteriorly or posteriorly depending on the individual patient's anatomy and the site of the fistula.

A vertical incision is made over the labia majora (Fig. 29-1). The fibrofatty bulbocavernosus fat pad is separated from adjacent structures using blunt and sharp dissection. The flap is usually based posteriorly, necessitating transecting the graft anteriorly and ligating the branches of the external pudendal artery and vein (Fig. 29-2). A tunnel is established beneath the labia minora and vaginal mucosa, and the graft is rotated underneath the tunnel to overlay the previously closed fistula site (Fig. 29-3). The fat pad is affixed in place using four corner stay sutures of 2−0 absorbable suture. If at all possible, the vagina is closed over the graft with a running absorbable suture. The graft space is

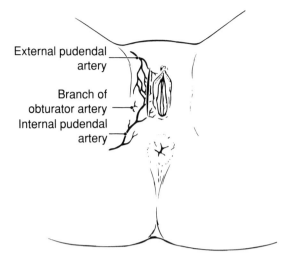

External pudendal artery

Branch of obturator artery

Internal pudendal artery

Figure 29-1. A vertical incision is made over the right labia majora. The dual major blood supply (internal and external pudendal arteries) and the less important lateral blood supply from branches of the obturator are demonstrated. (From Elkins TE, Delancey JOL, McGuire EJ. The use of modified martius graft as an adjunctive technique in vesicovaginal and rectovaginal fistula repair. Obstet Gynecol 1990;75:727.)

usually drained with either a Penrose drain or closed suction type of drain through a separate stab incision site, unless the graft bed is very dry. The labial incision is closed in a routine manner.

Most descriptions today differ from that of Martius' original one in which he employed the bulbocavernosus muscle itself. Use of the muscle requires a deeper dissection and is more likely to cause hemorrhage, which at times may be severe. The described technique is not only simpler and associated with much less bleeding, but also appears to be equally effective in bringing well-vascularized tissue over the fistula site. The blood supply of the graft is good, and the prominence of fibrous septa from the round ligament within the graft adds sufficient strength to afford rotation.[8]

Elkins and associates emphasize the following important observations: (1) It is possible to extend the graft dissection onto the mons pubis to obtain sufficient graft length to reach fistulous spaces at the apex of the vagina, which is the common site after hysterectomy, and (2) the graft readily forms granulation tissue and allows healing by secondary intention so it is not always necessary to close the vaginal mucosa over the fat pad. Disadvantages to leaving the vaginal incision open include a higher incidence of infection and vaginal scar formation and stricture. It is also stressed that use of the Martius flap is an adjunct to surgical repair and not curative for a fistula that cannot be closed completely because the fat pad is not capable of inducing closure of an incompletely closed fistula space, a fistula closed under tension, or one closed with non-viable tissue.[8]

Modifications of the Martius technique include use of a full-thickness island graft from the labia majora over an incompletely closed fistula.[9] Use of a full-thickness graft involving parts of both the labia minora and the labia majora has also been described.[10]

Excellent results have been reported using the Martius technique. Elkins and associates observed a 96% success rate in 25 patients who underwent repair of nonradiation-induced VVFs. In their series of five patients with radiation-induced fistulas, all were repaired successfully with the Martius technique.[8] Boronow reported a 50% success rate with this approach for VVFs and 84.2% success rate for rectovaginal fistulas.[7]

Complications attributed to the technique have generally been minimal. Blood loss is rarely more than a few hundred milliliters. Cellulitis associated with the graft has been noted in a small number of patients. Other complications include vaginal scarring and stricture formation, which may be severe enough to cause near obliteration of the vagina in some instances. Dyspareunia has also been observed.[8]

OMENTUM FLAPS

The omentum represents a valuable form of interposition pedicle material to be used in a variety of ways in the urinary tract, including closure of VVFs. The omentum appears to have unique properties that assist in the resolution of intra-

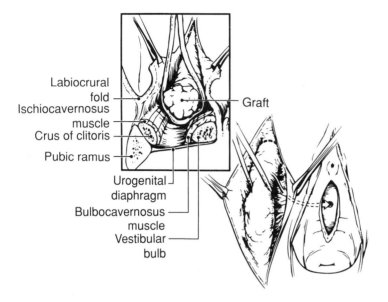

Labiocrural fold
Ischiocavernosus muscle
Crus of clitoris
Pubic ramus
Graft
Urogenital diaphragm
Bulbocavernosus muscle
Vestibular bulb

Figure 29-2. The bulbocavernosus fat pad is mobilized. Because most Martius flaps are based posteriorly, as depicted here, the graft is transected anteriorly after ligating the branches of the external pudendal artery and vein. (Inset) Anatomic structures adjacent to the graft. (From Elkins TE, Delancey JOL, McGuire EJ. The use of modified martius graft as an adjunctive technique in vesicovaginal and rectovaginal fistula repair. Obstet Gynecol 1990;75:727.)

abdominal infected processes while regaining its suppleness as healing is taking place.[11]

The healing potential of the omentum is derived from a combination of its blood supply and lymphatic drainage. Even though the omentum may not be particularly vascular in its resting state, it appears to have great potential to form neovascularity rapidly in response to inflammation. The omentum also represents the main site of lymphatic absorption in the abdominal cavity.[11] These properties enhance its value as pedicle material for correction of VVFs.

The omentum can be employed when using an abdominal approach for VVF repair or a combined abdominal and vaginal approach. If the surgeon contemplates using omentum, a longitudinal midline abdominal incision is made, which can be extended to the upper abdomen if

necessary to expose and mobilize the omentum sufficiently.

Depending on the individual's anatomy, a variety of omental flaps can be mobilized to gain adequate access to the pelvis.[12] The omental arterial supply comes from the right gastroepiploic artery, which is a branch of the gastroduodenal artery and the left gastroepiploic artery, a branch of the splenic artery (Fig. 29-4). The right and left omental arteries extend down their corresponding sides of the omentum, and there is a variable middle omental artery[12] (Fig. 29-5).

If the patient has a long omentum, an inverted L-shaped incision can be made in the omentum close to the transverse colon, basing the omental flap on either the right or left omental arteries (Fig. 29-6). If the omentum is short, it is necessary to mobilize the omentum from the

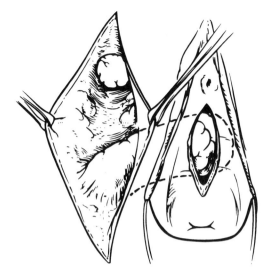

Figure 29-3. A tunnel is established beneath the labia minora and vaginal mucosa, and the graft is rotated medially to overlay the closed fistula site. (From Elkins TE, Delancey JOL, McGuire EJ. The use of modified martius graft as an adjunctive technique in vesicovaginal and rectovaginal fistula repair. Obstet Gynecol 1990;75:727.)

transverse colon and make the inverted L-shaped incision close to the stomach to gain sufficient omental length to reach the pelvis[12] (Fig. 29-7). This maneuver invariably requires extending the abdominal incision. Supposedly the right gastroepiploic artery is larger than the left in most patients. Therefore, it is preferable to base most omental flaps on the right gastroepiploic artery and its corresponding right omental artery.

Once the omental pedicle graft is established, it can be used in a variety of ways. After the bladder and vaginal sides of the fistula are repaired, it can be tacked into the pelvis between the vagina and bladder with several absorbable sutures. Whatever method one uses to repair the VVF, care should be taken to mobilize the bladder a centimeter or two below the fistula so the omentum can be tacked well below the bladder opening. The omentum should be fanned out as wide as conveniently possible to cover the fistulous area completely for a maximum distance. Additionally, in some instances, it is advisable to suture the omentum to the abdominal wall to

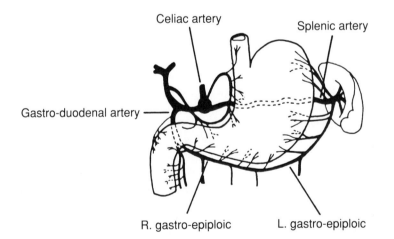

Figure 29-4. The origins of the right and left gastroepiploic arteries from which the omental blood supply arises. (From Petty WM, Lowy RO, Oyama AA. Total abdominal hysterectomy after radiation therapy for cervical cancer: Use of omental graft for fistula prevention. Am J Obstet Gynecol 1986; 154:1222.)

Normal length omentum

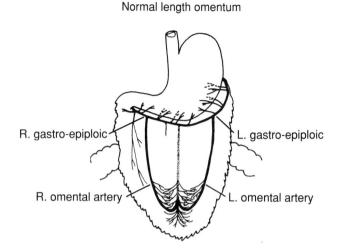

R. gastro-epiploic

L. gastro-epiploic

R. omental artery

L. omental artery

Figure 29-5. The right and left omental arteries represent the major blood supply of the omentum on which to design or base an omental flap. There is also a variable middle omental artery and a small accessory omental artery shown lateral to the right omental artery. (From Petty WM, Lowy RO, Oyama AA. Total abdominal hysterectomy after radiation therapy for cervical cancer: Use of omental graft for fistula prevention. Am J Obstet Gynecol 1986;154:1222.)

prevent torsion of the omentum after the abdomen is closed.

When using omentum during a combined abdominal and vaginal approach, the surgeon has a variety of options. The omentum can be fed into the vagina, where it is widely and loosely spread over the fistula, and sutured in position to the anterior and posterior margins of the vaginal dissection.[13] Alternately, the graft can be sutured between the bladder and vagina as described earlier.

An important role of omentum is its ability to serve as a framework for formation of new tissue. Experimentally in the rabbit bladder, rapid and complete regeneration of bladder epithelium has been noted when the bladder defect was plugged with an omental flap. The new epithelium on the periphery of the defect appeared to result not only from extension of bladder epithelium, but also from multipotential mesenchymal cells in the omentum. The formation of muscle bundles in the omentum was also demonstrated.[14]

In 52 patients in whom omentum was employed using an abdominoperineal approach, there were only 2 patients that had persistent incontinence, one of whom had stress incontinence that refused further operation.[13] Omentum has also been employed as a prophylactic measure to prevent fistula formation in patients who underwent total abdominal hysterectomy after radiation therapy for cervical cancer. No patients developed a VVF when this approach was used in a small series of five patients in this high-risk category.[12]

There are no particular complications associated with the use of omentum. When an abdominoperineal approach was used, one patient

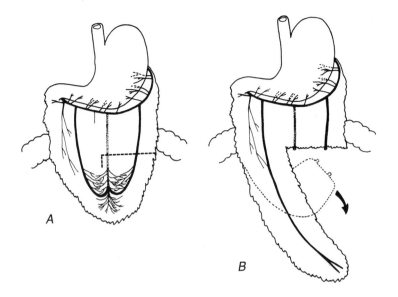

Figure 29-6. (A) If the patient has a normal length omentum, the omental flap is configured by making an L-shaped incision below the transverse colon. In this instance, the flap is based on the right omental artery, but either omental artery can be used. (B) The mobilized omental graft is rotated into the pelvis. (From Petty WM, Lowy RO, Oyama AA. Total abdominal hysterectomy after radiation therapy for cervical cancer: Use of omental graft for fistula prevention. Am J Obstet Gynecol 1986;154:1222.)

experienced a significant small bowel prolapse through the vagina.[13] Fortunately, the bowel was viable, and it was feasible to pull it back into the abdomen and repair the vaginal defect.

RECTUS ABDOMINIS MUSCLE FLAP

The rectus abdominis muscle is an excellent choice of tissue for repairing a number of pelvic defects, and when dealing with difficult VVFs, it may be the premier tissue. In general, muscle is extremely pliable, making it easy to work with. Well-vascularized muscle tissue is ideally suited for a number of reconstructive problems because it facilitates healing in the scarred areas that are being reconstructed and aids in biologic debridement.

The anatomy of the rectus abdominis has been well described.[15] The muscles are generally regarded as the abdominal flexors as well as the anterior stabilizers of the spine. The origin of each muscle extends from the apex of the costal margin laterally across the fifth, sixth, and seventh costal cartilages and arises just below the origin of the pectoralis muscle. The anterior fascia of the two muscles, the pectoralis and the rectus, are, in essence, contiguous. The tendinous insertion of the muscle is the medial aspect of the pubic rim. The rectus abdominis muscle is encased in a sheath consisting of the anterior and posterior rectus fascia. This fascia comes together in the midline to form the linea alba and laterally, where it then divides again to form the aponeurosis of the external oblique, internal oblique, and transverse abdominis muscles. There are three to four tendinous inscriptions within the muscle that result in segmentation of

Short omentum

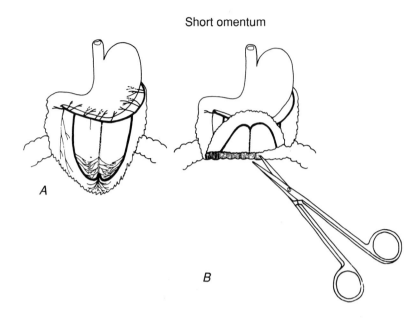

Figure 29-7. (A) Patient with a short omentum. (B) To gain sufficient length, it is necessary to dissect the omentum off the transverse colon before making the L-shaped incision below the stomach. (From Petty WM, Lowy RO, Oyama AA. Total abdominal hysterectomy after radiation therapy for cervical cancer: Use of omental graft for fistula prevention. Am J Obstet Gynecol 1986;154:1222.)

this long, straplike muscle. This segmentation increases the efficiency of muscle flexion.

The blood supply of the rectus muscle comes from three sources. Superiorly it is supplied by the superior epigastric artery, which is an extension of the internal mammary artery. The superior epigastric artery enters the muscle medially before fanning out under the upper one third of the muscle. Inferiorly the inferior epigastric artery originates from the external iliac artery and then passes medially through the transversalis fascia and into the rectus sheath. Encased in a fat pad, the artery proceeds medially and superiorly just above the posterior rectus sheath, entering the muscle from behind in the middle of the lower one third of the muscle. Segmental vessels represent the third source of blood to the muscle. These vessels, which accompany the segmental

motor nerves for the muscle (branches of the 7th to 12th spinal nerves), enter the rectus sheath laterally and pass underneath the lateral border of the rectus muscle and enter it posteriorly.

The venous drainage of the rectus abdominis muscle is by way of a large venae comitantes (paired veins on either side of each artery) that run with the superior and inferior epigastric arteries as well as the segmental vessels.

The rectus abdominis muscle is an excellent choice of tissue to interpose between the bladder and the vagina when repairing a VVF. This muscle can easily be dissected free from its bed and transected at its insertion on the symphysis. It can then be divided at any point at or above the umbilicus, leaving it attached to its lower pedicle, the inferior epigastric artery and veins. From its branching point off the iliac vessels, the muscle and its pedicle have a 360-degree arc of rotation that allows the muscle to reach any place in the pelvis.[16]

In the repair of VVFs, it is usually advisable to employ a midline incision. Therefore, access to the rectus abdominis muscle is accomplished by dissecting through the medial border of the rectus fascia. The anterior rectus fascia is elevated off the muscle, usually for about the lower two thirds of the length of the muscle (from above the umbilicus down to the symphysis). A similar dissection is carried out at the level of the posterior rectus sheath. In the area of the tendinous inscriptions, the dissection needs to be meticulous because the muscle is especially adherent to the anterior rectus sheath in these areas. Damage to this area can result in devascularization of distant muscle segments. Leaving the entire anterior rectus sheath intact and in continuity with overlying subcutaneous tissue and skin aids in both closure of the midline wound and preservation of the blood supply to the overlying tissue. Once the dissection of the rectus muscle has been completed to the lateral border, it can be divided superiorly and at the tendinous insertion on the pubic rim inferiorly. By lifting the muscle up, the inferior epigastric artery and associated veins are readily apparent. These vessels represent the vascular pedicle, which can be dissected out all the way to the external iliac vessels. Care should be taken to ligate the small branches that come off the pedicle as dissection progresses to the iliac vessels. Laterally along the course of the muscle the segmental arteries and nerves should be divided. This completely frees up the muscle and a complete vascular island flap based on one vascular pedicle, the inferior epigastric (Fig. 29-8).

A vertical 5- to 6-cm incision is made in the most lateral aspect of the posterior rectus sheath in the area where the inferior epigastric artery takes off from the iliac artery. This incision is carried through the peritoneum, and the muscle is passed through it into the abdominal cavity. The posterior rectus fascia is then repaired, leaving a small 1-cm opening for the pedicle. This hole should not be made so small that it will

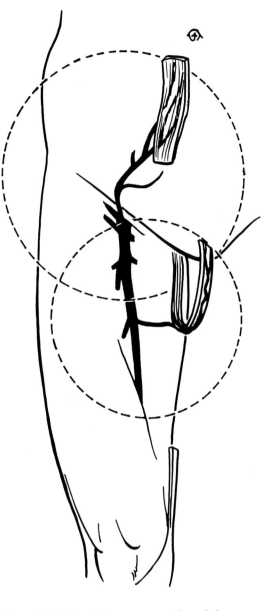

Figure 29-8. *Both the rectus muscle and the gracilis muscle, isolated on their respective pedicles, are illustrated. The wide arc of rotation of the gracilis muscle, the center of which is approximately 10 centimeters below the pubic bone, is also shown.*

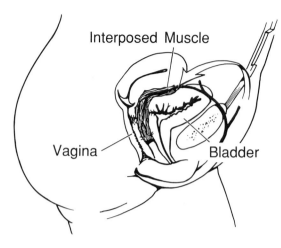

Interposed Muscle

Vagina

Bladder

Figure 29-9. A segment of rectus muscle isolated on the inferior epigastric vessel has been rotated down into the pelvis and interposed between the repaired bladder and vagina.

constrict the pedicle but also not so large that there is a possibility for a hernia.

The surgeon now has an excellent unit of highly vascularized tissue in the abdomen that can be passed down behind the bladder and sutured in between the repaired vagina and bladder to serve as interposition pedicle material (Fig. 29-9). The wide, thin nature of this muscle makes it ideally suited for this purpose. Closure of the incision in the rectus fascia can be performed either separately or incorporated into the midline abdominal wound closure.

It does not really matter whether the surgeon chooses to use either the left or right rectus muscles for this procedure. Obviously a muscle that has been operated through for any reason, such as a colostomy, should be spared and the opposite muscle used. If there is a history of an inguinal hernia repair on one side, it is suggested that the opposite side be used, although the inferior epigastric vessel is not commonly transected during herniorrhaphy.

Some of the advantages of using this muscle for repair of VVFs include minimal donor site morbidity, gravity tends to keep the tissue well

down in the lower portion of the pelvis because the muscle is delivered from above, and the muscle is in close proximity to the repair site. We have used this muscle in seven cases, all with excellent results. Menchaca and associates has reported three cases with successful repairs using the rectus abdominis muscle.[17] The long-term complications that might be expected are either an abdominal wall laxity in the area of rectus muscle sacrifice or a frank hernia. These complications, however, have not been observed to date.

The rectus abdominis muscle is an excellent muscle for reconstruction of VVFs. It is well vascularized, and its wide, relatively thin configuration makes it ideal for interposition between the bladder and vagina. There is minimal donor site morbidity, and the tissue is readily available. As Horton and colleagues state, it is a robust flap ideally suited for reinforcing both bladder and vaginal walls after repair.[18]

GRACILIS MUSCLE AND MYOCUTANEOUS FLAPS

The gracilis and its overlying fasciocutaneous tissues were once popular and frequently used for vaginal reconstruction and as interposition pedicle material for VVFs using a vaginal approach.[19] The gracilis muscle is a thin muscle in the medial aspect of the thigh. It takes its origin from the pubic tubercle of the pelvic rim and has a wide, flat muscle belly extending down for some 15 to 20 cm until it thins to form the gracilis tendon. The tendon inserts into the pes anserinus or "goose foot" tendon of the medial knee, which is attached to the medial aspect of the tibial plateau.

The muscle is innervated by a branch of the obturator nerve, whereas the blood supply comes from three sources. The first is the major pedicle, which is a branch of the profunda femoris. This vessel travels medially and posteriorly in a horizontal fashion underneath the adductor longus and enters the gracilis on its anterolateral side, 10 cm below the pubic rim. There are two to three other minor pedicles, branches of the femoral vessels superiorly and the saphenous artery inferiorly, which enter into the muscle further down on its belly. The third source of blood is from small vessels that accompany Sharpe's fibers at the origin of the muscle along the pubic rim.

The muscle gives two to three fasciocutaneous perforators from its belly, through the fascia to the overlying subcutaneous tissue and skin. This represents the blood supply for the cutaneous portion of a myocutaneous gracilis flap. Because there are only two to three fasciocutaneous perforators from the muscle, extra caution must be taken when planning to incorporate the overlying skin paddle into the flap to ensure that it is centered right over the muscle.

A common mistake is errant positioning of the skin incision for harvesting the gracilis muscle. When muscle alone is to be transferred, the incision should be over the middle of the muscle belly. With the patient's legs in the frog-leg position, a line drawn from the medial hamstring up to the medial pubic rim places the incision directly over the muscle body. This line should sag slightly, as does the muscle when the patient is positioned in this manner. When designing a myocutaneous flap, a skin paddle can be marked over top the body of the muscle that measures approximately 10×5 cm in an ellipse.

Mobilization of this muscle is initiated by dissecting down through the fascia. If a myocutaneous flap is to be elevated, the dissection on the anteromedial side should include the fascia and the septum that lies just anterior to the muscle itself, where at least two or three more perforators come up into the skin. Inclusion of these vessels increases the chances of having a viable skin flap or paddle. Dissection usually proceeds from inferior to superior by first isolating the tendon and transecting it. Thus, the muscle and overlying fasciocutaneous tissue, if it is being dissected with the muscle, can be elevated as a single unit. As one moves superiorly, it is advised that dissection be carried out higher on the posterior aspect until approximately 10 cm below the pubic rim, where there is often a small sentinel vessel entering the muscle opposite to the

main or major pedicle coming in anteriorly, which signals the entrance of the major pedicle. Once the major pedicle is visualized, the vascular pedicle is mobilized by dissection toward the femoral vessels. After the pedicle is free, a decision whether or not to transect the origin of the muscle must be made. The pedicle can vary in size. If it is thought to be sufficient to supply the muscle with blood adequately, the origin can be divided. This division of the origin facilitates a 180-degree rotation of the muscle to deliver the needed tissue to the reconstruction site in the perineum (see Fig. 29-8).

For the VVF repair being performed through the vagina, there is a ready-made incision for insertion of this flap to be interposed between the bladder and vagina. If the repair has been done through an abdominal approach, a labial incision is necessary to create a submucosal tunnel between the repair site and labial incision. Another tunnel from the labial incision down to the gracilis dissection site is also developed. These tunnels should be wide enough to facilitate unrestricted passage of the gracilis muscle along with the overlying subcutaneous tissue and skin, if it is included. In VVF repair, a skin paddle is not usually included, but if it is desired, it should be de-epithelialized to be completely buried up and around the vagina.

We have used this flap 12 times in 11 patients. One patient had a large, low fistula in which the first gracilis failed likely as a result of inadequate size after transfer, and a second procedure was required to achieve closure. A rectus abdominis muscle reconstruction was considered but was not an option owing to multiple prior abdominal procedures. In one instance, the procedure failed.

Ryan and associates have reported the use of this flap with good results; however, the reconstructions reported were generally low defects.[20] For the difficult higher fistulas, the gracilis muscle does not provide much tissue, which was undoubtedly the cause of our one failure.

The gracilis muscle has fallen out of favor for pelvic reconstruction because problems are inherent with its anatomy. It is limited at the 10-cm mark from the pubic rim, where the major pedicle enters. When the muscle is turned superiorly from this point, it is rare that there is enough length or bulk to interpose adequately between the two components of a VVF and get good coverage. The gracilis myocutaneous flap has a tenuous blood supply and is somewhat bulky. Because it is often necessary to maintain the origin of the muscle at the pubic rim intact owing to an inadequate major pedicle, the arc of rotation is severely limited, further hampering delivery of quality tissue to the reconstruction site.

FASCIOCUTANEOUS FLAPS

A much better alternative to the gracilis flap is a fasciocutaneous flap, with the base of the flap being centered between the vagina and the anus. This flap is essentially a finger of tissue with an 8-cm base running down the medial thigh. The length can be up to 30 cm. Because this flap is elevated in the subfascial plane, it includes the same tissue one would include in a gracilis flap. This long, thin flap, which is composed of subcutaneous tissue, fascia, and skin, is fairly well vascularized and has a rotation point just behind or beside the vagina. Therefore, the flap can be turned up into the vaginal area and de-epithelialized to reconstruct a number of areas. The donor site is often closed primarily. A major problem with this flap is that it leaves a redundant dog ear of tissue in the groin, at the point of rotation, which requires secondary revision. It is, however, much more reliable than a gracilis flap and can provide more soft tissue for interposition between the bladder and the vagina at a much higher level.

We have not used this flap for VVF repair but have employed it many times for a variety of perineal defects, including vaginal reconstruction. The main complication is the resultant dog ear from the rotation at its base. This has been easily dealt with by a secondary revision.

There are a number of other designs for fasciocutaneous flaps from the thigh. One is the posterior thigh flap, which can also be used for transposing tissue into the vaginal area. These flaps are more commonly used for repair of decubitus ulcers and other defects requiring reconstruction. None of them offer any advantages over either a medial thigh fasciocutaneous flap or a gracilis flap, as noted by Nahai.[19]

Summary

Complex VVFs, such as recurrent fistulas or those following radiation therapy, are particularly challenging surgical problems that generally require well-vascularized interposition pedicle material. The interposed tissue provides a seal that heals in place and helps achieve lasting repair.

Substantial scar tissue may be present in VVFs owing to the patient's propensity to form scar tissue around such deformities as fistulas, and multiple repairs and irradiation increase the likelihood of scar tissue. Scar tissue is associated with a general lack of stem cells that help promote good healing. Not only does fresh, well-vascularized tissue provide stem cells, but also it improves the blood supply of the poorly vascularized scar tissue. Additionally, the high vascularity of these tissues allows delivery of antibiotics and the components required for biologic debridement of the area.[21]

In our opinion, when the surgeon uses the vaginal approach to VVF repair, the Martius flap represents the preferred choice of pedicle material. When we use an abdominal approach, we prefer an omental flap for less complex fistulas and generally employ a rectus flap for complex recurrent or radiation-induced fistulas. It is also our opinion that flaps, such as the gracilis or medial thigh fasciocutaneous flap, are less than optimal and should be considered only as a last resort.

References

1. Little NA, Juma S, Raz S. Vesicovaginal fistulae. Semin Urol 1989;7:78.
2. McCall ML, Bolton KA, eds, transl. Martius'

Gynecological Operations: With Emphasis on Topographic Anatomy. Boston: Little, Brown, 1957:322.

3. Hibbart LT. Surgical management of rectovaginal fistulas and complete perineal tears. Am J Obstet Gynecol 1978;130:139.
4. Webster GD, Sihelnick SA, Stone AR. Urethrovaginal fistula: A review of the surgical management. J Urol 1984;132:460.
5. Morgan JE, Farrow GA, Sims RH. The sloughed urethra syndrome. Am J Obstet Gynecol 1978; 130:521.
6. Patchell RD, Bradford B. Transvaginal repair of rectal stricture utilizing martius bulbocavernosus pedicle graft. W Virg Med J 1977;73:124.
7. Boronow RC. Repair of radiation-induced vaginal fistula utilizing the martius technique. World J Surg 1986;10:237.
8. Elkins TE, DeLancey JOL, McGuire EJ. The use of modified martius graft as an adjunctive technique in vesicovaginal and rectovaginal fistula repair. Obstet Gynecol 1990;75:727.
9. Hoskins WJ, Park RC, Long R, et al. Repair of urinary tract fistulas with bulbocavernosus myocutaneous flaps. Obstet Gynecol 1984;63:588.
10. Symmonds RE, Hill LM. Loss of urethra: A report on 50 patients. Am J Obstet Gynecol 1978; 130:130.
11. Turner-Warwick R. The use of the omental pedicle graft in urinary tract reconstruction. J Urol 1976;116:341.
12. Petty WM, Lowy RO, Oyama AA. Total abdominal hysterectomy after radiation therapy for cervical cancer: Use of omental graft for fistula prevention. Am J Obstet Gynecol 1986;154:1222.
13. Orford HJL, Theron JLL. Repair of vesicovaginal fistulas with omentum. S Afr Med J 1985; 67:143.
14. Goldstein MB, Deardon FC. Histology of omentalplasty of the urinary bladder in the rabbit. Invest Urol 1966;3:460.
15. Mathes SJ, Nahai F. Clinical Atlas of Muscle and Musculocutaneous Flaps. St. Louis: CV Mosby, 1979:347.
16. McCraw JB, Arnold PG. McCraw and Arnold's Atlas of Muscle and Myocutaneous Flaps. Norfolk: Hampton Press, 1986.
17. Menchaca A, Akhyat M, Gleicher N, et al.: The rectus abdominis muscle flap in combined abdominovaginal repair in difficult vesicovaginal fistula. J Reprod Med 1990;35:565.
18. Horton CE, Sadove RC, McCraw JB. In: McCarthy J, ed. Reconstruction of female genital defects. Plastic surgery. Vol 6. Philadelphia: WB Saunders, 1990:4210.
19. Nahai F. Muscle and musculocutaneous flaps in gynecologic surgery. Clin Obstet Gynecol 1981; 24:1277.
20. Ryan JA, Gibbons RP, Correa RJ. Urologic use of gracilis muscle flap for nonhealing perineal wounds and fistulas. Urology 1985;26:456.
21. Taylor GI, Corlett RJ. The vascular territories of the body and their relation to tissue transfer. Plast Surg Forum 1981;4:113.

30

Radiation-Induced Vesicovaginal Fistulas

Christopher C. Fitzpatrick

Thomas E. Elkins

Incidence and Etiology

Vesicovaginal fistula formation represents the most serious form of radiation injury to the bladder and occurs in 0.5% to 2% of patients being treated for cervical cancer.[1-6] The overall incidence of serious bladder injury is 3% to 5%.[4,7-9] Fistulas also occur after radiotherapy for uterine cancer and other pelvic malignancies. External beam treatment is rarely responsible for fistula formation; the major cause is intracavitary radium. Although these fistulas are relatively uncommon, accounting for only 6% of all fistulas seen in one large series from the Mayo Clinic, they are notoriously difficult to treat, given the compromised nature of postirradiation tissues.[10] Hysterectomy following radiotherapy, particularly Wertheim's hysterectomy, significantly increases the risk of fistula formation.[4,11]

The majority of fistulas present within 1 to 3 years after treatment; they may, however, present after considerably longer intervals.[2,12] Up to 18% of radiation-induced bladder injuries present after 5 years; vesicovaginal fistula formation has been reported after 10, 19, and 28 years.[2,13,14] Presentation within 1 year is strongly associated with bladder invasion before treatment and recurrence of malignancy after treatment.[12]

The therapeutic effect of radiotherapy depends on the increased sensitivity of cancer cells to ionizing radiation and the ability of normal tissues to recover from injury. Optimum effectiveness requires a healthy microcirculation and effective cellular oxygenation. The dose of radiation required to treat pelvic malignancies often approximates the toxic dose to local tissues. In general, a total dose of 7000 rad is required for the treatment of cervical and uterine cancer. Although most bladders tolerate 6500 to 7000 rad over a period of 5 to 6 weeks, with morphologic changes appearing at approximately 8000 rad, there is no consistent relationship between the measured bladder dose and eventual fistula formation.[12,15] In a study of 500 patients with cervical cancer, Kottmeier and Gray reported a direct correlation between measured bladder and rectal radiation doses and subsequent complications.[16] In a similar study, Peckham and associates found no such correlation.[3] Lee and associates concluded that the dose rate rather than the treatment time is a critical factor in relation to tissue injury.[17] Hemorrhagic cystitis, vaginal vault necrosis, parametritis, previous pelvic inflammatory disease as well as malnutrition, hypertension, diabetes mellitus, occlusive vascular disease, and trauma appear to increase the risk of fistula formation in some patients.[5,9,14,18-20] In addition, individual variations in vaginal anatomy may distort the geometry of radium administration.[12]

Female Urology, edited by Elroy D. Kursh and Edward McGuire. J. B. Lippincott, Philadelphia, © 1994.

Histopathology

In 1933, Dean defined three phases of bladder response to radiotherapy: acute, subacute, and chronic.[21] The acute phase of injury usually commences 3 to 6 weeks after the start of treatment, subacute changes becoming evident at 6 months to 2 years.[12] The acute histologic findings include dilation and congestion of submucosal capillaries leading to submucosal and mucosal edema.[22] This is followed by degenerative epithelial cell changes characterized by cytoplasmic vacuolation and nuclear pyknosis. Perivascular lymphocytic cuffing and mucosal hemorrhage subsequently become evident. Epithelial inflammatory changes together with microcyst formation and syncytial clusters give way to desquamation and eventual ulceration. Focal vacuolar and hyaline changes are also noted in the muscularis.[22,23] Subacute changes include varying degrees of muscle fibrosis in addition to the persistence of acute changes and evidence of tissue recovery. At no time is there an absence of radiation-induced changes in exposed tissues, although a histologic steady state is usually reached after an interval of years.[14] Chronic vascular changes include proliferation and ectasia of capillaries in addition to obliterative endarteritis of arterioles and arteries, impaired fibrinolysis by endothelial cells being partly responsible for the latter process.[22,24–26] The resultant ischemia gives rise to mucosal atrophy, ulceration, and fistula formation together with fibrosis and hyalinization of connective tissue and smooth muscle. Epithelial debris may eventually calcify, and in cases of fistula formation, vaginal urea-splitting bacteria may form triple phosphate encrustations and actual calculi.[14,27]

Preoperative Assessment and Management

A thorough speculum and bimanual examination of the vagina, rectal examination, cystourethroscopy, and intravenous urography are recommended in all cases preoperatively. Fluo-rodynamics, with occlusion of the fistula orifice if necessary, may be of particular benefit in diagnosing associated problems, such as proximal urethral dysfunction, impaired bladder compliance, and vesicoureteral reflux. Creatinine clearance should be estimated if upper tract involvement is suspected. Instillation of methylene blue into the bladder may be helpful when fistula localization proves difficult. At cystoscopy, the site, size, and number of fistulas together with the state of the local tissues are carefully documented. Multiple biopsy specimens should be obtained to rule out recurrent malignancy. Other key points to notice include the presence of tissue edema, ulceration, slough, induration, infection, and calculi and the relationship of the fistula(s) to the urethra, bladder neck, and ureteral orifices. The classic locations of radiation-induced fistulas are the posterior part of the trigone and just behind the interureteral ridge.

The urine should be examined microscopically, cultured, and treated if infected. Associated local problems, such as rectovaginal fistula and stenosis of the ureter, rectum, and vagina as well as the presence of ammoniacal dermatitis and atrophic vaginitis, must be recognized and managed accordingly.

Postradiotherapy vesicovaginal fistulas do not close with catheter drainage alone.[12] Surgical repair should be postponed for at least 12 months after treatment so as to allow the radiation damage to run its course; occasionally longer intervals of time are required.[28] It is generally accepted that the greatest chance of success is with the first repair. The timing of surgery may be individualized based on cystoscopic evidence of arrested injury and healing.[29,30] There is no proven indication for the use of nonsteroidal anti-inflammatory agents or corticosteroids to facilitate earlier intervention.[31,32]

Patients awaiting surgical repair are in need of considerable support and reassurance. Problems such as distorted body image, loss of self-esteem, and psychosexual and social dysfunction as well as cancer phobias are often encountered and may require specialized management. Incontinence from small fistulas may be controlled with frequent voiding and the use of tampons, perineal pads, or silica-impregnated diapers. A contraceptive diaphragm with a watertight attachment to a urinary catheter can collect urine from large fistulas into a leg bag.[33] Long-term indwelling catheters are best avoided. Ammoniacal dermatitis is treated with sitz baths and zinc oxide barrier ointment; vaginal estrogen improves urogenital tissue integrity in postmenopausal or castrate women. In malnourished patients, a high-protein diet, vitamin and trace element supplements, and the correction of anemia are essential before surgical repair.

Surgical Repair

GENERAL SURGICAL PRINCIPLES

The majority of radiation-induced vesicovaginal fistulas can be closed transvaginally.[28] The major indication for abdominal repair is ureteral involvement; previous surgical failure(s), vaginal stenosis, and high vaginal location do not necessarily preclude a transvaginal approach.[28] Although partial colpocleisis, as described by Latzo, has been recommended by some, it is generally considered to be a less than satisfactory operation in the context of irradiated tissues.[12, 34, 35] Methods of suitable anesthesia include epidural, low spinal, and general. For proximal fistulas, Lawson's position may be used.[36] The patient is placed prone on the operation table with her knees apart and her ankles raised and supported in stirrups and with the table in reversed Trendelenburg tilt. Alternatively a jackknife position may be used in which the patient is placed prone with her hips well flexed and abducted, the table being "jackknifed" at this level.[37] For higher fistulas, an exaggerated lithotomy position is preferable.

Although prophylactic antibiotics are usually administered, the risk of infection is more significantly reduced by minimization of tissue trauma, obliteration of dead space, complete hemostasis, neovascularization, and effective bladder drainage postoperatively. Labial retraction

sutures and, if necessary, an episiotomy or Schuchardt's incision may improve exposure. Adequate light is essential; a headlight may prove helpful for fistulas located high in the vaginal vault. Appropriate instruments and materials are equally necessary. Instruments found to be most useful include Chassar Moir, Church, and Kelly fistula scissors; fine Allis forceps; Sims skin hooks; Sims and Breisky retractors; fine-tipped suction catheters; and long-handled scalpels with no. 11 and 15 blades. Lacrimal duct probes may be used to identify small fistula orifices. Although no one suture material has been shown to be superior, the use of 2–0 and 3–0 polyglycolic acid on CT-2 needles is favored by many for closure of the external layers of any multilayered fistula.

The placement of stay sutures close to the fistula margin and the insertion and inflation of a pediatric size Foley catheter through the fistula tract into the bladder helps to evert the fistula edge and improves descent and stability for dissection (Fig. 30-1). Infiltration of tissues with sterile normal saline may help in identifying the appropriate tissue planes; epinephrine should not be used in irradiated tissues. If the fistula encroaches on the ureteral orifices, they should be catheterized at the outset. If identification proves difficult, intravenous indigo carmine with or without furosemide may be helpful.

The classic method of fistula repair involves layered dissection, mobilization of tissues, and low tension closure. An inverted J incision is often used, the upper convex part circumscribing the fistula; anterior and posterior vaginal flaps are then developed. The subvaginal plane is dissected just above the level of the white pubocervical fascia, taking care to avoid overdissection, which may lead to local ischemia. If mobilization proves difficult, radial or circumferential incisions made at a distance from the fistula may facilitate mobilization and low-tension closure. Once hemostasis is achieved, these incisions may be left open. If the fistula tract is small, it can be excised; if large, the edges can be freshened. Overexcision should be avoided because this may result in the creation of a large defect.[36]

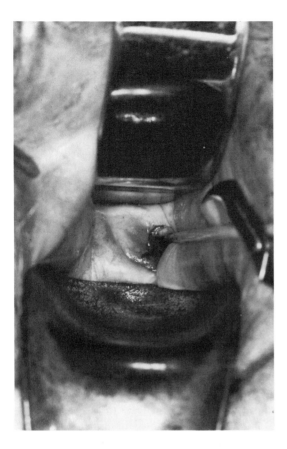

Figure 30-1. *Radiation-induced vesicovaginal fistula with Foley catheter* in situ.

The bladder is closed using submucosal interrupted Lembert sutures, placed 3 mm apart and a distance from the fistula edge. They should be knotted so as to coapt the tissues without strangulation. Figure-of-eight and pursestring sutures should be avoided because they may compromise the local blood supply.[38] A second layer of sutures is used to close the bladder muscle and to reduce the tension on the first. Bladder closure in the trigonal area should be in a transverse direction if possible; vertical closure may draw the ureteral orifices toward the midline and obstruct them. In view of the compromised blood supply in postirradiated tissues, the placement of a pedicled graft between the bladder and

vaginal suture lines is mandatory; this is discussed in the next section.

The integrity of the fistula repair may be tested on the completion of the repair by instilling methylene blue or indigo carmine into the bladder; care must be taken to avoid overdistention.

LABIAL GRAFTS

In 1928, Martius introduced the use of a pedicled unilateral ischiocavernosus/bulbocavernosus muscle graft for the repair of a large vesicovaginal fistula.[39] These muscles were exposed through a vestibular incision, detached from their origins, positioned beneath the bladder neck, and reattached to the contralateral pubic ramus. Martius proposed that this muscle graft would enhance continence by contributing both mechanical support and sphincteric activity to the region of the bladder neck. Betson outlined further possible advantages of this procedure; these included separation of bladder and vaginal suture lines, reduction of dead space, and neovascularization.[40] Later Martius modified the operation. Using a vertical incision over the labium majus, the bulbocavernosus muscle (and in certain descriptions just the overlying fibrofatty pad) was mobilized on a superior pedicle, tunneled subcutaneously, and secured to the site of fistula repair. With large fistulas, when low-tension closure of the vagina was not possible, Martius used the graft as a tissue substitute.[41,42] Although Birkhoff and co-workers recommended that this type of graft should be used in the repair of all fistulas, Martius argued that its use should be restricted to more complicated cases.[43]

Elkins and colleagues achieved an 86.5% success rate using a modified version of the Martius graft in the repair of 37 complex fistulas without significant morbidity.[44] All five patients with radiation-induced vesicovaginal fistulas were closed successfully and remained dry on short-term follow-up (4 months to 2 years). A rectovesical reservoir and colostomy were also created in one of these patients as a result of a large rectovesicovaginal fistula (cloaca); post-

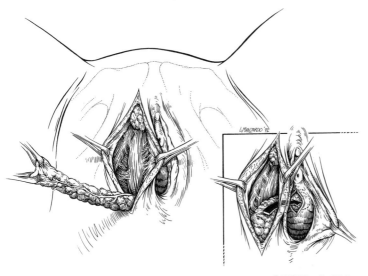

© 1992 University of Michigan

Figure 30-2. *Labial fibroadipose graft (with intact underlying bulbocavernosus).*

operatively she was continent of urine through her anal sphincter.

Cadaveric dissection of the graft used by Elkins and colleagues revealed it to be composed of fibroadipose tissue without any bulbocavernosus muscle fibers.[44] It is supplied by the external pudendal artery anteriorly and the internal pudendal artery posteriorly, these vessels forming a rich anastomosis in the graft. Symmonds had previously considered this well-vascularized fibroadipose pad to be the essential part of the transplant and not the bulbocavernosus muscle.[45] Excluding muscle from the graft reduces the risk of injury to the vestibular bulb and explains the low incidence of hemorrhage encountered during this procedure. Elkins and colleagues emphasize that the labial fibroadipose graft is an adjunctive repair technique and does not preclude the general principles of fistula repair (Fig. 30-2).

Hoskins and associates have reported on the use of myocutaneous labial grafts in the repair of two complex genitourinary fistulas associated with extensive tissue loss and fibrosis, one fistula being the result of radiotherapy for cervical carcinoma.[46] This technique involves the creation of a bulbocavernosus muscle flap with an overlying cutaneous island, which is tunneled subcutaneously and anchored to the site of fistula repair. The graft is then sutured to the surrounding vaginal mucosa. The authors emphasize the importance of securing the cutaneous island to the underlying fibroadipose pad and bulbocavernosus muscle so as to prevent avulsion of the delicate perforating vessels during the subcutaneous transfer. In cases with considerable tissue loss, requiring a large graft, the viability of the cutaneous island may be tested after mobilization and before grafting by the intravenous injection of fluoroscein dye with subsequent examination under Wood's light.

Although successful closure has been achieved using labial grafts even in fistulas presenting many years after treatment, the long-term integrity of these grafts remains questionable in irradiated tissues.[47,48]

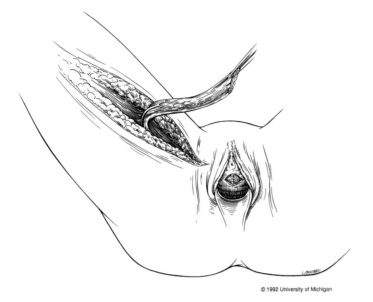

© 1992 University of Michigan

Figure 30-3. *Mobilization of gracilis muscle graft on its proximal vascular pedicle.*

GRACILIS MUSCLE GRAFTS

The gracilis muscle is one of the adductor muscles of the thigh. It passes from the lower border of the symphysis pubis and medial portion of the pubic ramus to the upper medial tibia. It adducts, flexes, and medially rotates the hip; it can, however, be sacrificed without a noticeable diminution in voluntary mobility because of the compensatory action of the other adductors (Fig. 30-3). The major arterial blood supply is derived from the profunda femoris or the medial circumflex femoral artery. The dominant artery or arteries together with the associated venae comitantes and sensorimotor branch of the obturator nerve enter the lateral border of the muscle approximately 7 to 12 cm from the pubic tubercle. A smaller artery enters the muscle 6 to 8 cm from the distal insertion.[49] In 1 out of 19 dissections, Ingelman-Sundberg discovered the latter to be the dominant arterial supply, thus rendering the muscle unsuitable for proximal grafting.[50] Doppler ultrasound may be used intraoperatively to localize these vessels. In the event of the

gracilis being unsuitable, the adductor longus or sartorious muscles may be used; there is, however, limited reported experience with these alternatives.[50,51]

In 1928, Garlock described the successful use of a gracilis muscle graft in the treatment of an intractable vesicovaginal fistula.[52] After mobilizing the bladder, a longitudinal incision was made on the medial side of the right thigh, exposing the gracilis muscle. The muscle was transected close to its insertion, sacrificing the distal vascular supply while maintaining the dominant proximal supply. The upper part of the thigh incision was then extended into the vaginal incision by cutting across the vulva transversely. The gracilis muscle was then positioned over the repaired fistula and secured in position with fine interrupted chromic catgut sutures (Fig. 30-4). The vaginal incision was then closed over the muscle graft.

Ingelman-Sundberg popularized this operation for the repair of radiation-induced vesicovaginal fistulas.[50] He modified the technique by transferring the gracilis muscle into the va-

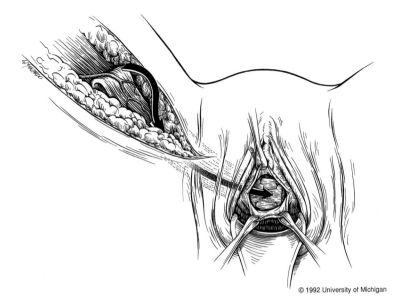

© 1992 University of Michigan

Figure 30-4. *Gracilis muscle graft positioned and anchored at the site of vesicovaginal fistula repair.*

gina through a perforation in the obturator membrane. He stressed the importance of avoiding trauma to the obturator nerve and vessels in addition to creating an opening in the membrane sufficiently large so as not to strangulate the graft blood supply. Hamlin and Nicholson subsequently simplified the operation by tunneling the reflected gracilis muscle subcutaneously from the apex of the thigh incision to the fistula site; this has become the standard operative technique for this type of graft.[53] Fleishman and Pincha have reported the use of the gracilis muscle graft in the abdominovaginal repair of fistulas, transferring the muscle into the space of Retzius by perforating the endopelvic fascial attachment to the pubic bone.[54]

A further modification of the gracilis graft involves the use of an overlying cutaneous island to close large defects. Using this technique, Heckler and colleagues achieved a cure in all five patients with large radiation-induced fistulas, in each of whom previous repair(s) had failed.[55]

Although breakdown of the skin wound occurred in three cases, the underlying repairs remained intact, protected by the muscle.

RECTUS ABDOMINIS MUSCLE GRAFTS

The blood supply of the rectus abdominis muscle is derived from the superior and inferior epigastric arteries. This muscle can be mobilized on an inferior vascular pedicle for the repair of genitourinary fistulas. It is exposed through an abdominal incision, transected across one of its tendinous intersections, mobilized, brought into the space of Retzius, and fixed to the site of fistula repair. Failure to anchor the graft securely may result in surgical failure owing to muscle retraction. Menacha and associates reported a successful outcome in three women with large intractable fistulas using this technique, two of the fistulas occurring after radiotherapy for carcinoma of the cervix.[56]

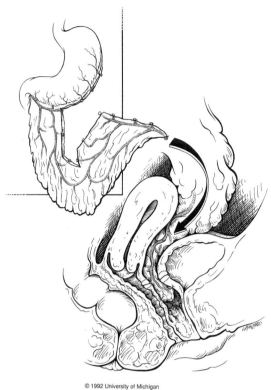

© 1992 University of Michigan

Figure 30-5. *Mobilization and anchoring of omental graft in transabdominal repair of vesicovaginal fistula.*

OMENTAL GRAFTS

The blood supply of the greater omentum comes from the right and left gastroepiploic arteries, which anastomose along the greater gastric curve. The omentum is mobilized by detaching it from the transverse colon and stomach (Fig. 30-5). The dominant right epiploic artery is most commonly used to form the vascular pedicle. Further lengthening is achieved by creating an omental J flap based on the arterial arcades. These flaps invariably reach the periurethral area.[57]

The use of omental grafts for the repair of fistulas was originally reported by Kiricuta and Goldstein in 1972.[58] They successfully closed all of 27 vesicovaginal fistulas, 22 of which followed Wertheim's hysterectomy and radiotherapy for cervical carcinoma. Using an abdominovaginal approach, Orford and Theron successfully repaired 52 of 59 fistulas using this technique also.[59] Turini and associates reported five genitourinary fistulas in women who had undergone radiotherapy followed by Wertheim's hysterectomy for carcinoma of the cervix.[60] The fistulas were repaired using a transperitoneal transvesical approach in conjunction with omentoplasty; ureteral reimplantation was required in two cases and a temporary colostomy in one. There were two failures in this group, one being associated with abdominal wound dehiscence and distal ureteral necrosis. In circumstances in which the vagina cannot be closed owing to extensive tissue destruction, the omentum can be used to patch the defect, epithelialization occurring over its surface.[61] There is some experimental evidence to support a similar role in extensive bladder defects.[61, 62] Omental grafts have also been used prophylactically in patients undergoing pelvic surgery who are at high risk of fistula formation. Petty and associates applied the graft between the vaginal vault and bladder base at the time of hysterectomy in five women who had previously undergone pelvic irradiation; no fistulas developed in this group, success being attributed to the graft-induced neovascularization.[63]

OTHER TECHNIQUES

For those patients with intractable vesicovaginal fistulas, an ileal conduit or continent diversion may be formed. Mannel and colleagues reported the successful use of the Indiana ileocecal pouch as a continent urinary reservoir in 10 women, 8 of whom underwent total pelvic exenteration for cervical carcinoma recurring after radiotherapy and 2 having urinary diversion for intractable postradiation vesicovaginal fistulas.[64] All patients achieved daytime continence between catheterizations. There were no significant postoperative complications in this series.

Mundy has described a complex technique for total substitution of the lower urinary tract in which a pedicled labial skin tube is anastomosed to a substitution cystoplasty.[65] The neourethra is tunneled subcutaneously in such a way as to provide a mechanical, nonmuscular continence mechanism. Mundy reported on six women having pelvic reconstruction for cloaca formation after radiotherapy for carcinoma of the cervix, three of whom had also undergone Wertheim's hysterectomy. Five of the six were continent between self-catheterizations. Kelemen and Lehoczky have reported the use of vulvocolpocleisis and colostomy, with the creation of a vesicovaginorectal reservoir for patients with cloacae after radiotherapy for gynecologic malignancy.[66] They achieved a successful outcome in all five cases, the patients voiding per rectum.

In the event of recurrent malignancy and short life expectancy, cutaneous ureterostomy or percutaneous nephrostomy may be performed.[67,68] A prerequisite for effective nephrostomy drainage is concomitant ureteral obstruction; this is achieved by ureteral ligation or by occlusion using hydrogel or cyanoacrylate.[68–70] Fistulas occurring a long time after treatment may be further complicated by small-capacity bladders and proximal urethral dysfunction. Augmentation cystoplasty and pubovaginal sling suspension may be required in addition to fistula repair.[47]

Postoperative Management

Effective bladder drainage is essential after surgery for 7 to 21 days, depending on the fistula size. For fistulas involving the lower trigone, bladder neck, and urethra, suprapubic drainage may be preferable. Overdistention from obstructing blood or mucus should be avoided by adequate hydration, regular monitoring of urinary output, and catheter irrigation when necessary. Prophylactic antibiotics are usually administered while the catheter remains in situ. A cystogram is recommended by some before removal of the catheter. Early leakage may respond to a more prolonged period of catheterization. Coitus is postponed for at least 6 weeks.

Prevention

The incidence of radiation-induced vesicovaginal fistulas may be further reduced by close attention to dose calculation and source application together with the effective management of acute radiation injuries. Vaginal vault necrosis, in particular, is a major risk factor for eventual fistula formation. It should be aggressively treated by careful removal of sloughed tissues, local toilet, vaginal estrogen, and appropriate antibiotics.[13]

Despite individualization of treatments based on computed dosimetry and dose fractionation, radiation injuries still occur and are probably inevitable in a small minority of patients, being independent of technical error and clinical mismanagement.[12] For patients with postirradiation fistulas, graft-induced neovascularization provides the key to successful repair.

References

1. Kottmeier HL. Complications following radiation therapy in carcinoma of the cervix and their treatment. Am J Obstet Gynecol 1964;88:854.
2. Cushing RM, Tovell HM, Liegner LM. Major urologic complications following radium and X-ray therapy for carcinoma of the cervix. Am J Obstet Gynecol 1968;101:750.
3. Peckham BM, Kline JC, Schultz AE, et al. Radiation dosage and complications in cervical cancer therapy. Am J Obstet Gynecol 1969;104:485.
4. Boronow RC, Rutledge F. Vesicovaginal fistula, radiation and gynecologic cancer. Am J Obstet Gynecol 1971;111:85.
5. Villasanta U. Complications of radiotherapy for carcinoma of the uterine cervix. Am J Obstet Gynecol 1972;114:717.
6. Obrink A, Bunne G. Gracilis interposition in fistulas following radiotherapy for cervical cancer: A retrospective study. Urol Int 1978;33:370.
7. Calame RJ, Wallach RC. An analysis of the complications of the radiologic treatment of carcinoma of the cervix. Surg Gynecol Obstet 1967;125:39.
8. Stockbrine MF, Hancock JE, Fletcher GH. Complications in 831 patients with squamous cell carcinoma of the intact uterine cervix treated with 3000 rads or more of whole pelvis irradiation. AJR Am J Roentgenol 1970;108:293.

9. Van Nagell JR, Parker JC, Maruyama J, et al. Bladder or rectal injury following radiation therapy for cervical cancer. Am J Obstet Gynecol 1974;119:727.

10. Lee RA, Symmonds RE, Williams TJ. Current status of genito-urinary fistula. Obstet Gynecol 1988;72:313.

11. Lawson J. The management of genito-urinary fistulae. Clin Obstet Gynecol 1978;5:209.

12. Buchsbaum HJ, Schmidt JD, Platz C, White AJ. Radiation cystitis, fistula and fibrosis. In: Buschbaum HJ, Schmidt JD, eds. Gynecologic and obstetric urology. 2nd ed. Philadelphia: WB Saunders, 1982:422–444.

13. Graham JB, Sotto SS, Paloueek FP. Carcinoma of the cervix. Philadelphia: WB Saunders, 1962.

14. Daly JW. Vesicovaginal fistula after radiation therapy. J Florida Med Assoc 1971;58:25.

15. Disaia PJ, Creasman WT. Clinical gynecologic oncology. 3rd ed. St Louis: CV Mosby, 1989.

16. Kottmeier HL, Gray KJ. Rectal and bladder injuries in relation to radiation dosage in cancer of the cervix: A 5 year follow up. Am J Obstet Gynecol 1961;82:74.

17. Lee KH, Kagan AR, Nussbaum H, et al. Analysis of dose, dose rate, and treatment time in the production of injuries by radium treatment for cancer of the uterine cervix. Br J Radiol 1976; 49:430.

18. Fletcher GH. Textbook of radio therapy. Philadelphia: Lea & Febiger, 1966.

19. Buchler DA, Kline JC, Peckham BM, et al. Radiation reactions in cancer of the cervix. Am J Obstet Gynecol 1971;111:745.

20. Joelsson I. Experience at radiuhemmet in treatment of carcinoma of the uterine cervix. Gynecol Oncol 1972;1:17.

21. Dean AL. Injury of the urinary bladder following irradiation of the uterus. Am J Obstet Gynecol 1933;25:667.

22. Hueper WC, Fischer CV, deCarvajal J, et al. The pathophysiology of experimental roentgen-cystitis in dogs. J Urol 1942;47:156.

23. Gowing NFC. Pathological changes in the bladder following irradiation. Br J Radiol 1960;33:484.

24. Watson EM, Herger CC, Sauer HR. Irradiation injuries in the bladder: Their occurrence and clinical course following the use of X-ray and radium treatment of female pelvic disease. J Urol 1947; 57:1038.

25. Lawson J. Vesical fistulae into the vaginal vault. Br J Radiol 1972;44:623.

26. Svanberg L, Astedt B, Kullander S. On radiation-decreased fibrinolytic activity of vessel walls. Acta Obstet Gynecol Scand 1976;55:49.

27. Graham JB. Painful syndrome of postradiation urinary-vaginal fistula. Surg Gynecol Obstet 1967;124:1260.

28. Zimmern PE, Hadley HR, Staskin DR, Raz S. Genitourinary fistulae: Vaginal approach for repair of vesicovaginal fistulae. Urol Clin North Am 1985;12:361.

29. Herbert DB, Vaughn ED. Vesicovaginal fistula: A therapeutic challenge. Infect Surg 1985; Feb:130.

30. Fearl CL, Keizure LW. Optimum time interval from occurrence to repair of vesicovaginal fistula. Am J Obstet Gynecol 1969;104:205.

31. Collins CG, Pent D, Jones FB. Results of early repair of vesicovaginal fistula with preliminary cortisone treatment. Am J Obstet Gynecol 1960; 80:1005.

32. Taylor JS, Henson AD, Rachow P, et al. Synchronous combined transvaginal-transvesical repair of vesicovaginal fistulas. Aust NZ J Surg 1980; 50:23.

33. O'Connor VJ. Review of experience with vesicovaginal fistula repair. J Urol 1980;123:367.

34. Latzko W. Postoperative vesicovaginal fistulae: Genesis and theory. Am J Surg 1942;58:211.

35. Graham JB. Vaginal fistulas following radiotherapy. Surg Gynecol Obstet 1965;120:1019.

36. Elkins TE, Drescher C, Martey JO, Fort D. Vesicovaginal fistula revisited. Obstet Gynecol 1988; 72:307.

37. Nichols DH, Randall CL. Vaginal surgery. 3rd ed. Baltimore: Williams & Wilkins, 1989.

38. Miller NF. The surgical treatment and postoperative care of vesicovaginal fistula. Am J Obstet Gynecol 1942;44:873.

39. Martius H. Die operative Wiederherstellung der volkommen fehlenden Harnrohre und des SchlieBmuskels derselben. Zentrabl Gynacol 1928;8:480.

40. Betson JR. The bulbocavernosus fat pad transplant for severe stress incontinence and vesicovaginal fistula: Rationale of the procedure, indications and technique. Am Surg 1961;271:129.

41. Martius H. Uber die Behandlung von Blasenscheidenfisteln, insbesondere mit Hilfe einer Lappenplastik. Geburtsh Gynakol 1932;103:22.

42. Martius H. Zur Auswahl der Harnfistel-und Inkontinenzoperation. Zentrabl Gynakol 1942; 32:1250.

43. Birkhoff JD, Wechsler R, Romas NA. Urinary fistulas; vaginal repair using a labial fat pad. J Urol 1977;117:595.

44. Elkins TE, DeLancey JOL, McGuire EJ. The use of modified Martius graft as an adjunctive technique in vesicovaginal and rectovaginal fistula repair. Obstet Gynecol 1990;75:727.

45. Symmonds RE. Loss of the urethral floor with

urinary incontinence. Am J Obstet Gynecol 1969;103:665.

46. Hoskins WJ, Park RC, Long R, et al. Repair of urinary tract fistulas with bulbocavernosus myocutaneous flaps. Obstet Gynecol 1984;63:588.

47. Zoubek J, McGuire EJ, Noll F, DeLancey JOL. The late occurrence of urinary tract damage in patients treated by radiotherapy for cervical carcinoma. J Urol 1989;141:1347.

48. Aartsen EJ, Sindram IS. The repair of the radiation induced rectovaginal fistulas without or with interposition of the bulbocavernosus muscle (Martius procedure). Eur J Surg Oncol 1988; 14:171.

49. Lacey CG, Stern JL. Gracilis flap vaginal substitution. In: Monaghan JM, ed. Rob and Smith's operative surgery: Obstetrics and gynaecology. 4th ed. London: Butterworths, 1987:238–243.

50. Ingelman-Sundberg A. Pathogenesis and operative treatment of urinary fistulas in irradiated tissue. In: Youssef AF, ed. Gynecology urology. Springfield, IL: Charles C Thomas, 1960:263–279.

51. Byron RL Jr, Ostergard DR. Sartorius muscle interposition for the treatment of the radiation-induced vaginal fistula. Am J Obstet Gynecol; 104:104.

52. Garlock JH. The cure of an intractable vesicovaginal fistula by use of a pedicled muscle graft. Surd Gynecol Obstet 1928;255:255.

53. Hamlin RHJ, Nicholson EC. Reconstruction of urethra totally destroyed in labour. BMJ 1969; 2:147.

54. Fleishman J, Pincha G. Abdominal approach for gracilis muscle interposition and repair of recurrent vesicovaginal fistulas. J Urol 1987;140:552.

55. Heckler WC, Holschneider AM, Kraeft H. Der Operative Verschluss recto-vaginaler, recto-urethraler und vesico-cutaner Fisteln durch Interposition des Musculus gracilis. Chiurg 1980; 51:43.

56. Menacha A, Akhyat M, Gleicher N, et al. The rectus abdominis muscle flap in a combined abdominovaginal repair for difficult vesicovaginal fistulae; a report of 3 cases. J Reprod Med 1990; 35:565.

57. Wein AJ, Malloy TR, Greenberg SH, et al. Omental transposition as an aid in genitourinary reconstructive procedures. J Trauma 1980;20:473.

58. Kiricuta I, Goldstein AMB. The repair of extensive vesicovaginal fistulas with pedicled omentum: A review of 27 cases. J Urol 1972;108:724.

59. Orford HJL, Theron JLL. The repair of vesicovaginal fistulas with omentum: A review of 59 cases. S Afr Med J 1985;67:143.

60. Turini D, Lunghi F, Nicita G. Our experience in the surgical treatment of complicated vesico-vaginal fistulas. Acta Urol Belg 1981;49:77.

61. Goldstein AMB, Deardon LC. Histology of omentoplasty of the urinary bladder in the rabbit. Invest Urol 1966;3:460.

62. Helmbrecht LJ, Goldstein AMB, Morrow JW. The use of pedicled omentum in the repair of large vesicovaginal fistulas: Experimental work in dogs. Invest Urol 1975;13:104.

63. Petty RM, Lowry RD, Oyama AA. Total abdominal hysterectomy after radiation therapy for cervical cancer: Use of omental graft for fistula prevention. Am J Obstet Gynecol 1986;154:1222.

64. Mannel RS, Braly PS, Buller RE. Indiana pouch continent urinary reservoir for treatment of complex vesicovaginal fistulas. Obstet Gynecol 1990; 75:891.

65. Mundy AR. A technique for replacement of the lower urinary tract without the use of a prosthesis. Br J Urol 1989;62:334.

66. Kelemen Z, Lehoczky G. Repair of fistulas in the vesicovaginal area by forming a urinary reservoir. Eur Urol 1986;12:389.

67. Krause S, Hald T, Steven K. Surgery for urologic complications following radiotherapy for gynecologic cancer. Scand J Urol 1987;21:115.

68. Janetschek G, Mack D, Hetzel MH. Urinary diversion in gynecologic malignancies. Eur Urol 1988;14:371.

69. Gunther R, Klose K, Alken P. Transrenal ureteral occlusion with a detachable balloon. Radiology 1982;1982:521.

70. Kinn AC, Ohlsen H, Brehmer-Andersson E, Brundin J. Therapeutic ureteral occlusion in advanced pelvic malignant tumors. J Urol 1986; 135:29.

VII

Urgency Frequency Syndromes

31

Interstitial Cystitis

C. Lowell Parsons

Interstitial cystitis (IC) is a diagnosis that has been used as a label for a rather severe and debilitating disorder of the bladder. This syndrome is traditionally characterized by severe urinary frequency, urgency, or lower abdominal or perineal pain. If a history is obtained from an individual afflicted with a severe form of this bladder dysfunction, it would be noted that the dysfunction usually has a gradual onset with an insidious progression (in most patients). The question could be posed: What is the diagnosis for an individual in an early phase of IC? To define this syndrome, it is important to consider this fact, especially because the early (mild) phase of this problem may be known by many names: urethral syndrome, trigonitis, urgency-frequency syndrome, pseudomembranous trigonitis. All these descriptions reduce to one common problem, urinary urgency, frequency, or pain in the absence of bacterial infection (or other definable pathology). This milder form of disease is present in perhaps 20% of individuals who are initially diagnosed as having recurrent urinary tract infection but who, in fact, have negative cultures. These are the people whose symptoms persist despite antibiotic therapy. Most resolve spontaneously after several weeks or months and go undiagnosed because they represent no major clinical problem (or the person will learn to "live with their symptoms"). It is difficult to put a distinct label on these patients. They would unlikely be deemed to have IC, but in fact they may indeed have a mild form or prodrome of this disorder.

This review of IC is based on the more liberal viewpoint that IC is a relatively heterogeneous disorder with a Poisson population distribution in regard to severity. Those at the extreme of the curve have traditionally been assigned this diagnosis, but in fact the majority of the patients fall in the middle with mild and moderate symptoms. In addition to a diagnostic dilemma, this disorder has been frustrating for the physician to treat because its cause is unknown, and therapy is consequently limited. Fortunately, there have been advances made in pathogenesis, diagnosis, and treatment, and these are reviewed.

There are many misconceptions concerning IC. Confusion exists as to what is normal bladder capacity under anesthesia, what an ulcer looks like, whether or not glomerulations exist, what is an abnormal voiding pattern, and what pathologic changes are found. These problems are also reviewed, first to help resolve them, second to provide some findings that may establish a clinical diagnosis, and third to promote better understanding of the pathogenesis and therapies of IC.

421

Female Urology, edited by Elroy D. Kursh and Edward McGuire. J. B. Lippincott, Philadelphia, © 1994.

Definition

The definition of IC has been changing significantly secondary to the marked interest in studying this disease. The expansion of the definition is controversial, but as clinical and epidemiologic data accumulate, this has been the steady trend. Historically it is widely accepted that patients with extremely small bladder capacities exhibiting the Hunner's ulcer (patch) and who also have severe bladder pain and urinary urgency represent the syndrome.[1,2] The controversy arises, however, when one asks the question: What diagnosis do you give to the individual who has a relatively short history (perhaps 5 to 7 months) of urinary urgency and frequency and perhaps some bladder-associated pain? These individuals may be diagnosed as having urgency frequency syndrome (UFS), urethral syndrome, urethrotrigonitis, and so on, but there is currently a growing tendency to place them into the category of mild forms of IC. This is a good term for this symptom complex because it suggests that there is involvement of layers deeper than the bladder epithelium, which is probably true.

In this chapter, a broad definition is used, and it includes patients who have urinary urgency and frequency or bladder pain in the absence of any demonstrable infection or other pathologic entity (*e.g.*, radiation or cancer) that might be inducing the problem. In addition, it is discussed here that the cause of this syndrome is probably not singular but represents several potential causes with a common result. The key word involving IC is that it is a *syndrome*, and there may be many stimuli that provoke the bladder and initiate symptoms. The bladder then responds with urgency, frequency, or pain, essentially its only response to noxious stimuli.

Another purpose for a broad definition of the syndrome is that the disorder is underdiagnosed. Many patients with milder forms could readily benefit from therapy if the diagnosis is considered. Treatment may be withheld if the physician reserves the diagnosis of IC for the more severe and classic symptoms.

Pathogenesis

Since the original description of the "elusive ulcer" of Hunner approximately 75 years, there has been slow progress in defining the cause of this disorder.[1,2] In part, this is because the severe form is relatively rare, making access to large numbers of patients for studies difficult. There have been many suggested causes, including lymphatic, chronic infection, neurologic, psychological, autoimmune disorders, and vasculitis.[3–11] Most of the proposed causes are hypothetical with little data to define the role of these mechanisms. Oravisto had suggested there were increased antinuclear antibodies in patients with IC.[10] It is difficult to know what this means because there is no obvious association with systemic autoimmune phenomena in these patients.

Currently several factors seem to play a causative role in IC. One of the more popular theories is that there is a defective bladder epithelium with loss of the *blood-urine barrier*, resulting in a leaky membrane.[12,13] An epithelium permeable to small molecules could then explain many of the symptoms associated with the complex. Chronic leak of small molecules could actually induce sensory nerves to depolarize, resulting in urgency frequency.[14,15] Diffusion of potassium across the membrane could be the ion that triggers the sensory nerve endings.[16] This latter concept is attractive, particularly because most of the patients do not have any significant signs of inflammatory responses in their bladder muscle, and no more than one third of the patients have mast cells to explain the sensory/urgency induced from their degranulation.[9,17–19]

EPITHELIAL LEAK

The more popular theory concerning pathogenesis, as noted previously, is that of an epithelial leak. There have been little data to support the concept that such a leak existed, and a subsequent study was unable to confirm the initial observation that both normals and IC patients had similar findings in their tight junctions relative to ruthenium red penetration.[12] A well-controlled study in 56 patients, however, has provided data to support the hypothesis that the bladder surface in patients with IC may indeed leak.[13] These investigators have currently developed an even more sensitive leak assay and believe that about 70% of patients with IC have a "leaky epithelium," whereas 30% do not. It is suggested that those who do not leak have some other problem, such as neurologic abnormality. They further emphasize that these findings support the concept that there are several causes of UFS.

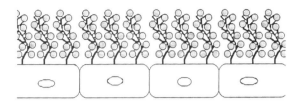

Figure 31-1. The concept of a biofilm layer at the bladder surface is schematically shown and demonstrates the location of the trapped water at the surface. Circles represent bound water, and the wavy lines represent the protein backbone.

GLYCOSAMINOGLYCANS: THE BLOOD-URINE BARRIER

Control of epithelial permeability in the bladder has long been thought to be due to tight junctions unique to the bladder epithelium and ion pumps.[12,20–26] Studies have provided data, however, to suggest that the bladder surface proteoglycans or glycosaminoglycans (GAG) may actually be the principal mechanism by which the epithelium maintains a barrier between the bladder wall and urine, the so-called blood-urine barrier.[13–15]

Surface proteoglycans (GAG, mucus) appear to have multiple roles in the bladder, including antiadherence and regulation of transepithelial solute movement.[15,27–29] The cell's external surface GAG are capable of preventing the adherence of bacteria, crystals, proteins, and ions, a function that is lost when this layer is removed with a dilute acid or detergent but restored when GAG is replaced by exogenous polysaccharides, such as heparin or pentosanpolysulfate (PPS).[27,30–32] The oxygen present on the sulfated polysaccharides is negatively charged and has a high affinity to bond ionically with water. This results in exclusion of urinary ionic solutes by a Donnan effect.[33] When GAG is present at a surface (the bladder), it in effect binds water molecules tightly to the oxygen of the sulfate groups in preference to calcium, barium, and even hydrogen ions.[34–36] Effectively

water molecules become trapped and interposed at the boundary between the cell surface (bladder) and the environment (urine) (Fig. 31-1). This bound molecular layer of water acts as a physical barrier such that urinary solutes, including urea and calcium, are not able to reach the underlying cell membranes, adhere to it, or move across it.[15]

Quaternary amines have a high affinity for sulfated polysaccharides and displace the water bound to the oxygen groups.[33,37,38] This concept is supported by the fact that when GAG chemically reacts with quaternary amines, it results in an increased entropy, reflecting the loss of water ordering around the sulfate groups.[33,39] It has been demonstrated both in animal and in human models that protamine sulfate inactivates native cell surface polysaccharides and results in increased epithelial permeability.[14,15] Damage to the transitional cells can be reversed by the addition of GAG, such as heparin.[14,15]

Based on these concepts, Parsons and colleagues proposed that the surface polysaccharide is functionally defective (not absent) in some patients with IC.[40] The cause for the deficiency could include reduced sulfation of the polysaccharides, diminished density or thickness of material, or the presence of a compound in urine such as a quaternary amine (known to inactivate GDG). It has been demonstrated that normal individuals who have their bladder surface challenged by the quaternary amine protamine lose

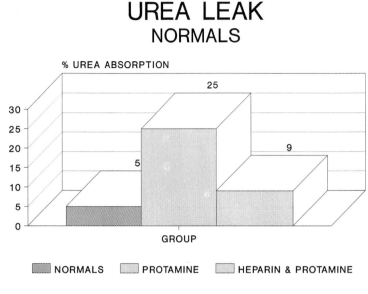

N=33

Figure 31-2. Results of urea movement across human epithelium. All subjects had three instillations of urea into their bladders. First, each person received urea, then they were exposed to protamine (2.5 mg/ml for 15 min) and had a second urea test (protamine). Next they had a heparin treatment and a third urea test (heparin). Protamine sulfate destroyed permeability barrier (polysaccharide) shown by increased urea uptake (25%). Heparin reduced the leak (9%).

the impermeability of the epithelium. The permeability to urea in normal individuals increases from 5% to 25%[14] (Fig. 31-2). When the blood-urine barrier is lost because of protamine treatment, all normal subjects experience urgency, frequency, and bladder pain, symptoms that are reversed with a subsequent treatment with heparin. These data are additionally supported by the fact that a synthetic polysaccharide similar to heparin is effective in ameliorating the symptoms of IC.[40–42] Based on these concepts, Parsons and colleagues measured the permeability of the normal bladder epithelium to a concentrated solution of urea and compared it with that of patients with IC.[13] Twenty-nine normal controls absorbed approximately 5% of the urea, whereas 56 patients with IC absorbed 25% (Fig. 31-3). It is proposed based on these obser-

vations that some patients with IC do have a leaky epithelium. The leak results in the urgency and frequency and potentially other secondary changes seen in the subepithelial tissues.

Controversy exists concerning the role of mast cells in this disorder. Mast cells have been reported by a number of investigators to be present in IC, whereas others believe they are also present in bladders not affected by IC.[9, 11, 18, 19] The central point of the controversy is whether or not mast cells play a causative or secondary role: causative in that they may be degranulating and producing the symptoms or that they represent a response to whatever is causing IC (*e.g.*, an epithelial leak) and be a type of defense mechanism that may ultimately become part of the problem.

There have been attempts at quantitating

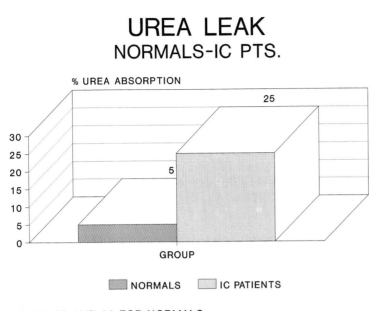

UREA LEAK
NORMALS-IC PTS.

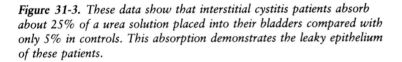

N=56 FOR IC AND 33 FOR NORMALS

Figure 31-3. These data show that interstitial cystitis patients absorb about 25% of a urea solution placed into their bladders compared with only 5% in controls. This absorption demonstrates the leaky epithelium of these patients.

mast cells (granulated and degranulated) both in the mucosa and in the subepithelial tissues.[43-45] Some investigators believe that mast cells are involved with IC, whereas others believe there is no increase of mast cells in IC when compared with their controls. Most of the controls studied, however, had bladder cancer and in fact are not normal.[43-45] Nonetheless, the presence of mast cells in one third of patients may result in degranulation and symptom aggravation. Control of this degranulation (even though the cells may be a defense mechanism) may be helpful therapy in some patients and is discussed later.

The role of inflammation and inflammatory mediators in IC is not known. Traditionally there has been a conception that inflammation is present in IC when this is probably not the case in most patients. Several points can be made that support the notion that inflammation plays little role in IC. First, on biopsy specimens, almost no inflammation is seen. Second, no systemic signs are found, that is, no leukocytosis.[46] Finally, no inflammatory mediators are found in the urine of more than 90% of these patients.[47] Patients with IC do not suffer from other generalized inflammatory diseases, such as collagen vascular diseases.[3,8] But there may be significant interplay between mast and inflammatory cells (their mediators), which is yet to be determined in subsets of patients.

IC has been suggested to be of psychosomatic origin, but this is rarely true. The majority of patients (especially with chronic pain) are secondarily affected by their disease and as a result may show signs of mild or moderate chronic depression. Those suffering from severe nocturia exhibit even more profound depression owing to sleep deprivation. In the author's experience, essentially no one has ever been cured of IC by psychotherapy. Earlier researchers reported similar findings.[4] Treating depression can improve overall sense of well-being for a patient and help the patient cope with the disease, but it does not cure the IC or reduce the number of daily voids. It is true that acute stress flares IC symptoms and stress reduction improves them, but the patient continues to have IC. It is important for rapport between the physician and the patient to remember that IC is not a psychological disorder.

Incidence and Epidemiology

Although IC was first identified in 1907 by Nitze, few epidemiological studies have been reported.[48] Oravisto, in a Finnish study of 103 people with IC, estimated an annual incidence of 1.2 cases per 100,000 and a prevalence of about 10 to 11 per 100,000.[49]

The incidence in the United States has been estimated from two sources. Held and associates estimated about 44,000 cases in the United States; the author's estimate extrapolated from San Diego County is placed at 40,000 to 60,000.[50] Held also estimated a worst case scenario in the United States at 450,000.[51]

DEMOGRAPHIC FACTORS

The previously mentioned studies reveal several risk factors. Sex, of course, is a risk factor, with a female to male ratio of about 9:1 in all reports.[50,52-54] Age is also a risk factor, with incidence generally limited to those older than 18 years of age, but there are reported cases in younger people.[55-58]

Median age of diagnosis is between 40 and 46 in most series with disease appearing several years earlier.[50,52,59] Race and ethnicity appeared to be a risk factor, with the disease occurring mostly in whites but also reported in blacks.[60-63]

In a review of 300 cases at the University of California, San Diego, it was also observed that those without diabetes (no diabetes seen) seem to be at a greater risk.[59] Finally, there was a 400% increased incidence seen in Jewish people. All these findings are similar to those seen in inflammatory bowel diseases.[52,64-69]

Pathology

One of the main diagnostic problems with IC is the lack of pathologic findings that are readily identified and quantified. Various descriptions have been proposed, but unfortunately there is nothing pathognomonic of IC in bladder biopsy specimens. The mast cell controversy has already been reviewed; approximately one third of these patients have increased mast cell infiltration of their bladder wall and mucosa (significance unknown). Light microscopy generally reveals a urothelium that is thinned, readily detached, and nearly absent in many areas.

In contrast to the normal six- or seven-layer thick epithelium, the mucosa is frequently only two to four cell layers thick. These changes are consistent with a dysfunctional epithelium.[13] A generalized pan cystitis with infiltration of the lamina propria by mononuclear and chronic inflammatory cells is seen.[70-73] These changes, however, are also consistent with the effects of hydrodilation. Most physicians obtain a biopsy specimen after the distention, and perhaps many of these changes are artifacts.

The distribution of collagen within the bladder wall is controversial.[74] One hypothesis suggests that as the disorder progresses, a fibrotic small end-stage type bladder develops. There are little or no data to support this theory. The author believes that this is untrue and instead that frequent low-volume voiding leads to a thinned epithelium with atrophic muscle bundles and the net result of a small bladder. Further, the only scarring present in the bladder wall is probably iatrogenic, stemming from prior biopsies because many of these patients undergo multiple biopsies over years, which causes it.[74] As the entire bladder shrinks from frequent low-volume voiding, this scar tissue takes on a disproportionate and artifactual enlarged total volume of the bladder wall. In the author's experience (more than 500 biopsies), scarring, in fact, is not identified when biopsy specimens are obtained from an area of the bladder not previously biopsied.

The main point relative to biopsy is that IC cannot be diagnosed by it. There is no way to rule in or out this disorder by pathologic examination of bladder tissue. Some of the changes, as mentioned previously, however, do support the diagnosis. Although it is rare that these patients are confused with those having carcinoma-*in-situ* of the bladder, the biopsy may be necessary to rule out cancer (reviewed by Burford).[75] A combination of cytologic evaluation of the urine and bladder washings plus the biopsy is necessary to exclude malignancy.

Signs and Symptoms

The primary symptom of IC is the presence of abnormal sensory urgency. From sensory urgency derives urinary frequency. In addition, most patients have associated bladder pain. One study has shown that of the patients presenting with IC, approximately 15% have little to no bladder pain, whereas 85% of patients presented with significant pain.[59] It is important to determine whether or not the pain is of bladder origin. To do this, ask the patient if the pain (despite being constantly present) worsens if the bladder is not emptied and improves (not disappears) with voiding. Bladder pain of IC is experienced suprapubically, in the perineum, vaginally, or in the low back.[4] Two thirds of patients do not experience dysuria.

Nocturia is variable, but in general, 90% of the patients complain of voiding at least one to two times per night.[59] Nocturia increases with the severity and duration of the disorder. The average patient voids approximately 16 times per day; a minimum for diagnostic purposes is eight voids per day.[76] The average voided volume is 105 ml (Table 31-1).

Between 85% and 90% of individuals with IC are female. Of those who are sexually active, the majority (75%) complain of exacerbation of the symptom complex associated with sexual intercourse.[59] The increase in symptoms may be felt during sexual activity, immediately after, or

Table 31-1. *Urinary Symptoms**

Nocturia	
Mean	4.7
90% cut-off level†	1.5 (1–2 voidings)
Range	0–13
1–2	41 (18%)
2–4	90 (40%)
4.5–8	63 (28%)
Daytime Frequency	
Mean	16.0
90% cut-off level	7
Range	5.5–40
Urgency	
Mild	8 (3.5%)
Moderate	63 (28%)
Moderate–severe	35 (15.5%)
Severe	119 (53%)
Pain	
None	41 (18%)
Mild	16 (7%)
Moderate	82 (36%)
Severe	86 (39%)

* Symptoms reported in 225 patients. Included are frequency distributions for symptom severity.
† Present in 90% of patients.

within 24 hours. In addition, most women who are still menstruating complain of a flare of symptoms at the time of the menstrual cycle.[4, 59]

The typical age of diagnosis in IC is between 40 and 46 years, with an average duration of symptoms for 3 to 4 years.[4, 59]

Evaluation

The physician has struggled to establish a diagnosis of IC primarily because no objective "blood test" existed. Evaluation of large numbers of patients with UFS reveals historical and clinical findings that help establish the diagnosis.

In August 1987, a group of investigators and patients interested in IC met at the National Institutes of Health and defined the NIDDKD (National Institute of Diabetes and Digestive and Kidney Diseases) criteria to establish the diagnosis for research purposes.[76] These criteria are a practical attempt to quantitate findings in IC. In part, they were based on a study reported by

Table 31-2. *Voiding Profiles of 186 Patients with Interstitial Cystitis*

	NUMBER OF VOIDINGS*	VOIDED VOLUMES (ml)	NOCTURIA
Average	16.4	106	4.7
90% Confidence limit†	10	160	1.5
Range	7–39	26–235	0–13

* Per day.
† 90% of patients had at least this level.

Table 31-3. *Changes Associated with Duration of Interstitial Cystitis*

	AVERAGE AT 1 YEAR*	AVERAGE AT >7 YEARS†
Number of patients	34	42
Voidings	15.2	17.3
Voided volume (ml)	128	105
Anesthetic capacity (ml)	711	518

* Represents patients with 1 year of symptoms.
† Represents patients with >7 years of symptoms.

Parsons in which the symptoms of more than 200 IC patients were measured and analyzed.[59] From Parsons' data, each variable was examined; the point that included 90% of the patients was the number taken for the NIDDKD criteria. For example, 90% of IC patients were found to void at least one to two times at night, complained of eight or more voidings during the day, and had moderate urinary urgency, but the presence of bladder pain was optional. The data on which these criteria were based are reported in Table 31-1. It is important to note that these criteria were developed to provide uniform criteria for researchers investigating IC. They were never meant to be a gold standard for diagnosis. Patients meeting this criteria have advanced disease. There are many patients with IC who do not meet this criteria but have the disease and benefit from therapy.

The most accurate assessment of number of daily voidings and average voided volume is determined from a 3-day voiding log in which each voiding is measured and recorded. From these data, it was found that the average patient voids 16 times per day with a capacity of 106 ml (Table 31-2). The voiding profile is a useful method to help establish the diagnosis of IC and may also be used subsequently to create a therapeutic plan and for follow-up care. As might be anticipated, patients with a longer disease history have a smaller functional bladder capacity, as reflected in the average voided volume and number of daily voidings (Table 31-3).

Duration of symptoms helps to define patients with IC versus those with UFS. The diagnosis of IC is more likely if the individual has experienced continuous symptoms for at least 6 months. Clinically to separate IC from UFS is worthwhile because UFS may need little or no therapy and the prognosis for the patient is good.

PHYSICAL EXAMINATION

There is one important part of the examination that helps confirm the diagnosis of IC. On physical examination, more than 95% of patients complain of a tender bladder base during the pelvic examination. Their discomfort is easily demonstrated by palpation of the anterior vaginal wall and the bladder.

Urine analysis on voided specimens is not useful in these patients because their low voided volumes make midstream collection impossible. One sees only vaginal secretions unless a catheterized specimen is obtained. A catheterized specimen examined under the microscope should show no bacteria, and most (90%) show no red or white blood cells. Urine should be sent for cytologic evaluation to rule out the possibility of carcinoma.

Urodynamics

The cystometrogram (CMG) is a valuable study to perform in patients with this syndrome because a normal CMG essentially excludes the diagnosis of IC. Because all patients complain of significant urinary urgency, this can usually be

Table 31-4. *Results of Cystometrograms in 75 Patients with Interstitial Cystitis**

Average capacity	220 ml ± 68
90% cut-off level	<350 ml
Postvoid residual >50 ml	5/75 (7%)
Number with increased sensory urgency†	71/75 (95%)
Patients with uninhibited contractions	4/75 (5%)
Detrusor myopathy	11/225‡ (5%)

* Average capacities and 90% cut-off levels are listed. Patients with uninhibited contractions did not respond to anticholinergic therapy.
† Patients with urgency at <100 ml. All had urgency at <125 ml.
‡ Detrusor myopathy is described by Holm-Bentzen *et al*;[77] all patients suspected had cystometrograms demonstrating increased sensory urgency, postvoid residuals >50 ml, and poor detrusor contractions. Detrusor volumes were >750 ml.

documented with cystometry. If gas is employed, patients have a sensation of significant urgency at less than 125 ml and with water less than 150 ml. If this portion of the CMG is normal, they probably do not have IC or only a mild form. In 75 patients with CMGs reported by Parsons, the average bladder capacity was 220 ml, with more than 90% of patients having a volume of less than 350 ml[59] (Table 31-4). There is an important caveat, however, relative to maximum bladder capacity. A small group of patients with significant IC develop detrusor myopathy (about 5%).[59,77] Individuals with this complication have large atonic bladders with little muscle present. They have moderate to severe sensory urgency, have large bladder capacities (>1000 ml), and usually carry residual urines (>100 ml). Detrusor function is poor or absent. Because most of the patients are females, they are able to void but primarily with a Valsalva maneuver. This subgroup represents approximately 5% (Table 31-4) of patients with IC.[59] Men with detrusor myopathy may require a program of intermittent catheterization as part of their treatment.

CYSTOSCOPIC EVALUATION

Cystoscopic evaluation of the bladder under anesthesia is both an important diagnostic and therapeutic maneuver. Examination under local anesthesia is to be discouraged because it offers little help in diagnosis and causes the patient severe discomfort. It is recommended that when IC is suspected, a cystoscopy be performed under anesthesia.

The cystoscopy under anesthesia is performed in a manner both to diagnose and to treat. The diagnosis depends on discovering one of two findings, a Hunner's ulcer or the presence of glomerulations or petechial hemorrhages. Not all patients, however, show these changes, so their absence does not exclude the diagnosis.

Cystoscopy

The cystoscopy should be performed in two phases. Phase one is the initial inspection. Here the physician should obtain specimens for cytology and urine for regular and tuberculosis culture (optional because almost never diagnosed). Visual examination of the bladder may reveal a true Hunner's ulcer (patch). The patch is a velvety red patch (Color Plate 1) present in only 8% of patients and is similar in appearance to carcinoma-*in-situ*.[59] It is not, however, a true ulcer. Biopsy at this part of the cystoscopy is not recommended. Prior biopsy site scars, which are frequently mistaken for ulcers, may also be seen.[74] Bladders with IC appear to heal poorly, and biopsy scars are frequently large but are recognized by the spoke wheel blood vessels that radiate from the central scarred portion (Color Plate 2). These scars frequently tear and bleed after distention and account for most so-called epithelial disruptions. Parsons reported as many as 75% of ulcers described at previous cystoscopy by other urologists to be biopsy site scars.[59]

The second phase of the cystoscopic procedure is hydrodistention to demonstrate glomerulations. Hydrodistention also induces a disease remission in 60% of patients. Hydrodistention is performed by filling the bladder slowly up to a maximum of 80 to 100 cm H_2O pressure. The urethra of the woman should be

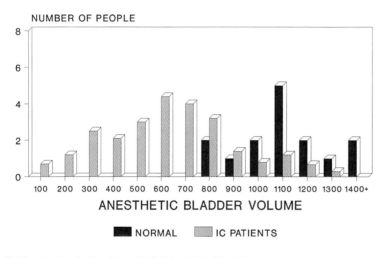

AVG= 1115 ml; N= 15   AVG IC= 579 N=261

Figure 31-4. *These data represent bladder capacities of patients with interstitial cystitis who had cystoscopy with general anesthesia. The mean capacity was 579 ml. Less than 1000 ml is considered abnormal. Normal bladders (patients undergoing cystoscopy who were incontinent) usually hold more than 1000 ml.*

manually compressed over the cystoscope to prevent leakage of fluid. After several minutes, the bladder is emptied and the volume measured and recorded. The last part of the effluent is usually bloody if glomerulations or ulcers are present. When the bladder is re-examined, the glomerulations should be demonstrated. They are diffusely located around the bladder, at least 10 to 20 per field of vision (Color Plate 3). Hemorrhages on the trigone or posterior bladder wall are irrelevant and do not constitute a positive finding because they probably represent cystoscope trauma.

What constitutes an abnormal bladder capacity under anesthesia is surprising to many physicians. A normal female bladder holds well over 1000 ml, whereas the IC bladder usually holds less than 850 ml.[59] The average anesthetic capacity for IC patients is between 550

and 650 ml (Table 31-1 and Fig. 31-4). Patients with a longer history of symptoms have smaller bladder capacities, suggesting the disease is slowly progressive.[59] This is also supported by the fact that patients with Hunner's ulcers have the worst symptoms and also have the smallest bladder capacities and the greatest epithelial leaks.[13,59]

BIOPSY

The last part of the cystoscopic procedure should be the biopsy. One should *never* obtain a biopsy specimen before hydrodistention because the bladder could tear at the biopsy site and may lead to a significant bladder rupture. If one is employing a caustic agent for therapy, *never* obtain a biopsy specimen before the solution is placed in the bladder. Should the solution extrav-

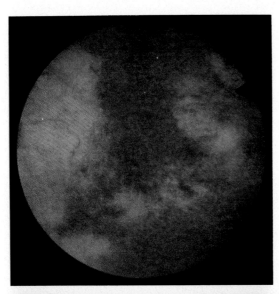

Color Plate 1. *Classic Hunner's ulcer (patch, not a true ulcer), a velvety red patch resembling carci-noma-in-situ.*

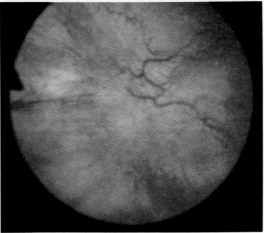

Color Plate 2. *Prior biopsy site scar. Recognized as a result of the presence of neovascularity with blood vessels radiating in a "spoke of the wheel" fashion.*

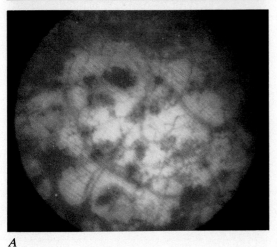

A

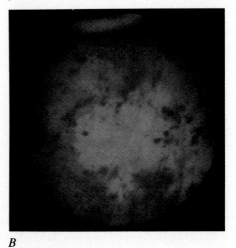

B

Color Plate 3. *Glomerulations or petechial hemorrhages that occur after hydrodistending a bladder in a patient with interstitial cystitis.*

asate through the biopsy site, severe tissue damage may occur.

The biopsy specimen itself is not diagnostic for IC but can rule out other diseases, such as carcinoma-*in-situ*. The findings on pathologic examination include the presence of mast cells (demonstrated by toluidine blue staining), inflammatory cells, and a thinned mucosa.[43,45] A normal biopsy result *does not* exclude IC and should not be used in diagnosis.

Although diagnosis of IC depends in part on abnormal cystoscopic findings, one cannot arbitrarily rule out the disease purely by the endoscopic findings. There are many patients who have IC without such findings who benefit from therapy. The physician needs to remember this disease complex is still primarily manifested by significant urinary urgency or frequency and perhaps few or no other findings.

Therapy

Few advances had been made in therapy for IC until recently. Most medications were employed empirically, and all were studied without controls. Drugs used for IC included anticholinergics, antihistamines, analgesics, and anti-inflammatories. Future drug efficacy studies must include controls to demonstrate whether therapy is active. Traditional and newer therapies that should aid the physician treating IC are reviewed.

When discussing therapy with the individual patient, it is important for the physician to point out that if the symptoms have been present for more than a year, no particular therapy is likely to be curative. Although the patient may have a significant remission of symptoms, in all probability relapse will occur. If patients are prepared for this eventuality, they are much less distressed when symptoms return and cope better with their disease. The physician–patient relationship is strengthened in terms of credibility if this area is addressed before treatment. Patients readily accept this explanation and overall appear to cope better with their disorder when they have a realistic outlook.

ANTIDEPRESSANT THERAPY

Chronic pain and sleep loss cause depression; thus it is valuable to place most IC patients on antidepressant medications. If tricyclic antidepressants are used, start with low doses (25 mg imipramine 1 hour before bedtime) and warn patients that they will be tired for the first 2 to 3 weeks of therapy. Once they become tolerant to this side effect, increase slowly to full dose. Imipramine, or amitriptyline, can be prescribed in doses beginning at 25 mg 1 hour *before* bedtime (aids in sleep and reduces tiring effect of medication). If fluoxetine (Prozac) is selected, use 20 mg/day and increase if needed to 40 mg.

Antidepressant therapy is an important adjunct to treatment. It does not cure IC, but patients function much better with their disabling symptoms if not depressed. In essence, they "feel better" even if they still void 20 times per day. Antidepressants, of course, do not cure IC, and it is important to emphasize this to the patient.

HYDRODISTENTION OF THE BLADDER UNDER ANESTHESIA

The report by Bumpus in 1930 of bladder hydrodistention improving the symptoms of IC has resulted in this procedure being a mainstay of therapy.[78] Few would question the activity of hydrodistention in ameliorating the symptoms in 60% of IC patients. The procedure must be performed under anesthesia because it is not possible to dilate a painful bladder without anesthesia. The procedure for hydrodistention has been described under diagnosis. Pressure dilatation of the bladder using a syringe is not recommended because it can result in bladder rupture; a maximum of 80 to 100 cm H_2O pressure is recommended.

The mechanism by which hydrodistention improves symptoms is unknown; several theories have been postulated. Neuropraxis induced by mechanical trauma may occur in some individuals. Few patients, however, awaken with decreased pain, to support the neuropraxis concept. Rather, most (80%) awaken from anesthesia with significantly worse pain that slowly improves over 2 to 3 weeks. This pain usually requires narcotic analgesia. Remission occurs over several weeks.

As a result of the increased pain, it is recommended that all patients receive belladonna and opium rectal suppositories immediately in the recovery room, or, better yet, instill 10 ml of 2% viscous lidocaine into the bladder at the end of hydrodistention. In addition, patients should be discharged with medication to control the increased pain.

Because most patients' symptoms are exacerbated by hydrodistention, we believe that this is due to epithelial damage by mechanical trauma. The disruption in the integrity of the mucosal cells increases the epithelial leak, causing symptoms to flare. Healing may occur over the next several weeks, which correlates with the time of clinical remission. Perhaps the epithelium regenerates and for a period of time is "healthy" and impermeable. Then whatever events initiate the disease continue, and relapse occurs.

Remission may persist between 4 and 12 months; hydrodistention may be repeated as needed. If no remission is obtained, repeat the dilation at least two more times because frequently in our experience patients respond to a subsequent dilation.

DIMETHYLSULFOXIDE

Dimethylsulfoxide (DMSO) was approved for use in IC in 1977.[79] Although no controlled clinical trials were ever conducted with DMSO, it does appear to induce remission in 34% to 40% of patients. The difficulty with DMSO is that it may induce an excellent remission in the first one or two cycles of therapy, but as an individual relapses and requires subsequent treatment, progressive resistance to its beneficial effects is seen.

For treatment, instill 50 ml of 50% DMSO into the bladder for 5 to 10 minutes. Longer periods are unnecessary because DMSO rapidly absorbs into the bloodstream. Instillations are performed on an outpatient basis, or the patient can be taught to perform it at home. The author recommends that patients receive six to eight weekly treatments to determine whether a therapeutic response is achieved. If the patient has moderate or worse symptoms, continue the therapy for an additional 6 to 12 months once every other week. Remember, once DMSO therapy is stopped, the patient is likely to become resistant to its use. Some patients experience a flare of symptoms when DMSO is placed into the bladder. This phenomenon may be related to DMSO's ability to degranulate mast cells and may occur primarily in patients who have significant bladder mastocytosis. Nonetheless, DMSO may be effective at treating these patients. Should the patient experience pain with DMSO, it is recommended that he or she receive intravesically 10 ml of 2% viscous lidocaine jelly 15 minutes before placing DMSO. If this is not successful, use an injectable narcotic or Toradol (ketorolac), 60 mg intramuscularly, before the intravesical instillation. The flare of symptoms associated with DMSO usually disappears over 24 hours. As these patients receive subsequent treatments, the pain tends to diminish.

Patients may also receive indefinite therapy using DMSO. As originally reported by Stewart and colleagues, patients have used DMSO weekly for several years without problems.[79] If a patient is on long-term therapy, it is recommended that he or she have a slit lamp evaluation at 6-month intervals. DMSO has been reported to be associated with cataracts in animals; however, this complication has not been reported in humans.

AMITRIPTYLINE

In an uncontrolled trial, amitriptyline was reported by Hanno and associates to ameliorate the symptoms of IC.[80] The patients were treated with 25 mg of amitriptyline 1 hour before bedtime for 1 week and then increased weekly by 25 mg to a 75-mg dose. Fifty percent of patients respond to this medication. The exact mechanism of action is unknown, although it may block H_1 histamine receptors and perhaps mast cell degranulation. More likely, the drug raises pain tolerance perhaps owing to its antidepressant activity. Antidepressant therapy has already been discussed.

ANTIHISTAMINES

Antihistamines have been tried in IC but without controlled studies. Antihistamines were chosen because of the possible role of mast cells.[70,72,81,82] In the author's experience, antihistamines are of little usefulness in the general management of IC. Some patients, however, respond to these medications, for example, diphenhydramine (Benadryl) or terfenadine (Seldane), especially if they have an allergic history and tend to have a symptom flare during allergy seasons.

STEROIDS

Because of the assumption that inflammation plays a role in this disorder, patients have received steroids. Badenoch found significant improvement in 19 of 25 patients treated with prednisone.[83] All were treated, however, following hydrodistention under anesthesia, which may have been responsible for most of the benefit. In this author's experience, steroids do not ameliorate the symptoms of this complex. As with most drugs, there have been no clinical trials conducted on the efficacy of steroids in IC.

INTRAVESICAL SILVER NITRATE

Intravesical silver nitrate was first reported in 1926 by Dodson.[84] Pool fashioned a treatment regimen in which bladder irrigations were begun under anesthesia with 1:5000 concentration.[86] This was followed subsequently by gradually increasing the concentrations on a daily basis, ultimately employing a 1% solution. Again this was done in an uncontrolled setting on patients who had had dilatation of the bladder under anesthesia. Pool reported good results in 89% of patients. There have been other uncontrolled studies reporting that this compound is helpful; nevertheless, it is not widely used today. One caution in

the use of silver nitrate: Never instill into the bladder after biopsy. If there is a perforation and this solution is placed into the bladder, intraperitoneal and extraperitoneal extravasation could occur, resulting in major tissue damage.

INTRAVESICAL SODIUM OXYCHLOROSENE (CLORPACTIN WCS-90)

Clorpactin is a highly reactive chemical compound that is a modified derivative of hypochlorous acid in a buffered base. Its activity is dependent on the liberation of hypochlorous acid and its resulting oxidizing effects and detergency.[86] It was reported by Wishard, who treated 20 patients with five weekly instillations of 0.2% clorpactin WCS-90 under local anesthesia.[86] Improvement was reported in 14 of the 20 patients, and follow-up was brief. Messing and Stamey, treating 38 patients with 0.4% Clorpactin, reported significant improvement in 72%.[54] Ureteral reflux is a contraindication to the use of Clorpactin. It is recommended that the compound usually be used under anesthesia.

HEPARIN

Heparin, when given by injection, has been reported to alleviate the symptoms of IC.[87] Again this was not in a controlled study. Long-term systemic heparin therapy cannot be employed because it results in osteoporosis in 100% of patients who use it for 26 weeks. In the author's experience, intravesical heparin has significant activity in approximately 50% of patients.[88] Here too the data were obtained in an uncontrolled investigation. Previous controlled studies by the author demonstrated a placebo effect of approximately 20%, suggesting possible activity for heparin.[41] The technique uses 10,000 units of heparin in 10 ml of sterile water, and this solution is instilled intravesically three to seven times per week. In moderate to severe patients, begin with daily therapy. If improvement is seen in 3–4 months, taper to treatment every other day. If symptoms increase, resume daily medication. This treatment can be carried on indefinitely. It takes 2 to 4 months to see improvements. The best improvements are noted after 1 to 2 years. Long-term therapy is recommended for patients with moderate or worse disease who respond to its use. Serum prothrombin time and partial thromboplastin time are monitored for several weeks after therapy begins to rule out the formation of an unusual antibody to heparin or systemic absorption. Heparin is not absorbed across the bladder mucosa. Patients are instructed in self-catheterization so this therapy can be performed at home.

PENTOSANPOLYSULFATE

Parsons and others first reported pentosanpolysulfate as active at ameliorating the symptoms of IC.[40–42, 89] Because pentosanpolysulfate (Elmiron) is a sulfated polysaccharide, theoretically it may augment the bladder surface defense mechanism or detoxify in urine agents that have a capacity to attack the bladder surface, for example, quaternary amines. In a controlled clinical study, 42% of patients were shown to have their symptoms controlled versus 20% for placebo.[89] This has been borne out in several subsequent studies, including a five-center trial in which 28% of patients versus 13% on placebo improved and a seven-center study of 150 patients, in which there was a 32% patient improvement versus 15% on placebo.[90] Additionally, an English-Danish study also found a significant reduction of pain in patients on drug compared with placebo.[19] Elmiron is not currently approved for use in the United States but may be available soon. It is employed in an oral dose of 100 mg three times per day. In patients with moderate disease, it appears to have about 40% to 50% activity. In the controlled clinical trials that were done on patients with severe disease, its activity was lower. Continued use of Elmiron for several years leads to long-term disease control in most of the drug responders. Response to therapy is first seen after 6 to 10 weeks. Patients do better after 6 to 12 months of therapy.

SURGERY

Approximately 3% of patients presenting with IC to the University of California, San Diego Medical Center have ultimately undergone some type of surgery for disease that is severe and refractory to all treatment. The question is the type of surgery to be performed.

CYSTOLYSIS

Attempts at surgical ablation of the bladder innervation by cystolysis are to be discouraged because most patients fail this and develop a neurogenic bladder with significant urinary pain.

BLADDER AUGMENTATION

A concept exists that these patients have small bladders and thus void frequently. Actually the reverse is true. They have sensory urgency, void frequently, and subsequently develop a small bladder. Hence attempts to augment the bladder with a patch of bowel are likely to fail. Patients then have a capacity that is large, have more difficulty emptying (usually requiring intermittent catheterization), and still retain all their sensory urgency and pain.[91]

URINARY DIVERSION ALONE

There are no controlled studies evaluating diversion alone, but studies suggest it is not effective.[92] The author, however, has removed two bladders in patients who had urinary diversions alone with persistent pelvic pain. The pain was eliminated by removal of the bladder. In counseling, one should tell patients that diversion alone may not be sufficient to control pain, and they may subsequently require a cystectomy. The patient can then decide whether or not he or she wants a risk of more than one surgery. It is the author's experience that almost no one elects for the potential of two surgeries.

Table 31-5. *Surgery for Interstitial Cystitis**

TREATMENT	PERSISTENT PAIN	NO PAIN
Cystectomy	1/25	24/25 (96%)

* Twenty-five patients underwent cystectomy for interstitial cystitis at UCSD. After 6 months, only one patient had persistent pelvic pain. That patient did not have "classic bladder pain" that increases with bladder filling but rather pelvic pain unrelated to voiding.

CYSTECTOMY AND DIVERSION

This is the mainstay of therapy for patients with *end-stage bladder.* It is successful, especially in today's environment of performing continent diversions. Pelvic pain presents after the procedure in 5% of patients (Table 31-5). In general, if patients have classic bladder pain associated with filling and relieved or partially relieved by emptying and have urinary frequency and urgency and stigmata of IC under anesthesia, they are likely to experience relief of their symptoms by cystectomy. Those individuals with severe pelvic pain not associated with classic parameters of IC and not exacerbated by bladder filling likely do not have their pain alleviated (Table 31-5).

BLADDER TRAINING

Whatever therapy is successful at alleviating the pain and sensory urgency of IC, the individual afflicted with the chronic form of the disorder has a small-capacity bladder that is in part based on sensory urgency and in part on frequent low-volume voiding. The author has discovered that in several controlled clinical trials, even with good remission of pain and urgency, there is almost no change in urinary frequency over a 12-week period. This issue must be addressed to obtain a functional recovery of the bladder. Persistent urinary frequency from a small bladder can be reversed after therapy has controlled urgency and pain. This is accomplished by training patients to undergo a program of progressively holding their urine to increase their bladder capacity.[93] This therapy can be directed by a urologic nurse. To begin this treatment, obtain a 3-day voiding profile from the patient (to include time of voiding and a measurement of volume). Determine the average time interval between voids, and gradually increase this interval monthly. For example, if the patient voids every hour, it is recommended that he or she attempt to void every hour and a quarter. At the end of 1 month increase the interval to an hour and a half. The patient should never progress too quickly because he or she will become discouraged and drop out. It takes 3 to 5 months of this protocol to see results. At the end of 3 to 4 months, the bladder capacity increases approximately 2 1/2 times, and there is a corresponding reduction in urgency and the number of voidings per day.[93]

We also discovered that in patients who have minimal or no pain associated with urinary frequency bladder training may be the only therapy required for improvement and in fact the only therapy that is effective. For more details concerning the employment of this protocol, the reader is referred elsewhere.[92]

Summary

IC is a syndrome in a state of rapid change in regard to the understanding of the pathogenesis and the development of therapy owing to a significant increase in research activity. These investigations will help the clinician quantitate the symptoms and clinical findings to diagnose the syndrome better and will simultaneously lead to new therapies that will result in symptom reduction (hydrodistention, DMSO, Elmiron, or heparin). In addition, bladder training methods can further rehabilitate the patient with the IC bladder. As reviewed herein, perhaps 75% to 85% of patients with moderate to severe IC can experience significant remission with conservative therapy and avoid the need for extirpative surgery.

References

1. Hunner GL. A rare type of bladder ulcer in women. Report of cases. Boston Med Surg J 1915;172:600.
2. Hunner GL. Elusive ulcer of the bladder: Further notes on a rare type of bladder ulcer with a report of 25 cases. Am J Obstet 1918;78:374.
3. Oravisto KJ, Alfthan OS, Jokinen EJ. Interstitial cystitis. Clinical and immunological findings. Scand J Urol Nephrol 1970;4:37.
4. Hand JR. Interstitial cystitis, a report of 223 cases. J Urol 1949;61:291.
5. Hanash KA, Pool TL. Interstitial and hemorrhagic cystitis: Viral, bacterial and fungal studies. J Urol 1970;104:705.
6. Oravisto KJ, Alfthan OS. Treatment of interstitial cystitis with immunosuppression and chloroquine derivatives. Eur Urol 1976;2:82.
7. Gordon HL, Rosen RD, Hersh EM, Yium JJ. Immunologic aspects of interstitial cystitis. J Urol 1973;109:228.
8. Silk MR. Bladder antibodies in interstitial cystitis. J Urol 1970;103:307.
9. Holm-Bentzen M, Lose G. Pathology and pathogenesis of interstitial cystitis. Urology 1987;29 (4 suppl):8.
10. Oravisto KJ. Interstitial cystitis as an autoimmune disease. A review. Eur Urol 1990;6:10.
11. Weaver RG, Dougherty TF, Natoli C. Recent concepts of interstitial cystitis. J Urol 1963;89:377.
12. Eldrup J, Thorup J, Nielsen SL, et al. Permeability and ultrastructure of human bladder epithelium. Br J Urol 1983;55:488.
13. Parsons CL, Lilly JD, Stein P. Epithelial dysfunction in non-bacterial cystitis (interstitial cystitis). J Urol 1991;145:732.
14. Lilly JD, Parsons CL. Bladder surface glycosaminoglycans: A human epithelial permeability barrier. Surg Gynecol Obstet 1990;171:493.
15. Parsons CL, Boychuk D, Jones S, et al. Bladder surface glycosaminoglycans: An epithelial permeability barrier. J Urol 1990;143:139.
16. Hohlbrugger G, Lentsch P. Intravesical ions, osmolality and pH influence the volume pressure response in the normal rat bladder, and this is more pronounced after DMSO exposure. Eur Urol 1985;11:127.
17. Lynes WL, Flynn SD, Shortliffe LD, et al. Mast cell involvement in interstitial cystitis. J Urol 1987;138:746.
18. Hanno P, Levin RM, Monson FC, et al. Diagnosis of interstitial cystitis. J Urol 1990;143:278.
19. Holm-Bentzen M, Jacobsen F, Nerstrom B, et al. Painful bladder disease: Clinical and pathoanatomical differences in 115 patients. J Urol 1987;138:500.
20. Englund SE. Observation on the migration of some labeled substances between the urinary bladder and blood in rabbits. Acta Radiol 1956; 135(suppl):9.
21. Kerr WK, Barkin M, D'Aloisio J, Merczyk Z. Observations on the movement of ions and water across the wall of the human bladder and ureter. J Urol 1963;89:812.
22. Lewis SA, Diamond JM. Active sodium transport by mammalian urinary bladder. Nature 1975; 253:747.
23. Fellows GJ, Marshall DH. The permeability of human bladder epithelium to water and sodium. Invest Urol 1972;9:339.
24. Hicks RM. The permeability of rat transitional epithelium. J Cell Biol 1966;28:21.
25. Hicks RM, Ketterer B, Warren RC. The ultrastructure and chemistry of the luminal plasma membrane of the mammalian urinary bladder: A structure with low permeability to water and ions. Phil Trans R Soc Lond B 1974;268:23.
26. Staehelin LA, Chlapowski FJ, Bonneville MA. Luminal plasma membrane of the urinary bladder. J Cell Biol 1972;53:73.
27. Parsons CL, Stauffer C, Schmidt J. Bladder surface glycosaminoglycans: An efficient mechanism of environmental adaptation. Science 1980; 208:605.
28. Parsons CL, Greenspan C, Mulholland SG. The primary antibacterial defense mechanism of the bladder. Invest Urol 1975;13:72.
29. Parsons CL, Greenspan C, Moore SW, Mulholland SG. Role of surface mucin in primary antibacterial defense of bladder. Urology 1979;9:48.
30. Gill WB, Jones KW, Ruggiero KJ. Protective effects of heparin and other sulfated glycosaminoglycans on crystal adhesion to urothelium. J Urol 1982;127:152.
31. Hanno PM, Parsons CL, Shrom SH, et al. The protective effect of heparin in experimental bladder infection. J Surg Res 1978;25:324.
32. Parsons CL, Mulholland S, Anwar H. Antibacterial activity of bladder surface mucin duplicated by exogenous glycosaminoglycan (heparin). Infect Immun 1979;24:552.
33. Menter JM, Hurst RE, Nakamura N, West SS. Thermodynamics of mucopolysaccharide-dye binding. III. Thermodynamic and cooperative parameters of acridine orange-heparin system. Biopolymers 1979;18:493.
34. Gryte CC, Gregor HP. Poly-(styrene sulfonic acid)-poly-(vinylidene fluoride) interpolymer ion-exchange membranes. J Polymer Sci 1976; 14:1938.
35. Gregor HP. Anticoagulant activity of sulfonate polymers and copolymers. In: Gregor HP, ed.

Polymer science and technology. Vol 5. New York: Plenum Press, 1975:51–56.

36. Gregor HP. Fixed charge ultrafiltration membranes. In: Selegny E, ed. Charged gels and membranes, part I. Holland: D Reider, 1976:235.

37. Hurst RE, Rhodes SW, Adamson PB, et al: Functional and structural characteristics of the glycosaminoglycans of the bladder luminal surface. J Urol 1987;138:433.

38. Bekturov EA, Bakauova KH, eds. Synthetic water-soluble polymers in solution. Basel: Hüthig & Wepf, Verlag, 1986:38–54.

39. Hurst RE. Thermodynamics of the partition of chondroitin sulfate-hexadecylpyridinium complexes in butanol/aqueous salt biphasic solutions. Biopolymers 1978;17:2601.

40. Parsons CL, Schmidt J, Pollen J. Successful treatment of interstitial cystitis with sodium pentosanpolysulfate. J Urol 1983;130:51.

41. Parsons CL, Mulholland S. Successful therapy of interstitial cystitis with pentosanpolysulfate. J Urol 1987;138:513.

42. Mulholland SG, Hanno P, Parsons CL, et al. Pentosan polysulfate sodium for therapy of interstitial cystitis: A double-blind placebo-controlled clinical study. Urology 1990;35:552.

43. Theoharides TC, Sant GR. Bladder mast cell activation in interstitial cystitis. Semin Urol 1991;9:74.

44. Lynes WL, Flynn SD, Shortliffe LD, et al. Mast cell involvement in interstitial cystitis. J Urol 1987;138:746.

45. Larsen S, Thompson SA, Hald T, et al. Mast cells in interstitial cystitis. Br J Urol 1982;54:283.

46. MacDermott JP, Miller CH, Levy N, Stone AR. Cellular immunity in interstitial cystitis. J Urol 1991;145:274.

47. Felsen D, Frye S, Bavendam T, et al. Interleukin-6 activity in the urine of interstitial cystitis (IC) patients. J Urol 1992;147:460A.

48. Nitze M. Lerbuch der Kystoscopie: Ihre Technik und Klinische Bedeuting. Berlin: JE Bergman, 1907:410.

49. Oravisto KJ. Epidemiology of interstitial cystitis: 1. In: Hanno PM, Staskin DR, Krane RJ, et al, eds. Interstitial cystitis. London: Springer-Verlag, 1990:25–28.

50. Held PJ, Hanno PM, Pauly MV, et al. Epidemiology of interstitial cystitis: 2. In: Hanno PM, Staskin DR, Krane RJ, et al, eds. Interstitial cystitis. London: Springer-Verlag, 1990:29–48.

51. American Foundation for Urologic Diseases. Research progress and promises. Baltimore: American Foundation for Urologic Diseases, 1980.

52. Oravisto KJ. Epidemiology of interstitial cystitis. Ann Chir Gynaecol Fenn 1975;64:75.

53. Walsh A. Interstitial cystitis. In: Harrison JH, Gittes RF, Perlmutter AD, et al. Campbell's Urology. 4th ed. Philadelphia: WB Saunders, 1978.

54. Messing EM, Stamey TA. Interstitial cystitis: Early diagnosis, pathology, and treatment. Urology 1978;12:381.

55. Farkas A, Waisman J, Goodwin WE. Interstitial cystitis in adolescent girls. J Urol 1977;118:837.

56. Bowers JE, Lattimer JK. Interstitial cystitis. Surg Gynecol Obstet 1957;105:313.

57. McDonald HP, Upchirch WE, Artime M. Bladder dysfunction in children caused by interstitial cystitis. J Urol 1958;80:354.

58. Lapides J. Observations on interstitial cystitis. Urology 1975;5:610.

59. Parsons CL. Interstitial cystitis: Clinical manifestations and diagnostic criteria in over 200 cases. Neurourol Urodynam 1990;9:241.

60. Pool TL. Interstitial cystitis: Clinical considerations and treatment. Clin Obstet Gynecol 1967; 10:185.

61. De Juana CP, Everett JC. Interstitial cystitis: Experience and review of recent literature. Urology 1977;10:325.

62. Hanno P, Wein A. Interstitial cystitis, Parts I and II. Update Series. Baltimore: American Urological Association, 1987.

63. Smith BH, Dehner LP. Chronic ulcerating interstitial cystitis (Hunner's ulcer). Arch Pathol 1972; 93:76.

64. Bures J, Fixa B, Komarkova O, et al. Nonsmoking: A feature of ulcerative colitis. BMJ 1982; 285:440.

65. Calkins B, Lilienfeld AM, Mendeloff AI, et al. Smoking factors in ulcerative colitis and Crohn's disease in Baltimore. Am J Epidemiol 1984; 122:498.

66. Cope GF, Heatley RV, Kelleher J, Lee PN. Cigarette smoking and inflammatory bowel disease: A review. Human Toxicol 1987;6:189.

67. Paulley JW. Ulcerative colitis: A study of 173 cases. Gastroenterology 1950;16:566.

68. National Center for Health Statistics. Health and nutrition examination survey, cycle II, 1976–1980. Washington DC: Government Printing Office, 1985.

69. Lilienfeld AM, Lilienfeld DE. Foundations of epidemiology. 2nd ed. New York:Oxford, 1980.

70. Larsen S, Thompson S, Hald T, et al. The distribution of mast cells within the bladder wall in interstitial cystitis. Br J Urol 1982;54:283.

71. Fall M, Johansson SL, Vahlne A. A clinicopathological and virological study of interstitial cystitis. J Urol 1985;133:771.

72. Smith B, Dehner LP. Chronic ulcerating interstitial cystitis. A study of 28 cases. Arch Pathol 1972;93:76.

73. Jacobo E, Stamler FW, Culp DA. Interstitial cystitis followed by total cystectomy. Urology 1974; 3:481.

74. Johansson SL, Fall M. Clinical features and spectrum of light microscopic changes in interstitial cystitis. J Urol 1990;143:1118.

75. Burford HE, Burford CE. Hunner ulcer of the bladder: A report of 187 cases. J Urol 1958; 79:952.

76. Gillenwater JY, Wein AJ. Summary of the National Institute of Arthritis, Diabetes, Digestive and Kidney Diseases Workshop on Interstitial Cystitis, National Institutes of Health, Bethesda, Maryland, August 28–29, 1987. J Urol 1988; 140:203.

77. Holm-Bentzen M, Larsen S, Hainau B, Hald T. Nonobstructive detrusor myopathy in a group of patients with chronic bacterial cystitis. Scand J Urol Nephrol 1985;19:21.

78. Bumpus HC. Interstitial cystitis. Med Clin North Am 1930;13:1495.

79. Stewart BH, Persky L, Kiser WS. The use of dimethylsulfoxide (DMSO) in the treatment of interstitial cystitis. J Urol 1968;98:671.

80. Hanno PM, Buehler J, Wein AJ. Use of amitriptyline in the treatment of interstitial cystitis. J Urol 1989;141:846.

81. Bohne AW, Hodson JM, Rebuck JW, Reinhard RE. An abnormal leukocyte response in interstitial cystitis. J Urol 1962;88:387.

82. Simmons JL. Interstitial cystitis: An explanation for the beneficial effect of an antihistamine. J Urol 1961;85:149.

83. Badenoch AW. Chronic interstitial cystitis. Br J Urol 1971;43:718.

84. Dodson AI. Hunner's ulcer of the bladder: A report of 10 cases. Va Med Monthly 1926;53:305.

85. Pool TL. Interstitial cystitis: Clinical considerations and treatment. Clin Obstet Gynecol 1967; 10:185.

86. Wishard WN, Nourse MH, Mertz JHO. Use of clorpactin wcs90 for relief of symptoms due to interstitial cystitis. J Urol 1957;77:420.

87. Lose G, Frandsen B, Hojensgard JC, et al. Chronic interstitial cystitis: Increased levels of eosinophil cationic protein in serum and urine and an ameliorating effect of subcutaneous heparin. Scand J Urol Nephrol 1983;17:159.

88. Parsons CL, Housley T, Schmidt JD, Lebow D. Treatment of interstitial cystitis with intravesical heparin. Br J Urol, in press.

89. Parsons CL, Mulholland SG. Successful therapy of interstitial cystitis with pentosanpolysulfate. J Urol 1987;138:513.

90. Parsons CL, Benson G, Childs SJ, Hanno P, Sant GR, Webster G. A quantitatively controlled method to study prospectively interstitial cystitis and that demonstrates the efficacy of pentosanpolysulfate. J Urol, in press.

91. Nielsen KK, Kromann-Andersen B, Steven K, Hald T. Failure of combined supratrigonal cystectomy and Mainz ileocecocystoplasty in intractable interstitial cystitis: Is histology and mast cell count a reliable predictor for the outcome of surgery? J Urol 1990;144(2 Pt 1):255.

92. Eigner EG, Freiha FS. The fate of the remaining bladder following supravesical diversion. J Urol 1990;144:31.

93. Parsons CL, Koprowski P. Interstitial cystitis: Successful management by a pattern of increasing urinary voiding interval. Urology 1991;37:207.

32

Urethral Syndrome

Richard Schmidt

The urethral syndrome is an exclusionary diagnosis that includes a variety of symptoms, all of which are difficult to explain and all reflective of inefficiencies of voiding behavior. Symptoms can be diverse, even paradoxical. There can be frequency or infrequency of urination; hesitancy or precipitancy in the initiation of voiding; a stream that is forceful or one that is slow, intermittent or terminated prematurely; urinary incontinence or urinary retention. There can be pain or no pain, symptoms may or may not be related to posture, and they may or may not be associated with stress or anxiety. The symptoms may be of recent onset, and at other times they have been present for many years. The severity of symptoms can vary tremendously from patient to patient and, to a lesser degree, in the same patient.

All of this can be quite confusing. It is difficult to treat, especially on a surgical level, a condition that is difficult to understand, let alone explain. There is an implication in the symptoms of a behavioral dysfunction of the urethral and pelvic floor striated muscle as well as a behavioral dyscoordination between the bladder and urinary sphincter.

Patients having the urethral syndrome present most commonly with some or all of the following irritative symptoms: urgency, frequency, nocturia, with or without discomfort; including generally pain in the suprapubic area, dysuria,

urethral sensitivity to catheterization, and even dyspareunia. Hesitancy in onset of a void and a slow, intermittent stream reflect a poorly coordinated relaxation effort on the part of the urinary sphincter and pelvic floor necessary in initiation and maintenance of the void. Incontinence may result from premature or precipitate relaxation of the sphincter.

A variety of abnormalities in behavior of the pelvic floor and urinary sphincter (high pressures, spasticity, dyssynergia, enhanced sphincter zone sensitivity) are identified when these patients are studied urodynamically.[1–4] Not uncommonly significant discomfort can be elicited when digital pressure is applied to the pelvic striated musculature (*i.e.*, especially the levator) on rectal examination. Therapy directed at this behavior often is successful in relieving the symptoms.

Thus, to qualify for this diagnosis, there should be a demonstrable absence of any overt pathologic process on the history, physical examination, and appropriate radiologic and neurophysiologic tests. Additionally, there should be an objective documentation of disturbed voiding patterns by a voiding diary, an abnormal uroflow study, and abnormalities on the urodynamic evaluation.

It is important to underscore the fact that these symptoms reflect a disturbance in the neu-

Female Urology, edited by Elroy D. Kursh and Edward McGuire. J. B. Lippincott, Philadelphia, © 1994.

rology of the lower urinary tract, in particular the behavior of the external sphincter. On examination, there is frequently poor pelvic muscle control on a volitional level as well as on an involuntary level. Urodynamic studies identify a variety of dysfunctional behaviors of the external urethral sphincter as well as an associated instability of the detrusor in 20% to 40% of patients.

Significance of Urodynamic Abnormalities

It is known that there are two layers to the pelvic floor as categorized by their innervation. The levator muscles have a distinct bellowslike movement, and their innervation source is the S-3 and S-4 nerve roots. The more superficial layers of the pelvic floor, which include the two sphincters of the urethra and anus, are innervated by the pudendal nerves, which derive most of their innervation from the S-2 segments. This superficial layer has a distinct clamplike movement. When patients with urethral syndrome are evaluated, discrepancies in the behavior of these two muscle groups are often apparent. These discrepancies can range from an inability to move the muscles at all (the so-called functionally frozen perineum) to discordant motions between the two muscle layers themselves, to underactivity or overactivity of both of these muscle groups. This type of behavior, if chronic, can create problems within the nervous system, leading to hypersensitivity and even inflammation. The similarities here are not too different from that of tennis elbow, or chronic shoulder syndrome from a sporting event abuse.

Urodynamic Changes

Urodynamically these patients demonstrate a spastic dysfunction of the external urinary sphincter with normal bladder compliance.[5,6] Although urethral spasticity is often not present during the filling phase, the vast majority demonstrate significant abnormalities either just before voiding or during the void itself. Even more striking is the functional disability evident in the pelvic floor; most of these patients are unable to exercise effective voluntary control over the striated muscles of the sphincter and pelvic floor. One can only speculate as to the neurologic consequences of such behavior. It is well established in many striated muscle systems that pain and soreness, even inflammation, develop if the muscle system is functionally abused (i.e., the tennis elbow, shin splints). Similar changes and symptoms can occur in the pelvic floor.

Why one patient develops symptoms of soreness and pain, whereas another with the same or similar behavior experiences only frequency, is not known. Such variations in response to injury is true of all skeletal muscle systems in the body. Some explanations are available, but others are not, including genetic factors that may be contributing to the evolution of the syndrome.

The different behaviors[6] can be subdivided into those that are seen during the fill phase (generally sustained high pressures in the sphincter and unstable contractions), those that are seen in the prevoiding phase (poor relaxation efforts resulting in either no void or delayed onset of the void, a spastic unsustained relaxation effort, and a spastic relaxation before the void), and finally, abnormalities that are seen during the voiding phase.

The fact that they exist as singular abnormalities independent of the bladder underscores the need for manometric studies of the sphincter during the various phases of cystometric evaluation.

FILL PHASE

Two types of behavior can be seen: sustained high pressures and clonic instability of the sphincter during the fill phase. The high-pressure sphincters are usually associated with discomfort, marked urge, or the triggering of detrusor instability with movement of the catheter. The high pressures generally preclude clonic spasticity because the sphincter muscle is near maximal recruitment. With lower basal sphincter pressure, however, clonic spasticity may be seen. Often the patient is unaware of the behavior in the early stages of filling.

PREVOID PHASE

Consistent with these patients' complaints of hesitancy is the difficulty for the sphincter to make a smooth transition from a storage-dependent behavior to one consistent with low-pressure detrusor evacuation. Three patterns of abnormal behavior were found in these patients in the attempt to initiate a void. (1) One pattern was a slow hesitant transition of the sphincter and levator to a relaxed posture. This would be associated with either a delayed onset of the void or a poor initial void because of a weak detrusor contraction. Neurologically this behavior would be consistent with ongoing inhibition of the detrusor or a failure in complete disinhibition of the detrusor. (2) A spastic, unstable relaxation behavior within the sphincter or (3) a spastic type of relaxation with a delayed onset of the void is another behavior pattern.

VOID PHASE

The efficiency of the void was affected by one of two types of behavior: an incomplete relaxation of the pelvic floor or urethral sphincter associated with a void. The stream would be slow because of the incomplete relaxation of the bladder outlet. The force of the detrusor contraction may have been suppressed because detrusor pressures were not excessively high. Alternatively, a normal or precipitous relaxation of the urethral sphincter could occur with the void periodically interrupted by the dyssynergic behavior of either or both the levator or urethral sphincter.

These observations suggest that investigation and treatment of the disorder may need to address inflammation and dysfunction of the striated muscles of the urethra and pelvic floor.[7–9] The fact that distinct behavioral abnormalities exist in these patients offers a therapeutic avenue for management of these patients. It also raises the question of whether or not a chronic behavioral abnormality can contribute to the onset of the symptoms.

Etiology

Very little is known of the response in deep muscle of the mechanisms that ultimately lead to fixed symptoms. The deep pelvic tissues are innervated by A (delta) and C afferent fibers. Several mechanisms enhancing transmission in these afferents are known to occur.[7,10]

1. The peripheral afferents can be lost through trauma or disease. This can result in increased spontaneous discharge from dorsal horn cells, which are involved in the transmission of pain within the spinal cord.
2. Selective loss of inhibitory input from the larger myelinated somatic afferents (A alpha) can occur. For example, a lack of dynamic fluctuation in pelvic floor tone might also result in a significant alteration in necessary afferent feedback. This could result from an organic event, such as nerve root pressure from a herniated disc or a pure functional imbalance in the muscle behavior.
3. Peripheral afferents can become sensitized by inflammation or muscle strain. They then maintain a higher level of spontaneous discharge activity than normal. Thus an acute or chronic irritation (*e.g.*, urinary tract infection and pelvic inflammatory disease or long-standing striated muscle dysfunction) may evolve into a pain syndrome through changes induced in pain afferents.

Experiments on damaged peripheral nerves have shown that changes occur in both the peripheral nerve and its central connections. The lower threshold level of response within a nerve can occur owing to repeated exposure to a noxious stimulus. The noxious stimulus can be simply that of chronic strain of the tissue through inappropriate behavior. As a result, progressively larger amounts of spontaneously recordable discharge activity result within the afferent feedback into the spinal cord. This aberrant afferent feedback to the spinal cord can subsequently trigger spastic reflexes or inhibition of behavior. The information is in the form of frequency of action potentials, and reflex adjustments can take place by gating mechanisms within the spinal cord. The central decoding (*i.e.*, Gates) is affected by the level of firing of visceral afferent nerves by afferent somatic input, by endogenous opioid and nonopioid analgesic systems,[11,12] and by central excitation or inhibitions from the brain stem, hypothalamus, and other superspinal areas. A similar concept leads to the neurobiologic theory of pain generation. Peptides can be released in an antidromic fashion from the dorsal root ganglia, and peripheral afferent fibers can be sensitized to release peptides by exposure to increased sympathetic afferent output.[10,11] This concept is embraced in the present neurobiologic view of inflammation, which has replaced the older immunobiologic view of inflammation.

Damaged afferents can demonstrate spontaneous activity near the dorsal root ganglia and increased mechanosensitivity at the regenerating ends. These are referred to as ectopic impulse sites. They are spontaneously active, sending information into the central nervous system that is disruptive and damaging to the integrity of reflex regulatory pathways. Repetitive noxious stimuli applied to the ends of a regenerating nerve lead to increasing intensity (*i.e.*, summation) and persistence of the pain response beyond the period of noxious stimulation. The ectopic impulse sites (axon bulbs or nodules) are thought to arise as a consequence of abnormal protein transport within the damaged afferent. They are sensitive to body movements and neuropeptides and catecholamines released as response to inflammation or injury. Because there may be several peptides, ectopic sites, or catecholamines, removing one may not produce a therapeutic benefit.

The characteristic ache of myofascial pain is consistent with an origin in ectopic neural pacemaker nodules formed where afferents cross spastic muscles (*e.g.*, paraspinal or urethral), or secondary spasticity may result from a mild strain or chronic discoordination in behavior of a dynamic and strong muscle.

Recommended Approach to Treatment

1. History and physical examination.
2. Urodynamic evaluation.
3. Biofeedback (counseling).
4. Drug therapy:
   a. Infection—antibiotic.
   b. Tricyclic medication—(amitriptyline [Elavil]).
   c. Voiding dysfunction
      —skeletal muscle relaxant (diazepam [Valium] or baclofen).
      —alpha blocker (prazosin [Minipress]) or agonist (clonidine).
   d. Anxiety—tranquilizer (haloperidol, methotrimezole, clorazepate [Tranxene]).
5. Nondestructive invasive therapies:
   a. Urethral dilatation.
   b. Mucosal blocks.
   c. Diagnostic nerve blocks.
   d. Acupuncture.
   e. Neural stimulation—vaginal, anal, superficial (transcutaneous electrical nerve stimulation [TENS]).
   f. Sacral root stimulation.
   g. Intrathecal baclofen.
6. Destructive therapies:
   a. Bladder neck or sphincter incision.
   b. Bladder neck or trigone alcohol injections.
   c. Peripheral chemoneurolysis using alcohol or phenol.
   d. Ureterolysis.
   e. Selective nerve rhizotomy.
   f. Diversion.

MODULATION THERAPY

One therapeutic modality useful in the management of this syndrome is that of neurostimulation. This technique takes advantage of gating principle wherein A alpha fibers can inhibit pain information from being transported by way of smaller C afferent nociceptive fibers. It has the potential to reverse aberrant release of peptides and to dampen central hyperexcitability, affecting the reflexes that determine the efficiency of lower urinary tract voiding.

Approximately 90% of afferent feedback through the sacral roots to the spinal cord is from striated muscle. Only 2% to 10% of the afferents arise from the viscera.[8] Increasing transmission of A alpha afferents' input to the spinal cord, through neural stimulation, can suppress pain transmission along the C fibers. The reverse is also true: The removal of A alpha input to the spinal cord can enhance the input of pain. Neurostimulation has a solid basis for treatment of spastic muscle dysfunction, with or without pain. Because many of the symptoms can be based on abnormal transmission within a nociceptive fiber, the most effective means of therapy is to modulate this transmission. Destructive approaches, such as injection of alcohol or phenol to the bladder neck, dissecting out the urethral nerves (urethrolysis), incision of the bladder neck or urethral sphincter, selective rhizotomies, diversion, or augmentations, are risky. They do not change the transmission of information along the nerve fibers and run a significant risk of leaving the patient with continued symptoms and additional alterations in lifestyle. Nondestructive therapies, such as biofeedback methods for re-education of voiding technique, simple urethral dilation, urethral vibration, mucosal blocks, nerve blocks, acupuncture, and neurostimulation, are not only less risky in that they do not permanently change the physiologic situation, but also make much more sense in that they do attempt to modulate the processing of information within the nervous system.

NEUROSTIMULATION

Neuromodulation is a nonspecific stimulus that causes both afferent and efferent impulses to be carried in the pelvic/somatic nerves.[3, 10, 13] These impulses are routed by way of interneurons to the detrusor motor nuclei and the pudendal nuclei. An inhibitory influence on the output from the pudendal nuclei to the external striated sphincter would decrease spasticity, thereby decreasing noxious painful pelvic sensation.

Stimulation of the levator muscle can produce immediate relief in the muscle soreness. This relief can be sustained by chronic stimulation by way of a permanently implanted electrode and pulse generator. The mechanism(s) is unknown, but known theories of endorphin enhancement or gating of neural input can be applied.[7] Properly applied, implantable neuroprosthetics are a safe, low-risk approach to the management of perineal or pelvic pain. Response to stimulation was most effective in those with urodynamically demonstrable pelvic floor dysfunction (instability, peak urethral pressures >100 cm H_2O, or poor sphincter relaxation with dyssynergic voiding). This relief, as a rule, is sustained only with continued neurostimulation, hence the need for a permanently implanted electrode and pulse generator.

These principles aside, the observation, visual or by urodynamics, of altered behavioral function within the pelvic floor should be addressed. Thus, biofeedback should be the integral part of all therapies of this disorder. One of the effective ways to re-educate patients into proper pelvic floor control is through direct stimulation of the sacral roots. This can be accomplished somewhat easily by introducing insulated needles into the sacral foramen and stimulating the sacral roots. By producing a strong, effective, pain-free contraction of the pelvic muscles, patients can learn to copy this behavior. In addition to the re-educational value of direct stimulation of the pelvic floor muscles, there is also the neural modulatory value of the technique. Enhancing the afferent input into the spinal chord along large A alpha afferent fibers can suppress the information within smaller C fibers contributing to symptoms.

IMPLANTED DEVICES

Implanted devices have specific advantages and are able to circumvent most of the disadvantages of TENS therapy.[3] Those patients who benefit from neurostimulation can be helped in a cosmetically acceptable manner, regardless of the time, place, need, or dependence on the neurostimulation. Inefficiencies in delivery of the current are minimized by direct application of current to a specific sacral nerve concerned with the painful tissue. Finally, direct nerve stimulation is the most efficient way to elicit muscle contraction, which, in turn, provides the best hope of relieving pain. Usually with stimulation of a sacral nerve, a pleasant pulling or tugging in the perineum is felt by the patient. With poor nerve coupling of the electrode, stimulation is experienced as a stinging, uncomfortably painful sensation.

A period of testing is required to determine if the proper set of nerve fibers can be found for long-term neurostimulation, then if the stimulation can be applied on a continuing basis. In this procedure, an insulated needle is positioned in one or more of the sacral foramen. Stimulation is applied gradually, by increasing (ramping) the current to a comfortable intensity. Usually the stimulation intensities are much higher and more comfortable when good muscle contraction is obtained. If it is not, the stimulation is unpleasant. When effective, the irritative and pain symptoms are greatly diminished, and tenderness is markedly reduced in pelvic muscles (*i.e.*, on rectal examination) during application of the stimulation.

Patients can be evaluated for the effectiveness of this therapy by leaving in temporary wires in the foramen for a period of 7 to 10 days. If they do well with this therapy but symptoms return on withdrawal of the stimulation, the electrode can be implanted permanently to help control their symptoms. Patients with urgency frequency disorders, dyssynergic voiding patterns, and even urinary retention can be helped through an insertion of a permanently implanted electrode either in the sacral foramen or around the pudendal nerve. Spastic, unstable activity within the urethral sphincter can be dampened down by stimulation. Also, the lability of reflexes within the pelvic floor can be controlled.

Response to stimulation was most effective in those patients who had urodynamically demonstrable pelvic floor dysfunction (instability, peak urethral pressures >100 cm H_2O, or poor sphincter relaxation and dyssynergic voiding). Neurostimulation was not helpful in the absence of spastic dysfunction in the pelvic striated muscle; benefit was obtained only if effective stimulation of the pelvic striated muscle was achieved.

The patient population, however, is a complicated one psychologically as well as physiologically, and as a result, therapeutic successes generally run in the range of 65% to 75%. It is a valuable approach in that it helps diagnose this disorder, can quantify the level of pelvic floor dysfunction (through comparative recruitment with stimulation as to voluntary hold), and allows evoked potential studies, which can quantitate neuromuscular integrity. Finally, there is the modulatory value by way of the gating principle of Melzach and Wall. It is safe and effective and does not obviate other approaches.

Conclusion

In general, urologists are encouraged to deal with pain on as conservative a level as possible. Emotional anxieties, difficult interpersonal relationships, or physical stresses in patients' environment should be carefully addressed, and every attempt should be made to enable the patient to understand that the chances for improving are better if such stresses can be minimized. Voiding dysfunction should then be corrected and pain dealt with through a variety of drug regimens. If pelvic muscle dysfunction is not corrected, the chances are against therapy being successful even with the help of medication.

Diagnostic nerve blocks, neurostimulation, or acupuncture would be the next level of therapy. As a last resort, in unusual circumstances, and only after exhaustive explanation of the consequences should surgical treatment be used. Often conservative therapies fail, but many patients benefit from such a stepwise approach.

References

1. Low JA, Armstrong JB, Mauger GM. The unstable urethra in the female. Obstet Gynecol 1989;74.
2. Raz S, Smith RB. External sphincter spasticity syndrome in female patients. J Urol 1976;15:443.
3. Schmidt RA. Applications of neurostimulation in urology. Neurol Urodynam 1988;7:585.
4. Schmidt RA. The urethral syndrome. Urol Clin North Am 1985;12:349.
5. Stamm WE, Running K, McKevitt M, et al. Causes of the acute urethral syndrome in women. N Engl J Med 1981;304:956.
6. Schmidt RA, Vapnek JM. Pelvic floor behavior and interstitial cystitis. Semin Urol 1991;19:154.
7. Fields HL. Pain. New York: McGraw-Hill, 1987.
8. Fields HL, Levine JD. Pain—mechanisms and management. West J Med 1984;141:347.
9. Schmidt R. Pelvic pain. In: Paulsen DF, ed. Prostate disorders. Philadelphia: Lea & Febiger, 1989;139–155.
10. Cervero F. Visceral nociception: Peripheral and central aspects of visceral nociceptive systems. Trans R Soc Lond [B] 1935;308:325.
11. LaMotte CC, De Lanerolle NC. Human spinal neurons: Innervation by both substance P and enkephalin, Neuroscience 1981;6:713.
12. Sweeney, MI, Sawynok J Evidence that substance P may be a modulator rather than a transmitter of noxious mechanical stimulation. Can J Physiol Pharmacol 1986;64:1324.
13. Campbell JN, Long DM. Peripheral nerve stimulation in the treatment of intractable pain. J Neurosurg 1976;45:692.

VIII   Other Conditions

33

Urethral Diverticula in the Female

Jenelle Foote

Gary E. Leach

History

In 1805, Hey reported the first case of urethral diverticulum in a woman.[1] A century later, Kelly described a single case in 1906.[2] Further interest in the diagnosis and surgical management as reflected in the gynecologic and urologic literature did not appear until the middle third of the 20th century, when Hunner reviewed a small series of women with urethral diverticula in 1938.[3]

Incidence

The incidence of urethral diverticulum in women has been estimated at 1.4% to 4.7% by a number of investigators. Aldridge and colleagues discovered urethral diverticula urethroscopically in 1.4% of 279 patients who were referred for a variety of indications. Hoffman and Adams obtained positive pressure urethrograms on 129 consecutive female patients without urinary symptoms and found an incidence of 4.7%.[5] Anderson diagnosed nine cases among 300 women with untreated carcinoma of the cervix, an incidence of 3%.[6] Davis and Robinson reported diverticula in 1.85% of female patients admitted to their urology services.[7] Serial experiences with urethral diverticula at the Cleveland Clinic, Mayo Clinic, and Johns Hopkins Hospi-

tal demonstrated that the reported incidence of the disease increased with the level of awareness at those institutions.[8-10]

Pathophysiology

There are two theories that have been proposed to explain the pathogenesis of urethral diverticula in women. Because of the occasional discovery of suburethral cysts in the newborn, a congenital cause has been proposed by some investigators, including Higgins and Runbousek, Pinkerton, and Ratner and Ritz.[11-13] Counseller and Gilbert and Cintron also thought that the diverticula were congenital with symptoms developing after trauma or nonspecific infections.[14,15] Nel postulated that congenital diverticula could arise in the following ways: (1) as remnants of Gartner's ducts, (2) from faulty union of primal folds, (3) from *cell rests*, (4) from vaginal wall cysts of müllerian origin, and (5) from congenital dilatation of periurethral cysts.[16]

Most authors favor the theory of an acquired nature of diverticula, however. Support for this opinion stems from the fact that urethral diverticula in women occur almost exclusively in young and middle-aged women, with the average age of diagnosis between 36 and 43 years.[17-20] It has been suggested that the trauma of child-

449

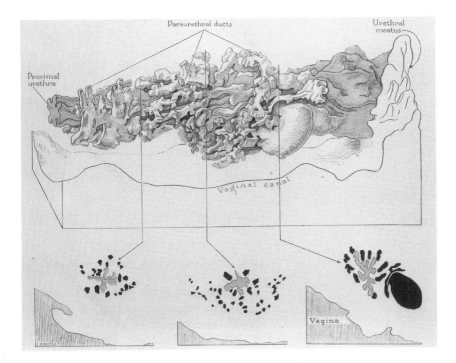

Figure 33-1. Huffman's 1948 drawing of a wax model of an adult female
urethra with its periurethral ducts and glands as seen in the right lateral view.
(From Huffman JW. The detailed anatomy of the paraurethral (sic) ducts in the
adult human female. Am J Obstet Gynecol 1948;55:86.)

birth may play a role in the cause of urethral
diverticula, although the percentage of nulli-
parity in this population ranges from 14% to
39%.[20–23]

An important contribution to the understanding of the pathogenesis of urethral diverticula and urethral anatomy is Huffman's work
in 1947, which detailed the anatomy of the periurethral glands and ducts. Wax castings of the
entire female urethra were made (Fig. 33-1). On
microscopic section, up to 31 periurethral glands
were seen throughout the length of the urethra,
with these glands and ducts being concentrated
in the middle and distal thirds of the posterolateral urethra.[24] The majority of urethral diverticula and their openings (or ostia) are also
located in the middle and distal thirds of the urethra, and most lie posterolaterally, between 3
and 9 o'clock. In a 1984 series of 204 patients

from the Mayo Clinic, only 9 patients had ostia
located anteriorly or anterolaterally.[9] Because
these findings are consistent with Huffman's anatomic work locating the periurethral glands in
this area, most authors support a theory describing a common origin of periurethral glands and
diverticula.

Routh postulated that infection and obstruction of the periurethral glands result in the
formation of retention cysts. Such obstruction
may be related to the trauma associated with
childbirth, instrumentation, or infection.[25] When
infected, the cysts, now abcesses, rupture into the
urethral lumen, establishing communication with
the urethra. In most histologic specimens, the
lining of the diverticulum shows squamous
metaplasia with ulceration and chronic inflammation.[26]

Peters and Vaughan suggested that gonococcus was the most common offending organism.[27] Lee's study, however, showed that *Escherichia coli* was the predominant organism, occurring in 13 of 19 patients cultured.[22] The site, method, and timing of collection were not specified. Other urinary pathogens are also associated with urethral diverticula, and mixed infections are frequent.[21] Because most diverticula harbor infection, perioperative antibiotic coverage is essential.

Associated Carcinoma

In a 1983 case report and review of the medical literature, Patanaphan and co-workers discussed 32 cases of cancer arising from urethral diverticula.[28] Adenocarcinoma was most common (19 cases); in the majority of cases, the cancer was localized in the midurethra. Other cancers were squamous cell carcinomas (four cases) and transitional cell carcinomas (nine cases). Transitional cell carcinoma occurred more commonly at the proximal urethra and appeared to be more aggressive. Common symptoms associated with carcinoma of the urethral diverticulum include a firm mass in the suburethral area, dysuria, and bleeding. The lack of a specific warning symptom, such as bleeding, may account for the advanced stage of presentation in some cases.[28]

Based on Patanaphan and co-workers' review of treatment regimens and results, the following recommendations were made: Diverticulectomy or radiotherapy alone is not generally curative. For limited disease, either radical surgery (*i.e.*, cystourethrectomy or anterior exenteration) or combined therapy in the form of diverticulectomy followed by curative irradiation is recommended. For advanced disease (*i.e.*, involvement of bladder neck, bladder, or inguinal lymph nodes), combined therapy, in the form of preoperative irradiation followed by radical surgery, is recommended.[28]

Adenocarcinoma of the urethral diverticulum can develop as the result of metaplasia of the epithelium, chronic irritation, or infection. In their 1983 case report, Evans and associates reviewed the presentation, management, and outcome of 12 reported cases of adenocarcinoma occurring in female urethral diverticula.[29] In contrast to Patanaphan and co-workers' review, in which several histologic types of cancer were summarized, Evans and associates limited their discussion to adenocarcinoma only. Evans and associates concluded that local excision alone is adequate when tumor appears localized to the diverticulum because two thirds of the patients treated with local excision were cured, and recurrences were effectively treated surgically (*i.e.*, with local excision or anterior exenteration), usually in combination with radiation therapy.[29]

After finding three metachronous adenocarcinomas in 20 cases of patients with diverticula in the proximal female urethra, Tesluk has recommended careful follow-up for patients who have had proximal diverticular surgery.[30] The adenocarcinomas developed at intervals of 8 months, 1 year, and 16 years after removal of pathologically benign diverticula.[30]

Symptoms

Some women with urethral diverticula are asymptomatic, with the diverticula being discovered serendipitously during routine pelvic examination. Women who are symptomatic from urethral diverticula have complaints that are nonspecific (Table 33-1). Because of this nonspecificity, the diagnosis is often not suspected and therefore delayed.[31] In fact, the duration of symptoms on presentation ranges from 1 to 15 years.[9] Symptoms may be subdivided into those that are irritative and those that are related to the mass effect of the diverticulum. The chronic irritative symptoms of frequency, urgency, and dysuria are common. Some patients describe a severe gripping, spasmlike pain after urination, with a sense of fullness in the region of the urethra that disappears after the spasm is gone or is relieved by pressure on the anterior vaginal wall.[9] Urinary tract infection is commonly present and is apt to be of a recurrent nature involving the same organism in serial cultures. In fact, urethral

Table 33-1. *Presenting Symptoms of Female Urethral Diverticula (% of patients)*

SERIES NO. PATIENTS YEAR	DAVIS AND TELINDE[10] 121 1958	MACKINNON ET AL[9] 204 1959	HOFFMAN AND ADAMS[5] 60 1965	KITTREDGE ET AL[65] 27 1966	DAVIS AND ROBINSON[7] 120 1970	PATHAK AND HOUSE[23] 45 1970	WOODHOUSE ET AL[66] 13 1980	ROZASAHEGYI ET AL[67] 50 1984	LEACH AND BAVENDAM[41] 37 1987
Vaginal Mass	—	12	45	—	—	18	15	—	16
Dysuria	63	73	58	52	32	47	31	80	10.8
Frequency Urgency	83	66	—	44	58	42	—	100	—
Recurrent Infections	—	46	—	—	33	—	23	80	40.5
Dyspareunia	24	14	20	15	12	13	—	70	19
Urethral Pain	—	29	—	—	30	26	—	45	—
Hypogastric Pain	—	—	25	4	—	—	—	60	—
Postvoid Pain/Dribbling	13	—	90	15	32	22	—	—	13.5
Hematuria	26	17	18	—	17	7	8	35	—
Incontinence	25	25	70	30	9	22	23	25	51
Stress Urge	—	—	—	—	—	4	—	—	35
Urethral Discharge	1.6	—	—	—	—	31	15	—	—
Asymptomatic	7.4	—	—	11	1.6	—	—	—	—

diverticula should always be suspected when urinary tract infections fail to respond to appropriate therapy or recur at frequent intervals.

Stewart interviewed a group of women with symptoms of "chronic cystitis" regarding the symptom of dyspareunia. Although the women in this group with the concomitant diagnosis of urethral diverticula had a 40% incidence of dyspareunia, the women without the diagnosis of urethral diverticula had a 50% incidence of dyspareunia. Thus, this study demonstrated that although dyspareunia is common to the evaluation of urethral diverticula, the symptom is nonspecific.[20]

Symptoms of urethral diverticula that may be secondary to its mass effect include dribbling, incomplete emptying, decreased force of stream, and the feeling of an anterior vaginal wall mass. In these patients, the distended diverticulum may cause enough distortion of the urethra to narrow its lumen. Postvoid dribbling, the third "d" of the classic triad of symptoms associated with urethral diverticula (*i.e.*, dysuria, dyspareunia, dribbling) is usually loss of a small amount of urine after voiding. The patient may report a mass in the anterior wall of the vagina that is associated with tenderness or the discharge of pus, urine, or blood when compressed.

Associated Incontinence

Urethral diverticula are frequently associated with bladder and urethral dysfunction. In a review of four studies (a total of 482 patients) by Bass and Leach, 32% of women with urethral diverticula presented with urinary incontinence.[32] In an attempt to decrease the risk of postoperative incontinence, 41 women with diverticula were evaluated urodynamically. All women underwent uroflow and multichannel cystometry and pressure-flow analysis. Twenty-five women (61%) had an abnormal urodynamic evaluation. Twelve had genuine stress urinary incontinence alone, eight had stress urinary incontinence with detrusor instability, and two had detrusor instability alone. Two patients had combined sensory and detrusor instability, and

one had myogenic decompensation. Based on the postoperative results (to be detailed later in this chapter), the authors concluded that preoperative urodynamics is useful in patients with urethral diverticula and that it greatly influences the choice of surgical procedure to maximize postoperative continence.[32]

Bhatia and others described a characteristic biphasic shape of the urethral pressure profile in six patients presenting with urinary incontinence who were subsequently found to have urethral diverticula.[33, 34] A significant decrease in the urethral pressure was observed at the anatomic location of the diverticular orifice (Fig. 33-2).[33, 34] Such a serendipitous finding in a patient undergoing urethral pressure profile should alert the operator to the possible presence of a urethral diverticulum.

Physical Examination

On physical examination, a midline bulge overlying the urethra is commonly seen (Fig. 33-3). When compression of the anterior vaginal wall bulge yields pus, blood, or urine from the meatus, a urethral diverticulum is likely to be present (Fig. 33-4). Palpation of a hard, irregular mass should alert the examiner to the possible presence of calculi or cancer.

In 1958, Davis and TeLinde reported that pus could be expressed from the external meatus on "stripping" the urethra in 63% of women with urethral diverticula.[10] Twenty-three years later, in 1981, Stewart and colleagues noted that the patients with diverticula had few physical signs other than localized anterior vaginal wall tenderness.[20] Although physical examination can be unremarkable, the authors are likewise impressed that the finding of a suburethral mass or tenderness is quite common and a sensitive indicator for the presence of a diverticulum.[6, 10, 35]

Differential Diagnosis

The differential diagnosis of an anterior urethral mass includes cystocele, Gartner's duct cyst,

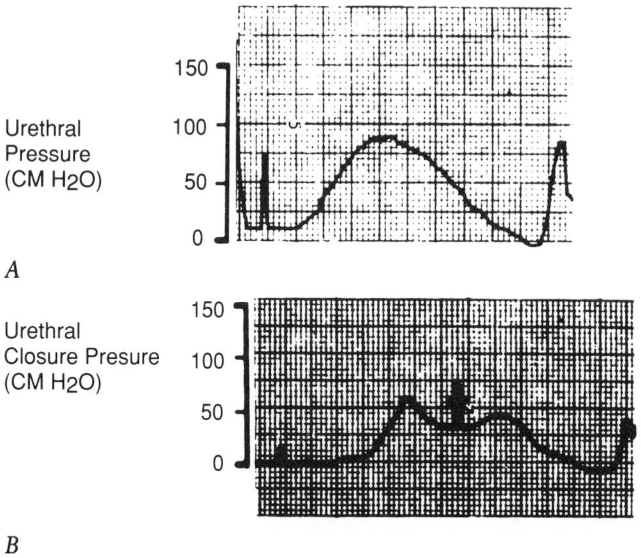

Urethral
Pressure
(CM H2O)

150
100
50
0

A

Urethral
Closure Presure
(CM H2O)

150
100
50
0

B

Figure 33-2. *(A) Normal urethral pressure profile. (B) Biphasic shape of urethral pressure profile with central depression* (arrow) *at diverticular communication site. (From Bhatia NN, McCarthy TA, Ostergard D. Urethral pressure profiles of women with urethral diverticula. Obstet Gynecol 1981;58:375.)*

vaginal inclusion cyst, urethral cancer, Skene's abscess, vaginal carcinoma, and ectopic ureterocele. An ectopic ureterocele can mimic a urethral diverticulum radiographically when only the dilated, prolapsed part of the ectopic ureterocele retains contrast material beneath the urethral meatus[36] (Fig. 33-5). Although ureteral ectopia is a relatively rare condition, 33% to 48% of these cases occur in adults, and nearly half of these patients have a history of nonspecific urinary tract infections without incontinence.[37] Blacklock and colleagues reported two cases in which marsupialization and excision of vaginal wall masses resulted in incontinence. The diagnosis of ectopic ureterocele was made postoperatively with intravenous pyelography and urethroscopy. Subsequent treatment with heminephrectomy and ureterectomy resulted in postoperative continence.[37]

Endoscopic Evaluation

Often the ostium or communication site between the diverticulum and the urethra can be located through the urethroscope. A blunt-tipped female urethroscope with a 0 or 30 degree lens provides optimal visualization of the urethral lumen. As previously noted, most openings are on the urethral floor (*i.e.*, posterior urethral wall) and are from 2 to 5 mm in diameter.[9] With the instrument in the distal urethra, massage of the suburethral area should be performed. This massage may cause the excretion of a stream of thick purulent material from the orifice of a diverticulum, at times resembling "toothpaste coming from a tube when it is being pressed."[9] The small size of the orifice as well as swelling and occlusion of the orifice may be responsible for the inability to demonstrate the orifice endo-

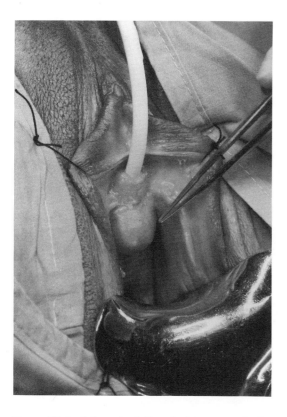

Figure 33-3. Suburethral diverticulum on vaginal examination. (From Leach GE, Bavendam TG. Female urethral diverticula. Urology 1987;30:407.)

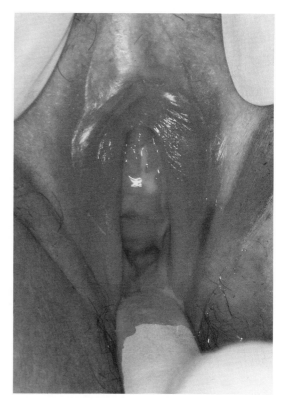

Figure 33-4. Pus expressed from urethral diverticulum on compression of anterior vaginal wall.

scopically. Both Davis and TeLinde and Butler reported the inability to visualize the orifices of known diverticula endoscopically approximately 40% of the time.[10,38]

Radiographic Studies

Approximately 6% to 10% of diverticula contain calculi[39,40] (Fig. 33-6). Presumably stasis of urine and chronic infection are responsible for the formation of these stones. The calculi can sometimes be detected on an abdominal or pelvic x-ray (Fig. 33-7).

Urethral diverticular sacs can be identified in the postvoid view of an intravenous pyelo-

gram (Fig. 33-8). It is essential that the films include the area several centimeters below the ischial tuberosities, however. Leach and Bavendam performed intravenous pyelograms in 36 of 37 women with urethral diverticula.[41] Although the diverticula were identified on eight postvoid views, the postvoid views were inadequate in 13 cases because of improper film position.[41]

A properly performed voiding cystourethrogram under fluoroscopic control is a sensitive radiographic study with which to demonstrate urethral diverticula.[42] In fact, Leach and Bavendam found that the voiding cystourethrogram confirmed the location and extent in 35 out of 36 women.[41] Only one woman required another radiologic study (double-balloon urethrogram,

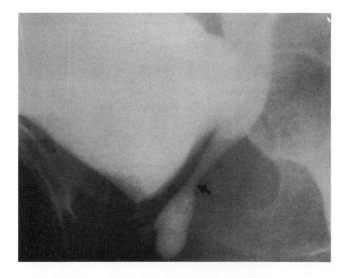

Figure 33-5. *Voiding cystourethrogram showing ectopic ureter (arrow) inserting into urethra. Note that the* pseudodiverticulum *is formed by the dilated prolapsed distal ureteral segment. (From Curry NS. Ectopic ureteral orifice masquerading as a urethral diverticulum. AJR Am J Roentgenol 1983;141:1325.)*

to be discussed later) to demonstrate the diverticulum.[41] Diverticula can be simple, multiple, or complex with multiple lobes (Fig. 33-9). An air-fluid level should alert the surgeon to the presence of a large diverticulum. Filling defects within the diverticulum may represent tumor, stones, or clots. The voiding cystourethrogram also permits the clinician to evaluate urethral hypermobility or rarely urethrovaginal fistulas, which may contribute to incontinence.

Although a well-performed voiding cystourethrogram is adequate to demonstrate urethral diverticula in the vast majority of patients, occasionally other radiologic diagnostic maneuvers are indicated. In 1959, Lang and Davis introduced positive pressure urethrography for the detection of diverticula in women.[43] They described the filling of the urethra using a closed system provided by a double-balloon catheter (Fig. 33-10). The purpose of the positive pressure technique is to occlude the urethra at both ends while filling it with contrast material under pressure.[43] Another study from the same institution reported how this technique dramatically improved the detection of urethral diverticula, resulting in as many new cases diagnosed in a 1-year period as had been detected in the previous 50 years.[10] No comment was made regarding the quality of less invasive studies (*i.e.*, voiding cystourethrogram), however. Stewart and colleagues evaluated 40 female patients with persistent urinary symptoms of cystitis with positive pressure urethrography. Sixteen were found to have urethral diverticula (an incidence of 40%), and 14 underwent diverticulectomy.[20]

Steinhardt and Landes described a variant of the retrograde urethrogram that uses countertraction as a means to elongate the female urethra.[44] An Allis clamp grasps the vaginal mucosa, and traction is applied away from the patient as the rubber olive tip of the Brodney device is applied snugly to the urethral meatus. Radiographs are obtained while the contrast medium is injected.[44]

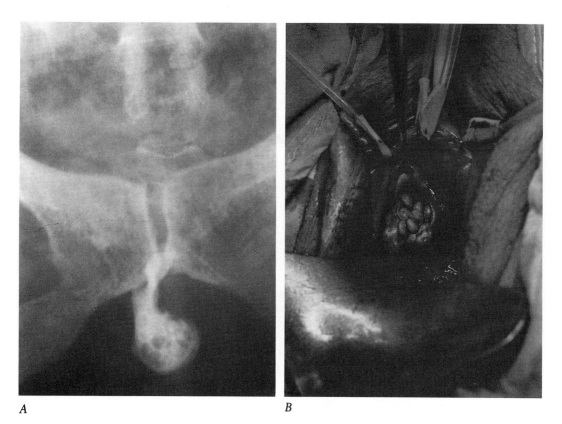

A *B*

Figure 33-6. *(A) Filling defects on postvoid view of cystourethrogram that represent calculi within a urethral diverticulum. (B) Diverticulum opened intraoperatively reveals multiple struvite stones. (From Leach GE, Bavendam TG. Female urethral diverticula.* Urology *1987;30:407.)*

Of historical interest, diverticula can be visualized by means of direct injection of contrast material into the ostium of the diverticulum by means of a 4 French urethral catheter passed through the endoscope. Although MacKinnon and associates were successful in making the diagnosis from this method in 53% of 203 cases, they state that the voiding cystourethrogram is more "reliable."[9]

Diverticula can also be visualized by percutaneous contrast material injection through the anterior vaginal wall. Using a 2-ml syringe with contrast media, the needle is advanced through the vaginal wall until the needle is in the diverticulum. The presence of urine or pus is confirmed by aspiration. By injecting the dye slowly into the suspected cavity, a diverticulum is demonstrated on anteroposterior and lateral x-ray films.[45] Potential complications of this type of approach include decompression of the sac, which may make subsequent attempts at excision difficult, and the creation of a draining sinus or fistula. Today with the availability of high-quality voiding cystourethrography, other more invasive attempts to visualize a suspected diverticulum, such as this, are usually unnecessary.

Wexler and McGovern examined three patients sonographically with known diagnoses of

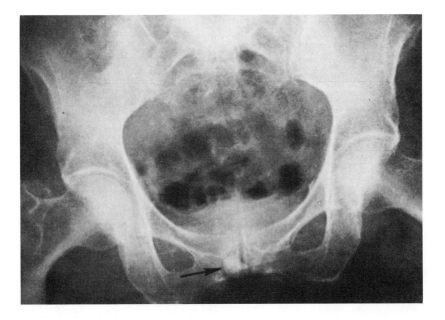

Figure 33-7. *Stone* (arrow) *in a urethral diverticulum demonstrated on a plain radiograph. (From Ward JN, Draper JW, Tovell HMM. Diagnosis and treatment of urethral diverticula in the female. Surg Gynecol Obstet 1967;125:1293.)*

urethral diverticula[46] (Fig. 33-11). All patients were scanned transabdominally in the supine position with a full bladder. Longitudinal scans of the pelvis were obtained with the transducer directed toward the base of the bladder to include the vagina. Transverse scans were performed with the transducer positioned in the midline just above the symphysis pubis. The authors state that the size and nature of the excised specimen conformed to the sonographic features, although pathologic details were not provided.[46] The incidental finding of cystic structures beneath the bladder base, therefore, should alert the ultrasonographer to the possible presence of a urethral diverticulum.

Treatment

Surgical treatment of female urethral diverticula may be subdivided into those methods that involve (1) ablation of the diverticular cavity; (2) marsu-

pialization of the cavity, either into the urethral lumen or into the vagina; and (3) removal of the diverticulum through a vaginal incision.

ABLATION OF THE DIVERTICULAR CAVITY

In 1957, Ellik described his experience with transvaginal diverticulectomy: "[S]urgical ablation is the usual treatment but may be accompanied by qualms, tedium and hazard on the part of the operator."[47] He then described seven women with urethral diverticula whose diverticular cavities were ablated with the packing of absorbable material. A stab incision was made through the anterior vaginal wall directly into the diverticulum. After the cavity was drained, the cavity was irrigated, and the lining was excoriated with a gauze sponge. The cavity was packed with absorbable hemostatic agents (*i.e.,* Oxycel or Gelfoam). The incision was then closed with interrupted chromic sutures. The author described symptomatic relief and the ab-

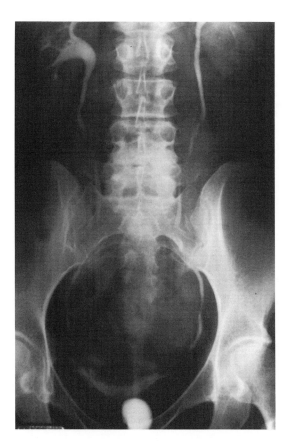

Figure 33-8. Postvoid view of an intravenous py-elogram showing filling of urethral diverticulum. (From Leach GE, Schmidbauer, CP, Hadley HR, et al. Surgical treatment of female urethral diverticulum. Sem Urol 1986;4:33.)

sence of a mass on palpation at 2 weeks follow-up. Ellik credited the success of this procedure to the absorbable material, which obliterated the cavity and sealed the urethral communication by the process of *fibrotic assimilation*.[47]

Mizrahi and associates reported a case involving the transvaginal periurethral injection of polytetrafluoroethylene (polytef) into a diverticulum with good results.[48] With urethroscopic inspection, a 17 gauge needle was inserted transvaginally and advanced periurethrally toward the diverticulum. The diverticulum collapsed after the injection of 5 ml of polytef. With 1 year

follow-up, the patient was free of symptoms, and a retrograde urethrogram revealed a normal urethra.[48] Potential complications with this approach include infection, which could lead to periurethral abscess, necrosis, and subsequent slough, as well as a granulomatous foreign body reaction, which could compromise future therapeutic procedures.

MARSUPIALIZATION OF THE CAVITY INTO THE URETHRAL LUMEN

In 1979, Lapides reported the treatment of six women with recurrent urethral diverticula.[49] The patients, who all had multiple diverticula in the mid or distal segments of the urethra, were treated with transurethral diverticulotomy with a resectoscope and knife electrode. The goal of this operation is to enlarge the mouth, or opening, of the diverticulum markedly into the urethra by incising the shared floor of the urethra and roof of the diverticulum. The technique involves urethroscopy and insertion of a knife electrode through the diverticular orifice. The entire tented roof of the diverticulum is divided with a cutting or blended current. This procedure may involve incising most of the length of the urethra (Fig. 33-12). Although Lapides stated that all patients were relieved of symptoms and infection during a period of follow-up of 1.5 to 7 years, the complication of incontinence was not discussed.[49]

Other transurethral procedures to treat small diverticula have been described, including resection of the diverticular roof and fulguration of the lining of the sac. The pocket can also be opened by the use of a Collings knife through a panendoscope.[9]

In 1989, Miskowiak and deLichtenberg reported two cases with a description of an "open" variant of this endoscopic procedure.[50] In this procedure, the ostium of the diverticulum is visualized and incised directly. These authors describe various techniques to aid in the localization of the ostium, including the expression of pus, the use of sound, and the performance of a meatotomy. When performed on diverticula lo-

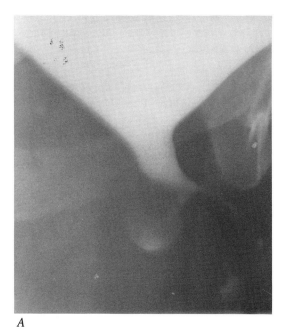

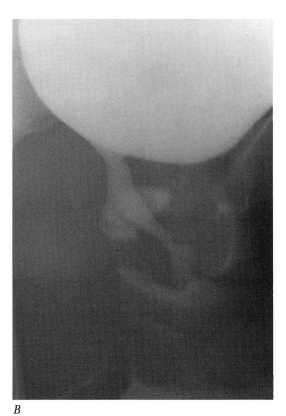

A

B

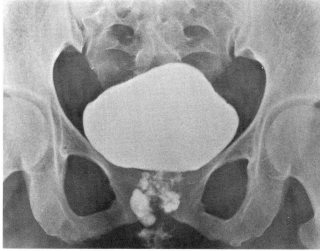

C

Figure 33-9. (A) Simple diverticulum demonstrated on voiding cystourethrogram. (B) Bilobed diverticulum that encircles the urethra. (C) Complex diverticulum with multiple lobes. ([A] from Bass JS, Leach GE. Surgical treatment of concomitant urethral diverticulum and stress urinary incontinence. Urol Clin North Am 1991;18:365. [B] from Leach GE, Bavendam TG. Female urethral diverticula. Urology 1987;30:407.)

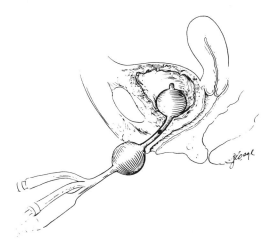

Figure 33-10. Trattner double-balloon catheter (CR Bard, Inc, Murray Hill, NJ): Proximal balloon occludes the bladder neck, and distal balloon occludes external meatus. Contrast material is injected into the urethra by way of a channel between the two balloons. (From Greenberg M, Stone D, Cochran ST, et al. Female urethral diverticula. AJR Am J Roentgenol 1981;136:259.)

cated in the middle and distal parts of the urethra, the authors suggest that these procedures are safe and easy to perform. Other suggested advantages are a short operating time and hospital stay with minimal risk of incontinence and urethrovaginal fistula.[50]

All marsupialization procedures have in common the division of the distal urethra. Continence subsequently depends on the functional integrity of the proximal urethra and bladder neck. The authors question the safety of such procedures for midurethral diverticula because up to 51% of continent perimenopausal women have open bladder necks on voiding cystourethrogram.[51] In these women, the level of continence is below the level of the bladder neck and is dependent on an intact midurethral "sphincter" mechanism. Owing to these concerns, the authors recommend that the performance of these marsupialization procedures should be limited to diverticula in the distal one third of the urethra only.

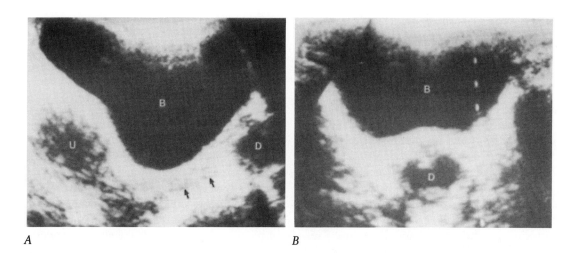

A *B*

Figure 33-11. (A) Longitudinal and (B) transverse angled pelvic sonograms. Diverticulum (D) filled with urine; base of bladder (B); uterus (U). (From Wexler JS, McGovern TP. Ultrasonography of female urethral diverticula. AJR Am J Roentgenol 1980;134:737.)

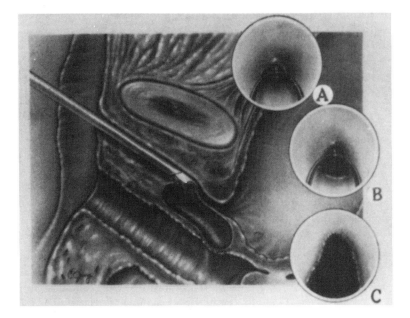

Figure 33-12. (A) After insertion of electrode into the diverticulum, the roof of the diverticulum is "tented" up. (B,C) The knife electrode is advanced until the entire roof of the diverticulum is divided. (From Lapides J. Transurethral treatment of urethral diverticula in women. J Urol 1979;121:736.)

MARSUPIALIZATION OF THE CAVITY INTO THE VAGINA

In 1970, Spence and Duckett published experience with nine women in whom urethral diverticula were treated with marsupialization into the vagina.[52] In this operation, division of the floor of the distal urethra between the external urinary meatus and orifice of the diverticulum is combined with a midline incision of the diverticulum proper and the underlying vaginal wall (Fig. 33-13). After the sac is saucerized, an absorbable suture is used to coapt the epithelial margins of the incised diverticulum and adjacent vagina. An indwelling urethral catheter and iodoform pack are placed for 48 hours. This technique was applied only to diverticula of the middle or distal third of the urethra for fear of iatrogenic incontinence or bladder injury.[52] Long-term follow-up of an adequate number of patients managed by the Spence and Duckett type of vaginal marsupialization is not available, especially with regard to the incidence of delayed complications, such as recurrent diverticula and postoperative urinary incontinence.

TRANSVAGINAL DIVERTICULECTOMY

Many variations of transvaginal urethral diverticulectomy have been described since Johnson first described the complete excision of the diverticular sac in five women in 1938.[53] These procedures have in common certain steps: (1) the incision of the anterior vaginal wall over the diverticulum, (2) the mobilization and excision of the diverticular sac, (3) the approximation of the urethra, and (4) the anterior vaginal wall closure. Different authors have proposed modifications of each of those steps.

Perioperatively consideration is given to ad-

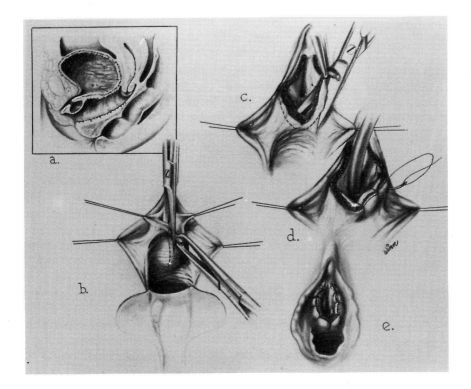

Figure 33-13. *Marsupialization of the urethra to the vagina as described by Spence and Duckett: (A,B) The urethral floor and diverticular sac are incised distal to the ostium of the diverticulum. (C) The redundant flaps are trimmed. (D, E) The margins of the trimmed sac and adjacent vaginal mucosa are approximated with a running locking suture. (From Spence HM, Duckett JW. Diverticulum of the female urethra. J Urol 1970;104:432.)*

equate bladder drainage, the prevention of infection, and excellent operative exposure. The authors use both a suprapubic tube and Foley catheter for perioperative bladder drainage because blockage of the Foley catheter postoperatively can lead to bladder spasm and a "blow out" of the diverticular repair. The suprapubic tube is placed early in the operative procedure with the aid of a Lowsley tractor. Patients receive anticholinergic medications postoperatively (*i.e.*, oxybutynin and imipramine every 8 hours; belladonna and opiate suppositories as needed) to prevent postoperative bladder spasms.

Oral antibiotics are given preoperatively to treat positive urine cultures. Patients perform antiseptic perineal scrubs and vaginal douches both the evening before and the morning of surgery and also receive a 10-minute iodophor perineal and vaginal preparation in the operating room. Broad-spectrum intravenous antibiotics are administered preoperatively and for 24 hours postoperatively. Patients are then maintained on oral antibiotics until after removal of the catheters, 10 to 14 days later.

The authors prefer the modified dorsal lithotomy position. Sasnett and colleagues have described the use of the jackknife prone position in five patients, however. As described, this position gives maximal exposure and allows the surgeon to work from a standing position.[54]

Incision of Anterior Vaginal Wall Over the Diverticulum

Wharton and TeLinde, Mackinnon and colleagues, Ward and colleagues, Benjamin and colleagues, and Lee have described making a vertical incision in the anterior vaginal wall to expose the underlying tissues.[9,19,22,55,56] In 1967, Ward and colleagues described exposure through the use of an inverted U-shaped vaginal flap.[56] Benjamin and colleagues, Boyd and Raz, and Leach and colleagues have subsequently described this type of incision as well[19,57,58] (Fig. 33-14). The advantage of this incision is the creation of a well-vascularized flap that covers the subsequent repair with nonoverlapping suture lines and thus minimizes the risk of postoperative urethral-vaginal fistula.

Although some authors proceed to the mobilization of the diverticular sac at this point, preservation and mobilization of a layer of periurethral fascia deep to the vaginal wall is extremely important.[55,56] Use of this layer reinforces the urethral reconstruction and decreases the risk of postoperative fistula and recurrence of the diverticulum. Mackinnon and associates and Lee describe making the incision in the periurethral fascia in a vertical fashion; Boyd and Raz and Leach and colleagues describe making this incision in a transverse fashion[9,22,57,58] (Fig. 33-15). The transverse incision is advantageous in that the suture line does not overlap the vertical urethral closure. The ease or difficulty with which the layers are separated depends on the amount of inflammatory reaction around the sac. Previous surgery and a history of radiation therapy in this area are both associated with scarring and a more difficult dissection.

Mobilization and Excision of the Diverticular Sac

Because a distended diverticulum is more easily mobilized, care should be taken not to massage the diverticulum and empty it prematurely during the preparation of the vagina. Although the authors only rarely encounter difficulty in keeping the diverticulum distended, a number of authors have described a variety of adjunctive means to keep the sac distended. Because of their experience in which "a prolonged search was frequently necessary to identify the diverticulum which was often thin walled and difficult to locate unless chronically inflamed and distended with pus," Stewart and co-workers described the insertion of the balloon of the Foley catheter into the diverticulum to facilitate dissection.[20] Sounds can be inserted into the diverticulum through the urethra, and catheters have been coiled into the sac to aid in identification. Methylene blue has been used to stain the walls of a multilobulated diverticulum to ensure complete excision of the sac. Hyams and Hyams have described packing the sac with gauze.[54] Moore has described a method in which a balloon is inserted into the diverticulum through a stab wound. The incision is closed with a pursestring suture, and the diverticulum is subsequently dissected.[17] Tancer and co-workers used a double-balloon catheter (Trattner, CR Bard Co, Murray Hill, NJ) to fill the diverticulum with water.[60] Hirschhorn injected a silicone and rubber mixture to distend the diverticulum. This material (*i.e.,* coagulum), on the addition of a catalyst, hardens to a rubbery white solid and aided in the dissection.[61] In the authors' experience, these maneuvers are rarely required because the diverticulum is usually easily identified after the vaginal flap is reflected off of the periurethral fascia.

Most authors describe mobilization of the entire diverticulum, identification of the urethra, and subsequent excision of the diverticular sac from the urethral wall[9,19,22,56,57,58] (Fig. 33-16). The diverticulum is completely excised, usually creating a large gap in the ventral urethra. All inflamed and fibrotic tissue at the communication site of the diverticulum is excised to minimize the risk of recurrent diverticulum formation. Tancer and colleagues described a 10-year experience with a method of *partial ablation* of diverticula, performed in 34 women.[60] In this method, the "easily excisable portion" of the sac is removed, without any effort made to remove the sac at its neck.[60] The authors believe, how-

(*continued on page 468*)

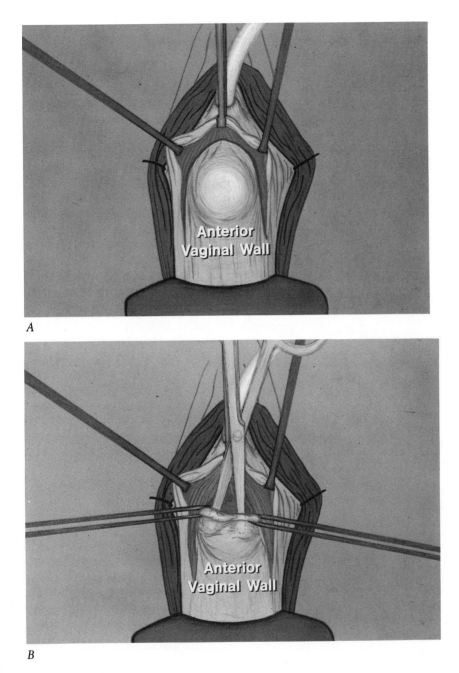

Figure 33-14. (A) An inverted U-shaped incision has been made after infiltrating the anterior vaginal wall with saline. (B) Dissection between the periurethral fascia and anterior vaginal wall facilitates mobilization of vaginal flap to the bladder neck. (From Leach GE, Schmidbauer CP, Hadley HR, et al. Surgical treatment of female urethral diverticulum. Sem Urol 1986;4:33.)

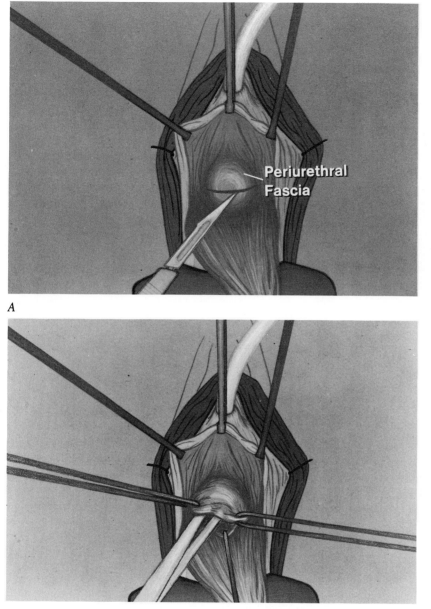

A

B

Figure 33-15. (A) The periurethral fascia should be incised transversely.
(B) Dissection between the periurethral fascia and the urethral diverticulum preserves the periurethral fascial layer for subsequent closure. (From Leach GE,
Schmidbauer CP, Hadley HR, et al. Surgical treatment of female urethral diverticulum. Sem Urol 1986;4:33.)

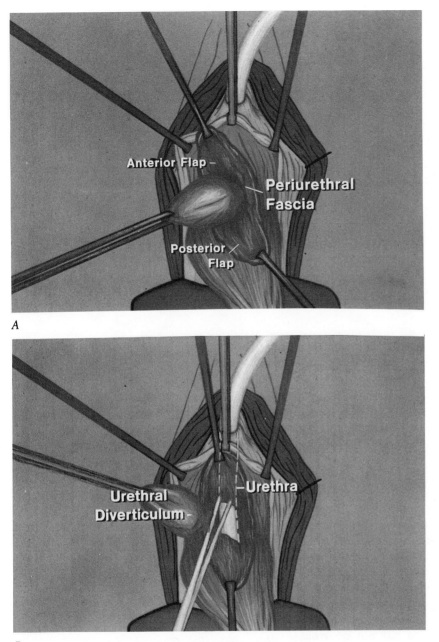

A

B

Figure 33-16. (A) Complete mobilization of the anterior and posterior flaps of the periurethral fascia exposes the diverticulum. (B) The diverticulum is completely excised after identifying the communication with the urethra. (From Leach GE, Schmidbauer CP, Hadley HR, et al. Surgical treatment of female urethral diverticulum. Sem Urol 1986;4:33.)

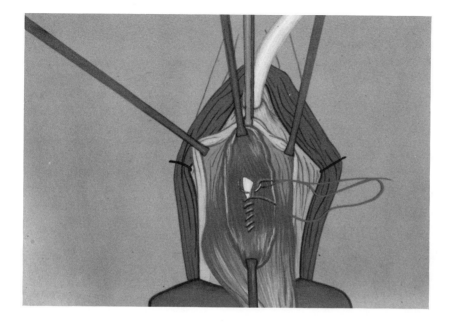

Figure 33-17. The urethral wall is closed with continuous absorbable suture over a 14 French Foley catheter. (From Leach GE, Schmidbauer CP, Hadley HR, et al. Surgical treatment of female urethral diverticulum. Sem Urol 1986;4:33.)

ever, that incomplete excision of the diverticular sac can compromise postoperative results and that complete excision of the sac should be accomplished.

Approximation of the Urethra

Most reports, including those of the authors, describe closure of the urethra in a lengthwise fashion with absorbable suture over a Foley catheter (Fig. 33-17). Closure over a 14 French Foley catheter does not compromise the urethral lumen. Ginsburg and Genadry thought it was best to close the urethral defect transversely to avoid stricture formation.[21] In the authors' experience, however, outlet obstruction has not occurred when the vertical closure is performed over a 14 French urethral catheter.

Closure of Periurethral Fascia and Anterior Vaginal Wall

After urethral closure, the anterior vaginal wall is closed in multiple layers. The authors close the periurethral fascia transversely and the anterior vaginal wall in a U fashion, thus avoiding overlapping suture lines (Fig. 33-18). The additional reinforcement of bulbocavernosus transplant or Martius fat pad graft (Fig. 33-19) has been described.[58, 60, 62] Such reinforcement is indicated when the layers of closure are poorly vascularized or atrophic (*i.e.*, after radiation therapy or secondary repair). These vascularized flaps of muscle or fat from the adjacent labia can provide a reinforcement for the urethral closure and thus aid healing.

Postoperative Care

Postoperatively anticholinergics and antibiotics are administered as described earlier. At 10 to 14 days postoperatively, the urethral catheter is removed, and a voiding cystourethrogram is performed under fluoroscopic control. The bladder is filled through the suprapubic tube. When

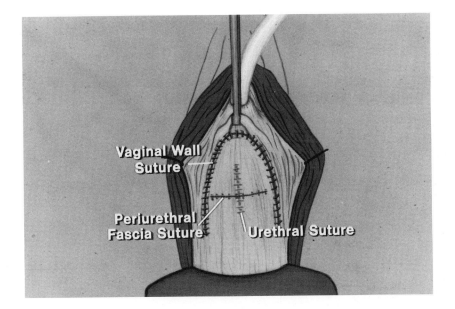

Figure 33-18. *Completed reconstruction demonstrates the lack of overlapping suture lines. (From Leach GE, Schmidbauer CP, Hadley HR, et al. Surgical treatment of female urethral diverticulum. Sem Urol 1986;4:33.)*

there is no extravasation from the urethral reconstruction site, the suprapubic tube is removed. When any extravasation is seen, the suprapubic catheter is placed to straight drainage (without replacement of the urethral catheter), and a voiding cystourethrogram is repeated in 1 week.

Results and Complications

Follow-up in most reported series of patients after transvaginal urethral diverticulectomy consists of history and palpation of the anterior vaginal wall. Postoperative radiographs are not obtained routinely. Success rates of 71%, 77%, 82%, and 100% have been reported in series involving 10, 34, 85, and 140 patients.[9,20,22,60]

The incidence of complications is quoted at 8% to 17%, with the rates of recurrence at 9% to 17%.[7,9,22,45,63] A 15% incidence of postoperative stress urinary incontinence has been reported[63] (Table 33-2). Complications of trans-

vaginal urethral diverticulectomy include bleeding, infection, urethral-vaginal fistula, ureteral injury, incontinence, persistence of bladder irritative symptoms, and persistence or recurrence of the diverticulum. Smaller sacs and loculations may be missed when the dissection is not meticulous. Lee suggested that "recurrence" of a diverticulum within a year in the same general location signifies that the original excision was incomplete. Conversely, the appearance of a diverticulum more than 1 year after an apparently successful resection, especially if it is in a different location, suggests that the "recurrent" diverticulum is new.[22]

Surgical Management with Bladder Neck Suspension

As already noted, a significant number of women present with voiding dysfunction and incontinence coincident with urethral diverticula. Lee

(continued on page 472)

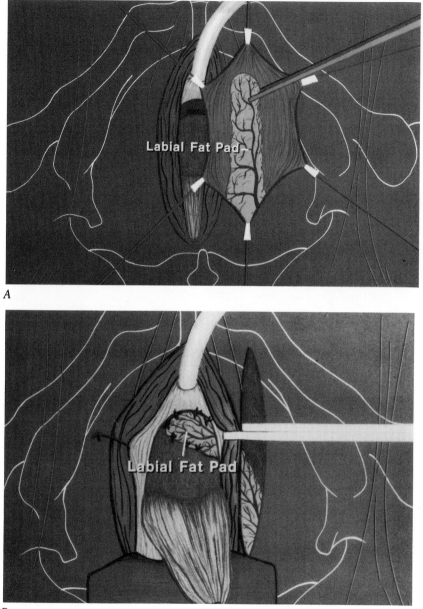

A

B

Figure 33-19. (A) A vertical incision over the labia majora exposes the labial fat pad. (B) The fat pad graft is tunneled medially and secured over the urethral reconstruction site. (From Leach GE. Urethrovaginal fistula repair with Martius labial fat pad graft. Urol Clin North Am 1991;18:409.)

Table 33-2. *Complications of Diverticulectomy (No. of patients)*

SERIES NO. PATIENTS YEAR	WHARTON AND TELINDE[55] 58 1956	DAVIS AND TELINDE[10] 84 1958	MACKINNON ET AL[9] 140 1959	BOATWRIGHT AND MOORE[69] 48 1963	HOFFMAN AND ADAMS[5] 60 1965	WARD ET AL[56] 24 1967	DAVIS AND ROBINSON[7] 98 1970	PATHAK AND HOUSE[23] 42 1970	LEE[22] 82 1983	LEACH AND BAVENDAM[41] 29 1987	TOTAL 665
Urethral-Vaginal Fistula	4	—	5	4	1	2	4	—	1	—	21 (3%)
Recurrence	—	10	2	—	—	7	1	—	8	1	29 (4%)
Stress Incontinence	1	—	*	2	4	3	—	—	13	6	29 (4%)
Stricture	3	—	—	1	1	—	—	—	—	—	2 (0.3%)
Recurrent Urinary Tract Infection	5	11	13†	—	—	—	—	3	2	—	34 (5%)

* "Several."
† 8–10%, according to the authors.

suggested that the urethral smooth muscle and the bladder neck can be damaged by both the expanding inflammatory mass and the trauma associated with surgery, thus resulting in stress incontinence.[22] In an attempt to improve the postoperative outcome, several authors have proposed treatment for stress incontinence at the time of diverticulectomy.

Lockhart and colleagues reported the treatment of six patients with proximal diverticula with a modified cystourethropexy.[64] A Stamey or modified Pereyra bladder neck suspension included plication of the periurethral fascia layers behind the bladder neck in all patients. Although all patients were cured of incontinence postoperatively (period of follow-up not specified), results with regards to the success of the diverticular repair were not mentioned.

Leach treated 31 women with urethral diverticula from 1982 through 1989. Eighteen women had urethral diverticula and concomitant stress urinary incontinence, severe urethral hypermobility, or diverticula extending beneath the proximal urethra and bladder neck. The women underwent transvaginal excision of the diverticulum with simultaneous bladder neck suspension. The bladder neck suspending sutures were placed before the diverticulectomy to preclude infection of the retropubic space from the chronically infected diverticular sac. The bladder neck suspending sutures were tied after the diverticulectomy. Postoperatively six of these women were incontinent, with a mean follow-up of 42 months. Five patients reported recurrent stress urinary incontinence, and one patient with cerebellar degeneration had severe detrusor hyperreflexia. In contrast, the 13 patients who did not fulfill the criteria for a simultaneous suspension procedure were treated with diverticulectomy alone. Only one was incontinent postoperatively, secondary to detrusor instability. There were no postoperative infections. The authors conclude that simultaneous bladder neck suspension in the presence of the aforementioned conditions facilitates postoperative continence and is not associated with major complications.[32]

Conclusion

The ability to diagnose urethral diverticula in women requires a careful history and physical examination as well as a high index of suspicion. Radiologic studies, especially a well-performed voiding cystourethrogram, is most helpful to diagnose and delineate the extent of urethral diverticula in the female patient. When the patient with urethral diverticulum complains of incontinence or other voiding symptoms, urodynamic evaluation can yield information essential to planning an appropriate surgical procedure. The ideal treatment of female urethral diverticula is transvaginal diverticulectomy with preservation of appropriate tissue layers to facilitate the urethral reconstruction. When indicated, the addition of a transvaginal bladder neck suspension at the time of diverticulectomy is both safe and efficacious.

References

1. Hey W. Practical Observations in Surgery. Philadelphia: Humphreys, 1805.
2. Kelly HA. Operative Gynecology. Vol 1. New York: Appleton, 1906:387.
3. Hunner GL. Calculus formation in a urethral diverticulum in women. Urol Cutan Rev 1938; 42:336.
4. Aldridge CW, Beaton JH, Nanzig RP. A review of office urethroscopy and cystometry. Am J Obstet Gynecol 1978;131:432.
5. Hoffman M, Adams W. Recognition and repair of urethral diverticula. Am J Obstet Gynecol 1965; 92:106.
6. Anderson M. The incidence of diverticula in the female urethra. J Urol 1967;98:96.
7. Davis BL, Robinson DG. Diverticula of the female urethra. J Urol 1970;104:850.
8. Engel W. Diverticulum of the female urethra. J Urol 1941;45:703.
9. Mackinnon M, Pratt PH, Pool TL. Diverticulum of the female urethra. Surg Clin North Am 1959; 39:953.
10. Davis HJ, TeLinde RW. Urethral diverticula. J Urol 1958;80:34.
11. Higgins C, Ranbousek E. Diverticula of the urethra in women. J Urol 1945;53:753.

12. Pinkerton J. Diverticulum of the female urethra. Br J Obstet Gynaecol 1956;63:76.
13. Ratner M, Ritz I, Siminovitch M. Diverticulum of the female urethra with multiple calculi. Can Med Assoc J 1949;60:510.
14. Counseller O. Urethral diverticulum in the female. Am J Obstet Gynecol 1949;57:231.
15. Gilbert C, Cintron F. The urethral diverticula in the female. Am J Obstet Gynecol 1954;67:616.
16. Nel J. Diverticulum of the female urethra. Br J Obstet Gynaecol 1955;62:90.
17. Moore TD. Diverticulum of the female urethra. J Urol 1952;68:611.
18. Herman L, Greene L. Diverticulum of the female urethra. J Urol 1944;52:599.
19. Benjamin J, Elliott L, Copper JF, et al. Urethral diverticulum in the female. Urology 1974;3:1.
20. Stewart M, Bretland PM, Stildolph NE. Urethral diverticula in the adult female. Br J Urol 1981;53:353.
21. Ginsburg DS, Genadry R. Suburethral diverticulum in the female. Obstet Gynecol Surg 1984;39:1.
22. Lee RA. Diverticulum of the female urethra. Obstet Gynecol 1983;61:52.
23. Pathak U, House M. Diverticulum of the female urethra. Obstet Gynecol 1970;36:789.
24. Huffman JW. The detailed anatomy of the paraurethral (sic) ducts in the adult human female. Am J Obstet Gynecol 1948;55:86.
25. Routh A. Urethral diverticula. BMJ 1890;1:361.
26. Wexler JS, McGovern TP. Ultrasonography of female urethral diverticula. AJR Am J Roentgenol 1980;134:737.
27. Peters WA III, Vaughan ED Jr. Urethral diverticulum in the female. Obstet Gynecol 1976;47:549.
28. Patanaphan V, Prempree T, Sewchand W, et al. Adenocarcinoma arising in female urethral diverticulum. Urology 1983;22:259.
29. Evans KJ, McCarthy MP, Sands JP. Adenocarcinoma of a female urethral diverticulum. J Urol 1981;126:124.
30. Tesluk H. Primary adenocarcinoma of the female urethral associated with diverticulum. Urology 1981;17:197.
31. Greenberg M, Stone D, Cochran ST, et al. Female urethral diverticula. AJR Am J Roentgenol 1981;136:259.
32. Bass JS, Leach GE. Surgical treatment of concomitant urethral diverticulum and stress urinary incontinence. Urol Clin North Am 1991;18:365.
33. Bhatia NN, McCarthy TA, Ostergard D. Urethral diverticula: Urethral closure pressure profile. Prog Clin Biol Res 1981;78:239.
34. Bhatia NN, McCarthy TA, Ostergard D. Urethral pressure profiles of women with urethral diverticula. Obstet Gynecol 1981;58:375.
35. Campbell J, Sniderman K. Urethral diverticula in adult females. J Can Assoc Radiol 1976;27:232.
36. Curry NS. Ectopic ureteral orifice masquerading as a urethral diverticulum. AJR Am J Roentgenol 1983;141:1325.
37. Blacklock ARE, Shaw RL, Geddes JR. Late presentation of ectopic ureter. Br J Urol 1982;54:106.
38. Butler WJ. The diagnosis of urethral diverticula in women. J Urol 1966;95:63.
39. Wharton LR, Kearns W. Diverticula of the female urethra. J Urol 1950;63:1063.
40. Kreiger JS, Poutasse EF. Diverticulum of the female urethra. Am J Obstet Gynecol 1954;18:706.
41. Leach GE, Bavendam TG. Female urethral diverticula. Urology 1987;30:407.
42. Zimmern P. The role of voiding cystourethrography in the evaluation of the female lower urinary tract. Prob Urol 1991;5:23.
43. Lang EK, Davis HJ. Positive pressure urethrography. Radiology 1959;79:401.
44. Steinhardt GF, Landes RR. Countertraction retrograde urethrography in females. J Urol 1982;128:936.
45. Ward JN. Technique to visualize urethral diverticula in female patients. Surg Gynecol Obstet 1989;163:278.
46. Wexler JS, McGovern TP. Ultrasonography of female urethral diverticula. AJR Am J Roentgenol 1980;134:737.
47. Ellik M. Diverticulum of the female urethra. J Urol 1957;77:243.
48. Mizrahi S, Bitterman W. Transvaginal, periurethral injection of polytetrafluroethylene (Polytef) in the treatment of urethral diverticula. Br J Urol 1988;62:280.
49. Lapides J. Transurethral treatment of urethral diverticula in women. J Urol 1979;121:736.
50. Miskowiak J, deLichtenberg MH. Transurethral incision of urethral diverticulum in the female. Scand J Urol Nephrol 1989;23:235.
51. Versi E, Cordozo SD, Studd JWW, et al. Internal urinary sphincter in the maintenance of female continence. BMJ 1986;292:166.
52. Spence HM, Duckett JW. Diverticulum of the female urethra. J Urol 1970;104:432.
53. Johnson CM. Diverticula and cysts of the female urethra. J Urol 1938;39:506.
54. Sasnett RB, Mims WW, Witherington R. Jackknife prone position for urethral diverticulectomy in women. Urology 1978;11:183.
55. Wharton LR, TeLinde RW. Urethral diverticulum. Obstet Gynecol 1956;7:503.

56. Ward JN, Draper JW, Tovell HMM. Diagnosis and treatment of urethral diverticula in the female. Surg Gynecol Obstet 1967;125:1293.
57. Boyd SD, Raz S. Female urethral diverticula. In: Raz S, ed. Female urology Philadelphia: WB Saunders, 1983:378.
58. Leach GE, Schmidbauer CP, Hadley HR, et al. Surgical treatment of female urethral diverticulum. Sem Urol 1986;4:33.
59. Hyams JA, Hyams MN. A new operative procedure for the treatment of diverticulum of the female urethra. Urol Cutan Rev 1939;43:573.
60. Tancer ML, Mouppan MMV, Pierre-Louis C. Suburethral diverticulum treatment by partial ablation. Obstet Gynecol 1983;62:511.
61. Hirschhorn R. New surgical technique for removal of urethral diverticula in the female patient. J Urol 1964;92:206.
62. Leach GE. Urethrovaginal fistula repair with Martius labial fat pad graft. Urol Clin North Am 1991;18:409.
63. Lichtman A, Robertson J. Suburethral diverticula treated by marsupialization. Obstet Gynecol 1976;43:203.
64. Lockhart JL, Ellis GF, Helal M, et al. Combined cystourethropexy for the treatment of type three and complicated female incontinence. J Urol 1990;143:722.
65. Kittredge R, Bienstock M, Finby N. Urethral diverticula in women. Am J Roentgenol Rad Ther Nucl Med 1966;98:200.
66. Woodhouse CRJ, Flynn JT, Molland EA, et al. Urethral diverticulum in females. Br J Urol 1980;52:305.
67. Rozasahegyi J, Magasi P, Szule E. Diverticulum of the female urethra. Acta Chir Hung 1984;15:33.
68. Boatwright D, Moore V. Suburethral diverticuli in the female. J Urol 1963;89:581.

34

Urinary Incontinence in the Older Woman

Neil M. Resnick

Urinary incontinence is common in elderly individuals, affecting 15% to 30% of those in the community, 30% to 35% of those in acute-care settings, and 50% to 60% of those in long-term care institutions.[1,2] Not only is it common, but also its burden is substantial. Medically, incontinent older individuals are predisposed to perineal rashes, pressure ulcers, urinary tract infections, urosepsis, falls, and fractures. Psychosocially, affected persons are frequently embarrassed, isolated, stigmatized, depressed, and regressed; they also are predisposed to institutionalization, although the extent remains undefined.[3,4] Economically, the costs of incontinence are startling. In the United States, more than $10 billion was devoted to the management of geriatric incontinence in 1987.[5] This figure exceeds the annual amount devoted to dialysis and coronary artery bypass surgery for all ages combined.

Despite its considerable prevalence, morbidity, and expense, however, incontinence in the elderly remains largely a neglected problem. Only the minority of incontinent individuals consult a health care provider, and frequently the problem is inadequately evaluated.[6-8] This is unfortunate because incontinence is abnormal at any age, and numerous studies have documented that, regardless of age, mobility, or mental status, incontinence is a highly treatable and often curable disorder, even in frail elderly.[2,9]

To formulate a logical and effective approach to the problem, the clinician must consider the impact that normal aging has on the genitourinary system and be aware of the theoretical and practical factors—both within and outside of the lower urinary tract—that can precipitate incontinence.

Impact of Age on Incontinence

At any age, continence depends not only on the integrity of lower urinary tract function, but also on the presence of adequate mentation, mobility, motivation, and manual dexterity. Although incontinence in younger patients is uncommonly associated with deficits outside the urinary tract, such deficits are frequently found in older incontinent patients. It is crucial to detect them, both because they exacerbate and occasionally even cause incontinence in the elderly and because design of an efficacious intervention requires that they be addressed.

In addition to recognizing the importance of factors outside the urinary tract, it is important to realize that the lower urinary tract itself changes with age, even in the absence of disease. Although there is still a dearth of data, bladder capacity, the ability to postpone voiding, and urinary flow rate appear to decline in both sexes, and maximum urethral closure pressure and urethral length probably decline in women.[2,10] Both the prevalence of uninhibited contractions and the postvoiding residual (PVR) volume

Female Urology, edited by Elroy D. Kursh and Edward McGuire. J. B. Lippincott, Philadelphia, © 1994.

likely increase, but the PVR volume probably increases to no more than 50 to 100 ml.[2, 10] Another important change is an alteration in the pattern of fluid excretion. Although younger individuals excrete the bulk of their daily ingested fluid before bedtime, many elderly people excrete the bulk of theirs during the night, even those who do not have peripheral venous insufficiency, renal disease, heart failure, or prostatism.[11] This fact, coupled with an age-associated increase in the prevalence of sleep disorders, leads to one to two episodes of nocturia in the majority of healthy elderly individuals.[12, 13]

Although none of these age-related changes causes incontinence, each predisposes to it. This predisposition, coupled with the increased likelihood that an older person will encounter an additional pathologic, physiologic, or pharmacologic insult, underlies the higher incidence of incontinence in the elderly. The corollary is equally important. *The new onset or exacerbation of incontinence in an older person is likely to be due to a precipitant outside the lower urinary tract that is amenable to medical intervention. Treatment of the precipitant(s) alone may be sufficient to restore continence*, even if there is a coexistent urinary tract abnormality. For instance, flare of hip arthritis in a woman with age-related detrusor overactivity may be sufficient to convert urinary urgency into incontinence. Treatment of the arthritis—rather than the uninhibited contractions—not only restores continence, but also lessens pain and improves mobility. These principles provide the rationale in the older patient for adding to the established lower urinary tract causes of incontinence a set of transient causes as well. Because of their frequency, ready reversibility, and association with morbidity beyond incontinence, the transient causes are discussed first.

Causes of Transient Incontinence

Transient incontinence is common in the elderly, afflicting up to one third of community-dwelling incontinent individuals and up to half of hospi-

Table 34-1. *Causes of Transient Incontinence*

Delirium/confusional state
Infection—urinary (symptomatic)
Atrophic urethritis/vaginitis
Pharmaceuticals
Psychological, especially depression
Excessive urine output (*e.g.*, heart failure, hyperglycemia)
Restricted mobility
Stool impaction

Adapted from Resnick NM. Urinary incontinence in the elderly. Med Grand Rounds 1984;3:281.

talized incontinent patients.[1, 2] Although most of the transient causes of incontinence in the elderly lie outside the lower urinary tract, two points are worth emphasizing. First, the risk of incontinence developing from a transient cause is increased if, in addition to physiologic changes of the lower urinary tract, the older person also suffers from pathologic changes; overflow incontinence is more likely to result from an anticholinergic agent in a woman with a weak bladder, and urge incontinence is more likely to result from a loop diuretic in a woman with detrusor overactivity or impaired mobility.[14, 15] Second, although termed *transient*, these causes of incontinence may persist if left untreated, and so they cannot be dismissed merely because the incontinence is of long duration.

The causes of transient incontinence can be recalled easily using the mnemonic DIAPPERS (misspelled with an extra 'P'; Table 34-1). In the setting of *delirium* (an acute confusional state due to virtually any drug or acute illness), incontinence is merely an associated symptom that abates once the underlying cause of confusion is identified and treated. The patient needs medical rather than bladder management.[2]

Symptomatic urinary tract *infection* causes transient incontinence when dysuria and urgency are so prominent that the older person is unable to reach the toilet before voiding. Asymptomatic infection, which is much more common in the elderly, is usually not a cause of incontinence.[2, 16] Because illness can present atypically in older patients, however, incontinence is occasionally the only atypical symptom of a urinary tract infection. Thus if an otherwise asymptomatic urinary tract infection is found on the initial evaluation, the bacteriuria should be treated and the result recorded in the patient's record to prevent future futile therapy.

Atrophic vaginitis is frequently a source of lower urinary tract symptoms, including incontinence. As many as 80% of elderly women attending an incontinence clinic have physical evidence of atrophic vaginitis, characterized by vaginal mucosal atrophy, friability, erosions, and punctuate hemorrhages.[17] Incontinence that occurs with this entity usually is associated with urgency and occasionally a sense of "scalding" dysuria, but both symptoms may be relatively unimpressive. In demented individuals, atrophic vaginitis may present as agitation.

The importance of recognizing atrophic vaginitis is that it responds to low-dose topical or systemic estrogen (*e.g.*, 0.3 to 0.6 mg conjugated estrogen/day). Moreover, similar to each of the causes of transient incontinence, treatment has other benefits as well; in the case of atrophic urethritis, treatment may also result in amelioration of dyspareunia and possibly reduction in the frequency of recurrent cystitis.[18, 19] Symptoms remit in a few days to 6 weeks, although the intracellular biochemical response takes much longer.[20] Although the duration of therapy has not been well established, one approach is to administer a low dose of estrogen on a daily basis for 1 to 2 months and then to taper it. Eventually most patients probably can be weaned to a dose given as infrequently as two to four times per month; after 6 months, estrogen can be discontinued entirely in some patients, although recrudescence of atrophy is common. Because the estrogen dose is low and given briefly, its carcinogenic effect is likely slight, if present at all. If long-term treatment with estrogen is required, however, a progestin probably should be added if the patient has a uterus. In addition, hormone treatment is contraindicated for women with a history of breast cancer; for those without such a history, mammography should be performed before initiating hormone therapy.

Pharmaceuticals are one of the most common causes of incontinence in the elderly, with several different categories of drugs implicated most often (Table 34-2).[2] Of note, many of these agents also are used in the treatment of incontinence, underscoring the fact that most medications used by the elderly are double-edged swords. The first category of relevant drugs is the long-acting sedative/hypnotics, such as diazepam and flurazepam, whose half-life can exceed 100 hours and which can cloud an older patient's sensorium. Loop diuretics, such as furosemide or bumetanide, by inducing a brisk diuresis, can also provoke leakage. Drugs with anticholinergic side effects are a particular problem and include major tranquilizers, antidepressants, antiparkinsonian agents (not L-dopa or selegiline but trihexyphenidyl and benzotropine mesylate), antihistamines, antiarrhythmics (disopyramide), antispasmodics, and opiates. By decreasing detrusor contractility, they can cause urinary retention and overflow incontinence. These agents are particularly important to ask about for two reasons. First, older patients often take more than one of them, and, second, these agents are contained in many nonprescription preparations (*e.g.*, antihistamines for colds or insomnia) that the elderly frequently take without consulting a physician.

Calcium channel blockers are another category of drugs that can cause incontinence. As direct smooth muscle relaxants, they may increase residual volume and may occasionally lead to overflow incontinence, particularly in women with detrusor weakness and a weak urethral sphincter.

This age-related decline in urethral length and sphincter strength also predispose to incontinence precipitated by two other categories of drugs. Angiotensin-converting enzyme (ACE) inhibitors—prescribed for patients with heart failure, hypertension, or recent myocardial infarction—commonly cause a persistent cough, which can lead to stress incontinence. Alpha-adrenoceptor antagonists (many antihypertensives), which block receptors at the bladder neck, may further reduce urethral resistance and also

Table 34-2. Medications that Can Potentially Affect Continence in Elderly Women

TYPE OF MEDICATION	EXAMPLES	POTENTIAL EFFECTS ON CONTINENCE
Potent diuretics	Furosemide, bumetanide	Polyuria, frequency, urgency
Anticholinergics	Antihistamines, trihexyphenidyl, benztropine, dicyclomine, disopyramide	Urinary retention, overflow incontinence, delirium, impaction
Psychotropics		
Antidepressants	Amitriptyline, desipramine	Anticholinergic actions, sedation
Antipsychotics	Thioridazine, haloperidol	Anticholinergic actions, sedation, rigidity, immobility
Sedatives/hypnotics	Diazepam, flurazepam	Sedation, delirium
Narcotic analgesics	Opiates	Urinary retention, fecal impaction, sedation, delirium
Alpha-adrenergic blockers	Prazosin, terazosin	Urethral relaxation
Calcium channel blockers	Nifedipine, verapamil, diltiazem	Urinary retention
Angiotensin converting enzyme (ACE) inhibitors	Captopril, lisinopril, enalapril	Cough leading to stress incontinence
Alcohol		Polyuria, frequency, urgency, sedation, delirium, immobility
Vincristine		Urinary retention

Adapted from Resnick NM. Urinary incontinence. In: Beck JC, ed. Geriatrics review syllabus. New York: American Geriatrics Society 1991: 141–154.

induce stress incontinence in older women.[21] Because hypertension affects approximately half of the elderly population and these agents are effective in its treatment, they will become more widely used now that recent clinical trials have proved that treatment of both diastolic and isolated systolic hypertension reduces the risk of stroke, heart attack, and death owing to cardiovascular disease.[22, 23] Thus, before considering other interventions for stress incontinence in a woman taking such a drug, substitution of an alternative agent should be tried, and the incontinence should be re-evaluated.

Psychological causes of incontinence have not been well studied in any age group but probably are less common in older individuals than in younger ones. Initial intervention is properly directed at the psychological disturbance, usually depression or lifelong neurosis. Once the psychological disturbance has been treated, however, persistent incontinence warrants further evaluation. *Excessive urine output* commonly contributes to or even causes geriatric incontinence, es-pecially in women with coexistent impairment of mobility or mentation. Causes include excessive fluid intake; diuretics (including theophylline-containing fluids and alcohol); metabolic abnormalities (*e.g.*, hyperglycemia and hypercalcemia); and disorders associated with fluid overload, including congestive heart failure, peripheral venous insufficiency, hypoalbuminemia (especially in malnourished debilitated elderly), and drug-induced peripheral edema associated with nonsteroidal anti-inflammatory drugs (NSAIDs) and some calcium channel blockers (*e.g.*, dihydropyridines such as nifedipine, isradipine, and nicardipine). Such conditions are likely to be present when incontinence is associated with nocturia.

Restricted mobility commonly contributes to incontinence in the elderly. It can result from numerous treatable conditions, including arthritis, hip deformity, physical deconditioning, postural or postprandial hypotension, claudication, spinal stenosis, heart failure, poor eyesight, fear of falling, a stroke, foot problems, drug-induced disequilibrium or confusion, or simply being restrained in a bed or a chair. A careful search often identifies these or other correctable causes. If not, a urinal or bedside commode may still improve or resolve the incontinence.

Finally, *stool impaction* is implicated as a cause of urinary incontinence in up to 10% of older patients seen in acute hospitals or referred to incontinence clinics;[2] the mechanism may involve stimulation of opioid receptors.[24] Patients usually present with either urge or overflow incontinence and typically have associated fecal incontinence as well. Disimpaction restores continence.

These eight reversible causes of incontinence should be assiduously sought in every elderly patient. In one series of hospitalized elderly patients, when these causes were identified, continence was regained by most of those who became incontinent in the context of acute illness.[2] Regardless of their frequency, however, their identification is important in all settings because they are easily treatable and contribute to morbidity beyond incontinence.

Established Incontinence

LOWER URINARY TRACT CAUSES

If leakage persists after transient causes of incontinence have been addressed, the lower urinary tract causes of established incontinence must be considered (Table 34-3). Excluding the rare extraurethral causes of incontinence (*e.g.*, fistula) and impaired detrusor compliance, the lower urinary tract malfunctions in much the same way as in younger patients except for a few notable differences.

Detrusor Overactivity

Detrusor overactivity is the generic term for uninhibited bladder contractions,[25] the leading lower urinary tract cause of incontinence in older individuals.[2] Although distinctions are commonly drawn between detrusor overactivity that is associated with a central nervous system lesion (detrusor hyperreflexia) and that which is not (detrusor instability), in older patients the distinction is often less clear because uninhibited contractions may occur incidental to normal

Table 34-3. *Lower Urinary Tract Causes of Established Incontinence in Elderly Women*

URODYNAMIC DIAGNOSIS	SOME NEUROGENIC CAUSES	SOME NONNEUROGENIC CAUSES
Detrusor overactivity	Stroke Parkinson's disease Alzheimer's disease Multiple sclerosis	Urethral incompetence/obstruction Cystitis Bladder carcinoma Bladder stone
Detrusor underactivity	Disc compression Plexopathy Surgical damage (*e.g.*, anterior-posterior resection) Autonomic neuropathy (*e.g.*, diabetes mellitus, alcoholism, vitamin B_{12} deficiency)	Idiopathic (common in women)
Outlet incompetence	Surgical lesion (rare) Lower motor neuron lesion (rare)	Urethral hypermobility (type 1 and 2 SUI) Sphincter incompetence (type 3 SUI)
Outlet obstruction	Spinal cord lesion with detrusor-sphincter dyssynergia (rare)	Large cystourethrocele Following bladder neck suspension

SUI = Stress urinary incontinence.
Adapted from Resnick NM. Voiding dysfunction and urinary incontinence. In: Beck JC, ed. Geriatric review syllabus. New York: American Geriatrics Society, 1991:141–154.

aging, a past stroke (which is clinically inapparent), or stress incontinence—even in a woman with Alzheimer's disease. To date, no reliable way to distinguish the source of such contractions has been devised.

Traditionally detrusor overactivity has been thought to be the primary urinary tract cause of incontinence in demented patients. Although this is true, it is also the most common cause in nondemented patients, and two studies have failed to find a definite association between cognitive status and detrusor overactivity.[26–27] Moreover, demented patients may also be incontinent owing to the transient causes already discussed. Thus it is no longer tenable to ascribe incontinence in demented individuals a priori to detrusor overactivity.

Recently detrusor overactivity in the elderly has been found to exist as two physiologic subsets—one in which contractile function is preserved and one in which it is impaired.[28] The latter condition has been termed *detrusor hyperactivity with impaired contractility* (DHIC), and it is the most common cause of established incontinence in frail elderly persons.[26] DHIC has several implications. First, because the bladder is weak, urinary retention develops commonly in these patients, and DHIC must be added to outlet obstruction and detrusor underactivity as a cause of retention. Second, even in the absence of retention, DHIC mimics virtually every other lower urinary tract cause of incontinence. For instance, if the uninhibited contraction is triggered by or occurs coincident with a stress maneuver, and the weak bladder contraction (often only 2 to 6 cm H_2O of pressure) is not detected, DHIC can be misdiagnosed as stress incontinence.[29] Alternatively, because DHIC is associated with urinary urgency, frequency, weak flow rate, significant residual urine, and bladder trabeculation, it may mimic prostatism in men. Third, bladder weakness often frustrates anticholinergic therapy of DHIC because urinary retention is induced so easily. Thus, alternative therapeutic approaches are often required (see discussion of therapy later).

Stress Incontinence

Stress incontinence is the second most common cause of incontinence in older women. As in younger women, it is caused most often by pelvic muscle laxity. A less common cause in older women is intrinsic sphincter deficiency (ISD) or type 3 stress incontinence.[30,31] Usually owing to operative trauma, a milder form of ISD in the elderly woman can also result from nothing more than urethral atrophy. In addition to leaking with stress maneuvers, women with ISD may dribble even when sitting or standing quietly; this is a helpful diagnostic and therapeutic point, because many such women become dry if bladder volume is kept below the leakage threshold (*e.g.*, 200 to 400 ml).

A third but rare cause of stress incontinence is urethral instability, in which the sphincter abruptly and paradoxically relaxes in the absence of an apparent detrusor contraction;[32] most older women who are thought to have this condition likely have DHIC instead. Finally, stress-associated leakage also can occur in association with urinary retention, but in this situation leakage is not due to outlet incompetence.

Detrusor Underactivity

Detrusor underactivity sufficient to cause urinary retention and overflow incontinence occurs in only about 5% to 10% of older women. Such pronounced bladder weakness is due to the same causes in older women as in younger women and presents in the same manner. As in younger women, symptoms of severe detrusor underactivity (*e.g.*, urgency, frequency, and nocturia) may mimic those of detrusor overactivity, and so exclusion of urinary retention is mandatory before initiating treatment for detrusor overactivity. Less severe degrees of bladder weakness occur commonly in older women. Although such a mild degree of weakness is insufficient to cause incontinence, when it occurs in association with other causes of incontinence, it can complicate their treatment (see discussion of therapy).

Outlet Obstruction

Frank outlet obstruction is as rare in older women as in younger women. When present, it is usually due to kinking associated with a large cystocele or to obstruction following bladder neck suspension; rarely bladder neck obstruction or a bladder calculus is the cause. With age, however, urethral elasticity decreases in most women, and in a small proportion of them—in whom it may be compounded by fibrotic changes associated with atrophic vaginitis—significant urethral stenosis may occur.

FUNCTIONAL INCONTINENCE

Of course, factors other than lower urinary tract dysfunction can contribute to established incontinence in the elderly woman because continence is also affected by environmental demands, mentation, mobility, manual dexterity, medical factors, and motivation. Although lower urinary tract function is rarely normal in such individuals, these factors are important to keep in mind because small improvements in each of them can result in marked amelioration of both incontinence and functional status. In fact, once one has excluded causes of transient incontinence and serious lesions of the urinary tract, attention to these factors often obviates the need for further investigation of the lower urinary tract.

Diagnostic Approach

The diagnostic approach has three purposes: to determine the cause of the incontinence; to detect related urinary tract pathology (Table 34-4); and to comprehensively evaluate the patient, the environment, and the available resources.[33] The extent and interpretation of the evaluation must be tailored to the individual and tempered by the realization that not all detected conditions can be cured (*e.g.*, invasive bladder carcinoma); that simple interventions may be effective even in the absence of a diagnosis; and that for many elderly

Table 34-4. *Serious Conditions that May Present as Incontinence*

Lesions of the brain and spinal cord
Carcinoma of the bladder
Bladder stones
Hydronephrosis
Decreased bladder compliance
Detrusor-sphincter dyssynergia

* Adapted from Resnick NM. Noninvasive diagnosis of the patient with complex incontinence. Gerontology 1990;36(suppl 2):8.

persons, diagnostic tests are themselves often interventions. Although optimal diagnostic and treatment strategies remain to be determined, the diagnostic approach outlined here is relatively noninvasive, accurate, easily tolerated, and detects most underlying pathology (Table 34-5). A modification of this approach is now mandated for residents of all U.S. nursing homes.[33a]

HISTORY

As for younger women, the first step is to characterize the voiding pattern and determine whether symptoms of abnormal voiding are present, such as straining to void or a sense of incomplete emptying. One must be careful in eliciting these symptoms, however, because many patients strain at the end of voiding to empty the last few drops. In contrast, many patients have been straining for so long that they fail to acknowledge it. Thus additional observations by the physician and family members are extremely useful.

Although the clinical type of incontinence most often associated with detrusor overactivity is urge incontinence, *urge* is neither a sensitive nor specific symptom; it is absent in 20% of patients with detrusor overactivity, and the figure is higher in demented patients.[26] Urge also is reported commonly by patients with stress incontinence, outlet obstruction, and overflow incontinence.

A better term for the symptom associated with detrusor overactivity is *precipitancy*, which

Table 34-5. *Clinical Evaluation of the Incontinent Older Woman*

HISTORY

Type (urge, reflex, stress, overflow, or mixed)

Frequency, severity, duration

Pattern (diurnal, nocturnal, or both; also, *e.g.*, after taking medications)

Associated symptoms (straining to void, incomplete emptying, dysuria, hematuria, suprapubic/perineal discomfort)

Alteration in bowel habit/sexual function

Other relevant factors (cancer, diabetes, acute illness, neurologic disease, urinary tract infections, pelvic or lower urinary tract surgery/radiation therapy)

Medications, including nonprescription agents

Functional assessment

PHYSICAL EXAMINATION

Identify other medical conditions (*e.g.*, congestive heart failure, peripheral edema)

Test for stress-induced leakage when bladder is full

Observe/listen to void

Palpate for bladder distention after voiding

Pelvic examination (atrophic vaginitis or urethritis, pelvic muscle laxity, pelvic mass)

Rectal examination (skin irritation, resting tone and voluntary control of anal sphincter, fecal impaction)

Neurologic examination (mental status and elemental examination, including sacral reflexes and perineal sensation)

INITIAL INVESTIGATION

Voiding/incontinence chart

Metabolic survey (measurement of electrolytes, calcium, glucose, and urea nitrogen)

Measurement of postvoiding residual volume

Urinalysis and culture

Renal ultrasound*

Urine cytology*

Uroflowmetry*

Cystoscopy*

* See text.
Adapted from Resnick NM, Yalla SV. Management of urinary incontinence in the elderly. N Engl J Med 1985;313:800. Reprinted by permission of the New England Journal of Medicine.

can be defined in two ways. For patients with no warning of imminent urination ("reflex" or "*unconscious*" incontinence[25]), the abrupt gush of urine in the absence of a stress maneuver can be termed *precipitant leakage*, and it is almost invariably due to detrusor overactivity. For those who do sense a warning, it is of less value to focus on the leakage because the presence and volume of leakage in this situation depend on bladder volume, the amount of warning, the accessibility of a toilet, the patient's mobility, and whether the individual can overcome the relative sphincter relaxation that accompanies detrusor contraction.[34] Instead precipitancy should be defined as the *abrupt sensation* that urination is imminent, *whatever the interval and amount of leakage that follows;* defined in these two ways, precipitancy appears to be both a sensitive and specific symptom.[35]

Similar to the situation for urgency, other symptoms ascribed to detrusor overactivity also can be misleading unless explored carefully in the older woman. Urinary frequency (>7 diurnal voids) is common[10] and may be due to preemptive voiding habits, overflow incontinence, sensory urgency, a stable but poorly compliant bladder, excessive urine production (*e.g.*, diabetes mellitus, hypercalcemia, or high fluid intake), depression, anxiety, or social reasons.[35] Conversely, incontinent women may severely restrict their fluid intake so that even in the presence of detrusor overactivity they do not void frequently. Thus the significance of urinary frequency—or its absence—can be determined only in the context of more information.

Nocturia is another common geriatric symptom that can be misleading unless it is first defined (*e.g.*, two episodes may be normal for the individual who sleeps 10 hours but not for one who sleeps 4) and then approached systematically (Table 34-6). The three general reasons for true nocturia—excessive urine output, sleep-related difficulties, and bladder dysfunction—can be differentiated by careful questioning and a voiding diary that includes voided volumes (Table 34-7). One first inspects the record of voided volumes to determine the functional

Table 34-6. *Causes of Nocturia*

VOLUME RELATED

Age-related
Excess intake/alcohol
Diuretic, caffeine, theophylline
Peripheral edema
    Congestive heart failure
    Hypoalbuminemia
    Peripheral vascular disease
    Drugs (*e.g.*, indomethacin, nifedipine)

SLEEP RELATED

Insomnia
Pain
Dyspnea
Depression
Drugs

LOWER URINARY TRACT RELATED

Small bladder capacity
Detrusor hyperactivity
Overflow incontinence
Decreased bladder compliance
Sensory urgency

Adapted from Resnick NM. Noninvasive diagnosis of the patient with complex incontinence. Gerontology 1990;36 (suppl 2):8.

bladder capacity (the largest single voided volume) and then compares this capacity with the volume of each nighttime void. For instance, if the functional bladder capacity is 400 ml, and each of three nightly voids is approximately 400 ml, the nocturia is due to excessive production of urine at night. If the volume of most nightly voids is much smaller than bladder capacity, nocturia is due either (1) to a sleep-related problem (the patient voids because she is awake anyway) or (2) to a bladder problem. Similar to excessive urine output, sleep-related nocturia may also be due to treatable causes, including age-related sleep disorders, pain (*e.g.*, arthritis), dyspnea, depression, caffeine, or a short-acting hypnotic (*e.g.*, triazolam). Bladder-related causes of nocturia are displayed in Table 34-6. Whatever the cause, however, the nocturnal component of incontinence is readily treatable.

Voiding Record

One of the most helpful components of the history is the voiding record kept by the patient or caregiver. Recorded for a 48- to 72-hour period, these charts note the time of each void or incontinent episode. Many incontinence records have been proposed; a sample is shown in Table 34-7.

To record the volume voided at home, an individual can use a measuring cup, coffee can, pickle jar, or other large container. Information regarding the volume voided provides an index of functional bladder capacity that, together with the pattern of voiding and leakage, can be quite helpful in pointing to the cause of the incontinence. For example, incontinence that occurs only between 8 a.m. and noon may be caused by a morning diuretic. Incontinence that occurs at night in a demented woman with congestive heart failure but does not occur during a 4-hour daytime nap in her wheelchair is likely due not to dementia but to the postural diuresis associated with the heart failure. A woman with volume-dependent stress incontinence may leak only on the way to void after a full night's sleep, when her bladder contains more than 400 ml, more than it ever does during her continent waking hours. A patient may also void frequently because of polyuria.

TARGETED PHYSICAL EXAMINATION

Similar to the history, the physical examination is essential to rule out transient causes and to evaluate comorbid disease and functional ability. In addition to the standard urologic examination, one should check for signs of neurologic disease more common in the older person, such as delirium, dementia, stroke, Parkinson's disease, cord compression, and neuropathy (autonomic or peripheral), as well as for atrophic vaginitis, functional impairment, and general medical illnesses, such as heart failure and peripheral edema. The rectal examination checks for fecal impaction, masses, sacral reflexes, and symmetry of the gluteal creases. Many neurologically unimpaired elderly patients are unable

Table 34-7. Sample Voiding Record

DATE	TIME	VOLUME VOIDED (ML)	ARE YOU WET OR DRY?	APPROXIMATE VOLUME OF INCONTINENCE	COMMENTS
4/5	3:50 p.m.	240	Wet	Slight	
	6:05 p.m.	210	Dry		
	8:15 p.m.	150	Dry		
	10:20 p.m.	150	Wet	15 ml	Running water
	10:30 p.m.	30	Dry		Bowel movement
4/6	3:15 a.m.	270	Dry		
	6:05 a.m.	300	Dry		
	7:40 a.m.	200	Dry		
	9:50 a.m.	?	Dry		
	11:20 a.m.	200	Dry		
	12:50 p.m.	180	Dry		
	1:40 p.m.	240	Dry		
	3:35 p.m.	160	Wet	Slight	
	6:00 p.m.	170	Wet	Slight	Running water
	8:20 p.m.	215	Wet	Slight	
	10:25 p.m.	130	Dry		

Voiding diary of an incontinent 75-year-old patient. Urodynamic evaluation confirmed a diagnosis of detrusor hyperactivity with impaired contractility (DHIC). Note the 24-hour urine output, however, of nearly 3 liters owing to the belief that drinking 10 glasses of fluid/day was "good for my health." (Patient did not mention this until queried about the voiding record.) Given the typical voided volume of 150 to 250 ml and a measured postvoiding residual volume of 150 ml, excess fluid intake was overwhelming the (normal) bladder capacity of 400 ml (150 + 250 ml). Although uninhibited bladder contractions were present, the easily reversible volume component of the problem—coupled with the risk of precipitating urinary retention with an anticholinergic agent—prompted treatment with volume restriction alone. After daily urinary output dropped to 1500 ml, frequency abated and incontinence resolved. (Adapted from DuBeau CE, Resnick NM. Evaluation of the causes and severity of geriatric incontinence: A critical appraisal. Urol Clin North Am 1991;18:243.)

to contract the anal sphincter volitionally, but if they can it is evidence against a cord lesion. The absence of the anal wink is not necessarily pathologic in the elderly, nor does its presence exclude an underactive detrusor (caused by diabetic neuropathy, for example).

Two other tests should be mentioned. The Q-tip test for pelvic floor laxity is of little value in determining the cause of a patient's leakage and has a high false-negative rate, especially in elderly women.[36] The second test is the Bonney (or Marshall) test, which is of limited usefulness in the elderly because vaginal stenosis is common and may lead to a false-positive result by precluding accurate finger placement. Furthermore, even if the test is performed correctly, a false-positive result may occur if the first episode of leakage was due to a cough-induced detrusor contraction, which, having emptied the bladder, does not recur during bladder base elevation.

Voiding

An observed void is part of the physical examination and reveals more about bladder and urethral function than any other component. When the patient feels full, she first should be asked to forestall voiding for several minutes to assess whether the sensation passes or is associated with precipitant leakage. While waiting, the examiner should explain the reason for observing micturition; if the patient will not allow it, one can assess the flow rate by using either a uroflow machine or an inexpensive portable audio monitor (used to monitor a baby's room at home) and then asking the patient to place a hand on the abdomen to check for straining during urination. Otherwise one accompanies the patient to the toilet, which has been equipped with a receptacle to allow measurement of the volume voided.

Instructions to the patient depend on the working diagnosis. If only stress incontinence is suspected and surgery is contemplated, straining should be searched for because if present it suggests detrusor weakness that might predispose to postoperative retention;[37] if pelvic muscle exercises are to be prescribed, the patient should be told that she will be asked to interrupt voiding midstream. If detrusor hyperactivity is suspected, one should try to trigger it by offering the patient fluids; by asking the patient to change posture, cough, or hop; or by jouncing the patient's heels (if she is unable to stand). If detrusor hyperactivity is precipitated, one should determine whether and how quickly the patient can interrupt the stream; rapid and complete interruption probably augurs well for bladder retraining.

The examination concludes with determination of the PVR volume. Adding the PVR volume to the voided volume provides an estimate of total bladder capacity and a crude assessment of bladder proprioception. A PVR volume above 50 to 100 ml suggests either bladder weakness or, rarely in women, outlet obstruction, but smaller values do not exclude either diagnosis, especially if the patient strained to void or double voided. Thus it is important to observe or listen to the voided stream. If straining is observed, one must ask the patient whether this is typical and take it into account when interpreting the PVR volume.

LABORATORY INVESTIGATION

Because easily reversible factors cause or contribute to urinary incontinence in most elderly individuals, one should measure electrolytes, blood urea nitrogen (BUN), and creatinine as well as obtain a urinalysis, urine culture, and PVR volume determination in all patients.[33,36,38,39] Electrolytes are checked for abnormalities of serum sodium that can produce altered consciousness. If the voiding record suggests polyuria, serum concentrations of glucose and calcium (and albumin, to allow calculation of free calcium levels in sick, malnourished patients) should be measured as well. When evaluating renal function, it is important to recognize that the age-associated decline in glomerular filtration rate (GFR)—30% by the eighth decade—is not associated with an increase in creatinine because of a concomitant decrease in muscle mass; thus normal creatinine levels do not imply a normal GFR.

A major caveat regarding urinalysis evaluation in the elderly is the high rate of asymptomatic bacteriuria, which occurs even in noncatheterized and community-dwelling individuals.[40] Asymptomatic bacteriuria does not cause incontinence, and treatment may lead to the selection of resistant strains.[40] Therefore bacteriuria should be treated only in the setting of otherwise unexplained new-onset incontinence, fever, leukocytosis, dysuria, or—particularly in demented or debilitated patients—inanition or agitation. Pyuria without bacteriuria raises the possibility of genitourinary tuberculosis because the elderly, especially those in nursing homes, are an unappreciated reservoir of this disease;[41] urinary culture for tuberculosis should be sent and an intermediate-strength purified protein derivative (PPD) checked with appropriate controls.

In any patient with sterile hematuria or suprapubic or perineal discomfort or in a patient at high risk for bladder carcinoma (*e.g.,* unexplained recent onset of urgency or urge incontinence), cystoscopy and urine cytology should be obtained.

URODYNAMIC TESTING

If the cause of the patient's incontinence still cannot be determined, urodynamic evaluation is the next step to consider. Although its precise role remains to be determined, urodynamic testing is probably warranted in older patients when diagnostic uncertainty may affect therapy, when empiric therapy has failed and other approaches would be tried, and when surgical correction is being contemplated.[33] Whatever its role, however, urodynamic evaluation of elderly patients is reproducible, safe, and feasible to perform, even in frail and debilitated individuals. In our series of more than 100 consecutively evaluated nursing home patients, whose mean age was 89 and all of whom received prophylactic antibiotics, only three cases of asymptomatic bacteriuria were induced; no cases of urosepsis, pyelonephritis, endocarditis, or cardiac ischemia were observed.[26] All but two patients were able to complete the examination at one sitting, and the original diagnosis was confirmed in all 30 patients in whom the examination was repeated.[42] It must be emphasized, however, that an extra person was employed whose sole job was to explain the procedure and comfort the patient during the test. Several modifications in the urodynamic suite were made as well.

Therapy

Similar to the diagnostic approach, treatment must be individualized because factors outside the lower urinary tract often have an impact on the feasibility and efficacy of the intervention. For instance, although both may have detrusor overactivity that can be managed successfully, a severely demented and bedfast woman must be treated differently from one who is ambulatory and cognitively intact. This section and Table 34-8 outline several treatments for each condition and provide some guidance for their use. It is assumed that serious underlying conditions and transient causes of incontinence have already been excluded or treated. It cannot be overemphasized that successful treatment of established incontinence, especially in the elderly, often must be multifactorial.

DETRUSOR OVERACTIVITY

The initial approach to detrusor overactivity is to identify and treat its reversible causes. Unfortunately, because many of its causes are not amenable to specific therapy, or a cause may not be found, treatment usually must be symptomatic. Simple measures, such as adjusting the timing or amount of fluid excretion (Table 34-7) or providing a bedside commode or urinal, are often successful. If not, the cornerstone of treatment is behavioral therapy. If the patient can cooperate, standard bladder training regimens, including instruction in techniques to suppress precipitancy, extend the voiding interval.[43-45] For instance, if the voiding record reveals that the patient is wet every 3 hours, she is asked to void every 2 hours and to suppress urgency in be-

tween. Once dry for 3 consecutive days, she can extend the interval by half an hour and repeat the process until a satisfactory result or continence is achieved. Patients need not follow this regimen at night; once they are dry during the day, they generally become dry at night. Biofeedback may be added, but its marginal benefit is unclear.[46]

If the patient cannot cooperate (*e.g.*, demented patients), *prompted voiding* is employed. With this technique, the patient is asked at regular intervals whether she needs to void, and if she responds affirmatively, she is escorted to the toilet. Positive behavioral reinforcement is employed, whereas negative reinforcement is avoided. Prompted voiding can reduce incontinence frequency in many nursing home patients by 25% to 45%.[47-49] Moreover, the 75% of such patients who will respond to prompted voiding can be identified within a few days. They are the patients who, when asked hourly, can appropriately recognize the intermittent need to void and can urinate into a toilet or commode at least half of the time. These patients can be divided further into two groups of roughly equal size according to the baseline frequency of incontinence. If they leak four times or less in a 12-hour daytime period, with prompted voiding they leak on average less than once; 60% of these patients (25% of all incontinent nursing home residents) actually become dry for 2 or more consecutive days. Fortunately, as the prompting interval is increased to 2 hours, improvement persists in most of these patients. For those who leak more than four times in the 12-hour baseline period, however, the frequency of incontinence generally decreases by approximately two episodes with prompted voiding, but they still are wet more than once daily. Unfortunately, increasing the interval in this group attenuates the benefit. Finally, for the 25% of patients who do not respond to prompting at baseline, little benefit can be obtained by further prompting. These results were obtained without medications and were said to be independent of simple cystometric findings, but few patients with stress or overflow incontinence were included.[49] Tailoring

Table 34-8. Treatment

CONDITION	CLINICAL TYPE OF INCONTINENCE	TREATMENT*
Detrusor hyperactivity with normal contractility	Urge	1. Bladder retraining or prompted voiding regimens 2. Bladder relaxant medication (anticholinergic, smooth muscle relaxant, calcium channel blocker) may be added, if needed and not contraindicated 3. Indwelling catheterization alone is often unhelpful because detrusor spasms often increase, leading to leakage around the catheter 4. In selected cases, induce urinary retention pharmacologically and add intermittent or indwelling catheterization
Detrusor hyperactivity with impaired contractility	Urge†	1. If bladder empties adequately with straining, behavioral methods (as above) with or without bladder relaxant medication (low doses; especially feasible if sphincter incompetence coexists) 2. If residual urine high (*e.g.*, >150 ml), augmented voiding techniques‡ or intermittent catheterization (with or without bladder relaxant medication). If neither is feasible, undergarment or indwelling catheter may be used. Urinary tract infection prophylaxis can be used for recurrent symptomatic infections if catheter is not indwelling
Stress incontinence	Stress	1. Conservative methods (weight loss if obese; treatment of cough or atrophic vaginitis; rarely use of pessary/tampon) 2. Pelvic muscle exercises with or without biofeedback/weighted intravaginal cones 3. Imipramine (or doxepin) or alpha-adrenergic agonists—with or without estrogen—if not contraindicated 4. Surgery
Underactive detrusor	Overflow	1. If duration unknown, decompress for several weeks and perform a voiding trial 2. If fails, or retention is chronic, try augmented voiding techniques with or without alpha-adrenergic antagonist, if any voiding possible; bethanechol is rarely useful unless bladder weakness is due to an anticholinergic agent that cannot be discontinued 3. If fails, or voiding is not possible, intermittent or indwelling catheterization

* These treatments should be initiated only after adequate toilet access has been ensured, contributing conditions have been treated (*e.g.*, atrophic vaginitis, heart failure), fluid management has been optimized, and unnecessary medications have been stopped. For additional details, recommendations, and drug doses, see text.
† But may also mimic stress or overflow incontinence.
‡ Augmented voiding techniques include Credé (application of suprapubic pressure) and Valsalva (straining) maneuvers and double voiding.
Adapted from Resnick NM. Voiding dysfunction and urinary incontinence. In: Beck JC, ed. Geriatric review syllabus. New York: American Geriatrics Society, 1991:141–154.

the regimen to the cause and pattern of incontinence may improve the outcome still further.

The voiding record can be helpful in another way. If incontinence is worse at night and the chart discloses a nocturnal diuresis sufficient to trigger uninhibited contractions, one must determine the cause of the diuresis (Table 34-6). If due to congestive heart failure, it should improve with diuretic therapy. If due to peripheral edema in the absence of congestive heart failure and hypoalbuminemia (*e.g.*, venous insufficiency), it should respond to pressure gradient stockings. If it is not associated with peripheral edema, it may respond to alteration of the pattern of fluid intake or administration of a rapidly acting diuretic in the late afternoon or early evening.[50] For the patient with DHIC whose voiding record and PVR volume reveal that uninhibited contractions are provoked only at high volumes, catheterization just before bedtime removes the residual urine, thereby increasing functional bladder capacity, and restores both continence and sleep.

Drugs can be added to augment behavioral intervention but not to supplant it because drugs generally do not abolish uninhibited contractions. There is a dearth of data regarding efficacy and toxicity in this population, and comparative or controlled trials are rare. Because those studies that are available generally show equivalent results (except for flavoxate, which fares poorly in controlled trials), the decision regarding which drug to employ (Table 34-9) is often based on factors unrelated to bladder function.[39] In the incontinent patient with dementia or taking other anticholinergic agents, propantheline is best avoided. In the patient with associated hypertension, angina pectoris, or abnormalities of cardiac diastolic relaxation, a calcium channel blocking agent may be preferred. Orthostatic hypotension often precludes the use of imipramine and nifedipine, but a tricyclic antidepressant may be preferred for an incontinent

Table 34-9. *Drugs for Detrusor Overactivity**

Smooth muscle relaxant
 Flavoxate, 300–800 mg/day†
Calcium channel blocker
 Diltiazem, 90–270 mg/day
 Nifedipine, 30–90 mg/day
Anticholinergic
 Propantheline, 15–120 mg/day‡
Combination smooth muscle relaxant and anticholinergic
 Oxybutynin, 5–20 mg/day
 Dicyclomine, 30–90 mg/day
Antidepressants
 Imipramine, 50–100 mg/day
 Doxepin, 50–75 mg/day

* Each drug is given in divided doses except for the antidepressants, which may be given as a single daily dose.
† Some uncontrolled reports suggest that doses up to 1200 mg/day may be effective with tolerable side-effects.
‡ Higher doses are occasionally tolerated and effective.

patient without orthostatic hypotension who also requires pharmacotherapy for depression. Medications with rapid onset of action, such as oxybutynin, can be employed prophylactically if incontinence occurs at predictable times. Occasionally combining low doses of two agents with complementary actions, such as oxybutynin and imipramine, maximizes benefits and minimizes side-effects. Intravesical application of several of these agents also appears to be effective but is useful only for patients in whom self-catheterization is feasible. Vasopressin, which appears to work in children, has demonstrated only limited efficacy in adults and none in elderly nursing home residents;[50a] given its expense and risk of inducing hyponatremia, its widespread use should await results of further studies.

Regardless of which medication is used, urinary retention may develop and the PVR volume and common indices of renal function (BUN, serum creatinine, and urine output) should be monitored, especially in DHIC, in which the detrusor is already weak. If subclinical urinary retention develops, functional bladder capacity may be reduced and may attenuate if not reverse the drug's effect; thus if incontinence worsens as the dose is increased, the PVR volume should be measured. (Anticholinergic-induced xerostomia—and the excess fluid ingestion it engenders—is another reason for incontinence exacerbation.) In contrast, inducing urinary retention and using intermittent catheterization may be a viable approach for patients whose incontinence defies other remedies (such as those with DHIC) and for whom intermittent catheterization is feasible. Other remedies for urge incontinence, including electrical stimulation (Chap. 10) and selective nerve blocks, are successful in selected situations but have not been studied extensively in the elderly.

Adjunctive measures, such as pads and special undergarments, are invaluable if incontinence proves refractory. A wide variety are now available, and most are included in an illustrated catalog available from the nonprofit organization Help for Incontinent People (P.O. Box 544, Union, SC 29379), allowing the recommendation to be tailored to the individual's problem.[51–53] For instance, for bedridden individuals, a launderable bed pad may be preferable, whereas for those with a stroke, a diaper or pant that can be opened using the good hand may be preferred. For ambulatory patients with large gushes of incontinence, a wood pulp–containing product is generally preferable to those containing a polymer gel because the polymer gel generally cannot absorb the large amount and rapid flow these individuals produce, whereas the wood pulp product can easily be doubled up if necessary. Optimal products for men and women also differ because of the location of the target zone of the urinary loss. Finally, one must know whether the patient has fecal incontinence as well so as to choose the most appropriate product.

Feasible external collecting devices have been devised for women only recently, but preliminary studies suggest that one such system already may be effective for debilitated women in nursing homes;[54] whether the device will adhere adequately in more active women remains to be determined. Indwelling urethral catheters are not recommended for detrusor overactivity because they usually exacerbate it. If they must be used (*e.g.*, to allow healing of a pressure sore in a patient with refractory detrusor overactivity), a small catheter with a small balloon is preferable to minimize irritability and consequent leakage around the catheter. Such leakage almost invariably results from bladder spasm, not a catheter that is too small. Increasing the size of the catheter and balloon often only aggravates the problem and, over time, may result in progressive urethral erosion and sphincter incompetence. If bladder spasm persists, agents such as oxybutynin can be employed. Especially in the elderly, alternative agents with more potent anticholinergic side-effects (*e.g.*, belladonna suppositories) should be avoided.

STRESS INCONTINENCE

The treatment of stress incontinence is covered in detail in Section III. Urethral hypermobility,

the most common cause of stress incontinence, may be improved by weight loss if the patient is obese; by therapy of precipitating conditions, such as atrophic vaginitis or coughing (*e.g.*, due to an angiotensin converting enzyme inhibitor); and (rarely) by insertion of a pessary. Pelvic floor muscle exercises are frequently effective,[45, 55, 56] especially if the patient also contracts the pelvic muscles at the time of stress. Many older women, however, are unable or unmotivated to follow these regimens; encouragement or biofeedback, if available, may be helpful.[46, 56] Experience with vaginal cones in older women is still limited.[39]

If not contraindicated by other medical conditions, treatment with an alpha-adrenergic agonist, such as phenylpropanolamine (50 to 100 mg/day in divided doses), may be added and is often beneficial for women, especially when administered with estrogen.[39] In fact, these two agents work for women with sphincter incompetence as well. Phenylpropanolamine is inexpensive, available without a prescription, and contained in many diet pills. The physician should prescribe the dose and guide the choice of preparation, because some capsules contain additional agents, such as chlorpheniramine, in doses that can be troublesome for elderly patients. Imipramine, with beneficial effects on the bladder and the outlet, is a reasonable alternative for patients with evidence of both stress and urge incontinence if postural hypotension has been excluded.

If these methods fail or are unacceptable, further evaluation of the lower urinary tract may be warranted. If urethral hypermobility is confirmed, surgical correction may be performed and is successful in the majority of selected elderly patients.[57–62] If sphincter incompetence is diagnosed instead, it too can be corrected, but a different surgical approach is often required, morbidity is higher, and precipitation of chronic urinary retention is more likely than with correction of urethral hypermobility. Conservative, nonpharmacologic treatment for type 3 sphincter incompetence consists of a toileting and fluid regimen that maintains bladder volume below the leakage threshold. This approach is often appropriate for the older woman, whose sphincter incompetence is more often due to atrophic changes than to repeated operations. If the volume threshold is less than 150 to 200 ml, however, this strategy is generally not feasible without the addition of medication. Other treatments for sphincter incompetence include periurethral injections and insertion of an artificial sphincter, although reported experience with these approaches in women older than age 75 is still limited.

If all other interventions fail, some collection devices are now available for elderly women.[52-54] As already discussed, pads and undergarments are employed as adjunctive measures, but in these cases, thin, superabsorbent polymer gel pads are frequently successful because the gel can more readily absorb the usually smaller amount of leakage. Some products consist of pads that can be flushed down the toilet, which is quite convenient for ambulatory women. Electrical stimulation is a promising alternative that is currently under investigation (Chap. 10).

OUTLET OBSTRUCTION

If a large cystocele is the problem, surgical correction is usually required and should include an outlet suspension if urethral hypermobility is also present. Prior urodynamic evaluation is helpful as well: If bladder neck incompetence or low urethral closure pressure (<10 cm H_2O) is observed, a different surgical approach may be required to avoid converting incontinence owing to obstruction into incontinence owing to sphincteric incompetence. Bladder neck obstruction is also corrected easily, in even the frailest patient. Distal urethral stenosis in women can be dilated and treated with estrogen. If meatal stenosis is present, more extensive intervention may be necessary; alternatively, dilation can be repeated at fairly frequent intervals. It should be noted, however, that most women who undergo dilation do not have urethral stenosis but rather an underactive detrusor; for these women, dilation is usually unhelpful and may be harmful.

UNDERACTIVE DETRUSOR

Management of detrusor underactivity is directed at reducing the residual volume, eliminating hydronephrosis (rarely present), and preventing urosepsis. The first step is to use indwelling or intermittent catheterization to decompress the bladder for up to a month (at least 7 to 14 days), while reversing potential contributors to impaired detrusor function (fecal impaction and medications). If an indwelling catheter has been inserted, it should be withdrawn (Table 34-10). If decompression does not fully restore bladder function, augmented voiding techniques (such as double voiding and implementation of the Credé [application of suprapubic pressure during voiding] or Valsalva maneuver) may help if the patient is able to initiate a detrusor contraction or if there is coexistent stress incontinence. Bethanechol (40 to 200 mg/day in divided doses) is occasionally useful in a patient whose bladder contracts poorly because of treatment with anticholinergic agents that cannot be discontinued (e.g., tricyclic antidepressant). In other patients, bethanechol may decrease the PVR volume if sphincter function and local innervation are normal, but evidence for its efficacy is equivocal, and residual volume should be monitored to assess its effect.[63,64]

If after decompression the detrusor is acontractile (and stress incontinence does not exist), these interventions are apt to be fruitless, and the patient should be started on intermittent catheterization or an indwelling urethral catheter. For individuals at home, intermittent self-catheterization is preferable and requires only clean, rather than sterile, catheter insertion. The patient can purchase two or three of these catheters inexpensively. One or two are used during the day, and another is kept at home. The catheters are cleaned daily, allowed to air dry at night, sterilized periodically, and may be reused repeatedly. Antibiotic or methenamine (Mandelamine) prophylaxis against urinary tract infection is probably warranted if the individual gets more than an occasional symptomatic infection or has an abnormal heart valve.[65,66] Intermittent cathe-

Table 34-10. *Removing an Indwelling Urethral Catheter*

Ensure that the bladder has been decompressed for at least several days and longer (7–21 days) if possible; the higher the residual volume, the longer the bladder should be decompressed

Correct reversible causes of urinary retention: fecal impaction; pelvic/perineal pain; and use of anticholinergic, alpha-adrenergic agonist, or calcium channel blocker medications. If an anticholinergic antidepressant/antipsychotic agent cannot be stopped, consider switching to one with fewer or no anticholinergic side-effects or consider adding bethanechol. Addition of an alpha-adrenoceptor antagonist may be helpful but is unproved in women

Treat delirium, depression, atrophic vaginitis, or urinary tract infection, if present

Record urinary output at intervals of 6–8 hr for 2 days

Pull catheter at a time that permits accurate recording of urine output and allows for postvoiding recatheterization; clamping the catheter before removal is not necessary

Reinsert catheter *only:*
1. After the patient voids, to determine postvoiding residual volume or
2. After the expected bladder *volume* (based on records of urine output)—not the time since the catheter was removed—exceeds a preset limit (*e.g.*, 600–800 ml) or
3. If the patient is uncomfortable and unable to void despite ensured privacy and maneuvers performed to encourage voiding (*e.g.*, running water, tapping suprapubic area, or stroking inner thigh)

If the patient voids and the postvoiding residual volume is:
1. >400 ml—reinsert the catheter and evaluate further, if appropriate*
2. 100–400 ml—watch for delayed retention and evaluate further, if appropriate*
3. <100 ml—watch for delayed retention

If the patient is unable to void, evaluate further, if appropriate*

---

* Further evaluation is appropriate when the patient and physician believe that if a surgically correctable condition were found (*e.g.*, urethral obstruction), an operation would be preferable to long-term catheterization or the other options described in the text. Modified from Resnick NM. Incontinence. In: Beck JC, ed. Geriatric review syllabus. New York: American Geriatrics Society, 1991:141–154.

terization in this setting is generally painless, safe, inexpensive, and effective and allows individuals to carry on with their usual daily activities. For debilitated patients who require caregiver assistance, however, intermittent catheterization is usually less feasible, although

sometimes possible.[67] If used in an institutional setting, sterile rather than clean technique should be employed until studies document the safety of the latter.

Unfortunately, despite the benefits and proven feasibility of intermittent catheterization, most elderly individuals choose indwelling catheterization instead. As for younger women, complications of chronic indwelling catheterization include bladder and urethral erosions, bladder stones, and bladder cancer as well as urosepsis.[66] Principles of catheter care are summarized in Table 34-11.

When indicated, indwelling catheters can be extremely effective, but their use should be restricted. They are indicated in the acutely ill patient to monitor fluid balance, in the patient with

Table 34-11. *Principles of Indwelling Catheter Care*

Maintain sterile, closed-gravity drainage system

Secure the catheter to the upper thigh or lower abdomen to avoid urethral irritation and contamination

Avoid frequent cleaning of the urethral meatus; washing with soap and water once daily is sufficient

Do not routinely irrigate the catheter

If symptomatic urinary tract infection develops, change the catheter before obtaining a culture specimen (cultures obtained through the old catheter may be misleading)

If catheter obstruction occurs frequently and urine cultures reveal *Providencia stuartii* or *Proteus mirabilis*, antibiotic treatment may reduce the frequency of obstruction but induces emergence of resistant organisms. In the absence of urea-splitting organisms, consider urine acidification if urine output is normal (at low output, acidification may increase blockage owing to uric acid crystals). If frequent blockage persists, consider using a silicon catheter

If bypassing occurs in the absence of catheter obstruction, it is likely due to a bladder spasm, which can be treated with a bladder relaxant medication

Surveillance cultures are unnecessary and potentially misleading

Infection prophylaxis (*e.g.*, with mandelamine or antibiotics) as well as treatment of asymptomatic bacteriuria is generally fruitless and usually leads to the emergence of resistant organisms

---

Adapted from Resnick NM. Voiding dysfunction and urinary incontinence. In: Beck JC, ed. Geriatric review syllabus. New York: American Geriatrics Society, 1991:141–154.

a nonhealing pressure ulcer, for temporary bladder decompression in patients with acute urinary retention, and in the patient with overflow incontinence refractory to other measures. Even in long-term care facilities, they are probably indicated for only 1% to 2% of patients.

References

1. Herzog AR, Fultz NH. Prevalence and incidence of urinary incontinence in community-dwelling populations. J Am Geriatr Soc 1990;38:273.
2. Resnick NM. Voiding dysfunction in the elderly. In: Yalla SV, McGuire EJ, Elbadawi A, Blaivas JG, eds. Neurourology and urodynamics: Principles and practice. New York: MacMillan, 1988: 303–330.
3. Herzog AR, Diokno AC, Fultz NH. Urinary incontinence: Medical and psychosocial aspects. Ann Rev Gerontol Geriatr 1989;9:74.
4. Wyman JF, Harkins SW, Fantl JA. Psychosocial impact of urinary incontinence in the community-dwelling population. J Am Geriatr Soc 1990; 38:282.
5. Hu T-W. Impact of urinary incontinence on health care costs. J Am Geriatr Soc 1990;38:292.
6. Ouslander JG, Kane RL, Abrass IB. Urinary incontinence in elderly nursing home patients. JAMA 1982;248:1194.
7. Herzog AR, Wein NH, Normolle DP, et al. Methods used to manage urinary incontinence by older adults in the community. J Am Geriatr Soc 1989;37:339.
8. Mitteness L. Knowledge and beliefs about urinary incontinence in adulthood and old age. J Am Geriatr Soc 1990;38:374.
9. Resnick NM, Yalla SV, Laurino E. Urinary incontinence among elderly persons. N Engl J Med 1989;320:1421.
10. Diokno AC, Brown MB, Brock BM, et al. Clinical and cystometric characteristics of continent and incontinent noninstitutionalized elderly. J Urol 1988;140:567.
11. Kirkland JL, Lye M, Levy DW, Banerjee AK. Patterns of urine flow and electrolyte excretion in healthy elderly people. BMJ 1983;287:1665.
12. Brocklehurst JC, Dillane JB, Griffiths L, Fry J. The prevalence and symptomatology of urinary infection in an aged population. Gerontol Clin 1968;10:242.
13. Diokno AC, Brock BM, Brown M, Herzog AR. Prevalence of urinary incontinence and other urological symptoms in the non-institutionalized elderly. J Urol 1986;136:1022.
14. Diokno AC, Brown MB, Herzog AR. Relationship between use of diuretics and continence status in the elderly. Urology 1991;38:39.
15. Fantl JA, Wyman JF, Wilson M, et al. Diuretics and urinary incontinence in community-dwelling women. Neurourol Urodyn 1990;9:25.
16. Boscia JA, Kobasa WD, Abrutyn E, et al. Lack of association between bacteriuria and symptoms in the elderly. Am J Med 1986;81:979.
17. Robinson JM. Evaluation of methods for assessment of bladder and urethral function. In: Brocklehurst JC, ed. Urology in the Elderly. New York: Churchill Livingstone, 1984:19–54.
18. Parsons CL, Schmidt JD. Control of recurrent lower urinary tract infection in the postmenopausal woman. J Urol 1982;128:1224.
19. Privette M, Cade R, Peterson J, Mars D. Prevention of recurrent urinary tract infections in postmenopausal women. Nephron 1988;50:24.
20. Semmens JP, Tsai CC, Semmens EC, Loadholt CB. Effects of estrogen therapy on vaginal physiology during menopause. Obstet Gynecol 1985; 66:15.
21. Mathew TH, McEwen J, Rohan A. Urinary incontinence secondary to prazosin. Med J Aust 1988;148:305.
22. Amery A, Birkenhager W, Brixko P, et al. Mortality and morbidity results from the European Working Party on High Blood Pressure in the Elderly trial. Lancet 1985;1:1349.
23. SHEP Cooperative Research Group. Prevention of stroke by antihypertensive drug treatment in older persons with isolated systolic hypertension. JAMA 1991;265:3255.
24. Hellstrom PM, Sjoqvist A. Involvement of opioid and nicotinic receptors in rectal and anal reflex inhibition of urinary bladder motility in cats. Acta Physiol Scand 1988;133:559.
25. Abrams PH, Blaivas JG, Stanton SL, Andersen JT. Standardization of terminology of lower urinary tract function. Neurourol Urodynam 1988; 7:403.
26. Resnick NM, Yalla SV, Laurino E. The pathophysiology and clinical correlates of established urinary incontinence in frail elderly. N Engl J Med 1989;320:1.
27. Dennis PJ, Rohner TJ, Hu T-W, et al. Simple urodynamic evaluation of incontinent elderly female nursing home patients. A descriptive analysis. Urology 1991;37:173.
28. Resnick NM, Yalla SV. Detrusor hyperactivity with impaired contractile function. An unrecognized but common cause of incontinence in elderly patients. JAMA 1987;257:3076.

29. Brandeis GB, Yalla SV, Resnick NM. Detrusor hyperactivity with impaired contractility (DHIC): The great mimic. J Urol 1990;143:223A.
30. McGuire EJ. Urinary incontinence. New York: Grune & Stratton, 1981.
31. Blaivas JG, Olsson CA. Stress incontinence: Classification and surgical approach. J Urol 1988;139:727.
32. McGuire EJ. Reflex urethral instability. Br J Urol 1978;50:200.
33. Resnick NM. Initial evaluation of the incontinent patient. J Am Geriatr Soc 1990;38:311.
33a. Resnick NM, Baumann MM. Urinary incontinence and undwelling catheter In: Morris JN, Hawes C, eds. Minimum data set training manual. Natick, MA: Elliot Press, 1991:F24–F31.
34. Dyro FM, Yalla SV. Refractoriness of urethral striated sphincter during voiding: Studies with afferent pudendal reflex arc stimulation in male subjects. J Urol 1986;135:732.
35. Resnick NM. Noninvasive diagnosis of the patient with complex incontinence. Gerontology 1990;36(suppl 2):8.
36. DuBeau CE, Resnick NM. Evaluation of the causes and severity of geriatric incontinence: a critical appraisal. Urol Clin North Am 1991;18:243.
37. Bhatia NN, Bergman A. Urodynamic predictability of voiding following incontinence surgery. Obstet Gynecol 1984;63:85.
38. NIH Consensus Development Conference. Urinary incontinence in adults. J Am Geriatr Soc 1990;38:265.
39. Agency for Health Care Policy and Research (AHCPR). Urinary incontinence in adults: Clinical practice guideline. US Government Printing Office: Department of Health and Human Services, 1992.
40. Baldassare JS, Kaye D. Special problems in urinary tract infection in the elderly. Med Clin North Am 1991;75:375.
41. Stead WW. Tuberculosis as an endemic and nosocomial infection among the elderly in nursing homes. N Engl J Med 1985;312:1483.
42. Resnick NM, Yalla SV, Laurino E. Feasibility, safety, and reproducibility of urodynamics in the elderly. J Urol 1987;137:189A.
43. Burgio KL, Burgio LD. Behavior therapies for urinary incontinence in the elderly. Clin Geriatr Med 1986;2:809.
44. Hadley E, Abbey J, Awad S, et al. Bladder training and related therapies for urinary incontinence in elderly people. JAMA 1986;256:372.
45. Fantl JA, Wyman JF, McClish DK, et al. Efficacy of bladder training in older women with urinary incontinence. JAMA 1991;265:609.
46. Burgio KL, Engel BT. Biofeedback-assisted behavioral training for elderly men and women. J Am Geriatr Soc 1990;38:338.
47. Hu T-W, Igou JF, Kaltreider DL, et al. A clinical trial of a behavioral therapy to reduce urinary incontinence in nursing homes. JAMA 1989;261:2656.
48. Engel BT, Burgio LD, McCormick KA, et al. Behavioral treatment of incontinence in the long-term care setting. J Am Geriatr Soc 1990;38:361.
49. Schnelle JF. Treatment of urinary incontinence in nursing home patients by prompted voiding. J Am Geriatr Soc 1990;38:356.
50. Pedersen PA, Johansen PB. Prophylactic treatment of adult nocturia with bumetanide. Br J Urol 1988;62:145.
50a. Dequeker J. Drug treatment of urinary incontinence in the elderly. Controlled trial with vasopressin and propantheline bromide. Gerontol Clin 1965;7:311.
51. Brink CA, Wells TJ. Environmental support for incontinence: Toilets, toilet supplements, and external equipment. Clin Geriatr Med 1986;2:829.
52. Snow TL. Equipment for prevention, treatment, and management of urinary incontinence. Top Geriatr Rehab 1988;3:58.
53. Brink CA. Absorbent pads, garments, and management strategies. J Am Geriatr Soc 1990;38:368.
54. Johnson DE, Muncie HL, O'Reilly JL, Warren JW. An external urine collection device for incontinent women. J Am Geriatr Soc 1990;38:1016.
55. Wells TJ. Pelvic (floor) muscle exercises. J Am Geriatr Soc 1990;38:333.
56. Burns PA, Pranikoff K, Nochajski T, et al. A comparison of effectiveness of biofeedback and pelvic muscle exercise treatment of stress incontinence in older community-dwelling women. J Gerontol: Med Sci 1993;48:M167–M174.
57. Stamey TA. Endoscopic suspension of the vesical neck for urinary incontinence in females. Ann Surg 1980;192:465.
58. Ashken MH, Abrams PH, Lawrence WT. Stamey endoscopic bladder neck suspension for stress incontinence. Br J Urol 1984;56:629.
59. Gillon G, Stanton SL. Longterm followup of surgery for urinary incontinence in elderly women. Br J Urol 1984;56:478.
60. Bavendam TG, Leach GE. Surgical management of female incontinence. Sem Urol 1987;5:94.
61. Griffith-Jones MD, Abrams PH. The Stamey endoscopic bladder neck suspension in the elderly. Br J Urol 1990;65:170.
62. Nitti VW, Bregg KJ, Sussman EM, Raz S. The Raz

bladder neck suspension in patients 65 years old and older. J Urol 1993;149:802.

63. Downie JW. Bethanechol chloride in urology—a discussion of issues. Neurourol Urodynam 1984; 3:211.

64. Finkbeiner A. Is bethanechol chloride clinically effective in promoting bladder emptying? A literature review. J Urol 1985;134:443.

65. Chawla JC, Clayton CL, Stickler DJ. Antiseptics in the longterm urological management of patients by intermittent catheterization. Br J Urol 1988;62:289.

66. Warren JW. Urine collection devices for use in adults with urinary incontinence. J Am Geriatr Soc 1990;38:364.

67. Hunt GM, Whitaker RH. A new device for self-catheterization in wheelchair-bound women. Br J Urol 1990;66:162.

35

Urinary Tract Infections and Infection Stones

W. Terry Jones

Martin I. Resnick

Urinary Tract Infections

DEFINITIONS

Although the prerequisite for diagnosing urinary tract infection (UTI) has traditionally been to find greater than 10^5 organisms per milliliter of urine, lower absolute numbers of colony-forming units (cfu) of bacteria in compromised hosts may still indicate significant infection. Pyuria must be present to classify bacteriuria as infection rather than colonization. Colonization denotes multiplication of microorganisms in the host without tissue invasion, whereas infection implies invasion of host tissues associated with an inflammatory response.[1]

UTI may be an isolated or a recurrent event. Recurrent infections are the result of either reinfection or relapse.[2] Reinfection is recurrent infection with an organism distinct from previous infecting organisms, and relapse is recurrent infection with an organism that has been isolated during a prior infection. Relapse is also called *persistent infection*.

PATHOGENESIS

Bacteria

Bacteria can invade and spread within the urinary tract by three possible routes: ascending, hematogenous, and lymphatic. Considerable clinical evidence suggests that the ascent of bacteria within the urethra represents the most common pathway of infection of the urinary tract, and for this reason the short urethral length and colonization of the entire urethra may explain the higher frequency of UTIs among women.[3] Massage of the urethra in women and presumably sexual intercourse can force bacteria into the bladder.[4-6] Longitudinal studies have shown that colonization of the vaginal introitus and urethra with organisms that cause UTI precede the onset of acute cystitis in women prone to urinary infection.[3,7-9] *Escherichia coli* is the most common uropathogen isolated in ascending UTI. Others, such as *Enterobacteriaceae* (including *Pseudomonas, Klebsiella*, and *Proteus*), *Staphylococcus saprophyticus*, and *Enterococcus*, are frequent uropathogens as well.

Infrequently, hematogenous or even lymphatic seeding of microorganisms within the urinary tract occurs. Urinary infection with *Salmonella* species, *Mycobacterium tuberculosis*, and *Histoplasma* results from hematogenous spread. Renal infection is not infrequently associated with *Staphylococcus aureus* bacteremia or *Candida* fungemia. Gram-negative infections of the kidney rarely occur by the hematogenous route because the unobstructed kidney is highly effective in eliminating the infection.[10]

Female Urology, edited by Elroy D. Kursh and Edward McGuire. J. B. Lippincott, Philadelphia, © 1994.

Once bacteria enter the urinary tract, the pathogenesis of bacteriuria is an interplay between bacterial virulence and host susceptibility. Virulence implies that bacteria associated with UTIs differ from the indigenous flora associated with colonization. Virulent strains that cause acute pyelonephritis differ from other strains in that they possess the ability to colonize the intestine, spread to and ascendingly infect the urinary tract, and induce symptoms in the host.[11] Several virulence factors have been described, including bacterial adherence (pili), lipopolysaccharide, capsular polysaccharide, hemolysins, and aerobactin.[11]

Bacterial adherence to uroepithelial cells is a specific process involving bacterial surface structures (adhesins) and complementary components on epithelial cells (receptors). The globoseries of glycolipids have been identified as the active component in certain epithelial cell receptors, whereas the chemical nature of mannose-containing receptors in the urinary tract has not been defined.[12-14] The adhesive capacity of *E. coli.* covaries with the expression of pili or fimbriae.[15] Adhesins, however, may also be expressed on the bacterial surface in the absence of fimbriae.[16] Mannose-sensitive strains tend to be associated with cystitis, whereas mannose-resistant strains tend to be associated with pyelonephritis. Included in the mannose-resistant strains are fimbriae associated with adherence to the P blood group antigen, the so-called P pili.[17]

The lipopolysaccharides of gram-negative bacteria consist of three components: the polysaccharide moiety providing the O antigen specificity, the core region, and the hydrophobic lipid A that anchors the molecule into the outer membrane. The lipid A moiety is toxic, highly inflammatory, and thought to account for many of the acute symptoms of UTI.[11] Capsular polysaccharides are classic virulence factors for bacteria by restricting the access of complement and phagocytes.[18] Hemolysins are cytotoxic proteins detected by their ability to lyse erythrocytes. The alpha-hemolysin of *E. coli* has been demonstrated to injure renal tubular cells and is thought to be a significant virulence factor.[19] The

ability to compete for free iron has been identified as an important virulence factor. Aerobactin and enterochelin are two siderophores identified that enable *E. coli* to compete for free iron.[20,21]

Host Susceptibility

Host susceptibility to urinary infection depends on the status of the natural defenses of the urinary tract and the presence of predisposing factors. The natural defenses of the urinary tract include the antibacterial properties of urine, antiadherence mechanisms, the mechanical effects of urinary flow and micturition, phagocytic cells, antibacterial properties of urinary tract mucosa, and immune mechanisms.[10] The most inhibitory properties of urine include high organic acid content, high urea content, high osmolality, and low pH. Multiple antiadherence mechanisms normally exist in the urinary tract and include bacterial interference, urinary oligosaccharides, uromucoid (Tamm-Horsfall protein), mucopolysaccharide lining, urinary immunoglobulins, spontaneous exfoliation of uroepithelial cells with bacterial attachment, and mechanical flushing of micturition.[10]

The natural defenses of the urinary tract may be overwhelmed in the presence of various factors known to predispose the host to the development of infection. Obstruction to urine flow at all anatomic levels of the entire urinary tract from the urethral meatus to the renal tubules is the most important predisposing factor to urinary infection. Urinary stasis permits adherence of bacteria and provides a pool of media suitable for bacterial growth and colonization. Calculi predispose to the development of infection by producing obstruction and facilitating the adherence and colonization of bacteria. Vesicoureteral reflux not only predisposes a patient to the development of infection, but also to the development of renal scarring, especially in the growing kidneys of children. Abnormal colonization of the female perineum, especially the periurethral region, with coliform bacteria predisposes to the development of recurrent UTIs even in the absence of anatomic abnormality.[8,22] Genetic factors may account for the increased epithelial cell receptivity to adherence and colonization by uropathogens among women with recurrent urinary infections.[23] Instrumentation and catheterization of the urinary tract predispose to the development of urinary infection by potential direct inoculation or provision of a pathway (intraluminal or extraluminal) for adherence and migration of bacteria.

EPIDEMIOLOGY

Acute infection of the urinary tract afflicts an estimated 10% to 20% of women at some point during their lifetime, and 3% experience recurrent infection.[24,25] The majority of infections in adult women probably are asymptomatic and clear spontaneously.[9,26] The phenotypes of asymptomatic bacteriuric strains are different from pyelonephritic strains, in that they rarely are adhering, often have lost the O and K surface antigen markers, and have a low frequency of hemolysin production. The eight O antigens, O1, O2, O4, O6, O7, O16, O18, and O75, constitute up to 80% of pyelonephritogenic E. coli.[11]

There are certain circumstances in which the patient is at increased risk of developing a UTI and suffering greater morbidity and mortality from the development of a UTI. For example, patients with indwelling catheters, diabetics, the elderly, pregnant women, and chronic renal failure patients all experience greater morbidity associated with the development of a UTI. The risk of acquiring a UTI following single catheterization is 0.5% to 1.0% in the healthy nonhospitalized population. In hospitalized patients, the incidence is 10% to 20% in women.[27] With an indwelling catheter, the infection rate increases with the duration of the catheterization. The cumulative risk ranges from 4% to 7.5% per day.[28] The urinary tract is the most common site of nosocomial infection, and approximately 80% of nosocomial UTIs are preceded by some form of urologic instrumentation, most often the indwelling catheter.[29,30] It is usually assumed that catheter-associated bacteriuria is asymptomatic and benign and resolves spontaneously

after removal of the catheter. It should be noted that in one study the acquisition of a UTI during indwelling catheterization was associated with a threefold increase in mortality among hospitalized patients.[31] Approximately 1% of patients with nosocomial UTIs experience bacteremia that causes or contributes to death in approximately 10%.[30,32]

There is an increased prevalence of asymptomatic bacteriuria among women with diabetes mellitus.[33] Diabetics are in part predisposed to UTIs because of poor bladder emptying from autonomic neuropathy. The risk of parenchymal damage, papillary necrosis, and perinephric abscess formation is greater among diabetic patients with pyelonephritis than nondiabetic patients with pyelonephritis. Emphysematous pyelonephritis occurs only in diabetics.

Aging is associated with an increase in the prevalence of bacteriuria. In young to middle-aged women, the prevalence of bacteriuria is less than 5%, whereas in women older than 65 years of age, the prevalence is greater than 20%.[34,35] Elderly subjects living at home are less likely to have bacteriuria than those living in nursing homes, who in turn are less likely to have bacteriuria than those in hospitals. Those who are mentally impaired are more likely to have bacteriuria than those who are mentally intact. The increased prevalence of bacteriuria among the aged is thought to be due to several different factors, including obstructive uropathy, increased perineal colonization with uropathogens, reduced antiadherence protective effect of uromucoid, and increased instrumentation of the urinary tract.[10] Bacteremia occurs more commonly in elderly women with uncomplicated pyelonephritis.[36] Bacteriuria in old age is associated with a reduction in survival of 30% to 50%.[1]

Pregnancy predisposes women to the development of symptomatic UTI when bacteriuria is present because of urinary stasis secondary to hydroureter of pregnancy and bladder hypotonicity. Right ureteral dilatation and associated hydronephrosis are usually worse than the left; 74% of cases of pyelonephritis are localized to the right side.[37] Only 2% of cases of pyelonephritis occur during the first trimester, 52% occur in the second trimester, and 46% occur in the third trimester.[37] Although the prevalence of bacteriuria in pregnant women is approximately that of nonpregnant women, the rate of symptomatic UTIs is three times higher.[39] The overall prevalence of bacteriuria in pregnancy is in the range of 4% to 7%; however, by culturing ureaplasmas and other fastidious organisms, the prevalence of bacteriuria has been reported to be as high as 25%.[39] Lower socioeconomic class, multiparity, and sickle cell trait are all associated with a higher prevalence of bacteriuria during pregnancy.[40–42] Bacteriuria seen during pregnancy reflects prior colonization rather than acquisition during the pregnancy itself.[43] Many complications of pregnancy have been attributed to UTIs during gestation, including preterm labor, low birth weight, and growth retardation. The association between acute pyelonephritis and premature delivery is well documented; however, the relationship of asymptomatic bacteriuria to prematurity, fetal mortality, maternal anemia, and maternal hypertension remain controversial issues.[43]

Patients with compromised renal function suffer greater frequency and morbidity from UTI. Azotemia, infrequent voiding, low urinary flow rates, and urinary concentration defects all contribute to bacteriuria. The incidence of UTIs differs depending on the primary renal disease: chronic glomerulonephritis, 12%; diabetic nephropathy, 13%; polycystic kidneys, 41%; and chronic pyelonephritis, 67%.[44]

CLINICAL MANIFESTATIONS

The term *UTI* embraces a variety of different clinical syndromes, each with its own unique diagnostic considerations, requirements for therapy, and prognosis. In general, UTIs can be divided into two main categories: upper and lower tract infections. Upper tract or renal infections represent a wide spectrum of diseases, including acute and chronic pyelonephritis, focal bacterial nephritis, renal and perinephric abscess, pyonephrosis, xanthogranulomatous and emphy-

sematous pyelonephritis, and renal tuberculosis. Lower tract infections are less diverse and include acute cystitis and emphysematous cystitis.

Acute Pyelonephritis

Clinically patients with acute bacterial pyelonephritis have the symptom complex of fever (38°C to 40°C), chills, malaise, nausea, vomiting, and flank pain, with or without the signs of lower tract infection. On physical examination, unilateral costovertebral angle tenderness is present. Urinalysis reveals bacteriuria, pyuria, and gross or microscopic hematuria. Often associated abdominal pain, distention, or ileus may occur, prompting consideration of intra-abdominal diseases, such as appendicitis, diverticulitis, or pancreatitis in the differential diagnosis. The classic syndrome of acute bacterial pyelonephritis is the typical presentation of renal infection in the otherwise normal host. In contrast, patients with compromising urologic or medical conditions who acquire renal infection often present atypically. Such cases of subclinical pyelonephritis may be associated with minimal symptoms of upper tract infection. Historical features suggestive of an increased likelihood of occult pyelonephritis in a patient with presumed acute cystitis include prior urinary tract abnormalities, diabetes mellitus, immunocompromising illnesses, a UTI before age 12, symptoms with the current episode for longer than 7 days, prior relapse following UTI therapy, and acute pyelonephritis in the past year.[45]

Chronic Pyelonephritis

The term *chronic pyelonephritis* has no clinical meaning. Chronic pyelonephritis instead implies prolonged or recurrent renal infection with progressive destruction of the parenchyma. The clinical course is variable, usually involving repeated episodes of illness with variable symptoms associated with costovertebral angle tenderness, bacteriuria, and pyuria.

Focal Bacterial Nephritis

Focal bacterial nephritis refers to acute renal infection limited to a single renal lobe and may also be known as focal pyelonephritis or acute lobar nephronia. This entity represents interstitial inflammation in a compartmentalized distribution. Symptoms are similar to, although more severe than, acute pyelonephritis.

Renal Abscess

Renal abscesses are characterized by a loculated collection of purulent material within the renal parenchyma. Perinephric abscesses penetrate beyond the capsule into the perinephric space and are usually secondary to a renal cause, such as renal calculi, ureteropelvic junction obstruction, or polycystic renal disease.[46] The clinical presentation of these two entities is variable. Generalized sepsis without symptoms referable to the kidney may occur. Frequently patients experience several weeks of fever, malaise, and vague abdominal pain with or without an abdominal mass.[47] Isolated from the collecting system within the parenchyma, the abscess may not cause bacteriuria, pyuria, or any urinary symptoms.

Pyonephrosis

Pyonephrosis refers to a hydronephrotic, poorly functioning collecting system filled with pus that is essentially an abscess. Ureteropelvic junction obstruction from a congenital anomaly, tumor, or calculus may result in this entity. The symptoms associated with pyonephrosis are variable but usually insidious in onset and vague as with a renal abscess.

Xanthogranulomatous Pyelonephritis

Xanthogranulomatous pyelonephritis represents an atypical form of chronic renal infection that mimics neoplastic and inflammatory parenchymal lesions. Typically women are afflicted in the fourth to sixth decade of life and have an associated history of prior calculous disease, diabetes mellitus, obstructive uropathy, or recurrent UTIs with incomplete treatment. The chronic symptoms include flank pain, fever, chills, persist urosepsis, malaise, and constipation.[47,49]

Emphysematous Pyelonephritis

Emphysematous pyelonephritis is considered a rare complication of acute pyelonephritis that occurs mainly in diabetics and reflects a severe necrotizing infection secondary to gas-producing organisms in the collecting system, parenchyma, and retroperitoneum.[47] The signs are usually those of persistent infection and deteriorating clinical status despite appropriate antibiotic treatment.

Renal Tuberculosis

Renal tuberculosis may progress for years before the onset of vague symptoms, including malaise, low-grade fever, night sweats, easy fatigability, and chronic suprapubic or flank pain. In addition, patients have chronic cystitis characterized by frequency, dysuria, and sterile pyuria with gross or microscopic hematuria.

Acute Cystitis

The classic symptoms of acute cystitis include frequency, dysuria, and suprapubic discomfort. Twenty percent to 30% of women with this symptom complex do not have a UTI, and 10% to 30% of women presenting with symptoms of cystitis have renal infection in addition to lower tract symptoms.[49,50] Additional symptoms of cystitis include urgency, voiding of small volumes, nocturia, foul-smelling urine, and incontinence. Suprapubic tenderness is a specific finding and is present in 10% of patients with cystitis.[51] The rare entity emphysematous cystitis is typically found in a poorly controlled diabetic or elderly debilitated patient with symptoms ranging from mild abdominal pain to fulminant sepsis.[47]

DIAGNOSIS

The practical foundations of diagnosis include a detailed history, physical examination, microscopic examination of urinary sediment, and quantitative urine culture. For women with symptoms suggesting genitourinary infection, the isolation of a single organism in a spontaneously voided specimen in quantitative counts greater than or equal to 10^5 cfu/ml is adequate for diagnosis of a urinary infection. For catheter specimens, quantitative counts of greater than or equal to 10^4 cfu/ml are indicative of true bacteriuria. With suprapubic aspiration, any number of potentially pathogenic organisms is considered diagnostic of bacteriuria.[52] UTI may be present with a quantitative count of less than 10^5 cfu/ml. This generally occurs in patients with frequency or diuresis when the urine remains in the bladder for too short a period of time to permit multiplication of the organisms. As many as one third of women with acute cystitis have quantitative counts less than 10^5 cfu/ml.[53] Certain fastidious organisms, gram-positive organisms, and yeast may not be able to multiply to quantitative counts as high as 10^5 cfu/ml in urine.[54]

Localization of infection to the bladder or kidney may be useful in determining the optimal management of women who are experiencing recurrent infections. Definitive methods for localization include direct culture of ureteric urine obtained at the time of cystoscopy and retrograde catheterization of the ureters, percutaneous aspirate of urine in the renal pelvis under ultrasound guidance, or Fairley's bladder washout method with an antibiotic solution.[55] The bladder washout method may not be valid in individuals with neurogenic bladders.[56]

In the setting of UTI, radiologic imaging studies often are obtained to evaluate for the presence of complicating conditions (obstruction, stones, or anatomic abnormalities) and on occasion to establish the appropriate diagnosis (emphysematous pyelonephritis or cystitis, lobar nephronia, renal or perirenal abscess). A wide array of imaging techniques are available (Table 35-1), including intravenous urography, voiding cystourethrography, ultrasonography, computed tomography (CT), magnetic resonance imaging (MRI), radionuclide imaging, and angiography. Appropriate use of radiologic studies is important to avoid excessive costs and redundant data collection.[57]

In the setting of acute pyelonephritis, intravenous urography may reveal renal enlargement or delayed or poor contrast excretion but usually is unremarkable. Similarly, ultrasonography most often is normal but may demonstrate renal enlargement or decreased cortical and medullary echogenicity. CT during acute pyelonephritis

Table 35-1. Imaging Studies

STUDY	ADVANTAGES	DISADVANTAGES	MISCELLANEOUS
Kidney, ureter, and bladder	Inexpensive screening tool	Inadequate visualization of kidney	Identifies gas and stones
Renal tomogram	Outlines renal masses	No assessment of function	Identifies stone size and position
Intravenous urogram	Assesses renal anatomy and function	Contrast allergy; contraindicated in renal failure	Identifies mass effect
Ultrasound	Rapid; inexpensive; no radiation	Operator dependent; obesity, bowel gas interference	Identifies fluid-filled structures
CT	Multiplanar image; assesses size and density of masses	Radiation; contrast allergy	Identifies fluid, gas, and stones
Radio-nuclide imaging (renal and gallium)	Accurately assesses blood flow and renal function	Nonspecific identification of inflammation	Detects renal obstruction and abscess
Arteriography	Evaluates renal masses and vascularity	Invasive; contrast allergy; contraindicated in renal failure	
MRI	Multiplanar image; assesses size and density of masses	Poor visualization of certain densities	

Modified from Benson M, LiPuma JP, Resnick MI. The role of imaging studies in urinary tract infection. Urol Clin North Am 1986;13:605.

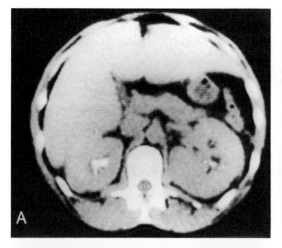
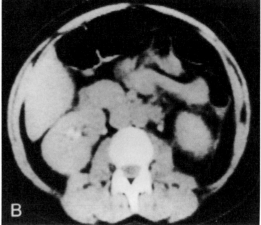

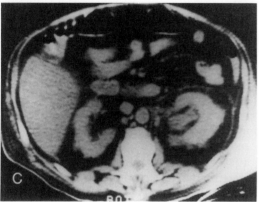

Figure 35-1. CT of acute pyelonephritis. Noncontiguous slides in a patient with acute pyelonephritis. (A), The left kidney is enlarged and demonstrates decreased excretion of contrast material in comparison to the right. (B) Inflammatory thickening of the renal fascia. (C) Another patient demonstrating slight increase in renal size in the left with associated mild dilation of the collecting system and renal fascial thickening. (From LiPuma JP, Haaga JR. The kidney. In: Haaga JR, Alfidi RJ, eds. Computed tomography of the whole body. St Louis: CV Mosby, 1983.)

(Fig. 35-1) also reveals generalized renal enlargement and may show decreased function, poor corticomedullary definition, thickening of Gerota's fascia, and focal decreased enhancement of renal lobes.[57]

Intravenous urography is more valuable in the assessment of chronic rather than acute pyelonephritis because of the anatomic changes associated with chronic or recurrent parenchymal infection. Focal diminished parenchymal thickness, generalized atrophy, and diminished function may be demonstrated by urography (Fig. 35-2). Ultrasonography and CT usually are not indicated because these studies provide essentially the same information as intravenous urography. On occasion, segmental scarring re-

sults in compensatory lobar hypertrophy, and in this situation ultrasonography and CT (Fig. 35-3) may help distinguish the resultant *pseudotumor* from renal carcinoma or abscess.[57]

Imaging is important in differentiating focal bacterial nephritis from renal abscess and tumor. In the setting of focal bacterial nephritis, intravenous urography may reveal caliceal distortion or decreased or delayed contrast excretion and may suggest a poorly defined renal mass. Ultrasonography demonstrates a vague hypoechoic mass, which may disrupt the corticomedullary junction. CT with intravenous contrast material (Fig. 35-4) typically reveals a wedge-shaped area of decreased enhancement. Radionuclide scanning with gallium provides correlation with

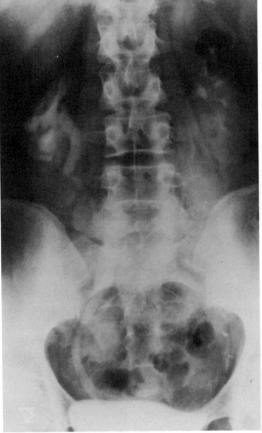

Figure 35-2. Urography of chronic pyelonephritis. *Most adults with acute pyelonephritis do not develop the morphologic changes of chronic pyelonephritis. These changes are associated with reflux nephropathy and infection occurring in infancy and childhood. Characteristically the kidney is normal in size or small. Focal scars overlie involved papillae, and underlying calicectasis is evident, or else the kidney is small with global loss of parenchyma and generalized calicectasis. The lesion may be unilateral or bilateral. If unilateral, compensatory hypertrophy in the opposite kidney is evident. In this case, the right kidney is small, with global loss of parenchyma and generalized calicectasis. Compensatory hypertrophy of the left kidney is evident. (From Benson M, LiPuma JP, Resnick MI. The role of imaging studies in urinary tract infection. Urol Clin North Am 1986;13:605.)*

increased uptake in the region of the lobar nephronia. Arteriography does not show hypervascularity in the focal region of the infection.[57]

Renal abscesses are usually evaluated and diagnosed by radiologic studies. Plain radiographic films such as kidney, ureter, and bladder films (KUB) reveal diffuse renal enlargement with distortion of renal contour, loss of psoas shadow, scoliosis with concavity toward the affected side, and renal fixation on inspiratory/expiratory films. A round, smooth-walled mass with low-amplitude echoes is the characteristic ultrasound appearance of a renal abscess (Fig. 35-5). CT is generally considered the imaging modality of choice for diagnosis and evaluation of renal abscesses. An abscess appears as a round mass of decreased attenuation surrounded by a rim of higher attenuation parenchyma known as the *ring sign* (Fig. 35-6). Thickening of Gerota's fascia and asymmetrical, ipsilateral psoas enlargement may also be demonstrated. Radionuclide scanning may be useful in differentiating renal abscesses from tumors. Arteriography seldom has a role in the evaluation of renal abscesses but if obtained typically reveals increased cortical vascularity of the surrounding viable parenchyma and avascularity of the abscess collection itself.[57]

Intravenous urography and CT cannot distinguish hydronephrosis from pyonephrosis (Fig. 35-7). Ultrasonography, however, is capable of this distinction. Hydronephrosis is characterized on ultrasound by dilated anechoic images of the renal pelvis and calices, whereas pyonephrosis is characterized by dilated images of the renal pelvis and calices filled with internal echoes consistent with debris (Fig. 35-8).[57]

Xanthogranulomatous pyelonephritis should be suspected when intravenous urography reveals a renal calculus associated with a nonfunctioning kidney possessing a mass (Fig. 35-9). Ultrasonography demonstrates renal enlargement, shadowing associated with calculi, and hypoechoic areas associated with parenchymal abscesses. CT suggests the diagnosis of xanthogranulomatous pyelonephritis when a calculus in the collecting system is seen in association with

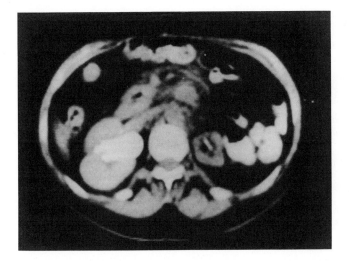

Figure 35-3. CT of chronic pyelonephritis. The left kidney functions but is markedly diminished in size, with global loss of parenchyma and increased renal sinus fat. The right kidney demonstrates compensatory hypertrophy but also evidence of focal scarring from previous infection immediately overlying a calix. (From LiPuma JP, Haaga JR. The kidney. In: Haaga JR, Alfidi RJ, eds. Computed tomography of the whole body. St Louis: CV Mosby, 1983.)

decreased contrast excretion and parenchymal masses with or without perirenal extension.[57]

Emphysematous pyelonephritis and cystitis are diagnoses established by plain radiographic films or intravenous urography that reveal air within the collecting system, renal parenchyma, or urinary bladder (Fig. 35-10). Ultrasonography reveals acoustic shadowing associated with the air/fluid interfaces present in these serious infections. CT is capable of providing the earliest and best images of gas with the renal parenchyma, collecting system, or bladder wall (Fig. 35-11).[57]

The radiologic diagnosis of renal tuberculosis is based primarily on plain radiographic films and intravenous urography. The findings on KUB include punctate renal calcifications and obliteration of the psoas shadow secondary to renal enlargement or perirenal abscess. Intravenous urography may reveal caliceal deformity secondary to ulceration with a moth-eaten or fuzzy appearance, infundibular stenosis, hydronephrosis, and ureteral beading from multiple strictures (Fig. 35-12). When renal tuberculosis is suspected, Ziehl-Neelsen staining of urinary sediment for acid-fast organisms may allow initiation of therapy while awaiting confirming cultures.[58] First-voided morning urine specimens are best for culturing mycobacteria, and multiple specimens should be obtained.[58]

TREATMENT

The appropriate treatment of UTIs is based on the location, severity, and chronicity of the infection. Medical treatment with antibacterial therapy alone is adequate for most UTIs; however, surgical intervention is required in certain circumstances to ensure recovery. Antibacterial therapy is categorized as curative, prophylactic, or suppressive based on the objectives of treatment.

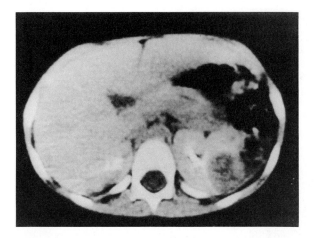

Figure 35-4. CT of focal pyelonephritis/nephronia. Homogeneous solid mass, demonstrating patchy enhancement after administration of contrast, without definable wall with overall decreased attenuation when compared with adjacent parenchyma in a patient with clinical evidence of pyelonephritis. (From LiPuma JP, Haaga JR. The kidney. In: Haaga JR, Alfidi RJ, eds. Computed Tomography of the Whole Body. St Louis: CV Mosby, 1983, with permission.)

Acute Cystitis

In the setting of acute cystitis, curative therapy is initiated after urine specimen collection for culture and sensitivity. An oral antibacterial agent with a broad spectrum of activity against gram-negative organisms that is excreted in high concentrations in the urine is empirically selected. First-line antibacterials include ampicillin, trimethoprim, trimethoprim/sulfamethoxazole, nitrofurantoin, and cephalexin. Specific therapy is used once culture and sensitivity results are available. The duration of treatment traditionally has been 7 to 14 days; however, this approach overtreats most patients.[59] Single-dose therapy is nearly as effective in women with acute cystitis, is less costly, and is associated with fewer side-effects.[60] Widespread adoption of single-dose therapy has not occurred because of slightly lower efficacy as compared with 7-day therapy and concern regarding its use in high-risk patients, such as pregnant women, diabetics, immunocompromised patients, patients with urinary tract abnormalities, and patients with occult upper tract infection. A 3-day course of therapy is associated with an incidence of adverse effects comparable to single-dose therapy and efficacy rates comparable to a 7-day course of therapy. Short-course therapy should be reserved for patients with presumed uncomplicated acute cystitis.[59] Posttherapy cultures can probably be safely omitted in cases of uncomplicated cystitis.[59]

Recurrent Cystitis

Women with recurrent cystitis may be managed with repeated courses of single-dose therapy.[61] Women with recurrent cystitis have an 85% reliability in identifying infection recurrence based on symptoms, and self-treatment is associated with a 90% cure rate.[61] In this setting, routine urine culture before therapy is not necessary, and

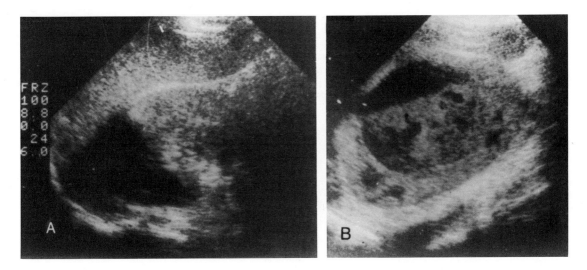

Figure 35-5. *Ultrasonography of renal abscess. The ultrasound picture of renal abscess is variable, depending on the stage of development. The picture can vary from a solid mass with irregular margins and slightly decreased echoes to the liquefactive stage with irregular margins and a hypoechoic to anechoic pattern depending on contained debris through transmission of echoes. As the necrotic material increases in the abscess, echogenicity increases and transmission decreases. (A) Hypoechoic mass in the upper pole. Note through transmission posteriorly and extension of the hypoechoic area beyond the kidney representing the perinephric extension of the abscess material. (B) A more mature renal abscess demonstrating a fluid-fluid level between denser necrotic material in the dependent portion of the abscess and simple fluid without necrotic material in the nondependent portion of the abscess. Note the hyperechoic nature of the necrotic material in the dependent portion of the abscess. (From Benson M, LiPuma JP, Resnick MI. The role of imaging studies in urinary tract infection. Urol Clin North Am 1986;13:605.)*

urine cultures need be obtained only if the patient relapses or fails to respond to single-dose therapy.[50] Prophylactic therapy is efficacious in the management of women with recurrent symptomatic cystitis, decreasing recurrences by 95%.[50] Prophylaxis is recommended if more than two symptomatic episodes occur within a 6-month period. The most widely and successfully used regimens are nitrofurantoin (100 mg), trimethoprim (50 mg) or trimethoprim/sulfamethoxazole (40 mg/200 mg) given once a day for 6 to 12 months. An alternate approach is to give single-dose postintercourse prophylaxis to women who identify intercourse as a precipitating factor in the development of infections.[62]

Acute Pyelonephritis

Patients with acute pyelonephritis can be divided into three categories: mild acute pyelonephritis that can be managed with outpatient antibacterial therapy; uncomplicated moderate to severe acute pyelonephritis that necessitates hospitalization for parenteral antibacterial therapy; and complicated acute pyelonephritis associated with catheterization, hospitalization, surgery, or urinary tract abnormalities that requires hospitalization for parenteral antibacterial therapy. Usually the patient is debilitated and unable to take adequate oral intake and is hospitalized for intravenous hydration, parenteral antibacterials,

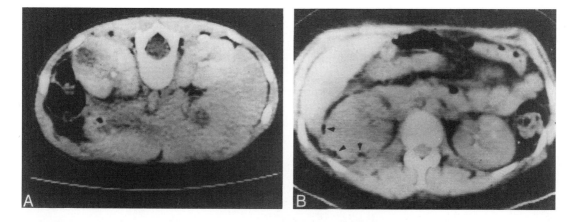

Figure 35-6. (A) CT of renal abscess. Mass effect posterolaterally in the left kidney. Following administration of contrast material, the mass is noted to have a relatively lucent center with an enhancing rim in a patient with clinical evidence of urinary tract infection. Lesion was drained percutaneously and resolved with surgical intervention. (B) CT of perinephric abscess. Right kidney is enlarged and demonstrates diminished function. Posteriorly the perinephric space is obliterated by purulent material with evidence of small collections of gas (arrowheads) in a patient with clinical evidence of a urinary tract infection. CT is the best method for detecting small amounts of gas in cases of suspect urinary tract infections. (From LiPuma JP, Haaga JR. The kidney. In: Haaga JR, Alfidi RJ, eds. Computed Tomography of the Whole Body. St Louis: CV Mosby, 1983.)

and parenteral analgesia if necessary. Initial choice of antibacterial therapy usually entails a combination of ampicillin or an extended-spectrum derivative penicillin (such as piperacillin or mezlocillin) with an aminoglycoside (such as gentamicin, tobramycin, or amikacin). Third-generation cephalosporins (such as ceftriaxone, cefotaxime, or cefoperazone) are also a reasonable initial choice until culture and sensitivity results are available. Parenteral agents are used until the patient is afebrile, symptomatically improved, and able to take fluids by mouth. The usual duration of therapy is 14 days. If relapse occurs after 14 days of therapy, retreatment with 6 weeks of an appropriate agent usually is curative.[2] In women with acute pyelonephritis, posttreatment cultures should be obtained 2 weeks after therapy.[63]

Asymptomatic Bacteriuria

The treatment of asymptomatic bacteriuria is controversial. There is currently no evidence to suggest that the presence of pyuria in association with positive culture in the absence of symptoms mandates antibacterial therapy.[50] The decision as to whether or not to treat is arbitrary and must be made on a case-by-case basis. Women with asymptomatic bacteriuria who undergo invasive genitourinary procedures should receive preprocedure antibacterial therapy to prevent sepsis. In general, asymptomatic UTIs are also treated in diabetics, severely immunocompromised patients, and renal transplant recipients.[50] In addition, pregnant women with asymptomatic bacteriuria should be treated because of the increased risk of development of symptom-

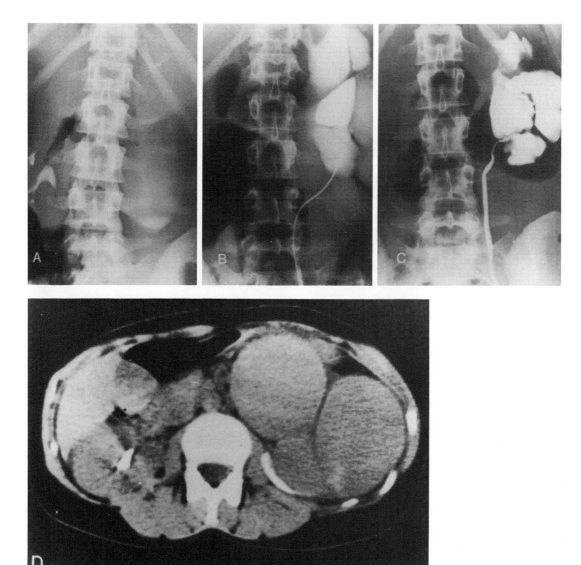

Figure 35-7. *(A) Urogram of pyonephrosis. (B) Retrograde pyelogram of pyonephrosis. This case illustrates some of the cardinal findings of pyonephrosis, with decreased function and poor visualization of the left renal unit, with marked dilation of the collecting system. The patient presented with fever, abdominal pain, and a palpable mass. The retrograde pyelogram shows the extent of caliceal expansion. (C) Retrograde pyelogram (following stent drainage) of pyonephrosis. Following decompression with a ureteral stent, follow-up retrograde studies indicated the probable cause, ureteropelvic junction obstruction. Although not apparent, a small calculus was also seen within the renal pelvis. (D) CT of Pyonephrosis. This CT scan of the same patient in (C) shows marked dilation of the caliceal system, with some variation in the density of the contents. The distinction between urine, blood, and pus, however, requires clinical correlation. (From Benson M, LiPuma JP, Resnick MI. The role of imaging studies in urinary tract infection. Urol Clin North Am 1986;13:605.)*

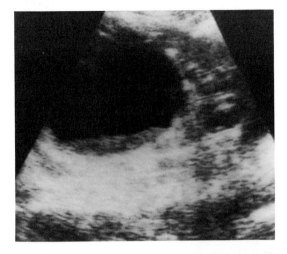

Figure 35-8. *Ultrasonography of pyohydronephrosis. Ultrasonography is valuable in establishing this diagnosis. The dilated, branching appearance of an obstructed collecting system containing increased echoes throughout the fluid or a fluid-debris level that shifts with changes in position of the patient is pathognomonic. In this case, the upper-pole moiety of a duplex system is obstructed, and a cystic structure with a fluid-debris level is identified in the upper pole. The central echo complex of the lower-pole moiety is noted to be normal. (From Benson M, LiPuma JP, Resnick MI. The role of imaging studies in urinary tract infection. Urol Clin North Am 1986;13:605.)*

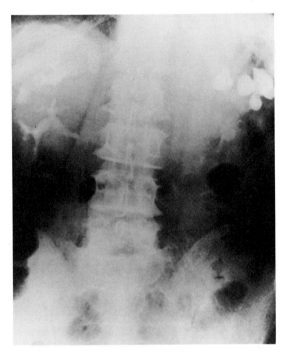

Figure 35-9. *Urogram of xanthogranulomatous pyelonephritis. Characteristic findings of xanthogranulomatous pyelonephritis include absence of function, staghorn calculus, and indistinct renal outline on the left. The clinical diagnosis was confirmed at the time of surgery, with intraoperative cultures positive for* Proteus. *The patient was an elderly black woman with diabetes mellitus. (From Benson M, LiPuma JP, Resnick MI. The role of imaging studies in urinary tract infection. Urol Clin North Am 1986;13:605.)*

atic UTI later during pregnancy. Approximately 70% to 80% of pregnant women treated with 7 to 10 days of antibacterials have elimination of bacteriuria. Ampicillin, nitrofurantoin, or sulfisoxazole are good first-line choices, although sulfisoxazole should be avoided late in pregnancy because of hyperbilirubinemia.[64] Follow-up culture should be done approximately 1 week after completion of therapy. If a patient fails to respond, a second course with a different agent is recommended. If this fails, suppression therapy with a single daily dose of nitrofurantoin is advised until delivery.[43] Likewise, successfully treated symptomatic acute pyelonephritis of pregnancy should be followed by suppressive therapy until delivery.[43]

Treatment of renal abscess usually is best carried out by surgical drainage in conjunction with parenteral antibacterial therapy, although percutaneous drainage in conjunction with parenteral antibacterials is a viable option. Medical therapy alone can on occasion succeed but usually requires long-term systemic administration of appropriate agents. Perinephric abscess also should be treated either by surgical or percutaneous drainage in conjunction with parenteral an-

(continued on page 512)

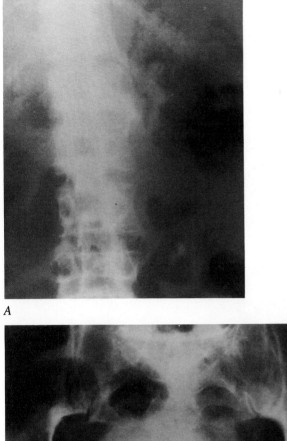

A

B

Figure 35-10. *Kidney, ureter, and bladder study of emphysematous pyelonephritis and cystitis. Diagnosis of emphysematous pyelonephritis is made on plain film that demonstrates radiolucent gas in and around enlarged kidney. Picture is created by the presence of gas in the renal parenchyma and collecting system and perinephric space. (A) This radiographic picture is diagnostic. Likewise, diagnosis of emphysematous cystitis is made on plain film that demonstrates radiolucent gas in the wall of the bladder. (B) This radiographic picture is diagnostic in patients with symptoms related to acute bladder infection. (From Benson M, LiPuma JP, Resnick MI. The role of imaging studies in urinary tract infection. Urol Clin North Am 1986;13:605.)*

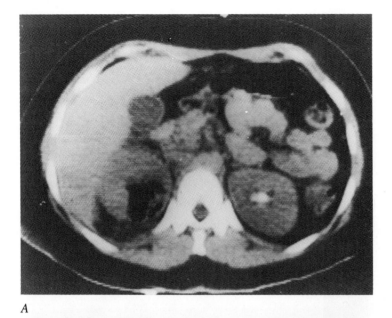

A

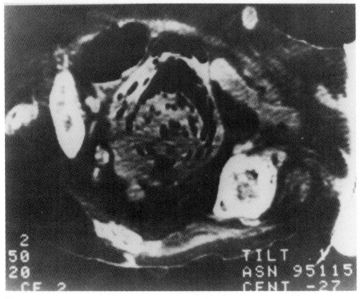

B

Figure 35-11. CT of emphysematous pyelonephritis and cystitis. (A) Note enlargement of the right kidney, nonfunction, and gas in the renal collecting system. There is extension of gas into the perinephric fat. (B) The air/tissue density contrast in evident in this case of advanced emphysematous cystitis, with pockets throughout the entire bladder wall. ([A] from LiPuma JP, Haaga JR. The kidney. In: Haaga JR, Alfidi RJ, eds. Computed tomography of the whole body. CV Mosby, 1983. [B] from Benson M, LiPuma JP, Resnick MI. The role of imaging studies in urinary tract infection. Urol Clin North Am 1986;13:605.)

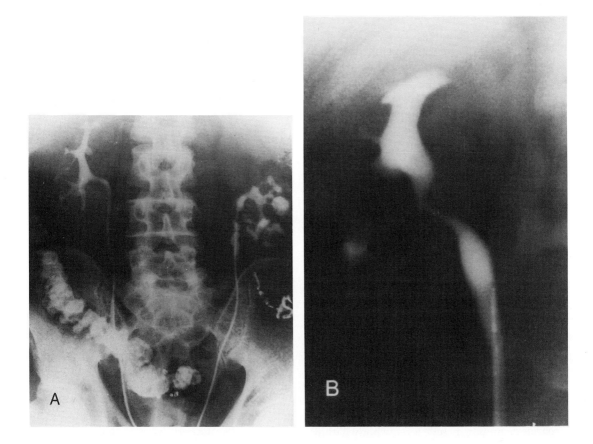

Figure 35-12. *Urogram of renal tuberculosis. The radiographic appearance of renal tuberculosis is varied. The disease is generally unilateral and can progress through several phases that may coexist. Early on, the kidney may appear normal. Later, medullary pyramid abscesses result in medullary cavities or areas of papillary necrosis and focal calcifications. The kidney may enlarge or be normal in size. The second phase demonstrates loss and scarring of tissue and associated infundibular stenosis and calicectasis. Strictures may also involve the ureteropelvic junction and result in obstruction. Finally, phase three can be thought of as autonephrectomy with extensive calcification in a kidney that is to close to normal in size or small (often called a* putty *kidney). (A) The earliest finding of renal tuberculosis is smudging of contrast material at the caliceal margin. This case represents the next phase of involvement, papillary necrosis. Note the multiple shaggy cavities involving the renal pyramids. (B) Elements of the second phase of renal tuberculosis include lower-pole infundibular stenosis and stricture of the renal pelvis. (From Benson M, LiPuma JP, Resnick MI. The role of imaging studies in urinary tract infection. Urol Clin North Am 1986;13:605.)*

tibacterial therapy and relief of the associated urinary tract obstruction.

Emphysematous pyelonephritis requires emergent nephrectomy in conjunction with parenteral antibacterial therapy. Pyonephrosis usually requires nephrectomy, although on rare occasions relief of obstruction along with appropriate antibacterial therapy suffices. Xanthogranulomatous pyelonephritis usually is diagnosed after nephrectomy, which is the treatment of choice.

Infection Stones

The term *infection stones* is synonymous with the terms *struvite stones, urease stones*, and *triple phosphate stones* and refers to calculi composed of magnesium ammonium phosphate and carbonate apatite that form as a result of infection with urea-splitting organisms. Infection stones account for 15 to 20 of all urinary calculi and occur more frequently in women at a 2 : 1 female-to-male ratio. Untreated renal infection stones grow and tend to assume a staghorn configuration completely filling the collecting system (Fig. 35-13). Predisposing factors to infection stone formation include foreign body within the urinary tract, neurogenic bladder, cutaneous urinary diversion, and the presence of a chronic indwelling urethral catheter. It is not yet known which comes first: the infection or the stone. Approximately one half of patients afflicted by infection stones, however, are found to have preexisting anatomic or metabolic abnormalities.[65]

PATHOGENESIS

Urea-splitting organisms produce urease, an enzyme that breaks down urinary urea into ammonia and carbon dioxide. Hydrolysis of the ammonia and carbon dioxide causes alkalinization of the urine, yielding increased concentration of carbonate and hydroxyl ions, which favors the supersaturation of magnesium ammonium phosphate, calcium phosphate, and carbonite apatite crystals. Urease production has been demonstrated in the following species of organisms:

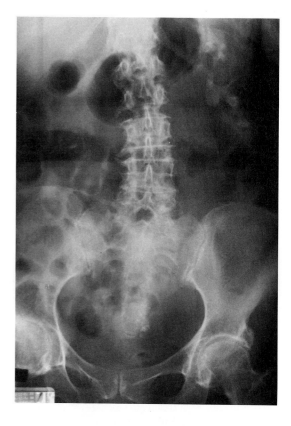

Figure 35-13. *Staghorn infection stone found in left kidney of this elderly white woman with associated right renal and proximal ureteral stones.*

Proteus, Klebsiella, Pseudomonas, Staphylococcus, Providencia, Ureaplasma urealyticum and *Enterococcus. E. coli* do not produce urease and when found in association with struvite stone most likely represent a superimposed infection.[65]

EVALUATION

A metabolic evaluation of all patients with infection stones should be performed in an effort to detect predisposing factors leading to stone formation. Measurement of serum and urinary creatinine, calcium, phosphorus, uric acid, oxalate, and electrolytes and the qualitative nitroprusside test for cystine may reveal that the patient has hyperparathyroidism, hypercalciuria, hyperuricosuria, renal tubular acidosis, cystinuria, or other metabolic causes of stone disease.

An essential step in the evaluation of any patient with stone disease is analysis of a stone passed or removed. Specific quantitative crystallographic analysis of stone material by x-ray diffraction and polarized microscopy can be performed by commercial laboratories. Analysis of the nucleus separate from the periphery of the stone often provides clues to the factors responsible for its formation.

Bacterial culture and antibiotic sensitivity studies of all organisms isolated from urine and stone specimens allow the appropriate choice of antibacterial therapy. At times, it may be of value to localize the UTI through the use of ureteral catheterization studies.

Accurate assessment of stone size and location within the kidney is imperative before treatment. Plain nephrotomography and intravenous urography with tomography and oblique views are useful radiographic studies that help identify small, poorly mineralized, nonopaque fragments and caliceal extensions. Retrograde pyelography is valuable for assessment of infundibular stenosis and caliceal dilation.

TREATMENT

A nonoperative approach to the management of infection stones should be condemned because of the significant morbidity and mortality associated with the resultant persistent UTI, perinephric diseases, and sepsis. Approximately 50% of these patients lose the unoperated kidney eventually because of persistent infection and obstruction from the stone. The overall mortality of untreated staghorn calculi ranges from 28% to 50% within 10 years of follow-up.[66-68]

Successful management of infection stones requires combined application of surgical and medical treatments with surgery serving as the primary modality and medical therapy serving as an adjunct. Specific antibacterial agents based on in vitro susceptibility results should be administered before, during, and after surgery. Usually penicillin or synthetic penicillin analogs

are given, although cephalosporins are an appropriate alternative choice. Potential nephrotoxic agents, such as aminoglycosides, should be avoided when open surgery is performed, especially during the immediate perioperative period if hypothermia and renal artery occlusion have been employed.

Urease inhibitors, such as acetohydroxamic acid and hydroxyurea, have been demonstrated to prevent growth of infection stones but have not proved to be capable of reducing stone size. Acetohydroxamic acid has been shown to inhibit *in vitro* urinary alkalinization and precipitation of magnesium ammonium phosphate and carbonite apatite in the presence of proteus infection.[69,70] These agents appear to be most useful in inhibiting the growth of residual stones when complete removal is not possible and in preventing new stone formation in patients with intractable UTIs.[65]

The objectives of surgical therapy for infection stones are as follows: (1) removal of all stones, (2) reconstruction of any strictured infundibula or obstructed calyces, (3) resolution of UTI, (4) preservation of all functioning renal parenchyma, and (5) prevention of recurrent infection and stone formation.

Open surgical options include nephrectomy, pyelolithotomy, and anatrophic nephrolithotomy. Nephrectomy should be performed only when severe obstruction and parenchymal damage have resulted in no significant salvageable renal function. Pyelolithotomy or extended pyelolithotomy may be undertaken when the stone is firm and caliceal extension is not significant, but other less invasive approaches (extracorporeal shock wave lithotripsy [ESWL] and percutaneous nephrostolithotomy) have essentially supplanted these techniques. Anatrophic nephrolithotomy is indicated for the removal of multiple, branched calculi, particularly when associated with infundibular stenosis or a dilated collecting system.[71,72] This procedure allows complete removal of all stone material in one setting and reconstruction of the collecting system, thereby ensuring optimal urinary drainage.

Percutaneous nephrostolithotomy is an option that is also appropriate for the removal of infection stones. Some advocate that all staghorn stones be treated in this manner, but others restrict the procedure to those patients with incomplete staghorn stones. Ultrasonic and electrohydraulic lithotripsy probes traditionally have been used for fragmentation, with the ultrasonic probe limited to use primarily in the renal pelvis because of its rigidity. The pulsed dye laser is an attractive alternative to either the ultrasonic or the electrohydraulic probes because the risk of trauma is significantly reduced with use of this form of energy for fragmentation.

ESWL may be used effectively as the primary modality of treatment on small or incomplete staghorn infection stones. Large staghorn infection stones can be fragmented with ESWL alone, but multiple treatments usually are required.[73] Usually large staghorn stones without associated infundibular stenoses can be managed with a combination of ESWL and percutaneous nephrostolithotomy.[73]

Acid solutions, such as hemiacidrin or Suby's G solution, can be successfully used to dissolve magnesium ammonium phosphate, calcium carbonate, and calcium phosphate stones.[74,75] Dissolution therapy appears to be best suited as an adjunct to surgical removal of infection stones by dissolving residual stone fragments too small to be seen radiographically.[76] When renal infection stones are to be dissolved, either a ureteral stent or nephrostomy tube is inserted. Antibacterial therapy must be used throughout dissolution therapy, and the urine must be sterile before infusing any solution. Initially normal saline is infused under low pressures (less than 25 cm H_2O) at a rate less than or equal to 120 ml/hour. If the patient tolerates this infusion without development of fever or flank pain, chemolysis is then started with close monitoring of intrapelvic pressures, temperatures, white blood cell count, and serum magnesium and creatinine levels. Infusion is stopped immediately if the patient develops flank pain, fever, elevated renal pelvic pressures, leakage around the nephrostomy tube, urinary infection, or hypermagnesemia.

FOLLOW-UP

Residual stone rates have been reported to range from 5% to 26%.[68,71,77,78] The stone recurrence rate approximates 30% within 6 years.[79] Only 60% to 80% of patients with infection stones are free of infections after open surgical removal of their stones.[65] These statistics emphasize the importance of long-term follow-up and re-evaluation of these patients. Initial follow-up should include urine cultures obtained at 1- to 2-month intervals for the first year and periodically thereafter. Intravenous urography with precontrast nephrotomography should be obtained approximately 3 months postoperatively.

References

1. Anderson RU. Urinary tract infections in compromised hosts. Urol Clin North Am 1986;13:727.
2. Turck M, Anderson KN, Petersdorf RG. Relapse and reinfection in chronic bacteriuria. N Engl J Med 1966;275:70.
3. Cox CE, Lucy SS, Hinman F Jr. The urethra and its relationship to urinary tract infection. II: The urethral flora of the female with recurrent urinary infection. J Urol 1968;99:632.
4. Bran JL, Levison ME, Kaye D. Entrance of bacteria into the female urinary bladder. N Engl J Med 1972;286:626.
5. Buckley RM, McGuckin M, MacGregor RR. Urine bacterial counts following sexual intercourse. N Engl J Med 1978;298:321.
6. Kelsey MC, Mead MG, Gruneberg RN, et al. Relationship between sexual intercourse and urinary tract infection in women attending a clinic for sexually transmitted diseases. J Med Microbiol 1979;12:511.
7. Cox CE. The urethra and its relationship to urinary tract infection: The flora of the normal female urethra. South Med J 1966;59:621.
8. Stamey TA, Timothy MM, Millar M. Recurrent urinary infections in adult women. The role of introital enterobacteria. Calif Med 1971;155:1.
9. Kunin CM, Polyak F, Postel E. Periurethral bacterial flora in women: Prolonged intermittent colonization with Escherichia coli. JAMA 1980;243:134.
10. Sobel JD. Pathogenesis of urinary tract infections—host defenses. Infect Dis Clin North Am 1987;1:751.
11. Svanborg Eden C, de Man P. Bacterial virulence

in urinary tract infection. Infect Dis Clin North Am 1987;1:731.

12. Kallenius G, Mollby R, Svensson SB, et al. The p^k antigen as receptor for the haemagglutination of pyelonephritic *E. coli*. FEMS Microbiol Lett 1980;7:297.

13. Leffler H, Svanborg Eden C. Chemical identification of a glycosphingolipid receptor for *Escherichia coli* attaching to human urinary tract epithelial cells and agglutinating human erythrocytes. FEMS Microbiol Lett 1981;8:127.

14. Ofek I, Mirelman D, Sharon N. Adherence of *Escherichia coli* to human mucosal cells mediated by mannose receptors. Nature 1977;265:623.

15. Svanborg Eden C, Hansson HA. *Escherichia coli* pili as possible mediators of attachment to human urinary tract epithelial cells. Infect Immun 1978; 21:229.

16. Orskov I, Birch-Andersen A, Duguid JP, et al. An adhesive protein capsule of *Escherichia coli*. Infect Immun 1985;47:191.

17. Parsons CL. Pathogenesis of urinary tract infections—bacterial adherence, bladder defense mechanisms. Urol Clin North Am 1986;13:563.

18. Kaijser B, Larrson P, Schneerson R. Protection against acute, ascending pyelonephritis caused by *Escherichia coli* in rats using isolated capsular antigen conjugated to a carrier substance. Infect Immun 1983;39:142.

19. Keane WF, Welch R, Gekker G, et al. Mechanism of *Escherichia coli* alpha-hemolysin-induced injury to isolated renal tubular cells. Am J Pathol 1987;126:350.

20. Braun V. *Escherichia coli* cells containing the plasmid Col V produce the iron ionophrone aerobactin. FEMS Microbiol Lett 1981;11:225.

21. Stuart SJ, Greenwood KT, Luke RKJ. Hydroxamate-mediated transport of iron controlled Col V plasmids. J Bacteriol 1980;143:35.

22. Stamey TA. The role of introital enterobacteria in recurrent urinary infections. J Urol 1973;109:467.

23. Schaeffer AJ, Jones JM, Dunn JK. Association of in vitro *Escherichia coli* adherence to vaginal and buccal epithelial cells with susceptibility of women to recurrent urinary tract infections. N Engl J Med 1981;304:1062.

24. Kass EH, Savage W, Santamarina BAG. The significance of bacteriuria in preventive medicine. In: Kass EH, ed. Progress in pyelonephritis. Philadelphia: FA Davis, 1965:3–10.

25. Sanford JP. Urinary tract symptoms and infection. Ann Rev Med 1975;26:485.

26. Nicolle LE, Harding GKM, Preiksaitis J, et al. The association of urinary tract infection with sexual intercourse. J Infect Dis 1982;146:579.

27. Turck M, Goffe B, Petersdorf RG. The urethral catheter and urinary tract infection. J Urol 1962; 88:834.

28. Fowler JE Jr. Nosocomial catheter-associated urinary tract infection. Infect Surg 1983;2:43.

29. Feingold DS. Hospital-acquired infections. N Engl J Med 1970;283:1384.

30. Stamm WE, Martin SM, Bennett JV. Epidemiology of nosocomial infections due to gram-negative bacilli: Aspects relevant to development and use of vaccines. J Infect Dis 1977;136(suppl):S151.

31. Platt R, Polk BF, Murdock B, et al. Mortality associated with nosocomial urinary tract infection. N Engl J Med 1982;307:637.

32. Stamm WE. Guidelines for prevention of catheter-associated urinary tract infections. Ann Intern Med 1975;82:386.

33. Forland M, Thomas V, Shelokov A. Urinary tract infections in patients with diabetes mellitus: Studies on antibody coating of bacteria. JAMA 1977;238:1924.

34. Kaye D. Urinary tract infections in the elderly. Bull NY Acad Med 1980;56:209.

35. Sobel JD, Kaye D. Urinary tract infections. In: Mandell GL, Douglas RG Jr, Bennett JE, eds. Principles and practice of infectious diseases, ed. 2. New York: John Wiley & Sons, 1985:426.

36. Gleckman RA, Bradley PJ, Roth RM, et al. Bacteremia urosepsis: A phenomenon unique to elderly women. J Urol 1985;133:174.

37. Duff P. Pyelonephritis in pregnancy. Clin Obstet Gynecol 1984;27:17.

38. Eykyn SJ, McFadyyen IR. Suprapubic aspiration of urine in pregnancy. In: O'Grady F, Brummfitt W, eds. Urinary tract infection. Oxford: Oxford University Press, 1968.

39. Gilbert GL, Garland SM, Fairley KF, et al. Bacteriuria due to ureaplasmas and other fastidious organisms during pregnancy: prevalence and significance. Pediatr Infect Dis 1986;5:S239.

40. Turck M, Goffe BS, Petersdorf RG. Bacteriuria of pregnancy: Relation to socioeconomic factors. N Engl J Med 1962;266:857.

41. Savage WE, Hajj SN, Kass EH: Demographic and prognostic characteristics of bacteriuria in pregnancy. Medicine 1967;46:385.

42. Pritchard JA, Scott DE, Whalley PJ, et al. The effects of maternal sickle cell hemoglobinopathies and sickle cell trait on reproductive performance. Am J Obstet Gynecol 1973;117:662.

43. Patterson TF, Andriole VT. Bacteriuria in pregnancy. Infect Dis Clin North Am 1987;1:807.

44. Saitoh H, Nakamura K, Hida M, et al. Urinary tract infection in oliguric patients with chronic renal failure. J Urol 1985;133:990.

45. Komaroff AL. Urinalysis and urine culture in women with dysuria. Ann Intern Med 1986; 104:212.

46. Salvatierra O Jr, Bucklew WB, Morrow JW. Perinephric abscess: A report of 71 cases. J Urol 1967;98:296.

47. Resnick MI, Older R. Diagnosis of genitourinary disease. New York: Thieme Stratton, 1982.

48. Smith DR, ed. General urology. Los Altos, CA: Lange Medical Publications, 1984.

49. Stamm WE, Wagner KF, Amsel R, et al. Causes of the acute urethral syndrome in women. N Engl J Med 1980;303:409.

50. Nicolle LE, Ronald AR. Recurrent urinary tract infection in adult women: Diagnosis and treatment. Infect Dis Clin North Am 1987;1:793.

51. Wong ES, Fennell CL, Stamm WE. Urinary tract infection among women attending a clinic for sexually transmitted diseases. Sex Trans Dis 1984;11:18.

52. Monzon OT, Ory EM, Dolson HL, et al. A comparison of bacterial counts of the urine obtained by needle aspiration of the bladder, catheterization, and midstream voided methods. N Engl J Med 1958;259:764.

53. Stamm WE, Counts GW, Running KR, et al. Diagnosis of coliform infection in acutely dysuric women. N Engl J Med 1982;307:463.

54. Andriole VT. Diagnosis of urinary tract infection by culture. In: Kaye D, ed. Urinary tract infection and its management. St Louis: CV Mosby, 1972: 28–42.

55. Fairley KF, Bond AG, Brown RB, et al. Simple test to determine the site of urinary tract infection. Lancet 1967;2:427.

56. Fairley KF, Grounds AD, Carson NE, et al. Site of infection in acute urinary tract infection in general practice. Lancet 1971;2:617.

57. Benson M, Li Puma JP, Resnick MI. The role of imaging studies in urinary tract infection. Urol Clin North Am 1986;13:605.

58. Narayana AS. Overview of renal tuberculosis. Urology 1982;29:231.

59. Johnson JR, Stamm WE. Diagnosis and treatment of acute urinary tract infections. Infect Dis Clin North Am 1987;1:773.

60. Fihn SD. Single-dose antimicrobial therapy for urinary tract infections: "Less is more"? Or "Reductio ad absurdum"? J Gen Intern Med 1986; 1:62.

61. Wong ES, McKevitt M, Running K, et al. Management of recurrent urinary tract infections with patient-administered single-dose therapy. Ann Intern Med 1985;102:302.

62. Vosti KL. Recurrent urinary tract infections: Prevention by prophylactic antibiotics after sexual intercourse. JAMA 1975;231:934.

63. Stamm WE. When should we use urine cultures? Infect Control 1986;7:431.

64. Dunn PM. The possible relationship between the maternal administrations of sulphamethoxpyridazine and hyperbilirubinemia in the newborn. Br J Obstet Gynaecol 1964;71:128.

65. Resnick MI. Evaluation and management of infection stones. Urol Clin North Am 1981;8:265.

66. Blandy JP, Singh M. The case for a more aggressive approach to staghorn stones. J Urol 1976; 115:505.

67. Priestley JT, Dunn JH. Branched renal calculi. J Urol 1949;61:194.

68. Singh M, Chapman R, Tresidder GC, et al. The fate of the unoperated staghorn calculus. Br J Urol 1973;45:581.

69. Griffith DP, Musher DM, Campbell JW. Inhibitor of bacterial urease. Invest Urol 1973;11:234.

70. Griffith DP, Musher DM, Itin C. Urease: The primary cause of infection-induced urinary stones. Invest Urol 1976;13:346.

71. Boyce WH, Elkins IB. Reconstructive renal surgery following anatrophic nephrolithotomy: Follow-up for 100 consecutive cases. J Urol 1974; 111:307.

72. Smith MJV, Boyce WH. Anatrophic nephrotomy and plastic calyraphy. Trans Am Assoc Genitourin Surg 1967;59:18.

73. AUA Committee on Percutaneous and Noninvasive Lithotripsy. Report of American Urological Association Ad Hoc Committee to Study the Safety and Clinical Efficacy of Current Technology of Percutaneous Lithotripsy and Non-invasive Lithotripsy. Baltimore: American Urological Association, 1985.

74. Mulvaney WP. A new solvent for certain urinary calculi: A preliminary report. J Urol 1959;82:546.

75. Suby HI, Albright F. Dissolution of phosphatic urinary calculi by the retrograde introduction of a citrate solution containing magnesium. N Engl J Med 1943;228:81.

76. Silverman DE, Stamey TA. Management of infection stones: The Stanford experience. Medicine 1983;62:44.

77. Marshall VF, Lavengood RW Jr, Kelly D: Complete longitudinal nephrolithotomy and the Shorr regimen in the management of staghorn calculi. Ann Surg 1965;162:366.

78. Wickham JA, Coe N, Ward JP. One hundred cases of nephrolithotomy under hypothermia. J Urol 1974;112:702.

79. Griffith DP. Infection-induced stones. In: Coe F, ed. Nephrolithiasis, pathogenesis and treatment. Chicago: Year Book Medical Publishers, 1978: 203–228.

36

Urinary Retention and Urethral Obstruction

Gary J. Faerber

Urinary Retention

Urinary retention can be defined as the inability to void. Urinary retention may be the result of increased outlet resistance, decreased bladder contractility, or a combination of both (Table 36-1). Painful stimuli from the pelvic or perineal region may be a cause of the inhibition of the normal bladder reflex mechanism of micturition, thus resulting in urinary retention. Examples of this occur in women who have undergone gynecologic surgery, orthopedic surgery involving the hip or knees, or intra-abdominal surgery. Women with painful herpetic lesions involving the perineum or the bladder itself may also develop urinary retention. Urinary retention associated with herpes progenitalis may be either the result of pain with inability to relax the external sphincter or the result of viral infection of the nerves causing temporary neurapraxias. Failure to empty the bladder may be the result of a muscular abnormality, neurologic abnormality, or both. Detrusor decompensation with poor bladder emptying can result from chronic over-distention secondary to volitional infrequent voiding, or it may be secondary to a sensory vesical defect, such as that encountered in diabetics. Fibrosis of the bladder wall may also interfere with bladder muscle effectiveness, and this in turn leads to poor emptying or retention. The most common cause of poor bladder contractility is probably neurogenic, such as that encountered in patients with spinal cord injury or those with peripheral neural lesions. Increased bladder outlet resistance is an additional cause of urinary retention, and this may be secondary to anatomic obstruction, which may be either congenital or acquired. Bladder outlet obstruction can also result from dysfunction of the urethra, in which there is failure of coordination between the detrusor and smooth or striated sphincter during a bladder contraction. Outlet obstruction is covered in some detail later in this chapter.

Urinary retention may be an acute, self-limiting problem or a chronic problem. Symptoms may vary depending on the cause. A thorough but orderly workup should be performed for any woman with urinary retention or for patients with voiding complaints and residual urine. As in any patient, the history and physical examination, with particular attention to the neurologic examination, are important and may help to form the diagnostic as well as therapeutic plan.

517

Female Urology, edited by Elroy D. Kursh and Edward McGuire. J. B. Lippincott, Philadelphia, © 1994.

Table 36-1. *Causes of Urinary Retention*

Bladder outlet obstruction
Primary vesical myopathy
Neurogenic
    Sensory denervated bladder
    Peripheral neural lesions
    Sacral cord, sacral root lesions
    Upper motor neuron lesions with detrusor sphincter
      dyssynergia
Psychogenic

HISTORY AND PHYSICAL EXAMINATION

The clinical history of patients with voiding complaints should be directed at the character of the urinary stream; the frequency of voiding; the presence of incontinence, nocturia, and dysuria; and suprapubic discomfort. Equally important is a prior surgical history, especially that of pelvic or prior anti-incontinence procedures. Prior pelvic or abdominal trauma, irradiation therapy, or any symptoms of neurologic disease should also be noted. Specific note of bowel dysfunction, including constipation and fecal incontinence, may assist in directing the evaluation to a somatic or autonomic dysfunction of the nerves serving the pelvic organs. A complete list of medications, both those prescribed and those purchased over the counter, should be compiled because many drugs adversely influence bladder function.

Overflow incontinence may develop in a patient with detrusor decompensation and is usually manifested by slow continuous leakage or leakage that occurs with a change in intra-abdominal pressure, and the latter mimics genuine stress urinary incontinence symptomatically. Retention of urine, secondary to outlet obstruction, may lead to frequency, nocturia, urgency, and urge incontinence related to the development of detrusor hyperreflexia associated with the obstructive process.

On physical examination, leakage of urine from the urethral meatus may be revealed. Su-
prapubic discomfort secondary to an overly distended bladder may be elicited with abdominal examination. Some patients may have no bladder sensation despite an easily palpable bladder. Normally the bladder cannot be percussed unless there is a volume of urine held in the bladder more than 150 ml. A bladder with a 500-ml volume can often be diagnosed by visible lower abdominal bulge.[1] Pelvic examination, paying special attention to the presence of a cystocele, the appearance of the urethral meatus, and palpation of the entire urethra and vesical neck region, should be performed. Bladder volume can be determined by direct catheterization or by bladder ultrasound. Once documentation of urinary retention is established, a through physical examination is required to ascertain the cause of the urinary retention. Special attention should be directed to the neurologic examination, including assessment of motor and sensory function, rectal sphincter tone, and upper and lower extremity reflexes as well as the bulbocavernosus reflex.

URINALYSIS

Urinalysis, routine urine cultures, and at times special urine cultures are essential because urinary tract infection can sometimes be the sole cause and in most instances a contributing factor to voiding dysfunction. Persistent or recurrent infection, despite appropriate antibiotic therapy, may be the first indication of urinary retention.

RADIOGRAPHIC STUDIES

Upper urinary tract evaluation at times may be indicated in patients with lower urinary tract dysfunction. Renal ultrasonography can determine the presence of hydronephrosis, renal calculi, and cortical thickness. Bladder ultrasonography has been shown to be accurate in assessing postvoiding residual urine volumes. Intravenous urography and voiding cystourethrography may at times be indicated.

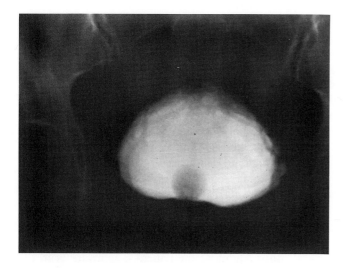

Figure 36-1. *Cystogram of a woman with outlet obstruction secondary to primary bladder neck obstruction. Note the severe bladder trabeculation.*

URODYNAMIC EVALUATION

Urodynamic testing can greatly assist in identifying factors that cause voiding dysfunction. It is important, however, that the urodynamic findings are consistent with the patient's symptoms and complaints. If discrepancies arise, certain portions of the evaluation may need repeating, or more sophisticated testing may be needed.

The normal adult bladder holds approximately 400 to 750 ml of urine with a mean rise in pressure of 6 cm H_2O on filling to that bladder volume; an increase of pressure greater than 15 cm H_2O for that volume, 400 to 750 ml, is abnormal.[2] Urinary retention secondary to decreased sensation, as commonly seen in diabetic patients, results in a large-capacity bladder with normal or increased compliance. Similarly, most female patients with chronic outlet obstruction develop large-capacity, high-compliance bladders. Only rarely in women does outlet obstruction result in trabeculation, diverticula formation, and so forth (Fig. 36-1). Cystoceles are usually asymptomatic; however, they can be associated with urinary retention, urgency, and frequency. Typically the larger the cystocele, the more likely it is associated with urinary retention.[3]

UROFLOWMETRY

Women have significantly higher flow rates than men when matched for age and voided volumes. An interrupted urinary stream on a flow rate may indicate abdominal straining or a voluntary or involuntary external sphincter contractility. The urodynamicist practitioner must be careful not to overinterpret urine flow studies. A normal uroflow does not, in women, necessarily rule out all obstructive processes.

A consistently increased postvoiding residual urine volume implies increased outlet resistance, decreased bladder contractility, or both. Postvoiding residual urine volume determination, either by direct catheterization or by ultrasonography, is accurate and quite reliable. An abnormal uroflow plus an elevated postvoiding residual urine implies obstruction; however, it does not provide an explanation of the cause of the obstruction. Poor urinary flow rates associated with poor reflex bladder contractility, as measured by pressure flow studies, may be related to vesical overdistention associated with longstanding obstruction or some primary vesical myopathy. These two conditions may be difficult or impossible to distinguish from one another in some instances. Intermittent catheterization, on a temporary or permanent basis, may be required and is the best method of management until an accurate diagnosis can be made.

CYSTOMETRY

Cystometry can provide information about the bladder only during filling and is not accurate as a study of the emptying phase of bladder activity. Compliance or the ability of the bladder to tolerate increasing volume with little or no change in pressure, the presence of uninhibited bladder contractions, and the patient's subjectivity to sensation during filling can be accurately assessed, but because up to 50% of patients are unable to initiate a voiding contraction volitionally during the performance of a cystometrogram, no comment can be made on the patient's ability or inability to void simply on the basis of failure to see a contraction at the time of a cystometrogram. The diagnosis, in other words, of detrusor areflexia cannot be established based on a cystometrogram that does not show a reflex bladder contraction.

VOIDING CYSTOMETROGRAMS WITH ELECTROMYOGRAPHY

Voiding cystometry with concomitant electromyography of the urethral sphincter allows the investigator to measure simultaneous external sphincter activity during the bladder contraction. In normal individuals, external sphincter activity should gradually rise as bladder volume rises. Before and all during a bladder contraction, sphincter activity should be markedly decreased or totally absent. If sphincter activity increases or does not decrease during a voiding contraction, this condition can be termed *detrusor sphincter dyssynergia*. True reflex detrusor sphincter dyssynergia is encountered only in patients with neurologic disease; however, there are some neurologically normal patients who exhibit what appears to be detrusor external sphincter dyssynergia, and some of these individuals demonstrate features of the nonneurogenic neurogenic bladder (Fig. 36-2). Although this condition was originally described in children, the entity also exists in adults. The supposition is that in patients who are otherwise neurologically normal, the appearance of dyssynergic sphincteric activity during bladder contractility is volitional, even though it may well be unconscious or the patient is unaware of it.

VIDEOURODYNAMICS

Probably the best method to diagnose the exact cause of urinary retention as well as many other complicated voiding disorders involves multichannel urodynamic studies with fluoroscopy or videourodynamics. These studies combine the simultaneous measurement of bladder and external sphincter pressures during bladder filling and bladder emptying with fluoroscopic visualization of the bladder and the urethra. It permits measurement of pressures anywhere along the urethra during both phases of bladder activity either at the sphincter or at any other point. Videourodynamic studies provide information that can permit the differentiation of retention resulting from outlet obstruction from that resulting from vesical dysfunction (Fig. 36-3).

URETHRAL PRESSURE PROFILOMETRY

Urethral pressure profilometry is not useful in a diagnosis of bladder outlet obstruction, either that secondary to a neurogenic or nonneurogenic cause.

ENDOSCOPY

Endoscopic evaluation is useful for the evaluation of bladder calculi, foreign bodies, urethral or bladder tumors, and the secondary effects of

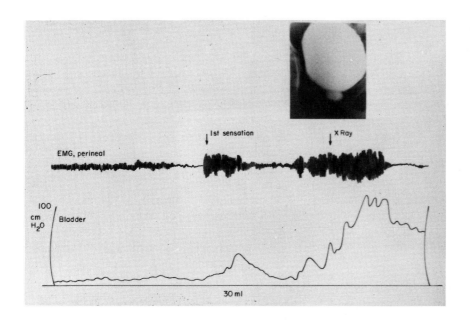

Figure 36-2. *Videourodynamic findings of detrusor sphincter dyssynergia showing simultaneous increase in external sphincter activity with a detrusor contraction.*

obstructive uropathy that include trabeculation and so forth, which are nonspecific changes. Endoscopy is not an accurate method of diagnosing or documenting obstructive uropathy.

PRIMARY VESICAL MYOPATHY

The treatment of urinary retention depends largely on the cause. Treatment to relieve bladder outlet obstruction is discussed later in this chapter. At present, there is no proven treatment that decreases residual urine secondary to myopathic disease by selectively improving detrusor contractile function. Lapides and others reported on the effectiveness of bethanechol chloride, an acetylcholinelike agent that is relatively selective to the bladder and gut and is cholinesterase resistant, in improving voiding in patients with atonic or hypotonic bladders.[4,5] The drug, given either subcutaneously in doses of 5 to 10 mg every 4 to 6 hours or orally in doses of 50 to 100 mg four times daily, was reported to decrease residual urine volumes. Other investigators have had disappointing results with the use of this same agent. Wein and co-workers reported no improvement in flow parameters or residual urine volumes after a 5-mg subcutaneous dose but did note that there was a corresponding increase in vesical pressures along the entire filling curve.[6] Barrett showed that there was no significant difference in residual urine volumes in a randomized, double-blind study in women with elevated postvoid residuals.[7] The combination of bethanechol chloride with phenoxybenzamine, an alpha-blocking agent, the latter given in hopes of inducing a simultaneous reduction in outlet resistance at the bladder neck, has also been studied with variable results.[8,9]

Prostaglandins, such as prostaglandin E_2, have been shown to have stimulating effects on the bladder. Direct installation of this agent into the bladder alone, or in combination with other agents, has been used to facilitate bladder contractility. Some investigators have noted favor-

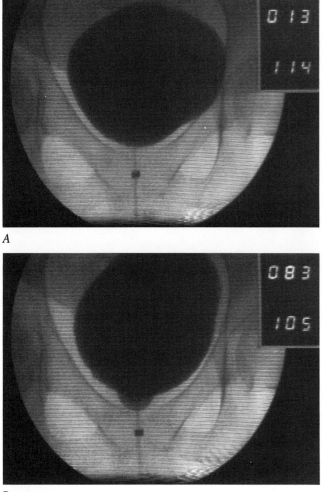

A

B

Figure 36-3. *(A) Videourodynamic study of a woman complaining of incontinence and weak, interrupted stream. At rest, patient has slightly increased detrusor and normal external sphincter pressures. (B) During voiding, same patient exhibits dyssynergia of the external sphincter with abnormal voiding pressures in excess of 80 cm H_2O.*

able results, whereas others have not.[10,11] Lepor and others reported that terazosin, a selective alpha$_1$ blocker, can decrease urethral outlet resistance in men with prostatic obstruction.[12,13] I am unaware of any studies using this agent, or similar agents, in women with an element of bladder outlet resistance.

Augmenting poor or absent bladder contractility by the Credé maneuver usually does not improve bladder emptying, unless urethral resistance is low enough to be associated with severe incontinence. Reduction cystoplasty, although it initially reduces bladder capacity, does not improve bladder emptying ability.

NEUROGENIC VESICAL DYSFUNCTION

Sensory neurogenic bladders, as, for example, those encountered in patients with diabetes or syphilis and tabes dorsalis, can develop tremendous residual urine volumes. This over time is associated with increasingly inefficient bladder contractility and the development of significant postvoid urinary residuals. Often these patients complain of urinary tract infections and a feeling of incomplete emptying and suffer from overflow incontinence. If these patients are placed on a strict timed voiding program with return to more physiologic bladder volumes, the retention can sometimes be alleviated. If the bladder has been severely damaged by chronic overdistention, these patients may require the initiation of self-intermittent catheterization for adequate bladder emptying and potential recovery of reflex bladder function.

Patients with neurogenic bladder dysfunction and elevated residual urine volumes most commonly demonstrate either an areflexic bladder or a reflex bladder associated with detrusor sphincter dyssynergia. Efficient bladder emptying can be accomplished by intermittent catheterization in either of these instances. If bladder compliance is poor or reflex, bladder activity occurs at relatively low volumes and anticholinergic agents can be used to provide for reasonable bladder volumes while maintaining intravesical pressures below 40 cm H_2O. If this cannot be accomplished, upper urinary tract damage results.[14]

At times, intermittent catheterization cannot be performed because of poor hand function, body habitus, or patient unwillingness. In these instances, a continent or incontinent ileovesicostomy can be performed. Experience with either the continent or incontinent ileovesicostomy at the University of Michigan involves 21 patients with a neurogenic bladder: 10 of whom were quadriplegics with little or no hand function, 8 patients with severe multiple sclerosis, and 3 paraplegics with a body habitus unsuitable for intermittent catheterization per urethram. Two patients underwent continent ileovesicostomy, whereas 19 underwent incontinent vesicostomy. All patients before surgery had upper urinary tract evaluations, with five showing evidence of hydronephrosis. All had elevated leak point pressures before their procedure with the exception of the two patients who underwent continent ileovesicostomy. All of the postoperative leak point pressures involving egress of urine across the incontinent ileovesicostomy were less than 20 cm H_2O and continued to remain low at follow-up. Renal function has been stable with no development of hydronephrosis at a mean follow-up of 4 years. The five patients with hydronephrosis preoperatively had resolution of that problem on postoperative follow-up evaluation.

In other cases, supravesical diversion, preferably into a low-pressure neoreservoir, may be required for adequate management of lower urinary tract dysfunction. Long-term Foley catheter drainage or suprapubic tube drainage is not recommended because of the complications associated with this type of bladder management. These include the formation of bladder calculi, urethral erosion, urethrovaginal fistula formation, hydroureteronephrosis, upper tract stone formation, and ultimately renal damage or loss.

PSYCHOGENIC RETENTION

Psychogenic retention is usually seen in young or middle-aged women and may either be acute or chronic in nature. Acute psychogenic retention is often temporally related to a traumatic psychological event in the patient's life. Urodynamic evaluation often reveals a normal or slightly increased compliance curve with bladder filling, absent or decreased bladder contractility, and maintenance of external sphincter pressures and activity throughout bladder filling even with "attempts of void." Possible causes for acute psychogenic retention include excessive stimulation of the pyramidal tract with resultant failure of relaxation of the external sphincter, which is volitional, or inhibition of the autonomic motor nucleus with resultant decreased bladder contractility.[15, 16] The diagnosis of psychogenic urinary retention, whether acute or chronic, must be one of exclusion. Appropriate neurologic and endocrine evaluation must be performed because subtle metabolic and neurologic diseases have been found in patients previously thought suffering from psychogenic retention.[17]

Acute psychogenic retention is usually self-limiting, with return of normal voiding with time. Intermittent catheterization is the preferred temporizing method of bladder management until resumption of normal voiding occurs. In those cases in which patients progress to a chronic state of urinary retention, overflow incontinence, recurrent urinary tract infection, and renal damage can occur. Urodynamic evaluation reveals an increased compliance curve with bladder filling as well as a markedly abnormal first sensation to void. It is not unusual for these patients to have no sensation of bladder fullness until they have reached large bladder volumes. Intermittent catheterization is the preferred method of bladder management; however, the other methods mentioned for neurogenic vesical dysfunction are also acceptable.

Bladder Outlet Obstruction

Bladder outlet obstruction characterized by high bladder pressure and low urinary flow rate voiding can be broadly classified as either mechanical or neurologic in origin (Table 36-2). Examples of mechanical obstruction include urethral strictures as a result of prior urethral trauma, for example, traumatic catheterization, overzealous urethral dilation, prior radiation for gynecologic malignancy. Other causes of mechanical obstruction include urethral tumor, transitional cell carcinoma, melanoma, squamous cell carcinoma, leiomyomata, foreign bodies, or extrinsic masses, including uterine fibromas, ovarian tumors, vaginal leiomyomas, and uterine prolapse obstructing either the bladder neck or the urethra. Bladder outlet obstruction due to primary causes either at the vesical neck or along the urethra, once thought to be common, is now considered to be relatively rare in women. The

Table 36-2. Bladder Outlet Obstruction

Mechanical
   Urethral stricture
   Postoperative obstruction after anti-incontinence procedures
   Primary bladder neck stricture
   Urethral tumors (transitional cell carcinoma, squamous cell carcinoma, melanoma)
   Urethral foreign bodies (vesical or urethral calculi)
   Extrinsic masses (uterine and vaginal masses, retroverted uterus)
Neurologic
   Detrusor external sphincter dyssynergia

traditional urologic practice, which was largely empiric, of urethral dilation for irritative vesical symptoms usually fails to achieve the desired effect, that is, absence of symptoms. A determination of the presence of reflex vesical contractility is required for establishment of the diagnosis of obstructive uropathy. One must be careful to delineate true voiding contractions from increases in bladder pressure, which are actually secondary to an increase in intra-abdominal pressure. "Voiding" by increasing intra-abdominal pressure and overcoming urethral resistance is within the capacity of some women. With reflex voiding, the vesical neck opens and funnels. If the bladder neck remains closed or is narrowed during a bladder contraction, this is reasonable indication of bladder neck obstruction. If, however, the bladder neck does not open but there is no voiding contraction, this is completely normal. Therefore it is imperative that bladder neck obstruction be diagnosed by the absence of normal opening of the bladder outlet during a true bladder contraction. That determination requires fairly sophisticated urodynamic equipment, including cystometry with rectal subtraction pressures, electromyography, and fluoroscopy.

Detrusor responses to outlet obstruction have been investigated extensively in animal models. Obstruction has been shown to induce smooth muscle hyperplasia and hypertrophy, collagen formation and deposition, and finally an alteration in smooth muscle function with resultant decreased bladder contractility.[18–20] Bladder hypertrophy and hyperplasia of the obstructive bladder seems to be reversible in some animal studies.[21] Nervous control of the bladder has also been shown to be affected by outlet obstruction. Intramural nerve terminal destruction, an increase in afferent input to the central nervous system, an increase in the threshold of the vesical stretch receptors, an increase in the muscarinic receptors, and the development of short latency spinal reflex have been reported to occur as a result of bladder outlet obstruction.[22–26] Experimental studies in animals involving urodynamic evaluation of obstructed bladders have consistently showed increased voiding pressures, increased voiding time, reduced ability to empty residual urine volumes, and unstable bladder contractions of lesser strength than normal bladders. Morphologic studies of human bladders with outlet obstruction have revealed smooth muscle hypertrophy and connective tissue infiltration similar to that reported in experimental obstruction on animals.[27]

URETHRAL STRICTURE

Congenital urethral stricture disease is rare (Fig. 36-4). Urethral meatal stricture is probably one of the most commonly overdiagnosed conditions in women presenting with voiding complaints. Previously the diagnosis of urethral meatal stricture was made by calibrating the urethral meatus with a bougie à boule. If on withdrawal of the instrument, there was either blanching of the meatal mucosa or any resistance, this was thought to be suggestive of a stricture. If this occurred in conjunction with any voiding symptoms, often these patients were treated with urethral dilation, urethral incision, or formal urethroplasty. Early results suggested that this type of therapy was successful in relief of symptoms; however, urodynamic verification of true urethral obstruction and improvement induced by the surgical procedures was not done. Tanagho and McCurry performed fluid dynamic studies with funnels mimicking the configuration of the vesical neck and urethra. In their

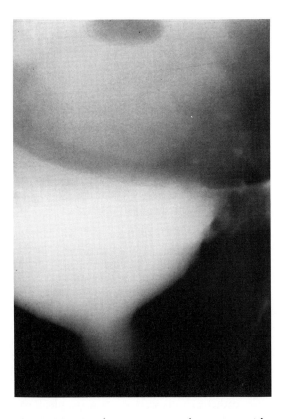

Figure 36-4. *Voiding cystogram of a woman with a documented distal urethral stricture secondary to a prior diverticulectomy.*

studies, they found that before a decrease in flow rate was observed, the outlet had to be less than 10 French diameter.[28] Rarely is the meatus or distal urethra less than 10 to 12 French, and therefore it is difficult to justify any procedure that would overdilate this region of the urethra beyond 12 French for presumed obstruction. The diagnosis of primary urethral meatal obstruction requires sophisticated, videourodynamic testing.

Iatrogenically caused urethral strictures may result from prior urethral diverticulectomy, prior urethral dilation, after previous meatoplasty, or after an anti-incontinence procedure. The diagnosis can be made in patients with symptoms by the demonstration of high voiding pressures associated with an area of fixed urethral narrowing. Treatment of urethral strictures can consist of urethrotomy either with an Otis urethrotome or under direct vision or Y-V plasty, depending on the location of the stricture.

POSTOPERATIVE OBSTRUCTION
AFTER ANTI-INCONTINENCE PROCEDURES

Postoperative urinary retention is one of the more common complications of anti-incontinence operative procedures. Early retention may be secondary to true bladder outlet obstruction from hyperelevation of the urethra; or it may be due to postoperative swelling and inflammation; or it may be functional, simply as a result of inhibition of a normal voiding pattern secondary to pain. In the latter two instances, normal voiding typically returns after resolution of the edema and pain. Interim treatment with self-intermittent catheterization has been shown to be successful. Some surgeons employ instead at the time of the anti-incontinence procedure a temporary suprapubic tube, which is removed after normal voiding has resumed.[29] Temporary Foley catheter drainage is also practicable. If true outlet obstruction is present, retention, either partial or complete, persists beyond the immediate postoperative period. Such patients, in addition to obstructive symptoms, may develop obstruction-induced detrusor instability with urgency and urge incontinence.

Both transabdominal and transvaginal anti-incontinence operative procedures can result in outlet obstruction. Marshall, Marchetti, and Krantz's original operation for stress incontinence used placement of sutures into the periurethral tissue with fixation of those sutures to the periosteum of the symphysis pubis.[30,31] Transient urinary retention has been reported in as many as 10% to 27% of patients undergoing this procedure, and this is thought to be secondary to urethral obstruction from the periurethral sutures[32] (Fig. 36-5). Burch modified the abdominal approach by using the vaginal wall to support the urethra rather than the periurethral tissue. The suspension sutures are placed much more laterally than those used for the Marshal-Marchetti-Krantz procedure.[33] Stamey in 1973 described a technique for the endoscopic needle suspension of the vesical neck by way of a transvaginal approach. In this technique, periurethral tissue is buttressed on either side of the urethra with a Dacron bolster, and under endoscopic visualization the sutures are lifted until the vesical neck closes. Constantinou and Stamey and Mundy have shown that the Stamey endoscopic bladder neck suspension induces some outflow obstruction.[34,35] Pereyra and Lebherz described a transvaginal approach to incontinence in 1967, which was later modified by Raz, wherein the urethral support is achieved by placement of the sutures into the pubocervical and paravaginal tissue rather than into the periurethral tissue as described by Stamey and Ruffins.[36,37] Leach and co-workers demonstrated urodynamically that the modified Pereyra needle suspension, as described by Raz, does not induce outflow obstruction.[38] Instead the Raz needle suspension appears to support and elevate the urethra rather than compress it; the latter effect can be seen in some patients who have undergone retropubic anterior urethropexy. McGuire and Lytton reported results using a pubovaginal sling in patients with a nonfunctional urethra described as Type III stress urinary incontinence.[39] Usually these are women who have failed previous anti-incontinence procedures and who have properly elevated, but poorly functioning internal urethral sphincter continence mechanisms. The sling improves urethral coadaptation without significantly increasing urethral pressures during voiding. Postoperative urinary retention was reported in 2 of 78 patients after slings, and this was thought to be secondary to excessive tension placed on the sling intraoperatively[40] (Fig. 36-6).

Patients who have undergone anti-incontinence procedures and are beyond the immediate postoperative period who have persistent voiding symptoms should be evaluated with urodynamic studies, preferably involving video-urodynamics. Outlet obstruction, as a cause of symptoms, must be distinguished from poor detrusor contractility or simple persistence of detrusor instability. Obstruction can be confirmed

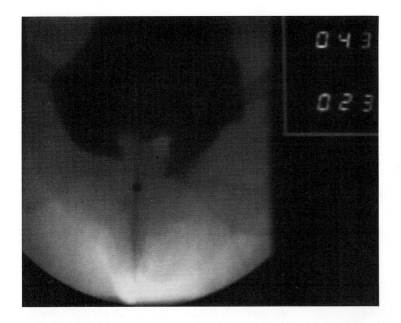

Figure 36-5. *Woman who underwent previous Marshall-Marchetti-Krantz urethropexy for stress urinary incontinence who developed postoperative obstruction. Note the configuration of the vesical neck and the high voiding pressure (greater than 40 cm H_2O).*

by an elevated pressure of 30 cm H_2O or more combined with some kind of documentation of increased urethral resistance or hyperelevation of the vesical neck and proximal urethra at the time of voiding.

Simple urethral dilation usually does not suffice to improve voiding symptoms in cases of obstruction of the urethra related to anti-incontinence procedures. Transurethral resection or incision have both been reported to improve patients thought to be obstructed after anti-incontinence procedures.[41,42] These methods, however, can result in severe incontinence. The preferred method of treatment for patients with postoperative urinary obstruction is a transvaginal urethrolysis. Patients who have undergone a previous anterior urethropexy can undergo vaginal urethrolysis and subsequent needle suspension without the risk of severe bladder injury that may occur during takedown of a retropubic

urethropexy by way of an abdominal approach. Bladder outlet obstruction after a needle suspension operation can be alleviated by transvaginal urethrolysis and cutting of one or both of the suspension sutures.[50] If both suspension sutures are cut, there is a risk, albeit small, of recurrent stress incontinence. Outlet obstruction after a pubovaginal sling can also be alleviated by loosening tension on the sling.

PRIMARY BLADDER NECK STRICTURE

Primary bladder neck obstruction is a rare occurrence in neurologically normal women. In the past, this entity was perhaps overdiagnosed in many women with voiding symptoms and a poor flow rate with urgency, hesitancy, and frequent bouts of cystitis. The diagnosis was usually based on uroflowmetry but sometimes simply on a postvoid residual urine and endoscopic find-

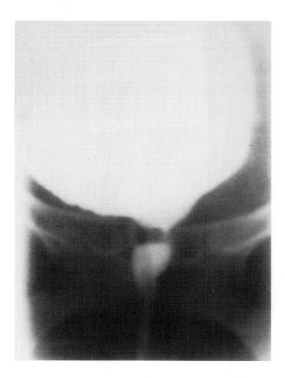

Figure 36-6. Woman with retention following a pubovaginal sling. Voiding cystogram indicates the sling is in proper position but too tight. This was further documented urodynamically. With loosening of the sling, the patient resumed normal voiding.

ings. Many women underwent transurethral incision or resection of the vesical neck, Y-V plasty of the vesical neck, or urethral dilation with variable results but with significant complications, including urethral stricture, intraoperative and postoperative hemorrhage, and urinary incontinence. With the advent of better urodynamic equipment and videourodynamic monitoring, the incidence of bladder neck obstruction was found to be actually quite rare. In an evaluation of 2500 women, Farrar and colleagues found 169 with outlet obstruction, or 7%. Four of these occurred at the level of the bladder neck and 165 within the distal urethra.[43] Abrams reported that 3.7% of 2124 female patients had bladder outlet

obstruction by a flow rate less than 15 ml per second as the only diagnostic instrument.[44] Diokno and associates reported on three cases of primary bladder neck obstruction that was well documented. All three patients had symptomatic and urodynamic improvement after transurethral incision.[45] Because these abnormalities are rare and the potential complications of surgical therapy relatively severe, urodynamic proof of true bladder outlet obstruction is a good idea before embarking on a surgical procedure (Fig. 36-7).

URETHRAL TUMORS

Urethral tumors in women present most commonly with bleeding, but symptoms of obstruction are also quite common. They constitute approximately 0.02% of all female genital cancers. In order not to miss the diagnosis, an awareness that the symptoms of urethral carcinoma mimic other benign diseases, such as urethral caruncles, polyps, or prolapse, and a high index of suspicion must be kept.[46] Urethral tumors often appear as violaceous lesions emanating from the urethral meatus or protruding from the meatus. Rectal, vaginal, and bimanual examinations are helpful in determining the extent of involvement. Endoscopic examination of the urethra and bladder with biopsies confirm the diagnosis. Proper treatment of the tumor usually results in alleviation of urethral obstruction.

EXTRINSIC CAUSES
OF URETHRAL OBSTRUCTION

Leiomyomas originating from the uterus, cervix, or anterior vaginal wall have been reported to cause obstructive voiding symptoms. Freed and colleagues reported on three women with vaginal leiomyomas with voiding difficulties who achieved symptomatic relief after suprapubic or transvaginal removal of these benign lesions.[47] Uterine diseases, including uterine prolapse and incarceration of the gravid uterus, have also been reported to cause outlet obstruction.[48] Vaginal

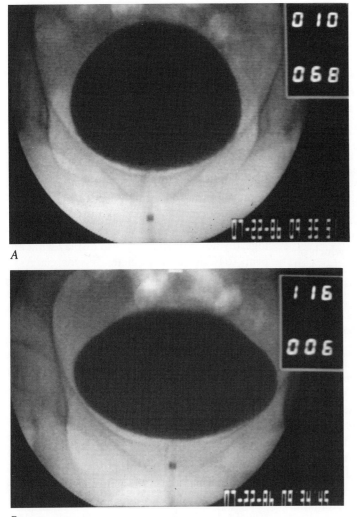

Figure 36-7. *(A) Primary bladder neck obstruction. Normal bladder and external sphincter pressures at rest. (B) Primary bladder neck obstruction. During voiding, note the high detrusor pressure (116 cm H$_2$O), absence of funneling of the vesical neck, and appropriate relaxation of the external sphincter.*

occlusion with resultant hematocolpos has been reported to cause outlet obstruction.[49] Vaginal occlusion can be congenital, or it can be secondary to postmenopausal atrophy, vaginal leiomyomas, radiotherapy for carcinoma of the cervix, or synechiae of the labia secondary to inflamma-tion. Pelvic malignancies, most notably uterine, cervical, and ovarian, can also cause bladder outlet obstruction. The most likely mechanism for all of the above-mentioned conditions caus-ing obstruction is mechanical compression of the vesical neck and proximal urethra.

FOREIGN BODIES

Foreign bodies can also cause obstruction. Often patients present with irritative symptoms plus dysuria and recurrent urinary tract infection. Vesical calculi both can cause bladder outlet obstruction and often form as a result of obstructive conditions. These calculi are usually associated with neurogenic bladder dysfunction with inadequate bladder emptying and recurrent urinary tract infection. The author recently evaluated a woman with multiple sclerosis who complained of dysuria and frequency, and on initiation of her stream, she would experience sudden abrupt cessation of stream. During fluorourodynamics evaluation, the patient was found to have a large vesical calculus, which on initiation of her stream, the stone acted like a ball valve at the vesical neck. The stone was removed with cessation of these symptoms. Calculi located in urethral diverticuli can become dislodged and cause urethral obstruction. Often these calculi are accompanied by symptoms of dysuria and can be diagnosed by physical findings on palpation of the urethra, by endoscopy, or by voiding cystourethrography. Any number of objects have been known to be inserted into the urethra either accidentally or intentionally. Q-tips, marbles, thermometers and thermometer probes, and paper clips have been recovered endoscopically from the urethra and bladder. Removal, either endoscopically or by way of open cystotomy, usually results in symptomatic relief.

NEUROLOGIC DETRUSOR EXTERNAL SPHINCTER DYSSYNERGIA

Outlet obstruction secondary to the lack of coordination between the detrusor and the external sphincter during a voiding contraction is often seen in patients suffering from spinal cord injury above the level of S-2. Although less common in women than in men, significant outlet obstruction secondary to the dyssynergic external sphincter, in combination with a poorly compli-

ant bladder, can lead to dramatic hydronephrosis and renal injury. Intermittent catheterization usually in conjunction with anticholinergic agents is successful in preventing further upper urinary tract damage. If the bladder volume/compliance curve cannot be shifted to the right with anticholinergics, patients may require either an augmentation cystoplasty or one of the other procedures that allow for low pressure urine storage. Although external sphincterotomies obviate high-pressure voiding in men, this type of procedure is discouraged in women because of the lack of an effective external collecting device.

There are other women who are neurologically normal who may also display what appears to be detrusor sphincter dyssynergia. As in women with detrusor sphincter dyssynergia secondary to a specific neurologic injury, these women may also complain of a weak, intermittent stream; urgency; urge incontinence; dysuria; and urinary tract infection. Whether they have true involuntary contraction of the external sphincter or whether this is some type of learned response to some prior noxious stimulus is unclear. It may be difficult or impossible to distinguish this group of women with *pseudodyssynergia* from those women with true dyssynergia based on proven neurologic disease. A thorough neurologic evaluation should be performed to rule out occult neurologic disease before labeling these women as dysfunctional voiders. Treatment, including skeletal muscle relaxants, biofeedback, paralysis of the detrusor with anticholinergics and intermittent catheterization, and even neurostimulation, has been tried with variable results.

An accurate, thorough history, with special attention to voiding patterns, prior surgery or trauma, and medication, in conjunction with a thorough physical examination is necessary when a woman presents with obstruction or has retention. Usually fairly sophisticated urodynamic studies are necessary to make the diagnosis of bladder neck or urethral obstruction in women.

References

1. Wyker AW. Standard diagnostic considerations. In: Gillenwater JY, Grayhack JT, Howards SS, et al, eds. Adult and pediatric urology. 2nd ed. St. Louis: Mosby, 1991:74.

2. Barrett DM, Wein AJ. Voiding dysfunction: Diagnosis, classification, and management. In: Gillenwater JY, Grayhack JT, Howards SS, et al, eds. Adult and pediatric urology. St. Louis: CV Mosby, 1987:868.

3. McGuire EJ, Gardy M, Elkins T, et al. Treatment of incontinence with pelvic prolapse. Urol Clin North Am 1991;18:349.

4. Lapides J. Neurogenic bladder: Principles of treatment. Urol Clin North Am 1974;1:81.

5. Sonda L, Gershon C, Diokno A, et al. Further observations on the cystometric and uroflowmetric effects of bethanechol chloride on the human bladder. J Urol 1979;122:775.

6. Wein AJ, Malloy T, Shafer F, et al. The effects of bethanechol chloride on urodynamic parameters in normal women and in women with significant residual urine volumes. J Urol 1980;124:397.

7. Barrett D. The effect of oral bethanechol chloride on voiding in female patients with excessive residual urine: A randomized double-blind study. J Urol 1981;126:640.

8. Khanna OP. Disorders of micturition: Neuropharmacological basis and result of drug therapy. Urology 1976;8:316.

9. Wein AJ. Pharmacologic treatment of lower urinary tract dysfunction in the female patient. Urol Clin North Am 1985;12:259.

10. Desmond A, Bultitude M, Hills N, et al. Clinical experience with intravesical prostaglandin E2: A prospective study of 36 patients. Br J Urol 1980; 53:357.

11. Delaere K, Thomas C, Moonen T, et al. The value of prostaglandin E2 and F2 in women with abnormalities of bladder emptying. Br J Urol 1981; 53:306.

12. Lepor H, Knapp-Maloney G, Sunshine H. Adose titrating study evaluating terazosin, a selective, once-a-day, alpha-blocker for the treatment of symptomatic benign prostatic hyperplasia. J Urol 1990;144:1393.

13. Lepor H. Role of long-acting selective alpha-1 blockers in the treatment of benign prostatic hyperplasia. Urol Clin North Am 1990;17:651.

14. McGuire EJ, Woodside JR, Borden TA, et al. The prognostic value of urodynamic testing in myelodysplastic patients. J Urol 1981;126: 205.

15. Lewin RJ, Dilland GU, Porter RW. Extrapyramidal inhibition of the urinary bladder. Brain Res 1967;4:3.

16. Bradley WE, Teague CT. Spinal cord organization of micturitional reflex afferents. Exp Neurol 1968;22:504.

17. Barrett DM. Evaluation of psychogenic urinary retention. J Urol 1978;120:191.

18. Brent L, Stephen FD. The response of smooth muscle cells in the rabbit bladder to outflow obstruction. Invest Urol 1975;12:494.

19. Levin RM, Memberg W, Ruggieri MR, et al. Functional effects of in vitro obstruction on the rabbit urinary bladder. J Urol 1986;135:847.

20. Malkowicz SB, Wein AJ, Elbadawi A, et al. Acute biochemical and functional alterations in the partially obstructed rabbit urinary bladder. J Urol 1986;136:1324.

21. Levin RM, Malkowicz SB, Wein AJ, et al. Recovery from short-term obstruction of the rabbit urinary bladder. J Urol 1985;134:388.

22. Gosling JA, Dixon JS. Detrusor morphology in relation to bladder outflow obstruction and instability. In: Hinman F, ed. Benign prostatic hypertrophy. New York: Springer-Verlag, 1983:666.

23. Reuther K, Aargaard J, Jenson KS. Lignocaine test and detrusor instability. Br J Urol 1983;55: 493.

24. Warwick RT. The symptoms of bladder outlet obstruction detrusor: Dysfunction and the myth of "prostatism." In: Hinman, F, ed. Benign prostatic hypertrophy. New York: Springer-Verlag, 1983:701.

25. Rohner TJ. Changes in adrenergic receptors in bladder outlet obstruction. In: Hinman F, ed. Benign prostatic hypertrophy. New York: Springer-Verlag, 1983:410.

26. Steers WD, DeGroat WC. Effects of bladder outlet obstruction on micturition pathways in the rat. J Urol 1988;140:864.

27. Gilpin SA, Gosling JA, Barnard RJ. Morphological and morphometric studies of the human, obstructed trabeculated urinary bladder. Br J Urol 1985;57:525.

28. Tanagho EA, McCurry E. Pressure and flow rate as related to lumen caliber and entrance configuration. J Urol 1971;105:583.

29. Stamey TA. Endoscopic suspension of the vesical neck for urinary incontinence. Surg Gynecol Obstet 1973;136:547.

30. Marshall VF, Marchetti AA, Krantz DE. The correction of stress incontinence by simple vesicourethral suspension. Surg Gynecol Obstet 1949;88:509.

31. Parnell JP, Marshall VF, Vaughan ED. Management of recurrent urinary stress incontinence

by the Marshall-Marchetti-Krantz urethropexy. J Urol 1984;132:912.

32. Zimmern PE, Hadley HR, Leach GE, et al. Female urethral obstruction after Marshall-Marchetti-Krantz urethropexy. J Urol 1984;132:912.

33. Burch JC. Cooper's ligament urethrovesical suspension for stress incontinence. Am J Obstet Gynecol 1968;100:764.

34. Constantinou CE, Stamey TA. Modification of urethral resistance and detrusor instability by endoscopic bladder neck suspension. Proceedings of the Third Joint Meeting of the International Continence Society, Boston, 1986.

35. Mundy AR. A trial comparing the Stamey bladder neck suspension with colposuspension for the treatment of stress urinary incontinence. Br J Urol 1983;55:687.

36. Pereyra AJ, Lebherz TB. Combined urethrovesical suspension and vaginourethroplasty for correction of urinary stress incontinence. Obstet Gynecol 1967;30:537.

37. Raz S. Modified bladder neck suspension for female stress incontinence. Urology 1981;17:82.

38. Leach GE, Yip CM, Donovan BJ. Mechanism of continence after modified bladder neck suspension. Urology 1984;29:238.

39. McGuire EJ, Lytton B. Pubovaginal sling procedures for stress incontinence. J Urol 1978;119:82.

40. McGuire EJ, Bennett CJ, Konnak JA, et al. Experience with pubovaginal slings at the University of Michigan. J Urol 1987;138:525.

41. Hellstrom P, Lukkarinen O, Konturri M. The treatment of incomplete bladder emptying in females by bladder neck incision. Ann Chir Gynecol 1987;76:124.

42. Choudhury A. Incisional treatment of obstruction of the female bladder neck. Ann R Coll Surg Engl 1978;60(5):404.

43. Farrar DJ, Osborne JL, Stephenson TP, et al. A urodynamic view of bladder outflow obstruction in the female: Factors influencing the results of treatment. Br J Urol 1976;47:815.

44. Abrams PH. Detrusor instability and bladder outlet obstruction. Neurourodynam 1985;4:317.

45. Diokno AC, Hollander JB, Bennett CJ. Bladder neck obstruction in females: A real entity. J Urol 1984;132:294.

46. Bracken RB, John DE, Miller LS, et al. Primary carcinoma of the female urethra. J Urol 1976;116:188.

47. Freed SZ, Haleem SA, Weiner I, et al. Bladder outlet obstruction caused by vaginal fibromyoma: The female prostate. J Urol 1975;113:30.

48. Swartz EM, Komins JI. Post obstructive diuresis after reduction of an incarcerated gravid uterus. J Reprod Med 1977;19:262.

49. Soloway MS, Rao MK, Kest L. Hematocolpos with urinary tract obstruction in an adult. J Urol 1977;117:811.

50. McGuire EJ, Letson W, Wang S. Transvaginal urethrolysis after obstructive urethral suspension procedures. J Urol 1989;142:1037.

37

Urologic Concerns in Endometriosis and Ovarian Remnant Syndrome

Christopher C. Fitzpatrick

Thomas E. Elkins

Definition

Endometriosis is defined as the presence of endometrial epithelium and stroma in an ectopic site excluding the myometrium; ectopic endometrium within the myometrium is termed *adenomyosis*.[1] Although adenomyosis has been referred to as endometriosis interna, this term is no longer used, endometriosis and adenomyosis being unrelated disorders.[1] Endometriosis was first described in 1860 by Von Rokitansky.[2] It is a major cause of gynecologic morbidity among women today.

Epidemiology

Estimates of the prevalence of endometriosis in the general population are purely speculative, based on direct visualization of the disease at laparoscopy or laparotomy. Prevalence rates are highly dependent on the nature of such surgical procedures. Strathy and co-workers observed endometriosis to be present in 20% of infertile women undergoing diagnostic laparoscopy and in 2% of women undergoing tubal ligation.[3] Using rates collated by the National Center for Health Statistics from all hospitals in the United States, Cramer found that endometriosis accounted for 4.5 of every 1000 hospital admissions among women aged between 15 and 44 years.[4] In the 44- to 64-year-old age group, the figure was 3.1; virtually no admissions occurred in females under 15 years old or over 64 years old. The prevalence at autopsy among women aged between 20 and 55 years is 0.3%; endometriosis was listed as a cause of death on only 3 of some 850,000 female death certificates.[5] Barbieri calculates the prevalence among women of reproductive age as between 1% and 7%.[6] The rise in prevalence over the past 10 years is in part due to an increased awareness of the disease, widespread use of diagnostic laparoscopy, and increasing recognition of atypical lesions.[7,8]

The initial diagnosis of endometriosis is usually made between the ages of 25 and 35 years; 50% to 65% of these women are nulliparous, the rest being of low parity. Endometriosis in teenage girls may be associated with congenital obstructive anomalies of the genital tract. Women with menstrual cycle lengths of 27 days or less are at increased risk of developing this disease as compared with women with longer cycle lengths and shorter durations of flow. The use of tampons, oral contraception, and delayed childbearing have not been shown to be influential.

Endometriosis is more prevalent among whites and Asians and higher socioeconomic groups. There appears to be a familial predisposition, with a 7% recurrence rate among first-

Female Urology, edited by Elroy D. Kursh and Edward McGuire. J. B. Lippincott, Philadelphia, © 1994.

degree relatives, making a genetic cause at least a consideration.[9]

Between 30% and 40% of patients with endometriosis are infertile; 5% to 15% of all cases of infertility are due to this disease. In rare instances, the disease has been described in men; it is well documented in female nonhuman primates.

Etiology and Pathogenesis

In 1927, Sampson proposed that endometriosis was caused by transtubal retrograde menstruation leading to implantation and cyclical proliferation of endometrial tissue.[10] This theory, however, does not explain extra-abdominopelvic or male endometriosis; retrograde menstruation is in fact a common innocuous event in menstruating women with patent fallopian tubes. Iatrogenic implantation of endometrial tissue, particularly at closure of episiotomy or cesarean section incisions, may occasionally give rise to focal endometriosis.

In 1952, Javert demonstrated the presence of benign endometrial cells within lymphovascular spaces and postulated a metastatic theory to explain the presence of endometriotic deposits in distant sites throughout the body (e.g., lung, bone, skeletal muscle, brain).[11] About 11% of patients with pelvic endometriosis have lymphatic involvement of pelvic lymph nodes.

The development of endometriosis through a process of metaplasia is consistent with the putative müllerian potential of pelvic mesothelium.[12] The rare occurrence of endometriosis in men is often taken as proof of this theory.[13–16] A review of the reported cases (four in total) reveals that all were receiving estrogen therapy for carcinoma of the prostate following local resection and orchiectomy. Stimulation of müllerian rest cells in the verumontanum seems a more plausible explanation.[17]

Peritoneal fluid in patients with endometriosis appears to contain increased amounts of prostaglandin $F_{2\alpha}$ and E_2, interleukin 1, and activated macrophages.[18,19] Increased local prostaglandins may adversely affect ovulatory function, uterotubal motility, fimbrial-oocyte pickup, and sperm penetration, whereas greater numbers of activated macrophages appear to curtail both sperm and embryo survival significantly. Interleukin 1 promotes fibrinogen synthesis and stimulates fibroblast proliferation and collagen deposition. Adhesion formation is further enhanced by the reduced tissue and peritoneal plasminogen activator activity found in patients with endometriosis.[20]

The presence of increased numbers of T and B lymphocytes in the peritoneal fluid and peripheral blood, a significant increase in the thyroxine-to-triiodothyronine (T_4:T_3) ratio, and the demonstration of circulating endometrial autoantibodies in patients with endometriosis further implies an underlying immune dysfunction.[21,22]

The cause of endometriosis-related infertility is multifactorial. In advanced disease, the ovaries may be encased in dense adhesions or destroyed by chocolate cyst formation. In addition, tubal mobility may be restricted and the normal tubo-ovarian anatomic relations grossly distorted; tubal patency is usually, however, preserved. Mild cases of endometriosis rarely involve mechanical factors. Many studies postulate that endometriotic implants generate a hostile pelvic milieu resulting in altered function or destruction of sperm, oocyte, and the early embryo. Reduced in vitro fertilization rates and increased rates of spontaneous abortion have been reported in women with endometriosis.[23,24] To date, there is no underlying theory to account for the protean nature of this disease.

Clinical Presentation

The predominant symptoms in women with endometriosis are abnormal uterine bleeding, secondary dysmenorrhea, chronic pelvic pain, dyspareunia, and infertility. Often there is poor correlation between the severity of symptoms and the extent of disease. Mild endometriosis may cause crippling dysmenorrhea; women with large endometriomas may be entirely asymptomatic.

Endometriosis involves the bowel in approximately 5% of cases.[25] The most common sites of involvement are the sigmoid colon and rectum.[25] Cyclical alterations in bowel habit, tenesmus, and rectal bleeding suggest enteric involvement.

The urinary tract is affected in approximately 1% of cases.[26] Of these, the bladder is affected in 85% and the ureter in 15%; renal involvement is rare.[26] Patients may present with cyclical suprapubic or groin pain, dysuria, and hematuria. Occasionally patients present with ureteral obstruction from endometriosis. Almost every organ in the body is a potential site for endometriosis; catamenial pneumothorax and epistaxis are well-recognized presentations. Physical findings suggestive of endometriosis include generalized pelvic tenderness, fixed uterine retroversion, enlarged ovaries, thickened uterosacral ligaments, and nodularity in the posterior cul-de-sac.

Diagnosis

Definitive diagnosis of endometriosis requires direct visualization of the disease. CA[125] assay, ultrasound, computed tomography, and magnetic resonance imaging are not diagnostic but may be useful in monitoring disease progression or regression. For patients with gastrointestinal or urologic symptoms, appropriate radiologic and endoscopic investigations are required; these are best performed during menstruation. With abnormal uterine bleeding, an endometrial biopsy or curettage is necessary to exclude co-existent endometrial pathology.

Laparoscopy, using a double-puncture technique with an additional intracervical manipulator, allows full visualization of the pelvis. The most common sites for endometriotic deposits in the pelvis, in order of frequency, are ovaries (60%), posterior broad ligaments, posterior cul-de-sac, uterosacral ligaments, and anterior cul-de-sac. Hemosiderin-stained peritoneal "powder burns" and ovarian chocolate cysts are the classic lesions described. Atypical lesions include red flame-shaped patches, strawberry nodules, white fibrotic plaques, translucent or bluish blebs, peritoneal puckering, or pocket formation. Suspected atypical lesions should be biopsied. The relevance of microscopic disease in biopsy specimens from macroscopically normal tissue remains unclear.[27]

Laparoscopic photography or video-recording may be helpful, if available. The extent of the disease should be classified according to the Revised American Fertility Society Classification of Endometriosis (i.e., stage I through IV: normal, mild, moderate, and severe).[28]

Treatment

Treatment of patients with endometriosis should be based on patient age, severity of symptoms, duration of infertility, and extent of disease. Minimal endometriosis, a diagnosis increasingly made among infertile women, does not necessarily warrant immediate treatment. At least 6 to 12 months may be allowed to pass before beginning therapy. This time should be used to exclude other causes of infertility. Well over 50% of these women conceive with expectant management alone.[29,30]

The range of therapies available for patients with endometriosis include (1) danazol, (2) progestogens, (3) gonadotropin-releasing hormone (Gn-RH) analogs, (4) human menopausal gonadotropin (hMG)–induced superovulation with intrauterine insemination (IUI), in vitro fertilization/embryo transfer (IVF/ET), gamete intrafallopian transfer (GIFT), and (5) surgery (laparoscopic, conservative, radical).

Danazol is a synthetic androgen derived from 17-ethinyltestosterone. It inhibits the preovulatory luteinizing hormone (LH) surge and also many of the enzymes involved in ovarian steroidogeneses; it displaces testosterone from sex hormone–binding globulin, thus increasing its bioavailability. The standard dose is 400 to 800 mg orally per day for 6 months. Side effects include weight gain, acne, hirsutism, deepening of the voice, muscle cramps, reduced breast size, hot flushes, and sweats. Of these, hirsutism and voice change are not always reversible.[31] Danazol may also cause a dose-related rise in hepatic transaminases and in the high-density lipoprotein–to–low-density lipoprotein ratio. It may cause virilization of the female fetus and is therefore contraindicated in pregnancy. Although danazol is highly effective in relieving pain, its role in the treatment of the associated infertility remains inconclusive.[31]

Progestogen-only regimens, such as medroxyprogesterone acetate, 10 to 30 mg orally per day, cause decidualization and eventual atrophy of endometriotic implants. Despite symptom relief, there is no convincing evidence of improved fecundity among infertile patients.[31] Troublesome side effects include breakthrough bleeding (50%), weight gain, fluid retention, and depression.

The most recent advance in the medical management of endometriosis is the development and use of Gn-RH analogs. Gn-RH is a hypothalamic decapeptide that stimulates the synthesis and release of follicle-stimulating hormone (FSH) and LH. It is secreted in a pulsatile fashion. By chemical modification at the 6 and 10 positions, a series of synthetic analogs have been created. Depot or bolus administration (by intranasal, subcutaneous, or intramuscular routes) induces a transient rise in FSH and LH followed by a profound hypogonadotropic hypogonadism brought about by pituitary receptor down-regulation. The castrate levels of estrogens result in glandular involution and stromal atrophy of endometriotic implants. Side effects include hot flushes, sweats, vaginal dryness, and trabecular bone loss. Almost complete osseous recovery seems to occur if the course of treatment is restricted to 6 months.[32] As with danazol and progestogens, Gn-RH agonists have not been shown to improve fecundity despite effective symptom relief.[31] They may also be used in superovulation programs as a prelude to hMG induction. Further research into this new therapeutic modality is required.

hMG-induced superovulation with ensuing IUI, IVF/ET, or GIFT is being increasingly used for the treatment of endometriosis-related infertility. Cycle fecundity rates of up to 18% have been reported in minimal and mild disease with IUI.[33] GIFT requires at least one patent tube; a recent report revealed a success rate of 23% per procedure.[34] IVF/ET is a therapeutic alternative in patients with severe adnexal disease as an alternative to or, more particularly, after failed laparoscopic or conservative surgery. In general, however, success rates are less than 10% per cycle among these patients.[23]

Laparoscopic ablation of endometriotic implants and pelvic adhesions can be effectively accomplished by carbon dioxide, argon, potassium-titanyl-phosphate (KTP) and neodymium: yttrium-aluminum-garnet (Nd:YAG) lasers. Small endometriomas can be removed completely without spillage; cysts greater than 8 cm in diameter are perhaps best removed at laparotomy. Adjunctive video control allows for more comfortable and refined surgery. Treatment at initial laparoscopic diagnosis is also feasible. Life-table analysis reveals that the monthly fecundity rate in patients treated for severe disease appears higher in patients treated laparoscopically rather than with danazol or conservative laparotomy.[35] In addition, the time interval between treatment and conception seems to be shorter with carbon dioxide laser than with other laparoscopic modalities.[35]

The indications for conservative surgery are failure to conceive after medical treatment, large endometriomas, extensive tubo-ovarian adhesions, operator preference, and the nonavailability of laser. Microsurgical techniques are essential to minimize adhesion reformation.[36] Adjunctive preoperative or postoperative medical treatment may improve the outcome of surgery.[36]

In patients for whom fertility is no longer an issue, total abdominal hysterectomy, salpingo-oophorectomy, and implantectomy are therapeutic options. A Maylard or Cherney incision together with retroperitoneal dissection is indicated in severe disease.[36] A preoperative intravenous urogram and intraoperative identification of both ureters are mandatory.

When complete oophorectomy is performed, estrogen-only replacement therapy can be given with a low risk of recurrent disease.[37] These patients, however, should be monitored closely.[37] Case reports suggest that after total hysterectomy and bilateral oophorectomy for endometriosis, residual or de novo endometriotic implants may undergo malignant transformation when stimulated with continuous estrogen-only replacement.[38] Although these cases are rare, Barbieri advises the addition of a cyclical progestogen (*e.g.*, medroxyprogesterone acetate, 10 mg orally per day for 12 days each month).[38]

More than 100 cases of ureteral obstruction owing to endometriosis have been reported.[17] The prognosis is serious; in one series of 62 patients, loss of renal function occurred in 46%, mainly as a result of delayed diagnosis.[39] In the majority of cases, the obstruction occurs in the distal third of the ureter; bilateral involvement is rare. Obstruction may be extramural or intramural, the former being more common. In extramural obstruction, the ureter is extrinsically compressed by ovarian endometriosis or encased in dense retroperitoneal fibrosis. In the intramural type, the ureteral wall/lumen is directly invaded. Intravenous or retrograde urography may confirm the type of involvement. Reversal of ureteral obstruction has been reported with use of progestogens, danazol, and Gn-RH analogs, but in several cases recurrence has occurred after discontinuation of treatment.[40–44] The primary management of this condition is surgery.[17] Both preoperative and postoperative medical treatment has proved disappointing in these cases.[17] For extrinsic obstruction, surgery consists of freeing the ureter from its fibrotic bed. Resection of the obstructed portion is necessary in cases of intrinsic obstruction with creation of either a ureteroneocystostomy or ureterureterostomy. Long-term radiologic or ultrasonic follow-up is mandatory.

As the recognized incidence of endometriosis increases, the reports of ovarian remnant syndrome (ORS) also increase. Ureteral obstruction by ovarian remnants was first reported by Major in 1968.[45] ORS is an unusual complication of oophorectomy in which remnants of ovarian cortex, left behind after surgery, or living independently from the ovary within the pelvis, become functional and occasionally cystic.[46] It is particularly associated with conditions that cause dense intrapelvic adhesions, for example, endometriosis, pelvic inflammatory disease, and inflammatory bowel disease.[47] As endometriosis becomes more common in society, ORS will become more common as well. The ORS is clearly distinct from the residual ovarian syndrome, in which an intentionally conserved ovary gives rise to symptoms or develops a pathologic process.[48] Patients with ORS often present with pain and dyspareunia with or without a definable pelvic mass; ureteral deviation/dilatation may be noted on an intravenous urogram.[47, 49] Premenopausal serum levels of gonadotropins and estradiol in the absence of hormone replacement therapy is suggestive of this syndrome; definitive diagnosis requires histologic confirmation.

Medical therapy may be used in symptomatic patients without ureteral involvement. Suppressive agents should be considered in those with small adnexal cysts; provocative therapy, using clomiphene citrate or hMG, may help localize small lesions before surgery, particularly when previous surgical localization and excision have failed.[51, 52] In view of the iatrogenic risk to the bowel at surgery, a preoperative bowel preparation is advisable. The risk of iatrogenic ureteral injury is minimized by a preoperative intravenous pyelography, cystoscopic insertion of ureteral stents, and lateral retroperitoneal dissection from the level of the pelvic brim.[53, 54] Retroperitoneal fibrosis may be prevented by covering the dissected ureter with omentum and areas of peritoneal denudation with an absorbable adhesion barrier, such as oxidized methyl cellulose.[55] This remains a significant risk, however, and postoperative evaluation of ureteral integrity is recommended 2 and 4 weeks after surgery.

For ORS resistant to medical and surgical treatments, low-dose radiotherapy may be useful with minimal risk to surrounding structures.[46] Routine intraoperative marking with radioopaque vascular clips may be helpful in this regard. Although ORS is rare, increasing numbers of cases are being seen; this probably relates to the increasing prevalence of endometriosis.[47,50]

Bladder involvement in endometriosis requires histologic confirmation and endoscopic or open resection. Medical treatment is reported to be temporarily beneficial, but recurrence is likely on cessation.[56]

Four cases of endometriosis occurring in men have been reported, three in the urinary bladder and one in the abdominal wall.[13-16] All were receiving postprostatectomy or postorchiectomy estrogen treatment for carcinoma of the prostate. Hematuria and pain were the most common presentations. Cystoscopy revealed polypoid lesions and ulceration. Symptoms subsided only after local resection and discontinuation of the estrogen treatment.

A total of 195 cases of malignancy arising in endometriosis have been reported.[57] The average age of presentation is 46 years. Before the diagnosis of cancer, 43 had been treated for endometriosis. The most common symptoms were abdominopelvic pain, pelvic mass, and abnormal vaginal bleeding. The ovary was involved in 80% of cases; the rectovaginal septum, colon, vagina, and pelvic peritoneum represented the majority of extraovarian sites of tumor development. Endometrioid adenocarcinoma was the most common histologic type, accounting for 70% of tumors in each group. Unopposed estrogenic stimulation may have been causative in 14 cases.

Conclusions

Despite recent diagnostic and therapeutic advances, endometriosis remains an enigmatic disease. Patients have variable symptoms and signs that do not necessarily correlate with the anatomic stage of the disease. Questions concerning cause, natural history, and the effect of treatment on fecundity remain, for the most part, unanswered. Ureteral obstruction from ovarian disease and ORS and malignant transformation at ovarian and extraovarian sites are increasingly recognized complications.

References

1. Clement PB. Endometriosis, lesions of the secondary mullerian system, and pelvic mesothelial proliferations. In: Kurman RJ, ed. Dr. Blaustein's Pathology of the Female Genital Tract. 3rd ed. New York: Springer-Verlag, 1987:516.
2. Von Rokitansky C. Ueber Uterusdrusen Niebildung um Uterus and Ovarialsarcomen. Zkk Geselbch d Aertze du Wien 1860;37:577.
3. Strathy JH, Monlgaard CA, Coulan CB, et al. Endometriosis and infertility: A laparoscopic study of endometriosis among fertile and infertile women. Fertil Steril 1982;38:667.
4. Cramer DW. Epidemiology of endometriosis. In: Wilson EA, ed. Endometriosis. New York: Alan R Liss, 1987:522.
5. Dreyfuss ML. Pathological and clinical aspects of adenomyosis and endometriosis. A survey of 224 cases. Am J Obstet Gynecol 1940;39:95.
6. Barbieri RL. Etiology and epidemiology of endometriosis. Am J Obstet Gynecol 1990;162:565.
7. Kirschen B, Poindexter AN, Fast J. Endometriosis in multiparous women. J Reprod Med 1989; 34:215.
8. Jansen RP, Russel P. Non-pigmented endometriosis: Clinical, laparoscopic and pathological definition. Am J Obstet Gynecol 1986;155:1154.
9. Simpson JL, Elias S, Malinak LR, et al. Heritable aspects of endometriosis: I. Genetic studies. Am J Obstet Gynecol 1980;137:327.
10. Sampson JA. Peritoneal endometriosis due to menstrual dissemination of endometrial tissue into peritoneal cavity. Am J Obstet Gynecol 1927;14:422.
11. Javert CT. The spread of benign and malignant endometrium in the lymphatic system with a note on coexisting vascular involvement. Am J Obstet Gynecol 1952;64:780.
12. Meyer R. Ueber endometrium in der Tube, soine uber die hieraustentstehenden wirklichen and veemantlechen Folgen. Zentrabe Gynacol 1927; 51:1482.
13. Oliker AJ, Harris AE. Endometriosis of the bladder in a male partner. J Urol 1971;106:858.
14. Pinkert T, Catlow C, Straus R. Endometriosis of the urinary bladder in a man with prostatic carcinoma. Cancer 1979;43:1562.
15. Schrodt GR, Alcorn M, Ibarez J. Endometriosis of the male urinary system. J Urol 1980;124:722.
16. Martin JD Jr, Hauck AE. Endometriosis of the male. Ann Surg 1985;51:426.
17. Mitchell GW. Extrapelvic endometriosis. In: Schenken RS, ed. Endometriosis: Contemporary concepts in clinical management. Philadelphia: JB Lippincott, 1989:307.

18. Badawy SZ, Marchall L, Cinenca V. Peritoneal fluid prostaglandins in various stages of the menstrual cycle: Role in infertile patients with endometriosis. Int J Fertil 1985;30:48.
19. Chacko KJ, Chacko MS, Anderson PJ, et al. Peritoneal fluid in patients with and without endometriosis. Prostaglandins and macrophages and their effect on the spermatozoa penetration assay. Am J Obstet Gynecol 1986;154:1290.
20. Ohtsuka N. Study of the pathogenesis of adhesions in endometriosis. Acta Obstet Gynecol Japon 1980;32:1758.
21. Badawy SZ, Cinenca V, Stezel A, et al. Immune Rosettes of T and B lymphocytes in infertile women with endometriosis. J Reprod Med 1987;37:194.
22. Wild RA, Shivers CA. Antiendometrial antibodies in patients with endometriosis. Am J Reprod Immunol 1988;8:84.
23. Seppala M. The world collaborative report on in-vitro fertilization and embryo replacement: current state of the art in January 1984. In: Seppala M, Edwards RG, eds. Fertilization and embryo transfer. Ann NY Acad Sci 1984;442:558.
24. Wheeler JM, Johnson BM, Malinak LR. The relationship of endometriosis to spontaneous abortion. Fertil Steril 1983;5:656.
25. Weid JC, Ray JE. Endometriosis of the bowel. Obstet Gynecol 1987;69:727.
26. Neto WA, Lopes RN, Curry M, et al. Vesical endometriosis. Urology 1984;24:271.
27. Murphy AA, Green R, De la Cruz I, et al. Unsuspected endometriosis documented by scanning electron microscope in visually normal peritoneum. Fertil Steril 1986;46:522.
28. Buttram VC. Evolution of the Revised American Fertility Society Classification of Endometriosis. Fertil Steril 1985;43:347.
29. Portuondo JA, Echanojaneregui AD, Herran C, et al. Early conception in patients with untreated mild endometriosis. Fertil Steril 1983;39:22.
30. Rodriguez-Escunero FJ, Neyro JL, Corcostegui B, et al. Does minimal endometriosis reduce fertility? Fertil Steril 1980;50:522.
31. Hurst BS, Rock JA. Endometriosis: pathophysiology, diagnosis and treatment. Fertil Steril 1989;44:297.
32. Dodin S, Lemay A, Maheux R, et al. Bone mass in endometriosis patients treated with GNRH agonist implants or danazol. Obstet Gynecol 1991;77:410.
33. Dodson WC, Whitesides DB, Hughes CL Jr, et al. Superovulation with intrauterine insemination in the treatment of infertility: A possible alternative to gamete intra-fallopian transfer and in-vitro fertilization. Fertil Steril 1987;48:441.
34. Schnenken RS, Riehl RM. In-vitro fertilization/ embryo transfer and gamete intra-fallopian transfer. In: Schnenken RS, ed. Endometriosis: Contemporary concepts in clinical management. Philadelphia: JB Lippincott, 1989:293.
35. Olive DL, Martin DC. Treatment of endometriosis-associated infertility with CO_2 laser laparoscopy: The use of one and two step parameter exponential models. Fertil Steril 1987;48:18.
36. duToit JP. Surgery for endometriosis. In: Monaghan J, ed. Operative surgery: Gynecology and obstetrics. 4th ed. London: Butterworths, 1983: 160.
37. Walters MD. Definitive surgery. In: Schnenken RS, ed. Endometriosis: Contemporary concepts in clinical management. Philadelphia: JB Lippincott, 1989:267.
38. Barbieri RL. Endometriosis 1990: Current therapeutic approaches. Drugs 1990;39:502.
39. Kane C, Dounin P. Obstructive uropathy associated with endometriosis. Am J Obstet Gynecol 1985;151:207.
40. Dick AL, Lang DW, Bergman RT, et al. Postmenopausal endometriosis with ureteral obstruction. Br J Urol 1973;45:153.
41. Gantt PA, Hunt JB, McDonough PG. Progestin reversal of ureteral endometriosis. Obstet Gynecol 1981;57:665.
42. Gardner B, Whitaker RH. The use of danazol for ureteral obstruction caused by endometriosis. J Urol 1981;125:117.
43. Freidman AJ, Barbrieri RL. Leuprolide acetate: Applications in gynecology. Curr Probl Obstet Gynecol Fertil 1988;11:207.
44. Rivlin ME, Muler JD, Krueger RP, et al. Leuprolide acetate in the management of ureter obstruction caused by endometriosis. Obstet Gynecol 1990;75:532.
45. Major FJ. Retained ovarian remnant causing ureteral obstruction. Report of two cases. Obstet Gynecol 1968;32:748.
46. Shemwell RE, Weed JC. Ovarian remnant syndrome. Obstet Gynecol 1970;36:299.
47. Pettit PD, Lee RA. Ovarian remnant syndrome: A diagnostic dilemma and surgical challenge. Obstet Gynecol 1988;71:580.
48. Christ JE, Lotze EL. Residual ovary syndrome. Obstet Gynecol 1975;46:551.
49. Webb MJ. Ovarian remnant syndrome. Aust N Z J Obstet Gynecol 1989;29:433.
50. Steege JF. Ovarian remnant syndrome. Obstet Gynecol 1987;70:64.
51. Kaminski PF, Sorosky JI, Mandell MJ, et al. Clomiphene citrate stimulation as an adjunct in locating ovarian tissue in ovarian remnant syndrome. Obstet Gynecol 1990;76:924.
52. Kosasa TS, Grifiths CT, Shane JM, et al. Diag-

nosis of a supernumerary ovary with human chorionic gonadotropin. Obstet Gynecol 1976;
47:236.

53. Berek JS, Darney PD, Lopkin C, et al. Avoiding
    ureteral damage in pelvic surgery for ovarian rem-
    nant syndrome. Am J Obstet Gynecol 1979;133:
    221.

54. Hajj SN, Mercer LJ. Retrograde dissection of the
    adnexa in residual ovarian syndrome. Surg Gyne-
    col Obstet 1987;165:451.

55. Interceed Adhesion Study Group. Prevention of
    post surgical adhesions by Interceed (C7-7), an
    absorbable adhesion barrier: A prospective ran-
    domized multicenter clinical study. Fertil Steril
    1989;51:933.

56. Weinberg RW. Vesical endometriosis. Urology
    1978;11:72.

57. Heaps JM, Nieberg RH, Berek JS. Malignant neo-
    plasms arising in endometriosis. Obstet Gynecol
    1990;75:1023.

38

Vaginal Infections

Nancy A. Little

This chapter presents an overview of vaginal infections, with practical information for the clinician. It is not meant to be an exhaustive review of basic science. Appropriate references are made to direct those who wish more in-depth reading.

A review of vaginal infections cannot be performed without a review of sexually transmitted diseases (STDs). The presentations of many of these diseases are quite different in the female patient, and many are asymptomatic. Each disease is reviewed by presentation of epidemiology, etiology and pathogenesis, clinical presentation, laboratory diagnosis, and treatment.

Vaginal infections are extremely common in clinical practice and are often dismissed as inconsequential by the physician. Vaginal discharge, however, is among the 25 most common reasons for consulting physicians in private office practice in the United States. In women attending STD clinics, vaginitis has been found in 28% to 33%. It is the most frequent complaint in self-referred patients in gynecologic clinics, and approximately 40% of these women have some type of vaginitis. Vaginitis in adult women can lead to marked discomfort and irritation. Thus it is the responsibility of the clinician to make an accurate diagnosis by systematic evaluation rather than relying on shotgun therapy.[1]

As in the evaluation of any patient with a genitourinary complaint, a detailed history must be obtained, including a description of the duration and nature of symptoms. A description of the vaginal discharge should include duration, odor, consistency, and color. A thorough sexual history, including recent change of sexual partner, past infections and response to therapy, and type of contraception, must be obtained.[1]

Physical examination should begin at the introitus with inspection and palpation of the vulva and vaginal vestibule. Focal vulvitis or vestibulitis may be missed if this area is overlooked. A speculum is then placed intravaginally, and the vaginal walls and cervix are studied for erythema, petechiae, ulceration, edema, atrophy, and adherent discharge. The pooled vaginal secretions are also evaluated for color, consistency, and volume. After inspection, the pooled vaginal secretions are swabbed to obtain a valid specimen suitable for rapid pH estimation. Swabs are also obtained for saline and 10% potassium hydroxide (KOH) microscopic examination as well as for immediate performance of a 10% KOH amine elaboration test (whiff test).

Bacterial and fungal cultures may be required in selected cases. In the presence of possible cervicitis, cervical specimens should also be obtained for identification of *Chlamydia trachomatis, Neisseria gonorrhoeae*, and herpes simplex virus. Saline microscopy aids in identi-

Female Urology, edited by Elroy D. Kursh and Edward McGuire. J. B. Lippincott, Philadelphia, © 1994.

fication of clue cells, trichomonads, and yeast or hyphae, and in evaluation of whether polymorphonuclear cells are present and whether they are increased. A ratio of polymorphonuclear cells to epithelial cells of 1 or less is deemed to be normal by most investigators. Exfoliated vaginal epithelial cells are analyzed to assess for an increase in basal or parabasal cells, which may be due to a relative estrogen deficiency or reflect an inflammatory reaction in the vaginal wall. Vaginal flora are also examined, paying close attention to the intercellular spaces. Normally vaginal flora consist of unclumped rodlike organisms in moderate numbers. This configuration is maintained in vulvovaginal candidiasis but changes in both trichomoniasis and bacterial vaginosis. In these two infections, normal flora are lost and replaced by large numbers of clumped coccobacillary organisms. Gram's stain examination of vaginal secretions is not dictated on a routine basis and adds little to the saline and KOH examination. The saline examination has low sensitivity in detecting *Candida* species, and therefore a 10% KOH microscopic examination should always be performed. Mixed infections are common, mandating both the saline wet mount and KOH examination to identify additional causes of vaginitis.[1]

The vagina is composed of nonkeratinizing squamous epithelium that undergoes cyclic growth that is related to hormonal status. Colonization of organisms on the vaginal epithelium is controlled by binding sites; nutritional status; and other factors, such as pregnancy, diabetes mellitus, steroids, and immunosuppression.[2] The dominant organism in normal women is *Lactobacillus* species, accounting for more than 95% of the vaginal organisms.[3] Colonization by *Candida* species and lactobacilli increases throughout pregnancy. This is thought to be due to hormonal influences. The normal vaginal pH is 4.0 to 4.5. Hormonal changes lead to an increase in vaginal pH, which increases adherence of *Candida albicans*. The increase in *Candida* vaginitis before menses is also related to this increase in vaginal pH.[2] The glycogen content of the vaginal epithelium is also hormonally de-

pendent and thus is important in the colonization of yeast. During pregnancy or with the use of oral contraceptives, hormonal concentration, glycogen content, and pH are all increased. Similarly, the rate of yeast isolation in postmenopausal women was found to be nearly five times higher in those receiving estrogen replacement therapy.[2]

Ninety percent of the cases of vaginitis are accounted for by vulvovaginal candidiasis (VVC), trichomoniasis, and bacterial vaginosis (BV). BV is the most common infection (30% to 50%) followed by VVC (20% to 25%) and trichomoniasis (10% to 20%). Fifteen percent to 20% of these patients have a mixed infection caused by two or more agents. Another pathogen, *Chlamydia*, has had a marked increase in incidence, may be asymptomatic, and causes significant morbidity. The remaining 10% encompasses atrophic vaginitis, ulcerative vaginitis due to *Staphylococcus aureus*, toxic shock syndrome, and other causes.[1]

In most patients, a thorough history; careful physical examination; and the use of pH, saline wet mount, and KOH test give the diagnosis. In a small percentage, diagnosis requires further testing, specifically cultures. Care must be taken to avoid the traps that may lead to a missed diagnosis, such as failing to examine the patient, examining the patient without a thorough vaginal and cervical examination, assuming that the pathogen remains the same in subsequent infections or that a positive culture for *Gardnerella vaginalis* presumes the presence of bacterial vaginosis, failing to perform basic laboratory tests in the office, treating normal flora such as *Escherichia coli* and enterococcus as pathogens, and using shotgun therapy.

Bacterial Vaginosis

EPIDEMIOLOGY

BV, also called *nonspecific vaginitis*, is the most common form of vaginal infection in women of childbearing age.[1,4] *Gardnerella vaginalis* has been recovered in 0% to 50% of asymptomatic women and 70% to 95% of women with a diagnosis of BV.[5] *Gardnerella* is significantly associated with symptoms of vaginitis and yet presents in a considerable proportion of asymptomatic women.[3, 6–8]

The exact prevalence of bacterial vaginosis is unknown, but one author has reported its presence in 15% of women at a university student gynecology clinic, 10% to 25% of pregnant women, and 37% of women attending a STD clinic. Fifty percent of women are asymptomatic.[3] Another investigator diagnosed BV in 17% to 19% of women seeking gynecologic care in family practice or student health care clinics, 16% to 29% of pregnant women, and 24% to 37% of symptomatic women in STD clinics. The prevalence reaches 50% to 60% in some at-risk populations. *Gardnerella vaginalis*, however, has been isolated in 10% to 31% of virgin adolescent girls.[1] Yet another investigator found *Gardnerella vaginalis* in 53% of adult women who consulted general practitioners for symptoms of vaginitis and in 22% of a control group consisting of women who presented for cervical smears and family planning checks.[6] In the community, the prevalence of asymptomatic *Gardnerella* has been estimated between 10% and 33%.[6]

Gardner maintained that most women whose sexual partner remained untreated become reinfected. The theory of BV as a STD is supported by its lower prevalence in sexually inactive women. In addition, one report states that *Gardnerella vaginalis* has been isolated from the urethra of 80% to 90% of partners of women with BV, but not in male controls.[5]

BV has been reported as a possible risk factor for pelvic inflammatory disease, including endometritis, salpingitis, and posthysterectomy fever.[3, 4] New epidemiologic findings also suggest that BV in pregnancy appears to be causally related to postpartum endometritis, amnionitis, and preterm rupture of membranes with consequent prematurity. These findings have been confirmed by other investigators.[3] *Gardnerella* organisms have been isolated in amniotic fluid infection, chorioamnionitis, postpartum endometritis, and bacteremia.[1, 9]

ETIOLOGY AND PATHOGENESIS

In 1955, Gardner and Dukes defined a condition they designated *Haemophilus vaginalis* vaginitis. The name then evolved to *Corynebacterium vaginale*, and now the organism is *Gardnerella vaginalis*.[5]

The term *bacterial vaginosis* has recently been advocated for this syndrome, in place of the original term *nonspecific vaginitis*, to reflect the complex alteration of the vaginal bacterial ecosystem and to indicate the presence of increased discharge without apparent inflammatory reaction or true tissue infection. Many diverse facultative anaerobic bacteria as well as *Gardnerella vaginalis*, *Mobiluncus* species, and *Mycoplasma hominis* are present in the vaginal flora of these patients.[1, 4, 10]

The issue of whether BV is a sexually transmitted infection is controversial. The age of infected women and history of previous genital infections and previous sexual contacts suggest that BV is sexually transmitted. In addition, male sex partners of women with BV have a higher rate of *Gardnerella vaginalis* and anaerobes isolated from the urethra than male controls. Nevertheless, because *Gardnerella vaginalis* can be isolated from 15% of virgin prepubertal girls, these findings do not prove sexual transmission.[3] Other nonsexual risk factors have been associated with BV. Oral contraceptives and barrier methods protect against BV, and intrauterine devices increase the risk for infection with BV. Factors that seem to be unrelated to BV include frequency of intercourse, oral or rectal sexual contact, tampon use, douching, and antibiotic use. The cause for this massive overgrowth of anaerobes is unknown.[1, 3]

The normal vaginal flora is usually *Lactobacillus* species, which accounts for more than 95% of all the organisms in the vagina. In contrast, *Lactobacillus* has been found in only 25% to 65% of women with BV and at a 100-fold to 1000-fold decrease in bacterial counts. *Gard-*

nerella vaginalis counts in bacterial vaginosis are 100-fold to 1000-fold higher than in normal vaginal flora. The lactobacilli isolated also appear to be of species other than those found in normal vaginal flora and include organisms incapable of producing hydrogen peroxide.[3, 8]

This disturbance in the vaginal microbial ecosystem is accompanied by a massive overgrowth of *Gardnerella vaginalis, Bacteroides* species, anaerobic cocci, *Mycoplasma hominis, Mobiluncus* species, and peptostreptococci. BV is better characterized as an increased concentration of bacteria rather than an increased prevalence of organisms, although both properties are present.[3]

Gardnerella vaginalis is a fastidious, gramvariable, coccobacillary organism.[8] It lacks decarboxylases and is not thought to produce polyamines but may elaborate catabolic products, which facilitate growth of anaerobes.[3] Increased concentrations of putrescine also furnishes an excellent vehicle for growth of *Mycoplasma hominis*. The critical mechanism that results in the drop in lactobacilli and the overgrowth of the anaerobes and *Gardnerella vaginalis* remains unknown.[1, 3]

CLINICAL PRESENTATION

As previously stated, up to 50% of women with BV may be asymptomatic. The principal symptom described by the patient is vaginal malodor, often described as fishy and often emerging after intercourse. Patients do not often relate an abnormal vaginal discharge, pruritus, dysuria, abdominal pain, or dyspareunia, as may be seen in vulvovaginal candidiasis or trichomoniasis. *Gardnerella vaginalis*, however, has also been detected in high numbers in the urine of patients with acute urinary symptoms and reflux nephropathy and in the urine of pregnant women. Examination reveals a thin, grayish white adherent discharge that may be evident on the labia and introitus.[1, 11]

Attendant with the anaerobic bacterial overgrowth in BV is the increased production of amines by these anaerobes aided by microbial de-

carboxylases. In the presence of increased vaginal pH, amines volatilize to produce the typical abnormal fishy odor. This malodor is also produced when 10% KOH is added to vaginal secretions. The aromatic amines, putrescine and cadaverine, were initially thought to be responsible for the malodor, but trimethylamine has been implicated as the dominant abnormal amine in BV. Bacterial polyamines produced together with the organic acids found in the vagina in BV are cytotoxic, contributing to the discharge by causing exfoliation of vaginal epithelial cells. *Gardnerella vaginalis* attaches to exfoliated epithelial cells, particularly at the alkaline pH above 5 found in BV. The *Gardnerella* organisms adherent to the exfoliated epithelial cells produce the pathognomonic *clue* cells.[1, 3]

DIAGNOSIS

The clinical diagnosis of bacterial vaginosis is defined by a composite of four criteria. The findings must satisfy at least three of the four criteria: (1) increased grayish white, homogeneous, adherent vaginal discharge; (2) vaginal pH greater than 4.5; (3) detection of clue cells in vaginal secretions at microscopy representing more than 20% of observed vaginal epithelial cells; and (4) a malodorous discharge with a positive amine test—release of fishy amine odor on mixing the discharge with 10% KOH. To reiterate, it must be kept in mind that mixed infections also frequently occur.[3, 4, 5, 8, 12, 13]

The saline wet mount examination is mandatory because it allows detection of clue cells; exclusion of *Trichomonas;* assessment of polymorphonuclear cells, which are typically absent in these cases; and assessment of the background bacterial flora with predominant coccobacillary organisms.[1, 3]

The presence of clue cells is the single most reliable indicator of BV. Clue cells are exfoliated vaginal squamous epithelial cells covered with *Gardnerella vaginalis*, giving the cells a granular or stippled appearance with a loss of defined cell borders. This adherence is optimal at the high pH above 5 associated with BV. Not all clue cells are composed exclusively of adherent *Gardnerella vaginalis* because microscopic observation occasionally reveals clue cells composed mainly of curved rods consistent with *Mobiluncus* species. These cells have been termed *comma cells*.[1,3,5,6]

Gram's stain is emerging as the best diagnostic test for BV. Some investigators have found that Gram's stain criteria for BV correlate better with the presence or absence of clue cells and composite clinical criteria than results of semiquantitative cultures for *Gardnerella vaginalis*.[4,7]

Use of vaginal culture for the diagnosis of BV is controversial. This is due to the fact that although cultures for *Gardnerella vaginalis* are positive in almost all cases of BV, *Gardnerella vaginalis* is also detected in 50% to 60% of women who fail to meet the diagnostic criteria for BV.[1]

MEDICAL TREATMENT

The basis for successful therapy is oral metronidazole. Most studies report use of 800 to 1200 mg/day for 1 week in divided doses. This regimen resulted in immediate clinical cure rates in excess of 90% and approximately 80% at 4 weeks. Shorter oral treatment regimens with a single 2-dose of metronidazole or for 2 to 3 days appear to achieve comparable immediate clinical response rates, but higher relapse rates have been reported. The beneficial effect of metronidazole results predominantly from its antianaerobic activity and because *Gardnerella vaginalis* is susceptible to the hydroxymetabolites of metronidazole. Although *Mycoplasma hominis* is resistant to metronidazole, the organism is usually not detected at follow-up visits of successfully treated patients. Similarly, *Mobiluncus curtsii* is resistant to metronidazole but usually disappears after therapy.[1,8,9,14,15] Several authors have reported highly successful therapy of BV with topical and oral clindamycin. Oral clindamycin (300 mg twice daily) or topical 2% cream or suppository (once daily for 7 days) has excellent anaerobic activity as well as moderate activity against *Gardnerella vaginalis* and *Mycoplasma hominis*. Clindamycin is the first equally effective alternative to metronidazole, especially in women who are pregnant, allergic to metronidazole, or cannot tolerate metronidazole.[1,8,14,15] Metronidazole intravaginal sponges (250 to 100 mg for 3 days) or chlorhexidene pessaries may also be effective in the treatment of BV.[6,8]

Amoxicillin or ampicillin (500 mg orally three or four times daily for 7 days) is less effective than metronidazole or clindamycin but may be useful during pregnancy, when metronidazole is contraindicated.[8,14,15] Despite indirect evidence of sexual transmission, treating the sexual partner to prevent reinfection remains controversial. Although the genital organisms associated with BV are commonly found in male sexual partners and are transmissible by intercourse, the factors that lead to disease may still be endogenous.[8] Several studies, including a randomized, double-blind clinical trial using metronidazole or placebo, have failed to demonstrate a substantial improvement in symptoms or microbiologic cure or recurrence rates by treatment of the sexual partner. Approximately 30% of initially responding patients have recurrence of identical signs and symptoms within 3 months. It remains unclear whether this is due to reinfection, failure to correct vaginal flora disturbance, or failure to re-establish the normal *Lactobacillus*-dominant flora. The current consensus is apparently to restrict treatment of partners to those situations in which intractable or recurrent BV is a problem.[1,3,5,8]

The usefulness of barrier methods of contraception to prevent reinfection is also controversial. Some authors find that oral contraceptives and barrier methods protect against and intrauterine devices increase the risk of infection, whereas others state that barrier methods do not affect the subjective or clinically diagnosed cure rates.[3,5]

The use of metronidazole during pregnancy is limited. Amoxicillin and ampicillin, in the doses described, are less effective than metronidazole but may be useful during pregnancy when metronidazole is contraindicated. Clinda-mycin, in the doses described, has also been shown effective.[1,3,8]

In the past, it was not routine to treat asymptomatic BV because patients often improved spontaneously over a period of months. If BV has the potential to cause upper genital or urinary tract disease, especially in pregnancy, a change in management procedure is necessary. Additional results of recent epidemiologic studies need to be corroborated.[1]

Candidiasis

EPIDEMIOLOGY

In the United States, after BV, the most common cause of vaginal infection is the yeast *Candida albicans*. Candidal vaginitis infection occurs at least once in at least 75% of women during the childbearing period. Forty percent to 50% of these women also have a second infection. Fewer than 5% of the adult female population suffers from repeated or recurrent VVC.[1,16]

Candida may be isolated from the genital tract of approximately 20% of asymptomatic, healthy women of childbearing age. Many women carry low concentrations of *Candida albicans* in the vagina without subjective symptoms. Several factors have been associated with increased rates of asymptomatic vaginal colonization with *Candida* and *Candida* vaginitis, including pregnancy, high estrogen–content oral contraceptives, uncontrolled diabetes mellitus, corticosteroid therapy, decreased cellular immunity, tight-fitting synthetic underclothing, antimicrobial therapy, intrauterine device, increased frequency of coitus, candy binges, obesity, and women frequenting STD clinics. Others, however, have reported no association of VVC with any particular birth control method; direction wiped following toileting; menstrual protection; use of feminine hygiene products; wearing tight clothing, hose, or synthetic underwear; diet; or stress.[1,16–19]

Candida is rarely isolated in premenarchal girls, and *Candida* vaginitis has a lower prevalence after menopause, emphasizing the hormonal dependence of the infection.[1] Reducing vaginal estrogen decreases recurrence, probably by influencing adherence of spores to the vaginal epithelium. Protection from osteoporosis by the use of estrogens may lead to an increased incidence.[16] Some authors have suggested that *Candida* can be sexually transmitted. One study found that patients with candidiasis were twice as likely as controls to have been sexually active in the past 4 weeks and that the odds increased with increasing frequency of sexual intercourse. Others, however, have found no relationship between new or multiple sexual partners in the past 4 weeks and an increased incidence of candidiasis.[18]

ETIOLOGY AND PATHOGENESIS

Between 65% and 90% of yeasts isolated from the vagina are strains of *Candida albicans*. The remainder are due to nonalbicans strains of *Candida* species. The most common of these are *Torulopsis glabrata* and *Candida tropicalis*. One investigator evaluated 175 patients and found that 65% were infected with *Candida albicans*, 23% with *Candida tropicalis*, and only one with *Torulopsis glabrata*.[20] *Candida albicans* adheres to the vaginal epithelial cells. It may then cause cell damage and inflammation by direct hyphae invasion of the epithelial tissue. The characteristic curdy vaginal discharge consists of an aggregate of hyphae and exfoliated epithelial cells with a few polymorphonuclear cells.[1]

Meticulous evaluation of women with recurrent candidal vaginitis rarely reveals a precise precipitating or causal factor. The repository theory maintains that there is a repository of infection that continually "seeds" the vagina. The gastrointestinal tract has been implicated as this source. This intestinal reservoir theory is founded on the report of retrieval of *Candida* from rectal culture in almost 100% of women with VVC. Nonetheless, concurrent treatment of both the gastrointestinal tract and the vaginitis has not eliminated chronic candidiasis.[1,19]

The immune status of the host may also play a role in candidal infections. The carbohydrate mannan secreted by the candidal organism causes immunosuppression in the host, possibly by induction of specific suppressor T lymphocytes. This suggests that recurrent or chronic candidal infection may be sheltered by a lack of immune response in the host.[19]

Sexual transmission of *Candida* has also been implicated in the pathogenesis of candidal infections. The species of *Candida* found in the vagina is often the same species found in the oral cavities of both partners and in the male ejaculate. Penile carriage in the circumcised male equals that in the uncircumcised male. A reservoir of infection may be in the seminal vesicles. Support for this theory are the finding of *Candida* organisms in ejaculate specimens; the absence of yeast organisms in prostatic fluid; the presence of yeast organisms in the seminal ejaculate; and the high fructose concentration in the seminal vesicles, which may nourish these organisms. Despite this inferred evidence, verification that sexual transmission occurs is still deficient, and the contribution of sexual transmission to the cause of VVC remains unknown.[1, 19]

CLINICAL PRESENTATION

The most common presenting complaint in acute VVC is vulvar pruritus, which is present in almost all symptomatic patients. Along with pruritus, vaginal discharge is also a frequent complaint, but neither is specific to VVC. Vaginal discharge is not always present and is frequently minimal. The vaginal discharge is typically described as cottage cheese–like in character but may vary from watery to thick and homogeneous. Vaginal tenderness, vulvar burning, dyspareunia, and dysuria are common. Odor, if present, is minimal and nonoffensive. Of the associated symptoms, only pruritus is consistently reported in *Candida* vaginitis. Characteristically symptoms are exacerbated in the week before the onset of menses, with some alleviation noted with onset of menstrual flow.[1, 10, 21]

Physical examination can range from showing only mild erythema of the labia minora with a white creamy discharge to a bright erythema, superficial skin erosions, and swelling often with satellite pustules of the labia and vulva. Pustules erode in intertriginous areas, leaving the characteristic erosions with a whitish collar of scale. On vaginal examination, white adherent "thrush" patches of exudate are seen on the erythematous, inflamed vaginal mucosa. The cervix is usually normal.[1, 21, 22]

It is important to keep in mind that history and physical examination are not invariably predictive of the presence of this organism, even with a history of oral contraceptive use, recent use of antibiotics, or pregnancy.[12]

DIAGNOSIS

Although a correct diagnosis often can be made based on clinical features alone, laboratory confirmation is necessary because even the most experienced physician may be mistaken. Many studies have verified the lack of specificity and sensitivity of signs and symptoms, and therefore diagnostic tests are mandatory even for uncomplicated *Candida* vaginitis. Further, patients often present with mixed infections that require simultaneous treatment. If the vaginal secretion is curdled, white, or slate colored; has a normal pH and no odor; and is of normal volume, the patient likely has a normal vaginal secretion.[10, 22] The pH of vaginal secretions, a saline wet mount, and a KOH preparation are the simplest, quickest, and most useful office procedures for identifying *Candida*.[22]

A saline wet mount preparation should routinely be done and has a sensitivity of 40% to 60%. Using the saline wet mount, the three most common causative organisms usually can be easily identified. *Candida* species is recognized by spores, *Trichomonas vaginalis* by motile trichomonads, and *Gardnerella vaginalis* by clue cells.[1, 22]

The 10% or 20% KOH preparation is remarkably valuable and even more sensitive than the saline wet mount in revealing the presence of pseudohyphae, spores, and budding yeast cells.[1,22] The KOH slide preparation provides a sensitivity in the range of 40% to 80%.[10,17,21]

A vaginal pH within normal range (4.0 to 4.5) is generally found with *Candida* vaginitis and essentially eliminates the possibility of trichomoniasis or *Gardnerella vaginalis* vaginitis. The finding of a vaginal pH in excess of 5.0 should alert the physician to the possibility of BV, trichomoniasis, or a mixed infection. *Candida*, however, can occasionally be present at all pH ranges.[1,22]

The cervical smear can also be a useful means of quickly identifying *Candida albicans* when blastospores and pseudomycelia are present. *Torulopsis glabrata* demonstrates budding or nonbudding yeast without pseudohyphae.[22]

The definitive diagnosis of acute *Candida* vaginitis in women with acute symptoms is made by the presence of symptoms and signs compatible with acute *Candida* vaginitis, a vaginal pH less than 4.5, positive saline microscopy, positive KOH preparation, a positive culture for *Candida* species, and exclusion of other causes of vaginitis.[10]

The microscopic identification of budding yeast or pseudohyphae is the best office test for identifying *Candida* organisms, but the lack of these is not evidence that the organism is absent. Microscopic examination of vaginal secretions, including saline and KOH preparations, is widely used but has been criticized for lack of sensitivity.[10,12]

Culture is the most sensitive method for detecting the presence of yeast. Isolation of vaginal yeast by culture, however, is expensive and requires at least 24 hours before results are available. Another pitfall of culture is that it fails to distinguish between *Candida* vaginal colonization and infection. The need for routine cultures is controversial, but certainly vaginal cultures should be performed in the presence of negative saline and KOH preparations. The most reliable means of culturing *Candida* is provided by use of Sabouraud medium. This medium reveals a large number of pseudomycelia or true mycelia with blastospores. The finding of chlamydospores is also striking and supposedly pathognomonic of *Candida*.[1,10,22]

A useful alternative for the rapid diagnosis of *Candida* vaginitis is the detection of *Candida albicans* antigens in vaginal secretions.[10] Many physicians lack the time, expertise, and equipment for microscopic examination. A new method for rapid, dependable diagnosis of *Candida* vaginitis uses a slide latex agglutination technique. This technique employs polystyrene latex particles that are coated with purified immunoglobulins from antiserum raised in rabbits against partially purified cell wall fractions of *Candida albicans* serotypes A and B and *Torulopsis glabrata*. One study revealed a sensitivity of 81% and a specificity of 98.5%. These results, however, could not be verified by others, and thus the rapid slide test offers no advantage over standard microscopy. In addition, the cost of office microscopy is approximately $0.10 versus $1.00 to $2.00 for the slide latex agglutination test.[1,10]

MEDICAL TREATMENT

Imidazoles are able to destroy a yeast organism only if the cell wall of the organism depends on ergosterol synthesis. To kill an organism that has a large amount of ergosterol in its cell wall, an increased concentration of an imidazole is necessary. Pyrimidines are converted into the chemotherapeutic agent 5-fluorouracil in the cell nucleus, where they destroy DNA or RNA.[20]

There is little evidence that the formulation of the topical antimycotic influences clinical efficacy, so the patient's preference can dictate which vehicle is used. Anticandidal creams may be preferable to suppositories because the cream can be shared by the patient with her partner. Extensive vulvar inflammation dictates local application of cream. Antifungal agents that have been used in the topical treatment of *Candida* vaginitis are listed in Table 38-1.[14,17,21]

Candida tropicalis and *Torulopsis glabrata* species are more difficult to eradicate because of the ineffectiveness of imidazole compounds on

Table 38-1. Topical Therapy of Vaginal Candidiasis

DRUG	FORMULATION	DOSAGE
Butoconazole (Femstat)	2% cream	5 g × 3 days
Clotrimazole	2% cream	5 g × 7–14 days
(Gyne-Lotrimin)	10% cream	5 g single application
(Mycelex-G)	100-mg vaginal tablet	1 tablet × 7 days
	100-mg vaginal tablet	2 tablets × 3 days
	500-mg vaginal tablet	1 tablet once
Miconazole	2% cream	5 g × 7 days
(Monistat 3)	100-mg vaginal suppository	2 suppository × 7 days
	200-mg vaginal suppository	2 suppository × 3 days
	1200-mg vaginal suppository	1 suppository once
Tioconazole	2% cream	5 grams × 3 days
	6.5% cream	5 g single application
Terconazole (Terazol)	2% cream	5 g × 3 days

the cell wall of these organisms. *Candida tropicalis* lacks ergosterol in its cell wall and thus is not killed by drugs designed to interfere with ergosterol synthesis. A tenfold increase in dose is necessary with drugs such as nystatin and miconazole to eliminate these organisms. One exception to this principle is butoconazole. This agent's spectrum of activity includes the *Candida tropicalis* organism. Butoconazole nitrate is a newer imidazole, and the cures gained with a 3-day course of butoconazole 2% cream have been reported to be comparable to those obtained with a 6-day course of miconazole nitrate 2% cream or a 3-day course of clotrimazole vaginal tablets (200 mg/day).[19, 20, 23]

Management of recurrent and chronic VVC remains troublesome, with approximately 25% of women with symptoms of VVC not responding to first-line therapy. The first step is to confirm the diagnosis of VVC with culture. Thereafter, predisposing factors must be eliminated. The majority of women with recurrent VVC do not have identifiable predisposing factors and require long-term maintenance suppressive prophylaxis. Because of the requirement for long-term therapy, the convenience of oral treatment is evident, and the best suppressive prophylaxis has been achieved with daily low-dose ketoconazole, 100 mg daily over 6 months. Despite

this, the benefits of suppressive therapy must be weighed against the potential toxicity of oral antifungal agents. Low-dose ketoconazole is surprisingly free of dose-dependent side-effects but is not free from idiosyncratic toxic reactions, such as hepatitis. The role of newer agents, such as fluconazole, requires further investigation. In addition, none of these agents have been specifically approved by the Food and Drug Administration (FDA) for use in VVC. Improvement in response to therapy may also be influenced by modifying the method of sexual contact, using barrier contraceptive methods, using barrier protection in underwear to keep the area dry and uncontaminated, prescribing specific antimycotic therapy directed at the site of infection in both partners, and, when feasible, changing the use of systemic broad-spectrum antibiotics.[1, 16, 19, 22] In resistant cases, painting the vagina, cervix, and vulva with 1% gentian violet daily for 3 to 4 days gives rapid relief of symptoms. It is efficacious despite being messy and causing permanent stains in clothing.[13]

There has been a significant trend toward short-course therapy with progressively higher antifungal doses, ultimately leading to single-dose therapeutic regimens. The formulation of these agents, together with the high doses inserted, results in persistence of active compounds in inhibitory concentration for several days. Single-dose and short-course therapy may be feasible in patients with occasional mild or moderate infections in pregnant and nonpregnant women.[1]

None of the oral antimycotic agents have been specifically approved by the FDA for use in VVC. Nonetheless, ketoconozole (400 mg daily for 5 days), itraconazole (200 mg daily for 3 days or 400 g single dose), and fluconazole (150 mg in a single dose) have all proved efficacious in attaining clinical and mycologic cure in acute VVC. Clinical results of oral therapy are equal, if not superior, to conventional topical antimycotic therapy. Several studies have apparently indicated that most women prefer oral therapy if given the choice. Again the advantages of oral therapy must be weighed against the possible side-effects and toxicity. Hepatotoxicity occurs in approximately every 10,000 to 15,000 patients treated with oral ketoconazole therapy. Other side-effects include gastrointestinal upset in 10% and rarely anaphylaxis. The side-effects of itraconazole and fluconazole seem to be much less frequent.[1]

Because clinical response tends to be protracted and recurrences more frequent, the treatment of VVC during pregnancy is more troublesome. Most topical antifungal agents are effective when prescribed for periods of 1 to 2 weeks. Although systemic absorption of topical antifungals is minimal, the potential risk of vaginal antimycotic therapy to the developing fetus during the first trimester of pregnancy must be weighed against the benefit gained by the patient. Although longer duration of therapy may be required to eliminate the yeast infection, single high-dose therapy with clotrimazole has been shown to be effective in pregnancy.[10]

Trichomonas

EPIDEMIOLOGY

Trichomonas vaginalis is the only organism in this species regarded to be pathogenic. Humans are its only natural host. It is considered the predominant nonviral STD. In women of reproductive age, *Trichomonas* is the second most common cause of bacterial vaginitis, second only to BV. The prevalence of trichomoniasis is related to the level of sexual activity of the specific group being evaluated. The incidence of *Trichomonas* varies from 2% in private offices to 56% in STD clinics. Trichomoniasis has been reported in approximately 5% of women in family planning clinics, 13% to 25% of women visiting gynecology clinics, 50% to 75% of prostitutes, and 7% to 35% of women in STD clinics.[1] Based on some authors' reports, if a conservative estimate of 5% prevalence in the general population is given, at least 6 million women and their partners are infected annually in the United States. Peak incidence is between ages 16 and 35.[1,24]

Trichomoniasis can be documented in at least 85% of female partners of infected men consistent with the known high transmission rate. Cure rates for women are increased with simultaneous treatment of their male sexual partners. There is also a high prevalence of gonorrhea in women with trichomoniasis.[1]

Nonsexual transmission is theoretically possible although poorly documented. The agent is site-specific. Live organisms have been found in urine and in semen specimens after exposure to air for several hours. The *Trichomonas* organism can also survive for hours on damp towels and clothing used by infected women. Use of nonbarrier contraception is significantly related to transmission. Oral contraceptives may decrease the prevalence of trichomoniasis.[1,24] The clinical development of trichomoniasis in pregnancy is the same as that seen in nonpregnant women, and there is no satisfactory evidence that trichomoniasis is associated with premature rupture of membranes and prematurity. Perinatal transmission does occasionally occur.[1]

ETIOLOGY AND PATHOGENESIS

Trichomonas vaginalis is thought to be the first recognized STD. It is a unicellular flagellate that generally appears pyriform or ovoid because of ameboid movement. In fresh preparations, it is recognized by its jerky, swaying movement. It is an extracellular parasite, reproduces by binary fission, attaches to epithelial cells of mucous membranes, and is a strict anaerobe. The organism exists only in the genitourinary tract on the squamous epithelial cells lining the anterior fornix of the vagina, Skene's glands, and urethra in women and in the urethra, prostate gland, and under the foreskin in uncircumcised men. Because urogenital trichomoniasis is a multicentric infection in women, systemic treatment is mandatory for cure.[1, 8, 10, 24]

CLINICAL PRESENTATION

Most concerning is that 10% to 50% of infected women are asymptomatic. Approximately one third of these asymptomatic women become symptomatic within 6 months. Symptomatic women may have the acute onset of profuse, yellow vaginal discharge; abnormal vaginal odor; vulvar pruritus; cystitis; dysuria; and mild dyspareunia. Fewer than 10% have an erythematous vulva. Symptoms may exacerbate during or immediately after menstruation. The most common symptom, increased vaginal discharge, is found in more than half of the symptomatic cases. Pruritus occurs in 25% to 50% of patients and is often severe. About half of infected women relate some degree of dyspareunia. Some patients have lower abdominal discomfort, but *Trichomonas* has not be shown to cause pelvic inflammatory disease. It is noninvasive so lymphadenopathy is rare. Trichomoniasis is strongly associated with BV because *Trichomonas* creates an anaerobic environment, allowing the overgrowth of anaerobic bacteria. In any case, other STDs should always be suspected.[1, 24, 25]

Although controversial, the incubation period is estimated to range from 3 to 28 days. Vaginal discharge is reported in 50% to 75% of women with trichomoniasis. The classically described green, frothy, malodorous discharge, however, is related in only about 10% of symptomatic infected patients. The discharge is gray in about 75% of patients. Frothiness is seen more commonly in BV. *Trichomonas* infection usually elicits an acute inflammatory response leading to the profuse vaginal discharge, which contains large numbers of polymorphonuclear cells. In general, the number of polymorphonuclear cells correlates with the intensity of the symptoms.[1, 24]

Physical findings represent a spectrum of findings. Diffuse vulvar erythema is seen in 10% to 33%. The vaginal walls are also erythematous and granular appearing in severe cases. Colpitis macularis or punctate cervical hemorrhages (strawberry spots) are apparent to the naked eye in only 2% of cases but can be seen on colposcopy in 45% of patients.[1, 24, 25]

Recurrent trichomonal infections are common, indicating that a clinically significant protective immunity does not appear to occur. An immune response to *Trichomonas*, however, does develop as manifested by low titers of serum antibody.[1]

DIAGNOSIS

The sensitivity of symptoms and signs associated with trichomoniasis is low. Careful history, physical examination, wet mount preparation, and wider use of more sensitive tests for subclinical infection, such as culture or direct immunofluorescent staining of vaginal fluid, may lead to improved detection and control of this infection.[12, 25]

Vaginal pH is generally elevated above 5. On saline wet mount preparation, an increase in polymorphonuclear cells is almost always present, although their absence does not exclude trichomoniasis. Optimally patients should be advised not to douche for 2 days before their examination because douching lowers the number of viable organisms, making it more difficult to detect trichomonads. Vaginal secretions should be collected on cotton swabs from the anterior and lateral vaginal fornices, not the endocervical area. To perform a wet mount preparation, a swab containing secretions is placed into a small amount of saline, and this suspension is placed onto a slide, covered, and examined under the microscope. The ovoid parasites are slightly larger than polymorphonuclear cells and are best recognized by their jerky mobility. The saline wet mount preparation, however, is positive in only 40% to 80% of cases. The false-negative rate for this technique is 50%.[1,24,26,27]

Culture is currently considered the most sensitive method for detecting *Trichomonas vaginalis*, with 95% sensitivity. The false-negative rate for culture is 5%. Swabs from the infected area are placed directly into suitable medium, such as Kupferberg, Feinberg-Whittington, or Diamonds culture. The major disadvantage of culture is the length of time for diagnosis, 2 to 7 days. When properly performed, both saline wet mount and culture are close to 100% specific.[1,24,26,27]

Two new staining methods have used monoclonal antibody technology. Sensitivity and specificity are claimed to be similar to that of culture. To stain trichomonads selectively, *Trichomonas* direct enzyme immunoassay and fluorescent direct immunoassay employ peroxidase-labeled and fluorescent-labeled solutions of monoclonal antibodies to various *Trichomonas vaginalis*, structures such as membrane, cytoplasm, nuclei, and flagella. This method has several advantages over both wet mount examination and culture. It is more sensitive than wet mount because nonmotile trichomonads can be detected, and results can be available within 1 hour, permitting both diagnosis and treatment at a single clinic visit. One report demonstrated that monoclonal antibody staining detected 86% of positive specimens. The false-negative rates for direct immunofluorescence techniques, however, are reported at 36%.[24,26,27]

Thus wet mount studies were insensitive but quick and readily available. Culture is the most sensitive but requires a several day waiting period for diagnosis. Direct immunofluorescence with monoclonal antibodies holds promise as a sensitive and specific alternative to cultures for rapid detection of *Trichomonas vaginalis* in the future.[26]

MEDICAL TREATMENT

The cornerstone of therapy is the 5-nitroimidazole group of drugs—metronidazole, tinidazole and ornidazole. Only metronidazole is available in the United States. Oral therapy is preferred to local topical therapy primarily because infection of the urethra and periurethral glands is a source for endogenous reinfection.[1]

Standard therapy consists of oral metronidazole (250 mg three times daily for 7 days). The cure rate is 95%. Comparable results have also been obtained with a single oral dose of 2.0 g of metronidazole, with cure rates in the range of 82% to 88%. Because patient compliance is highest with single-dose therapy, this regimen is preferred clinically. The cure rate increases to more than 90% when sexual partners are treated simultaneously. Additional advantages of single-dose therapy include better patient compliance, lower total dose, shorter period of alcohol avoidance, and, perhaps, decreased ensuing *Candida* vaginitis from a less disruptive effect on the vaginal ecosystem. A disadvantage of single-dose therapy is the need to insist on simultaneous treatment of the sexual partner. Occasionally patients fail to respond to conventional metronidazole therapy. Patients who do not respond to the initial course often respond to a second standard course of 7-day therapy.[1,14,15,24,28]

Most strains of *Trichomonas vaginalis* are susceptible to metronidazole, although resistant strains are rarely isolated. When highly resistant infections occur, increased dosages of metronidazole may be needed for the drug to cure the infection. Concomitant intravaginal treatment with metronidazole tablets or suppositories may be helpful.[8] Resistance is relative and varies from mild to severe. Susceptibility data should be obtained before treatment of intractable cases. Intravenous metronidazole is used only for patients who cannot tolerate high oral doses required for cure. Most treatment failures appear to result from reinfection from untreated partners or poor compliance with taking medication. Other medications may alleviate symptoms. Clotrimazole, an imidazole without the 5-nitro group, eradicates symptoms with topical vaginal use but does not eradicate the infection as effectively as oral metronidazole. It may serve a role in relieving symptoms in cases refractory to metronidazole and in the first trimester of pregnancy.[8, 14, 15, 24, 28]

A metallic taste in the mouth, headache, dizziness, darkening of the urine, and nausea (10%) are common dose-related side-effects of metronidazole therapy. Self-limited leukopenia (7.5%) has been rarely reported but has not been associated with single-dose therapy. When combined with alcohol, metronidazole may produce a disulfiramlike reaction. Other adverse reactions have included a variety of generalized skin reactions, potentiation of warfarin activity, and neurologic reactions in those receiving long-term therapy. There appears to be no antagonism between metronidazole and other antibiotics.[1, 8]

The primary reason to treat *Trichomonas vaginalis* is to relieve discomfort from inflammation of the Bartholin's and Skene's glands and stop further sexual transmission. *Trichomonas vaginalis* by itself is not associated with severe sequelae. It should serve as an alarm, however, to the possible presence of other STDs. Partners of infected women should be treated empirically. In addition, it changes the normal vaginal environment, with increase in pH and promotion of facultative and anaerobic bacterial growth, which can ultimately lead to BV. This bacterial overgrowth can lead to serious sequelae as discussed earlier, including pelvic inflammatory disease, ectopic pregnancy, infertility, and preterm labor.[24]

Neonatal transmission of *Trichomonas* can occur at delivery. Metronidazole is contraindicated in the first trimester of pregnancy because it readily crosses the placenta, may have teratogenic effects, and fetal levels equal that of the mother. Although many clinicians administer this medication in the second and third trimester and no teratogenic actions have been reported in humans, its safety in the rest of pregnancy has not been established. No other adequate therapy exists, however. For patients with severe symptoms after the first trimester, treatment with 2 g of metronidazole in a single dose may be considered. Clotrimazole topical therapy may also serve a role in relieving symptoms in the first trimester of pregnancy. Pregnant women probably should be treated to prevent sequelae caused by bacterial proliferation and subsequent upper genital tract infection. Treatment can be delayed until the second trimester with no adverse effects. Metronidazole reduces the number of anaerobic bacteria as well as eliminating *Trichomonas vaginalis*, allowing normalization of the vaginal ecosystem.[1, 14, 15, 24, 28]

If *Neisseria gonorrhoeae* is found on Gram's stain or culture of endocervical, urethral, or vaginal discharge, the treatment regimen should be the same as that recommended for uncomplicated gonorrhea in adults, including cotreatment for chlamydial infection (see later).[14]

Differentiation of Vulvovaginal Candidiasis, Bacterial Vaginosis, and Trichomonas Vaginitis

Although many of the symptoms and signs of these three infections are similar, several of the features of each can help in differentiation. The normal vaginal pH is 4.0 to 4.5 and remains in normal range in VVC. With BV and *Trichomonas*, the pH is generally elevated above 5.0. Although discharge may vary in consistency, volume, odor, and color for all three entities, BV and *Trichomonas vaginalis* commonly have a more offensive odor. The amine test is performed by adding 10% KOH to a sample of the vaginal secretions. BV liberates a fishy odor. This may also occasionally be present in *Trichomonas* infection. It is not found in candidiasis.

Saline microscopy reveals normal flora, blastospores, and pseudohyphae in VVC. Clue cells, coccobacillary flora, and absence of polymorphonuclear leukocytes are noted in bacterial vaginosis. Motile trichomonads, numerous leukocytes, and no clue cells or abnormal flora are noted in trichomoniasis. Ten percent KOH microscopy shows pseudohyphae and spores in candidiasis but is negative in BV and trichomoniasis.

Chlamydia trachomatis

EPIDEMIOLOGY

Chlamydia trachomatis is currently the most common STD in the United States. There are an estimated 3 to 5 million new cases each year, and the incidence is increasing. The incidence of *Chlamydia trachomatis* in sexually active women at risk is reported between 6% and 23%. It is two to five times more prevalent than *Neisseria gonorrhoeae*, and co-infection with *Chlamydia trachomatis* and *Neisseria gonorrhoeae* is common. The lack of a widely available diagnostic test; nonspecific symptoms of *Chlamydia* infection; lack of partner notification; and the requirement for multiple dose, several day therapy have been major factors contributing to increasing incidence.[29–33]

Women aged 16 through 25 are reported to account for 81.7% of all chlamydial infections. Females younger than 16 or older than 35 accounted for only 2.4% of all infections. The incidence is especially high in adolescents, approximately 40%. It is estimated that 20% to 40% of all sexually active women have been exposed to *Chlamydia trachomatis* and have positive antibodies to the organism. *Chlamydia* cases are more likely to be white than their gonorrhea counterparts. In women attending a STD clinic, one author reported that 17% had positive cervical cultures, with an incidence of 13% in whites, 7% in married women, none in those using a diaphragm, and 38% in those also positive for *Neisseria gonorrhoeae*. Black women are more likely to be infected than white women, and unmarried pregnant women have higher infection rates than married pregnant women.[29,31,33–37]

Eighty percent of women are asymptomatic, and most cases are identified through screening or contact tracing.[34] The asymptomatic patients are obviously more likely to suffer from long-term consequences of the infection. The risk of chlamydial infection among asymptomatic persons is increased in those with multiple sexual partners, a new sexual partner in the preceding 2 months, or a sexual partner with a chlamydial infection. There is some evidence that oral contraceptives increase the risk of chlamydial infection as compared with women using no birth control methods, but it is unclear whether this relationship is causal or simply related to sexual behavior. Therefore routine testing for *Chlamydia trachomatis* is recommended for asymptomatic persons at high risk of infection.[31,33,35,37]

Chlamydia is transmitted by sexual contact. Between 25% and 50% of patients with STD are infected by *Chlamydia trachomatis*. The incidence of simultaneous infection by *Neisseria gonorrhoeae* and *Chlamydia trachomatis* has been reported as 9.2%. Nonetheless, the same investigator reported that among 63 patients with *Neisseria gonorrhoeae* infection, 26 (41.3%) were also infected by *Chlamydia trachomatis*. Among patients infected by *Chlamydia trachomatis*, 10.6% also had positive cultures for *Neisseria gonorrhoeae*.[29] Another investigator reported that *Neisseria gonorrhoeae* and *Chlamydia trachomatis* are found co-infecting an individual in approximately 60% of cases.[33,35]

The Centers for Disease Control have recommended routine chlamydial testing in asymptomatic persons who attend STD or family planning clinics and for those who otherwise would not receive antichlamydial therapy and are in high-risk groups. *Chlamydia* is the causative agent in about half of cases of mucopurulent cervicitis. It is estimated that chlamydial infections are responsible for 25% to 50% of the 1 million cases of pelvic inflammatory disease reported annually in the United States. Pelvic inflammatory disease is an important cause of infertility and ectopic pregnancy. Unexplained pyuria or culture-negative cystitis in sexually active women should suggest the possibility of chlamydial infection. Chlamydial infections are estimated to cost between 1 and 2.2 billion dollars per year. It appears to becomes cost-effective to screen for *Chlamydia* in populations in which the prevalence of infection exceeds 6%.[30–33,37]

Approximately 8% to 12% of pregnant women have cervical chlamydial infections. Infection during pregnancy can produce postpartum endometritis, and *Chlamydia trachomatis* is transmitted to the infant in more than half of deliveries. More than 155,000 infants are born to mothers with chlamydial infections every year. Neonatal infection can result in ophthalmia neonatorum conjunctivitis, nasopharyngeal colonization, and pneumonia. Therefore pregnant women in high-risk groups should at least be tested at their first prenatal visit. The American College of Obstetricians and Gynecologists recommends chlamydial culture not only at the first prenatal visit, but also during the third trimester in this group.[31,37]

Infections and complications caused by *Chlamydia trachomatis* include pelvic inflammatory disease, obstructive infertility, perihepatitis, ectopic pregnancy, bartholinitis, urethritis, cervicitis, salpingitis, preterm labor and birth, low birth weight, premature rupture of membranes, stillbirth, chorioamnionitis, and postpartum or postabortal endometritis.[30,33,35,37,38]

ETIOLOGY AND PATHOGENESIS

The name *chlamydozoa* comes from the Greek word for "cloak."[38] Chlamydiae are obligate intracellular bacteria that use intracellular biochemical products produced by the host cell. The phagosome enlarges as the organism replicates, ultimately filling the cell's cytoplasm and displacing the nucleus to one side. This developing phagosome is referred to as an *inclusion*.[33,37]

The primary target cells for the nonlymphogranuloma venereum *Chlamydia trachomatis* infections are columnar epithelial cells. These cells line the surfaces of the conjunctivae, urethra, endocervix, endometrium, and fallopian tubes, which partially explains the association with certain clinical disease syndromes caused by these organisms. A classic acute inflammatory response with polymorphonuclear leukocytes is not seen in recurrent infections, but rather a mononuclear cell response is seen. This implies that recurrent chlamydial infection may be less likely to be symptomatic while causing damage to the upper genital tract.[33,37]

CLINICAL PRESENTATION

Most cases of *Chlamydia trachomatis* genital tract infections are asymptomatic. Many patients appear not to experience symptoms in the acute phase of infection. One author reported a large series of more than 3000 patients in which only 24% were symptomatic.[29] The most common complaint in this group was vaginal discharge with or without pain. If a patient related symptoms of vaginal discharge or pelvic pain, she was almost twice as likely to have a positive culture for *Chlamydia trachomatis* than if she were asymptomatic. Common symptoms are vaginal discharge, bleeding, lower abdominal pain, or dysuria. These are nonspecific, however, similar to *Neisseria gonorrhoeae*, *Chlamydia trachomatis* frequently infects the urethra (25% to 50%), rectum (25%), cervix (40% to 75%), salpinx (10% to 20%), and abdomen causing Fitz-Hugh-Curtis syndrome (30% to 80%). Because 30% to 50% of women with cervical gonococcal infection have simultaneous chlamydial infections, identification of gonorrhea distinguishes a group of women at high risk for chlamydial infection and its sequelae.[29,30,33,37,39]

The endocervix is the most common female organ infected by *Chlamydia trachomatis*. The majority of these infections, however, are asymptomatic and thus detectable only by screening. Cervicitis is the most common finding during pelvic examination. The presence of specific signs attributed to mucopurulent cervicitis makes the diagnosis of *Chlamydia* likely. These signs include a green or yellow mucopurulent cervical discharge, cervical ectopy, edema in the area of ectopy, and easily produced endocervical mucosal bleeding. Clinically the presence of green or yellow mucopus on a swab that has been inserted into the cervical os or 10 or more polymorphonuclear leukocytes per oil immersion field of a cervical Gram's stain smear in non-menstruating women strongly suggests chlamydial endocervical infection.[29,30,33,37]

Although most *Chlamydia trachomatis* urethral infections are asymptomatic, an acute urethritis that mimics a cystitis is sometimes seen. Pyuria with a negative urine culture in a young, sexually active woman with a new sexual partner and these symptoms should alert the physician to possible chlamydial infection.[30]

Chlamydia trachomatis is an important cause of pelvic inflammatory disease, causing up to one third of all cases. The clinical presentation of chlamydial pelvic inflammatory disease is similar to that of other organisms, although the symptoms may be less severe than those manifested in women with gonococcal pelvic inflammatory disease. There may be less fever or leukocytosis. The most common presenting complaint is lower abdominal pain. Fever and increased vaginal discharge may be present. Commonly symptoms begin at the time of menstruation. On examination, uterine tenderness with cervical motion is present in addition to unilateral or bilateral abdominal pain. Enlarged fallopian tubes are not always palpable but when present are highly suggestive of the disease. A large adnexal mass indicates the presence of a tubo-ovarian abscess or possibly an ectopic pregnancy.[30,33,37]

Perihepatitis, known by the eponym Fitz-Hugh-Curtis syndrome, used to be caused primarily by *Neisseria gonorrhoeae* but now is more commonly caused by *Chlamydia trachomatis*. It is conjectured that organisms run over from the tubal ostium into the pelvic cavity and gain access to the right upper quadrant by following the flow of the peritoneal fluid to the diaphragm. The clinical presentation is the same as pelvic inflammatory disease, with right upper quadrant pain and tenderness, nausea, vomiting, and fever in a young, sexually active woman. Fitz-Hugh-Curtis syndrome may occur with or without clinical evidence of pelvic inflammatory disease.[33,37]

DIAGNOSIS

The gold standard test for the diagnosis of *Chlamydia trachomatis* infection is culture in mammalian cell lines. The McCoy cell culture assay is most commonly used.[29] It is expensive (approximately $15 per test), however, and requires multiple steps and 6 to 7 days to complete. Special precautions must be taken to collect and transport specimens properly.[37] Specimens must be refrigerated and transported at 4°C to the laboratory within 24 hours to maintain viability of the *Chlamydia* organism.[30] Culture is the most sensitive and specific test for detecting chlamydial infection in asymptomatic patients. Urethral and endocervical cultures have a sensitivity of 80% to 90% and specificity of 100%.[28,31,33]

When obtaining endocervical samples, a small wire brush, originally designed to obtain endocervical cell samples for cytologic studies, may be better than swabs. The goal is to obtain a good sample of endocervical lining cell with minimal contamination by vaginal secretions. When serial samples are procured, the best specimen for *Chlamydia trachomatis* isolation is the last one obtained. Simultaneously culturing urethra and endocervix increases the yield of culture-positive women by as much as 20%.[37]

Two advances in cell culture techniques have simplified these methods. These include the use of cell monolayers grown in 96-well microtiter plates and fluorescein-conjugated monoclonal antibodies to identify chlamydial inclusions in infected monolayers. This increases the sensitivity of initial inoculation and makes a second passage needless. Thus the results are available after 3 days, and the cost of the culture is decreased. Despite these advances, the strict transport conditions required to maintain viability and the small number of laboratories equipped to perform these cultures have limited this testing to larger, centralized laboratories. Thus noncultural methods for detection of *Chlamydia* antigen have been developed.[30]

There are two general approaches to antigen

detection. These are the direct immunofluorescence staining of specimens using monoclonal antibodies (DFA) and elution from swabs with measurement by enzyme-linked immunosorbent assay (ELISA) methods.[28, 30, 33]

Chlamydia-specific monoclonal antibodies conjugated to fluorescein isothiocyanate have become accessible for rapid staining of *Chlamydia trachomatis* elementary bodies in specimens. This test requires preparation of a meticulously obtained endocervical or urethral specimen on a glass slide. The slide is air dried and fixed at the bedside with methanol or acetone that is supplied with the collection kit. An advantage of this method is that fixed slides can be held at room temperature for several days until transport to the laboratory. Using a one-step procedure in the laboratory, slides are stained with conjugated monoclonal antibody reagent. In high-risk populations with 15% to 26% prevalence of infection, this test is similar in sensitivity (90%) and specificity (95%) to culture. In populations with a lower prevalence, between 9% and 11%, however, the sensitivity drops to 77%.[30] Theoretically this test could be performed in the physician's office or clinic while the patient waits for the results. A high-quality fluorescent microscope equipped with special objectives is required, however, and makes the technique difficult in most office settings. In addition, a well-trained, experienced microscopist is necessary to detect the elementary bodies, which may be present in only small numbers.[28, 31, 33, 37]

Chlamydia antigen detection by ELISA also has become increasingly available over the last several years. Specimens are collected and placed in a special transport medium that is provided with the diagnostic kit. Transport conditions are not as strict as for cultures, but specimens still must be delivered to the laboratory within a few days of collection. Results are available within 24 hours of procuring the specimen. Neither sensitivity nor specificity is 100%, however. The sensitivity of the ELISA test is similar to that of the DFA test in high-risk groups of women and higher than the DFA test in groups of women

with intermediate prevalence range.[30] An advantage of the ELISA method over the DFA method is that the result for a positive test is objective, so specially trained personnel and instruments are not required.[37] Fluorescent antibody microscopy and ELISA may be useful where culture is unavailable or too expensive.[28, 31, 33]

MEDICAL TREATMENT

The principal problem in treating *Chlamydia trachomatis* infection is diagnosis. To date, emergence of antimicrobial resistance has not been reported.[30]

The drug of choice for *Chlamydia trachomatis* infection in adults is tetracycline or its derivatives. Success rates for tetracycline (500 mg orally four times a day for 7 days) are greater than 90%. Doxycycline and minocycline are equally effective. They both have the advantage of twice-daily dosing. Minocycline, however, has been reported to cause inner ear toxicity and is not used extensively. Doxycycline (100 mg twice daily for 7 days) has become the actual drug of choice for most chlamydial infections because of the simplicity of twice-daily dosing and the availability of a generic form. The failure rate of therapy is approximately 5% in most studies.[14, 15, 29, 33, 37, 40]

Erythromycin is recommended as the drug of choice in patients who are intolerant or allergic to tetracycline and in pregnant patients. With the large number of cases of *Chlamydia trachomatis* and the incidence of drug intolerance, allergies, and contraindications, the availability of alternative medications is important. Up to one third of patients complain of gastrointestinal and other side-effects when given tetracycline, doxycycline, or erythromycin.[9] Other alternative drugs include sulfisoxazole (1 g orally four times daily for 7 days or 500 mg orally four times daily for 10 days) or amoxicillin (500 mg orally four times daily for 7 days).[9, 14, 15, 29, 33, 37]

One investigator reported a protocol that compared clindamycin with erythromycin for *Chlamydia* infection. Fifty-six patients enrolled in the clindamycin arm and 57 in the erythromycin arm of the protocol. Forty-seven of 56 (83.9%) completed clindamycin therapy and had microbiologic cures. Only 25 of 57 (43.9%) women, however, completed erythromycin therapy. The number of side-effect failures for erythromycin was 22 of 57 (38.6%). The number of side-effect failures for clindamycin was only 4 of 56 (7.1%) The adverse reactions most commonly experienced were nausea and vomiting with or without abdominal pain. A rash developed in one patient in each arm of the protocol, and one patient developed esophageal ulcers with clindamycin therapy.[29]

Chlamydia may sometimes persist despite what appears to be adequate therapy. Azithromycin is the prototype azalide antibiotic chemically related to erythromycin and seems to be effective in the treatment of uncomplicated *Chlamydia trachomatis* infections. Single-dose therapy with azithromycin (1 g orally) may be particularly useful in circumventing compliance problems and is as effective as a standard 7-day course of doxycycline. Other STDs that can be treated with azithromycin include *Neisseria gonorrhoeae, Treponema pallidum,* and *Haemophilus ducreyi.* Azithromycin develops high and prolonged tissue concentrations, allowing once-daily dosing with shorter courses of therapy of 1 to 5 days.[40,41]

Ofloxin (300 mg twice daily for 7 days) has also been found effective in eradicating endocervical *Chlamydia trachomatis* infection and for treatment of mixed infection caused by *Chlamydia trachomatis* and *Neisseria gonorrhoeae.*[42,43]

Chlamydia trachomatis infection is a STD. Therefore it is extremely important that both sex partners be treated to prevent reinfection. Partners of patients with chlamydial disease are usually asymptomatic. It is particularly important to relate this fact in counseling infected women because asymptomatic men often deny that they might have a STD.[37]

Chlamydia infection often silently coexists with gonorrhea and may go undetected until sequelae occur. Therefore both diseases should be treated simultaneously.[39] In clinical settings in which routine testing for *Chlamydia* is not available, treatment is often prescribed based on clinical signs or as cotreatment for gonorrhea.[14] *Chlamydia* infections, however, are not treated by ceftriaxone, which is used for gonorrhea, and additional treatment is necessary if *Chlamydia* is present concurrently.[44]

Tetracyclines must be avoided in pregnant women and in children younger than 9 years of age owing to tooth staining. Erythromycin (500 mg orally four times daily for 7 days) is the treatment of choice for pregnant women. Nonetheless, pregnant women may be intolerant to erythromycin, especially during the first trimester. Lowering the dose to 250 mg four times daily and extending the total treatment period to 2 weeks is one way to circumvent this problem. This regimen, however, has not been studied extensively. Erythromycin ethylsuccinate, 800 mg orally four times a day for 7 days, or erythromycin ethylsuccinate, 400 mg orally four times a day for 14 days, may be better tolerated. Erythromycin estolate is contraindicated during pregnancy because drug-related hepatotoxicity can result. Alternative drugs are sulfisoxazole and amoxicillin. Sulfisoxazole should be avoided near the time of delivery because the sulfonamides interfere with bilirubin binding to albumin in neonates. Amoxicillin (500 mg orally three times daily for 7 days) should be used only after all other approaches have been attempted. In addition, one should remember that beta lactam antibiotics of the cephalosporin class have absolutely no effect on *Chlamydia trachomatis.*[14,15,33,37]

Chlamydia Trachomatis (Lymphogranuloma Venereum Immunotypes)

EPIDEMIOLOGY

Lymphogranuloma venereum (LGV) is an uncommon disease in the United States, with fewer than 100 cases reported annually.[37,45]

ETIOLOGY AND PATHOGENESIS

LGV immunotypes of *Chlamydia trachomatis* are more virulent than those described earlier. Progressive infection of cell monolayers results in microscopically discernible cytopathic effects.[37]

CLINICAL PRESENTATION

The most pronounced clinical characteristic of this disease is enlarged, painful inguinal lymphadenopathy. Lymphadenopathy is the result of multiple enlarged, matted nodes. These are generally unilateral but may be bilateral in occasional cases. Approximately one third of patients manifest enlarged lymph nodes above and below the inguinal ligament (Groove sign). This finding is said to be pathognomonic for this disease. The Groove sign, however, has also been reported to be seen in patients with chancroid. Lymph nodes are often extremely tender and may coalesce to form buboes that suppurate and produce draining cutaneous sinuses.[14, 37, 45]

Systemic symptoms of fever, chills, myalgia, and malaise are frequently seen in patients with LGV, and some patients have systemic lymphadenopathy.[37]

The primary infection may occur in the posterior third of the vagina or in the cervix, and these patients may present with pelvic pain and symptoms of proctitis. These areas are primarily drained by the pelvic lymph nodes. Primary proctitis resembling Crohn's disease may be seen in homosexual men and women who practice passive anal intercourse.[37] Ulceration is found in fewer than 30% of women. When present, the ulcer of LGV is a transient, shallow, painless ulcer, which antedates the inguinal lymphadenopathy by 7 to 30 days.[45]

Without adequate treatment, fibrosis of the inguinal lymphadenopathy occurs and leads to lymphatic obstruction and lymphedema of the external genitalia. *Chlamydia trachomatis* is rarely cultured from the lesions at this late stage. Rather secondary infections with other organisms, including anaerobes, ensue. Extensive reconstructive surgery may be needed at this phase.[37]

DIAGNOSIS

In general, the diagnosis is made based on serologic criteria with a chlamydial complement fixation titer of greater than 1:64 and clinical characteristics of LGV. Titers of this magnitude, however, may occasionally be seen with more commonly occurring non-LGV serotypes of *Chlamydia trachomatis*.

Specific diagnosis of LGV requires culture of *Chlamydia trachomatis* with immunotyping or the use of microimmunofluorescence serology, which can differentiate type-specific serologic responses. Microimmunofluorescence, however, is available only in particular research laboratories in the United States.[45]

MEDICAL TREATMENT

The drug of choice for this disease is doxycycline (100 mg orally twice a day for 21 days). Tetracycline (500 mg orally four times daily for 21 days), erythromycin (500 mg orally four times daily for 21 days), sulfisoxazole (500 mg orally four times daily for 21 days), or an equivalent sulfonamide are all effective alternative regimens in the management of LGV. Buboes should be drained by needle aspiration rather than formal incision and drainage because the latter procedure may increase the risk of generating chronic lymphocutaneous fistulas.[14, 28, 37]

Atrophic Vaginitis

ETIOLOGY AND PATHOGENESIS

Clinically significant atrophic vaginitis is unusual, and the majority of women with atrophic vaginal mucosa are asymptomatic and without inflammation. The symptomatic patient demonstrates inflamed, atrophic vaginal mucosa. The epithelium becomes thin and lacks glycogen because of reduced endogenous estrogens. This leads to reduced lactic acid production and increased vaginal pH to 6.5 to 7.5. The elevated pH encourages the overgrowth of nonacidophilic coliform bacteria and the dissipation of *Lactobacillus* species. Symptoms are usually absent, especially in the absence of intercourse.[1, 13]

CLINICAL PRESENTATION

Characteristic symptoms include vaginal soreness, dyspareunia, and infrequent spotting or discharge. Burning or vaginal soreness is frequently precipitated by intercourse. The vaginal mucosa is thin with diffuse redness and occasional petechiae and shows lack of vaginal folds. Vulvar atrophy may also be present. Discharge, if present, may vary from a blood discharge to thick or watery, and the pH ranges from 5.5 to 7.0.[1]

DIAGNOSIS

On microscopic examination of the vaginal secretions, increased polymorphonuclear cells associated with small, round epithelial cells and bacteria are observed.[13] These round, parabasal cells represent immature squamous cells that have not been exposed to adequate estrogen. The *Lactobacillus*-dominated flora are replaced by mixed flora of gram-negative rods. Bacterial cultures in these patients are not necessary and can be misleading.[1, 13]

TREATMENT

The treatment of atrophic vaginitis is predominately topical vaginal estrogens. If systemic symptoms are noted, oral estrogens may be considered. One half to one applicatorful of conjugated estrogens (Premarin) cream used nightly for 1 to 2 weeks is usually sufficient to alleviate atrophic vaginitis.[1] Some of our own patients are actually maintained on small amounts of topical estrogen applied to the vaginal introitus nightly.

Neisseria gonorrhoea

EPIDEMIOLOGY

Approximately 2 million persons acquire gonorrhea every year in the United States. The re-

ported incidence of gonorrhea increased markedly from the mid 1960s to the mid 1970s, leveled off to about 1 million cases per year through 1981, and then started to decrease. This trend essentially continued until 1989, when a new endemic steady state emerged. The most powerful elements influencing the incidence of gonorrhea from 1982 to 1989 have been the concern about acquired immunodeficiency syndrome (AIDS) and the contrasting but growing behavior of sex-for-drugs. The gonorrhea epidemic in the United States has condensed down around heterosexual, poor, urban minorities who have high rates of illicit drug use and prostitution.[31, 46]

Forty percent to 50% of heterosexual women with gonorrhea infection have coexisting chlamydial infection. Postgonococcal cervicitis occurs in 30% of women treated with a single dose of penicillin, amoxicillin, other beta lactam antibiotic, or spectinomycin because of failure to eliminate coexisting chlamydial infection. Thus, as previously stated, gonorrhea treatment regimens that simultaneously eradicate *Chlamydia* would be of great benefit.[9] Approximately 25% of women who have had gonorrhea are unable to conceive. Sixty percent to 90% of women who have vaginal intercourse with an infected man become infected.[46] Pregnant women with active gonococcal infection are at increased risk of obstetric complications, and infants born to these mothers may develop gonococcal conjunctivitis (ophthalmia neonatorum), which can produce blindness if untreated. The incidence of gonorrhea is highest in young adults under age 25, unmarried persons, persons of low socioeconomic status, and persons with multiple sexual contacts.[47]

ETIOLOGY AND PATHOGENESIS

Gonorrhea is an old disease, and humans are the only natural hosts for the species *Neisseria gonorrhoeae*. *Neisseria gonorrhoeae* can infect or colonize a broad range of columnar or transitional epithelial cell membranes.[46]

CLINICAL PRESENTATION

The proportion of patients with symptoms during cervical infections is quite variable. If nonspecific symptoms, such as vaginal discharge, dyspareunia, metrorrhagia, and lower abdominal discomfort, are included, up to 60% to 70% are symptomatic. Regardless, only 10% to 20% of infected women have a noticeable endocervical mucopurulent discharge or a purulent vaginal discharge that conclusively comes from the cervix. This makes it difficult to determine an exact incubation period. Some untreated infections are probably indolent and remain undiagnosed for months. Gonococcal salpingitis usually occurs early in the course of infection and during or shortly after menstruation. The proportion of infected women who develop salpingitis is variable and is influenced by many factors, such as early diagnosis and treatment, diagnostic criteria used for salpingitis, use of oral contraceptives, and types of infecting strains.[46] Nonetheless, gonorrhea infection is evidence of unsafe sexual behavior and the companion risk of acquiring human immunodeficiency virus (HIV).[46]

DIAGNOSIS

The gold standard for diagnosis of *Neisseria gonorrhoeae* is culture in inoculated selective media, such as Thayer-Martin media. It is the most sensitive and reproducible test. In the clinical setting, a Gram-stained smear often demonstrates the organisms. Gram-stained smears, however, can be time-consuming, difficult to interpret and have a low sensitivity of 30% to 60%. Nonetheless, they should be used in high-risk patients. Early diagnosis and treatment in these cases may prevent sequelae and further spread of infection. A variety of new methods are being developed, such as antigen detection and genetic probes.[46,47]

The American College of Obstetricians and Gynecologists recommends obtaining endocervical cultures for *Neisseria gonorrhoeae* in all pregnant women during their first prenatal visit, and a second culture is recommended late in the third trimester for women in high-risk groups.[47]

MEDICAL TREATMENT

Ceftriaxone (125 or 250 mg intramuscularly as a single dose) is the drug of choice in the treatment of uncomplicated urethral, endocervical, or anorectal gonococcal infection. It is a third-generation cephalosporin.[44] Ceftriaxone is the only single-dose regimen that is active against CMRNG (chromosome-mediated resistant *Neisseria gonorrhoeae*), PPNG (penicillinase-producing *Neisseria gonorrhoeae*), and TRNG (tetracycline-resistant *Neisseria gonorrhoeae*), and that has been proved to cure all forms of uncomplicated gonorrhea. Important considerations in treatment are single-dose efficacy and possible coexisting chlamydial infection, which occurs in up to half of the cases in some high-risk populations. Until widespread, simple, inexpensive testing for *Chlamydia* becomes available, persons with gonorrhea should also be treated for presumptive chlamydial infections. This is likely the most cost-effective approach to control *Chlamydia* at this time.[15,46]

For patients who cannot take ceftriaxone, the alternative drug of choice is spectinomycin (2 g intramuscularly single dose). Newer alternatives for the treatment of resistant *Neisseria gonorrhoeae* are limited. The fluorinated quinolones (norfloxacin, ciprofloxacin, and ofloxacin) are active against resistant strains and have a different mechanism of action. Ofloxin seems to be as effective as ceftriaxone for gonorrhea and may be given as single dose or multiple day therapy.[48] It is also useful for mixed infections with *Chlamydia trachomatis*.[43] The two major concerns about the quinolones have been their tendency to induce neurotoxicity and resistant bacteria formation. Some quinolones also have activity against *Chlamydia trachomatis* so one drug therapy can be given.[15,46]

Plasmid-mediated beta-lactamase production in *Neisseria gonorrhoeae* strains has become a universal problem. This cannot be ascertained with simple laboratory techniques because mutational resistance generally accords a relative but not absolute antibiotic resistance.[9] The molecular mechanism of this chromosomal mediated resistance is reduced permeability of the cell membrane. Until recently, chromosomal resistance usually could be overcome by increasing dosage.[9,15,46]

Chancroid

EPIDEMIOLOGY

Chancroid occurs sporadically in the United States and has been more commonly encountered in the past decade. In 1988, 5001 cases were reported. The disease is centered in particular areas, especially New York City. Approximately three out of every five cases is reported from this city. Most of the cases occur in men.[9,45,49]

Chancroid is endemic in many developing countries, but in the United States most cases are associated with contact with an infected prostitute. Most patients are young, black and Hispanic men. Chancroid and other ulcerative genital diseases, along with the use of sex-for-drugs behavior, are major factors contributing to the heterosexual transmission of the HIV virus. Patients with HIV may not respond to therapy for chancroid.[17,50]

ETIOLOGY AND PATHOGENESIS

Haemophilus ducreyi, a gram-negative streptobacillus, is responsible for chancroid and has not been isolated from nonhuman sources. It has the ability to acquire plasmids, which confer antibiotic resistance. The bacteria are believed to require a break in integrity of the skin to induce disease.[9,50,51]

CLINICAL PRESENTATION

In women, chancroid has a variable presentation. The incubation period has not been well delineated but is probably similar to that in men,

being 4 to 7 days. Women may be asymptomatic and generally present later than men.[50,51]

Chancroid usually presents as one or a few exquisitely painful ulcers. The pain is probably related to the depth of the ulcers, which tend to be reddened, purulent, and foul smelling with an irregular undermined border. The ulcers can enlarge to the size of a quarter. The base is usually indurated with a gray exudative membrane. The ulcers of chancroid may occasionally be shallow, with an appearance similar to genital herpes. The most common presentation in women is the appearance of these ulcers on the vulva or perirectal area. Only 7% of asymptomatic women with the disease have ulcers on the vaginal wall or cervix, although they may have a vaginal discharge. Ulceration is commonly more extensive in women but supposedly heals faster than it does in men.[17,45,51]

Lymphadenitis is less common in women than in men, probably because lymphatic drainage from the posterior two thirds of the vagina is to sacral nodes. Lymphadenitis, however, was noted in 35% of Kenyan women with chancroid. These tender buboes appear a few days after the primary ulcer and can lead to scarring, fibrosis, and lymphedema.[17,45,51]

DIAGNOSIS

Most cases of chancroid are diagnosed clinically. Gram's stain shows gram-negative coccobacilli in parallel rows or in a clustered, "school of fish" appearance. Some investigators have reported that Gram's stain may have low sensitivity and specificity, although others have reported a sensitivity of 62% and a specificity of 99%. Culture is definitive, and selective media are effective in isolating these organisms. More than one type of medium should be used because some isolates selectively grow on one medium and not another. Nonetheless, culture itself is difficult and has low sensitivity. Even in dedicated research laboratories, *Haemophilus ducreyi* is recovered from at most 80% of clinically suspected cases.[9,45,51]

The differential diagnosis of any genital ulcer includes chancroid, genital herpes, and syphilis. Therefore diagnosis based only on clinical evidence may be inaccurate. Evaluation of patients with genital ulcers should include cultures for *Haemophilus ducreyi* and herpes simplex virus as well as serologic tests for *Treponema pallidum.*[17,51]

MEDICAL TREATMENT

Antibiotic resistance has developed owing to a lack of effective single-dose regimens and failure to treat coexisting infection, such as syphilis and gonorrhea. Antibiotic resistance to ampicillin and amoxicillin is globally extensive. Several plasmid-mediated beta-lactamases have been identified that control this resistance.[9]

Ceftriaxone (250 mg intramuscularly single dose) is the treatment of choice for uncomplicated chancroid or gonorrhea.[44] Erythromycin (500 mg orally four times daily for 7 days) may also be used.[51,52]

One alternative is trimethoprim-sulfamethoxazole (160/800 mg orally twice daily for 7 days). Trimethoprim-sulfamethoxazole resistance has occurred, however, especially outside the United States, and single-dose trimethoprim no longer has the efficacy of other regimens.[15,53] Another alternative is oral amoxicillin with clavulanic acid (500 mg/125 mg three times daily for 7 days). If relapse occurs in a properly treated patient without re-exposure, a culture should be obtained to rule out emergence of bacterial resistance. If resistance is suspected initially, sensitivity testing is performed with alternative antibiotics before retreating. HIV testing should be done when indicated by the history and presentation.[17] Yet another alternative is ciprofloxacin (500 mg orally twice daily for 3 days). Quinolones are contraindicated during pregnancy and in children under age 16 years.[14,51,52]

Symptoms usually improve within 3 days of beginning therapy, and lesions improve within 7 days. Lymphadenopathy resolves slowly, and aspiration may be necessary. Sexual partners, whether symptomatic or not, should be examined and treated.[14,17,51,53]

Syphilis

EPIDEMIOLOGY

Between 1981 and 1989, the rates of primary and secondary syphilis in the United States increased markedly. In 1989, almost 20,000 cases of primary syphilis were reported, with approximately 80% occurring in men.[45] In blacks, the incidence of primary and secondary syphilis more than doubled between 1985 and 1989. In the United States, 32,000 new cases occur yearly, and it is estimated that only 1 of 10 cases is reported. Thus there may be more than 300,000 new cases yearly.[54] The incidence in whites and persons of Asian or Pacific Island origin continued to be low and declined. Rates in Hispanics were stable, being between those in blacks and whites. The incidence in Native Americans and male homosexuals has declined.[55] At this time, the incidence of syphilis in the United States is highest in large metropolitan areas with large minority populations.[56] Sexual contact with an infected person bears a 1 in 3 to 1 in 10 chance of transmission.[17,57]

Genital ulcer disease facilitates HIV transmission and is a marker of high-risk activity. Sex-for-drugs behavior also facilitates transmission. Patients with genital ulcer disease should receive a recommendation to be tested for HIV infection as well as being tested for other STDs. It has also been suggested that screening is warranted in high-risk populations.[14,45,57–65]

ETIOLOGY AND PATHOGENESIS

Treponema pallidum subspecies is a member of the family of Spirochaetaceae. It has a phospholipid-rich outer membrane with few surface-exposed proteins. This characteristic may facilitate evasion of host-mediated immune defenses.[56]

Syphilis is a STD, and about one third of individuals exposed to a sexual partner with infectious syphilis acquire the disease. Other possible routes of transmission include transfusion of infected blood and perinatal transmission.[56]

Syphilis is called "the great imitator," so

other venereal diseases must be ruled out, such as herpes simplex, Reiter's syndrome, and any other genital ulcerative disease.[57]

CLINICAL PRESENTATION

The incubation period of syphilis is approximately 3 weeks. Most patients note a papule or macule at the site where the ulcer develops. Primary syphilis is distinguished by the classic chancre. Up to one half of cases may have more than one ulcer. The ulcers are painless and have smooth margins with firm, indurated borders and a clean, indurated base that has serous exudate. Nevertheless, atypical ulcers are common. In women, the external genitalia is the most common site for ulcers. Ulcers may also occur in the vagina, and up to 21% of female patients have been noted to have primary syphilis with ulcers on the cervix. Up to 80% of patients have inguinal adenopathy, which is small and rubbery in consistency and in general bilateral.[17,45,56]

The initial response to infection is a local infiltrate of polymorphonuclear leukocytes at the site of inoculation. This is followed by cutaneous ulceration and invasion of the lesion with lymphocytes and plasma cells. The primary lesion soon heals, but the immune responses that develop do not prevent dissemination of the spirochete or development of secondary manifestations.[56]

The Jarisch-Herxheimer reaction is an acute febrile response with symptoms of headache and myalgia that may occur after any therapy for syphilis. Patients should be made aware of this possible reaction. Jarisch-Herxheimer reactions are more common in patients with early syphilis, and pregnant patients should be warned about the possibility of early labor. Antipyretics may be helpful but are not proven to prevent this reaction.[14]

DIAGNOSIS

Definitive diagnosis of Treponema pallidum requires dark-field or fluorescence microscopy of ulcer material. Most microscopes can be fitted with a dark-field condenser, making immediate clinical diagnosis accessible. The spirochetes demonstrate a characteristic corkscrew morphology, with flexing and hairpin motility. The best specimens for dark-field examination are serous fluid expressed from the base of the lesion after cleansing with sterile saline.[56] Fluorescent antibody microscopy also provides a sensitive test for detection of Treponema pallidum in clinical specimens. This technique uses either direct or indirect fluorescence. One advantage of this method over dark-field microscopy is that it does not require live organisms and therefore can be performed on fixed slides in the laboratory. Another advantage of this method is that it requires less expertise than dark-field microscopy because of the high specificity of the antibody reagents. Disadvantages are that results may not be immediately available and that it is not widely available.[14,17,45,56,66]

Serology only provides evidence that infection has occurred. A positive titer cannot discriminate present from past infection. A rapid plasma reagin (RPR) or Venereal Disease Research Laboratory (VDRL) test should be done in every case of genital ulcer disease. These so-called nontreponemal tests measure antibody directed against cardiolipin rather than measuring specific treponemal antibody. Cardiolipin constitutes 10% of the cell lipids of Treponema pallidum. These nontreponemal tests are positive in about 80% of cases of primary syphilis, and the RPR is slightly more sensitive than the VDRL. All positive nontreponemal tests should be verified by a specific treponemal test. These include the fluorescent treponemal antibody–absorbed (FTA-ABS) test or microhemagglutination–Treponema pallidum (MHA-TP) test.

False-positive test results appear in approximately 1% of the general population and 6% to 9% of intravenous drug users and in acute viral infections, such as genital herpes, some vaccinations, and autoimmune diseases.[14,17,45,56,66]

MEDICAL TREATMENT

The drug of choice for treating all stages of syphilis is still parenteral penicillin G benzathine (2.4

million units intramuscularly single dose). Alternatives include doxycycline (100 mg orally twice daily for 2 weeks) or ceftriaxone (250 mg intramuscularly once daily for 10 days).[15,67] In nonpregnant patients with penicillin allergy, currently recommended alternative regimens include erythromycin or tetracycline for 2 weeks. These regimens, however, have not been studied adequately and cause side-effects in at least one third of patients, leading to poor patient compliance. Management of patients with histories of penicillin allergy should probably include skin testing and desensitization.[9,14,17,56,57]

Pregnant women should be screened early in pregnancy. In high-risk patients, screening should be repeated in the third trimester and at the time of delivery. Seropositive pregnant women should be considered infected unless previous treatment history and sequential serologic antibody titers are documented to show an appropriate response. Pregnant women should be treated in doses appropriate to the stage of disease. Tetracycline and doxycycline are contraindicated in pregnancy. Erythromycin carries a high risk of treatment failure in the fetus. Pregnant women with histories of penicillin allergy should first have a detailed history about the allergy. If necessary, they should then have skin testing and either be treated with penicillin or referred for hospitalization and desensitization. Women who are treated in the second half of pregnancy are at risk for premature labor if Jarisch-Herxheimer reaction occurs. They should be advised to seek medical attention if they notice any change in fetal movements or have any contractions. Stillbirth is a rare complication of treatment. Nonetheless, therapy is necessary to prevent further fetal damage, and the possibility of stillbirth should not delay treatment.[14,56,57]

Patients should have clinical and serologic follow-up at 3, 6, and 12 months to assess response to treatment. If nontreponemal antibody titers have declined fourfold or more by 3 months with primary and secondary syphilis, this is generally considered an adequate response. Failure of titers to fall or persistent signs and symptoms should be considered treatment failure, although reinfection should be considered. Patients should then have a cerebrospinal fluid examination and be retreated appropriately.[14,56]

Several studies have shown an association between genital ulcer diseases and HIV infection as well as treatment failure of benzathine penicillin in early syphilis in HIV seropositive patients.[15] Transmission of either disease may be potentiated by the presence of the other. The presence of a genital ulcer could predispose an exposed individual to HIV infection by providing an area of entry for HIV. HIV transmission by a person with both a genital ulcer disease, such as syphilis, and HIV infection might be more capable owing to shedding of HIV-infected white blood cells directly from the base of a chancre during sexual activity. There has also been conjecture that altered host response owing to HIV infection might vary the clinical manifestations of syphilis, and immunosuppression may increase the risk of neurosyphilis.[56,66,68]

HIV and AIDS

EPIDEMIOLOGY

As stated earlier, an association between genital ulcer disease, which breaks down the mucosal barrier, and HIV infection has been noted. These genital ulcer diseases include syphilis, chancroid, *Trichomonas*, herpes, *Candida*, endocervical *Chlamydia*, and gonorrhea. Lack of circumcision and prolongation of genital ulceration owing to advanced stage of HIV infection have also been found to have an association with increased risk of transmission. STDs not only act as cofactors in HIV transmission, but also, conversely, HIV infection seems to modify the natural history and response to therapy, promoting disease progression and treatment failure. Condoms augment natural skin barriers and thereby reduce the risk of HIV transmission.[14,69–71]

Control of other STDs, such as *Chlamydia trachomatis*, has been given low priority compared with funding for AIDS control programs.

This lack of support not only allows for increasing transmission of AIDS through association with other STDs, but it puts women at a considerable risk. Not only are they at increased risk of infertility, but also at increased risk of HIV infection, owing to the ulceration and cervicitis created by these STDs.[70]

There is a several month to 15-year latency period between infection and development of AIDS. It is estimated that the risk of transmission in each male/female sexual encounter in which one of the partners has the HIV virus is 1%. Women who participate in anal intercourse with an infected partner are more likely to acquire infection than women who have only vaginal intercourse or oral-genital contact. Transmission does occur in both directions.[14,17,70,72]

At this time, the only way to prevent AIDS is to prevent the infection with the HIV virus. This can be guaranteed only by sexual abstinence or contact with sexual partners who are not infected. A large number of HIV-infected persons, however, are asymptomatic and unaware that they are infected.[14]

In the United States, the fraction of AIDS cases that are ascribed to heterosexual contact is approximately 5%. This heterosexual transmission accounts for about 1% of cases in men and 30% of cases in women. Blacks and Hispanics account for a significantly higher proportion of heterosexually transmitted AIDS cases. Transmission occurs in both directions, and there seems to be no difference in the risk of transmission in either direction. The fraction of sexual partners infected varies widely depending on the group reviewed. This fraction was lower for hemophilia or transfusion recipients than for other risk groups. This risk appears higher for intravenous drug abusers, bisexual men, or mixed risk groups. Risk is also increased with the increasing practice of sex-for-drugs.[70,71]

Voluntary, confidential testing and counseling should be encouraged in those with other STDs. Positive test results may affect the recommended diagnostic evaluation, treatment, or follow-up of their disease.[14]

ETIOLOGY AND PATHOGENESIS

AIDS was first described in 1981. It is transmitted by interchange of infected cells or body fluids. Penetrating sexual intercourse is the predominant route of transmission. HIV is found in semen and cervical secretions.[17]

CLINICAL PRESENTATION

AIDS is a late manifestation of infection with HIV. Most people infected with HIV remain asymptomatic for months to 15 years.[14,17]

A prodromal-type illness of generalized lymphadenopathy, fever, night sweats, weight loss, and diarrhea (the AIDS-related complex) may occur. This generally progresses with the development of opportunistic infections and at times the cutaneous malignancy Kaposi's sarcoma.[17]

DIAGNOSIS

HIV infection is diagnosed by HIV antibody tests. Detectable antibody is usually generated within 3 months of infection. A negative antibody test result does not rule out infection from recent exposure. If antibody testing is being performed for correlation to a specific exposure, the test should be repeated at 3 and 6 months. ELISA is the screening antibody test used to detect HIV. If this screening test is positive, a more specific test, the Western blot assay, is used. Positive results from screening tests must be confirmed before being considered conclusive.[14] Depletion of T_4 helper-inducer lymphocytes is the immunologic hallmark of AIDS.[17]

MEDICAL TREATMENT

The drug of choice in the treatment of AIDS is zidovudine (ZDV). This drug was previously known as azidothymidine. It is believed to suppress viral replication by inhibiting the activity of reverse transcriptase. It is used in persons with AIDS-related complex or full-blown AIDS and a CD4 (T_4) count of less than 200/mm^3. Therapy with zidovudine prolongs survival, decreases the frequency and severity of opportunistic infections, and appears to delay progression to full-blown AIDS in patients who have AIDS-related complex. Dosage is generally 300 mg/day.[14, 17] Serious side-effects usually consist of anemias and cytopenias and have been common during ZDV therapy. Therefore patients taking ZDV require careful follow-up.[14]

Genital Herpes

EPIDEMIOLOGY

Primary infections of genital herpes simplex occur in 200,000 to 700,000 Americans each year, and 20,000,000 episodes of recurrent genital herpes are estimated to occur annually. The incidence of primary genital herpes infection is about equal in men and women, but women are more likely to return to their physician for subsequent attacks.[45, 47]

The incubation period is 2 to 10 days, and sexual contact with infected patients who have active or inactive disease puts a person at risk of herpes simplex virus (HSV) infection. In couples in which one partner is known to have genital herpes, several studies have estimated the annual risk of sexual transmission of genital herpes to be about 10%.[17, 47, 74]

With acute and suppressive therapy, the annual recurrence rate has dropped from greater than 12 to 1.0 to 1.4 in the third year. Daily suppressive acyclovir therapy was effective and well tolerated, and no serious side-effects were noted.[75]

Approximately 4% of symptomatic primary episodes require hospitalization, and genital herpes is estimated to cost $500 million per year in the United States.[64]

ETIOLOGY AND PATHOGENESIS

HSV, types 1 and 2 (HSV-1 and HSV-2), can cause genital infection; however, 75% to 80% are caused by type 2 virus, and genital infection is more common than oral infection.[17]

Both types are part of the human herpesvirus family of DNA viruses. There is roughly 50% base sequence homology between HSV-1 and HSV-2. Typing of isolates, however, can now be done in most clinical laboratories using monoclonal antibodies.[74]

The HSV inoculates and replicates in the dermis and epidermis. Viral particles are then transported to the neuronal nucleus. Infection leads to viral replication and cell death in vulnerable cells in the dermis and epidermis. The status of the virus in neurons, known as latency, is not well understood.[74]

CLINICAL PRESENTATION

Genital herpes is distinguished by a prodrome of paresthesia 12 to 48 hours before the appearance of vesicles. Grouped vesicles or pustules on an erythematous base are the hallmark of genital herpes. These rupture, leaving multiple, shallow, painful ulcerations. Adjacent vesicles may coalesce to form large areas of ulceration. These ulcerations then progress to crusting and healing. Without treatment, groups of new lesions form in the second week and all lesions heal by the end of the third week. Tender, generally bilateral lymphadenopathy usually accompanies primary lesions.[17, 45, 74]

The severity of the first episode of genital herpes varies, depending on whether the patient has previously been exposed to HSV. Primary infection is severe in persons without pre-existing antibody to HSV. Painful vesicles linger for 10 to 12 days before forming ulcerations, which last an additional 1 to 2 weeks. In persons with pre-existing antibodies to HSV, the first episode is more mild, and subsequent attacks of recurrent genital herpes are even more mild, with a total duration of about 10 days. In first-episode genital herpes, lesions are usually bilateral or midline. With subsequent infections, lesions tend to be unilateral. Systemic symptoms are more common in the first episode and consist of fever, myalgia, and headache.[17, 45]

HSV can be cultured from the cervix in 88%

of women with primary disease, 65% to 70% with first-episode, nonprimary disease, and 12% to 20% with recurrent disease. The cervix is visibly abnormal, with erythema and erosions in 90% of instances when HSV-2 is cultured. Viral cultures from the cervix are also positive in 80% with primary HSV-1.[45,74]

The mean duration of viral shedding from lesions in untreated, primary genital HSV-1 or HSV-2 infections is 11 days compared with 7 days in untreated, nonprimary genital herpes. The duration of viral shedding from cervical lesions is similar in primary and nonprimary infections.[74]

Many patients, especially women, have difficulty urinating owing to dysuria. Urinary retention, however, is uncommon. This severe dysuria can usually be managed by having patients urinate while immersing their perineums in a warm tub of water to decrease the pain of contact between undiluted urine and lesions. When urinary retention occurs in the absence of lesions or dysuria, however, the cause may be autonomic nervous system dysfunction or rarely transverse myelitis. Severe autonomic dysfunction occurs in fewer than 1% of primary episodes. Intermittent catheterization may be required for several days to 4 to 8 weeks.[74]

DIAGNOSIS

HSV is the most common cause of genital ulcers in patients seen in STD clinics in the United States. The diagnosis of genital herpes is more probable when there are multiple rather than single ulcers, when ulcers are painful, when they are recurrent or preceded by a prodrome of paresthesia, and when lymphadenopathy is tender.[74]

Although genital herpes is generally distinct enough to be diagnosed clinically, confirmation of clinical diagnosis with culture should be obtained. All tests for HSV are most sensitive during the vesicle stage; however, tissue culture isolation is the most sensitive and specific. Viral isolation rates are approximately 90% from ves-

icles and pustules but less than 30% from crusted lesions. Preferably the culture should be obtained within 7 days of lesion onset in a first episode or within 2 days in recurrent disease to obtain the highest rate of viral recovery.[17,45,73,74]

Alternatives to standard viral culture include cytologic diagnosis by Papanicolaou or Tzanck smears and viral antigen or DNA detection. Overall, these nonculture tests are about 80% as sensitive as culture.[45,74]

The Tzanck smear is an easily performed cytologic test. The Tzanck smear detects multinucleated giant cells that are formed as a result of infection with herpesviruses. The test is performed by scraping the base of the vesicle, placing the material on a slide, staining the slide (Wright's stain), and looking for the characteristic multinucleated giant cells on light microscopy. The sensitivity of the Tzank smear has been reported as 50% to 80% in the vesicle stage. The specificity has been variably reported up to 94%. This may be due to the experience of the person reading the slides.[17,45,73,74]

MEDICAL TREATMENT

No known cure exists for genital herpes infection. Acyclovir (Zovirax) is the drug of choice for genital herpes infection. The drug acyclovir does hasten healing but does not affect the risk, frequency, or severity of recurrences if discontinued. It is an acyclic analog of guanosine. The triphosphate form of acyclovir is a competitive inhibitor of the nucleotide deoxyguanosine triphosphate and inhibits HSV DNA polymerase.[14,17,74]

For the first clinical episode, acyclovir (400 mg orally three times daily or 200 mg orally five times daily for 7 to 10 days or until clinical resolution) is used. Topical therapy with acyclovir is considerably less effective than oral therapy.[14,15,74]

For recurrent infection, acyclovir (200 mg orally two to five times daily for 5 days or 800 mg orally twice a day) is used. Patients who have relentless or regular recurrences can be given oral acyclovir suppressive therapy (200 mg orally two to five times daily or 400 mg twice daily). Daily treatment reduces frequency of recurrences by at least 75% in patients with more than six recurrences per year. Safety and efficacy have been demonstrated in patients taking daily therapy for up to 3 years. After 1 year of continuous suppressive therapy, acyclovir should be discontinued to assess the patient's recurrence rate. Acyclovir, oral or intravenous, shortens the duration of pain, viral shedding, and systemic symptoms in primary herpes simplex infection.[14, 15, 17, 74]

For severe disease, intravenous acyclovir (5 mg/kg of body weight every 8 hours for 5 to 7 days or until clinical resolution) is used.[14, 15, 74]

Acyclovir-resistant strains of HSV have been isolated from persons receiving suppressive therapy, but they have not been connected to treatment failure in immunocompetent patients. At this time, there are no safe, efficacious alternatives to acyclovir for treatment of genital herpes infections in the normal host.[14, 74]

Patients with clinical immunodeficiency have a more severe clinical course of genital herpes than do immunocompetent hosts. Some physicians use increasing doses of acyclovir as well as suppressive therapy for immunocompromised patients. The efficacy of this regimen, however, has not been conclusively established.[14]

The safety of acyclovir therapy in pregnant women has not been established. Intravenous acyclovir is probably helpful in the presence of life-threatening, disseminated maternal HSV infections with encephalitis, pneumonitis, and hepatitis. It is not recommended in pregnant women without life-threatening infection, such as recurrent genital herpes episodes or as suppressive therapy. At the commencement of labor, all women should have a careful history and physical examination. Women without symptoms or signs of infection or prodrome may proceed with vaginal deliveries. Cultures of the birth canal at the time of delivery may be helpful in neonatal management if treatment becomes necessary.[14]

Genital Warts

EPIDEMIOLOGY

Human papillomavirus (HPV) infections are not invariably easy to diagnose but were reported to account for 1,150,000 outpatient visits in 1984. These infections are not reportable to public health departments. Most of these patients are young, between the ages of 15 and 30, and more women seek treatment than men. The true incidence of HPV infections of the genital tract is thought to be strikingly higher than estimated.[76]

ETIOLOGY AND PATHOGENESIS

There are numerous types of HPV. Exophytic genital and anal warts and condyloma acuminatum are caused most commonly by types 6 and 11. Types 16, 18, 30, 31, 33, 34, and 35 seem to have oncogenic potential and are associated with genital dysplasia and carcinoma. Malignancies of the genital epithelium in women often contain HPV DNA sequences. Therefore biopsy is required in all cases of atypical, pigmented, or persistent warts. All women with anogenital warts should have an annual Papanicolaou smear.[14, 17, 76]

CLINICAL PRESENTATION

HPV lesions are identified by large, soft, fleshy, cauliflowerlike lesions that arise on the external genitalia, oral, and anal regions.[17] Vulvar condyloma acuminatum are soft, whitish, sessile tumors, with fingerlike projections. They are found in moist areas, such as the introitus and labia. On the skin, these lesions take on a more keratotic appearance. These vulvar condyloma acuminatum may also take the form of small smooth papules, which may or may not be pigmented. Large areas of disease coalesce. HPV types 16 and 18 are recovered from vulvar papules that histologically show epithelial dysplasia. Vulvar carcinoma is associated with HPV in 80% of cases. Subclinical HPV infection of the vulva or vagina can be recognized by application of dilute acetic acid followed by colposcopic examination.

Condyloma acuminatum of the vagina occurs in at least one third of women who have vulvar condylomata. Multiple lesions are commonly seen. Most are asymptomatic, although vaginal discharge, pruritus, and postcoital bleeding may occur. HPV types 6 and 11 are usually discovered. Again HPV infection is identifiable by acetic acid staining of the vaginal mucosa followed by colposcopic examination. Vaginal malignancy has been reported in association with HPV infection.

Condyloma acuminatum of the cervix develops in one of five women with HPV infection in other locations of the genital tract. These are usually caused by HPV types 6 and 11 and appear as papillary epithelial proliferations in the cervical transformation zone. Subclinical cervical HPV infection is much more common than cervical condyloma acuminatum. Cytopathic effects are found in up to 3% of routine cervical Papanicolaou smears, including koilocytosis, atypia, and multinucleation. Application of dilute acetic acid to the cervix may demonstrate the presence of flat acetowhite plaques. Subclinical HPV infection of the cervix may progress to cervical intraepithelial neoplasia and microinvasive carcinoma. Malignant cervical lesions have been reported in association with HPV types 16, 18, or 31.[76]

DIAGNOSIS

Subclinical cases are diagnosed by Papanicolaou smear, colposcopy, and application of acetic acid. The diagnosis is usually made on clinical appearance. Biopsy with typing, however, is the definitive method for diagnosis.[17]

To make the diagnosis clinically, the skin of the genital area is soaked in 3% acetic acid for 5 minutes and then examined directly or under magnification. A shiny, white appearance of the skin occurs, called *acetowhiting*. Acetowhiting displays foci of epithelial hyperplasia. When intraepithelial neoplasia is present, these lesions may have a dull gray or dull white color.

Cytology and histology are readily available to most physicians. The koilocyte is a large cell with a hyperchromatic nucleus and perinuclear clear ring in the cytoplasm, which is virtually diagnostic of HPV-induced lesions. Lack of these cellular changes, however, does not guarantee freedom from papillomavirus infection.

In the research setting, the most extensively used method for detecting HPV is based on DNA hybridization, and this is currently the only method that allows differentiation among the 60 HPV types. The principle of DNA hybridization is that a DNA molecule that contains a radioactive affinity label can be placed under conditions in which it will bind or hybridize with a second DNA molecule that is similar.[76]

MEDICAL TREATMENT

HPV is refractory to treatment, and no modality completely eradicates the infection. Patients must understand that they are still infectious to their sexual partners. Condoms, however, decrease the risk of transmission. Oral warts may also be found. HPV has been demonstrated in neighboring tissue after laser treatment of cervical intraepithelial neoplasia associated with HPV infection and after extensive laser vaporization of the anogenital area. The benefit of treating subclinical HPV infection has not been proved, and recurrence is common. The effect of treatment on HPV transmission is unknown. Thus the goal of treatment is removal of exophytic warts and relief of signs and symptoms, not the eradication of HPV. HPV infection of the female lower genital tract is a multicentric disease. All patients with evidence of HPV infection should have colposcopic examination of the entire genital tract.[14, 17, 77, 78]

For warts on the external genitalia or perianally, the treatment of choice is cryotherapy with liquid nitrogen or a cryoprobe. Cryotherapy is nontoxic, requires no anesthetic, and does not result in scarring. Alternatives include electrofulgeration, carbon dioxide laser ablation, podophyllin (10% to 25% in a compound tincture of benzoin—contraindicated in pregnancy), trichloroacetic acid (80% to 90% solution), fluorouracil (Efudex), or alpha interferon (Intron A, Roferon A, Alferon A). Treatment with interferon is not recommended because of its relatively low efficacy, high incidence of toxicity, and high cost. Nonetheless, podophyllin remains the most widely used treatment for genital warts, even though the cure rate is low.[14,15,17,76]

Podophyllin should be limited to a total volume applied of less than 0.5 ml per treatment session. It should be thoroughly washed off in 1 to 4 hours. Less than 10 cm^2 should be treated at each session. Applications may be repeated at weekly intervals. Mucosal warts are more likely to respond than highly keratinized warts on the penile shaft, buttocks, and pubic areas. Trichloroacetic acid should be applied only to warts and then powdered with talc or sodium bicarbonate to remove the unreacted acid. Applications may be repeated at weekly intervals. Carbon dioxide laser and conventional surgery are useful in managing extensive genital and perianal warts, especially for those who have not responded to cryotherapy. Similar to other treatments, these modalities do not eradicate HPV.[14,76]

For vaginal warts, first-line therapy is liquid nitrogen cryotherapy. Use of a cryoprobe is contraindicated because it risks vaginal perforation and fistula formation. Carbon dioxide laser may also be used. Alternatives are trichloroacetic acid and podophyllin. The treatment regimen is similar to that already discussed. When podophyllin is used, the treatment area must be dry before the speculum is removed. Less than 2 cm^2 should be treated per session. Podophyllin is contraindicated in pregnancy.[14,17,76]

The treatment of choice for intraurethral warts is cryotherapy with liquid nitrogen. Alternatives include podophyllin and sometimes fluorouracil cream, delivered by a urethral catheter once a week until lesions disappear (not FDA approved).[14,17,76]

When cervical warts are found, dysplasia must be excluded before treatment is begun. Thus management should be carried out in consultation with an expert.[14,17]

Cesarean delivery and routine screening for prevention of transmission of HPV infection to the newborn has not been of proven benefit. HPV can cause laryngeal papillomatosis in infants, but the route of transmission is unknown.[14]

It must be noted that one author states that podophyllin should not be used on the cervix, vagina, urethral meatus, anal mucosa, or buccal mucosa owing to systemic reactions and local reactions.[76]

Scabies

EPIDEMIOLOGY

Scabies infestation of the skin can be sexually transmitted by prolonged body-to-body contact. Some authorities have noted that epidemics of scabies occur in 30-year cycles. Mites can survive off the host for as long as 34 hours at normal room temperature.[15,17,79]

ETIOLOGY AND PATHOGENESIS

Scabies is caused by *Sarcoptes scabiei*, the human itch mite. Fertilization in the human itch mite takes place on the host. The female mite physically forces her way between the corneocytes and tunnels through into the live stratum granulosum to gain nourishment. Intracellular fluid from these deeper skin areas may leak into the burrows and into the mite's mouth. This fluid provides a medium for antigens from the mite's body, including secretions and feces, that stimulate an inflammatory and immune response in the dermis. Eggs are deposited at a rate of one to two a day and require 3 to 4 days to hatch.[79]

CLINICAL PRESENTATION

There is a 4- to 6-week latent period from the time of infestation to symptom manifestation. There may be less than 100 mites on the body at this time. Scabies then manifests itself by a severe allergic reaction with severe pruritic dermatitis.

This begins an itch-scratch-itch cycle. This allergic reaction actually kills many of the mites, leaving fewer than the initial number. Skin lesions are characterized by erythematous papules or nodules with a central crust. The predominant areas of the body include the finger webs, wrist folds, genital area, axillary folds, nipples, navel, under the breasts in females, between the buttocks, and flexor surfaces. Both the rash and burrows are rarely found above the neck or on the palms or soles. Nodules can persist for months after successful treatment.[17,79]

DIAGNOSIS

The definitive diagnosis of scabies infestation is made by covering the lesions or burrows with mineral oil, scraping with a scalpel blade, and examination under a microscope. Identification of mites, mite eggs, or fecal pellets is required. The mite is found at the blind end of the burrow and can be removed by using a needle, swabbing the skin with ether, or applying clear cellophane tape and quickly removing the tape.[17,79]

MEDICAL TREATMENT

Lindane (Kwell), 1% permethrin (NIX), or pyrethrins with piperonyl butoxide (RID) are effective topical treatments for scabies. Topical lindane has been the traditional treatment, but a new preparation of permethrin (Elimite) may be confirmed to be the drug of choice.[15]

Lindane (1%—1 oz of lotion or 30 g of cream) is applied thinly to all areas of the body from the neck down after showering. It is washed off 8 hours later, and the application is repeated. After the application, a low or medium strength topical corticosteroid can be applied for the pruritus. Treatment is repeated after 1 week if clinical improvement does not occur. The patient's sexual partner and household contacts must also be treated. Clothing and bed linen that have been used in the past 2 days must be washed and dried in hot cycles or dry cleaned. Insecticide sprays are effective for killing mites on furniture. Pruritus may continue for 4 to 8 weeks after successful treatment.[14,17,79]

The first reported case of lindane-resistant scabies occurred in Panama. A reported 25% treatment failure rate was noted. Permethrin 5% cream may be a safe and effective alternative for the treatment of lindane-resistant scabies. Permethrin does not have the potential central nervous system toxicity of lindane.[80,81]

The use of lindane for treatment of pregnant women is controversial. Lindane is a neurotoxin, causing seizures, when used in large amounts. One author reports the use of lindane in children, pregnant and nursing mothers, and patients with epilepsy without untoward effects.[82] An alternative for infants, children 2 years of age or less, and pregnant and lactating women is crotamiton (10%), applied from the neck down on two successive nights, then washed off 24 hours after the second application.[17]

References

1. Sobel JD. Vaginal infections in adult women. Med Clin North Am 1990;74:6.
2. Galask RP. Vaginal colonization by bacteria and yeast. Am J Obstet Gynecol 1988;158:4.
3. Sobel JD. Bacterial vaginosis—an ecologic mystery. Ann Int Med 1989;111:7.
4. Eschenbach DA, Hillier S, Critchlow C, et al. Diagnosis and clinical manifestations of bacterial vaginosis. Am J Obstet Gynecol 1988;158:4.
5. Vejtorp M, Bollerup AC, Vejtorp L, et al. Bacterial vaginosis: A double-blind randomized trial of the effect of treatment of the sexual partner. Br J Obstet Gynaecol 1988;95:920.
6. West RR, O'Dowd TC, Smail JE. Prevalence of Gardnerella vaginalis: An estimate. BMJ 1988;296:1163.
7. Mengel MB. Diagnostic criteria for bacterial vaginosis. J Fam Pract 1989;29:4.
8. Lossick JG. Treatment of sexually transmitted vaginosis/vaginitis. Rev Infect Dis 1990;12:6.
9. Stamm WE. Problems in the treatment of bacterial sexually transmitted diseases. Am J Med 1987;82:4A.
10. Sobel JD, Schmitt C, Meriwether C. A new slide latex agglutination test for the diagnosis of acute Candida vaginitis. Am J Clin Pathol 1990;94:3.

11. Lam MH, Birch DF. Survival of *Gardnerella vaginalis* in human urine. J Clin Microbiol 1991;95:2.
12. Reed BD, Huck W, Zazove P. Differentiation of *Gardnerella vaginalis, Candida albicans,* and *Trichomonas vaginalis* infections of the vagina. J Fam Prac 1989;28:6.
13. Foreman A, Smith CB. Vaginitis. Systematically solving a bothersome problem. Postgrad Med 1990;88:5.
14. Centers for Disease Control. 1989 sexually transmitted diseases treatment guidelines. MMWR 1989;38:S-8.
15. Treatment of sexually transmitted diseases. Med Lett Drugs Therap 1990;32(810) p. 5.
16. Friedrich EG. Vulvovaginal candidiasis: Current perspectives in candidal vulvovaginitis. Am J Obstet Gynecol 1988;4:985.
17. Finkbeiner AE, Kuhn R. How to treat sexually transmitted disease. Contemp Urol 1991;9:29.
18. Foxman B. The epidemiology of vulvovaginal candidiasis: Risk factors. Am J Pub Health 1990;80:3.
19. Horowitz BJ, Edelstein SW, Lippman L. Sexual transmission of Candida. Obstet Gynecol 1987;69:6.
20. Horowitz BJ. Antifungal therapy in the management of chronic candidiasis. Am J Obstet Gynecol 1988;158:996.
21. McKay M. Cutaneous manifestations of candidiasis. Am J Obstet Gynecol 1988;158:4.
22. Kaufman RH. Establishing a correct diagnosis of vulvovaginal infection. Am J Obstet Gynecol 1988;158:4.
23. Adamson GD. Three-day treatment of vulvovaginal candidiasis. Am J Obstet Gynecol 1988;158:4
24. Thomason JL, Gelbart SM. Trichomonas vaginalis. Obstet Gynecol 1989;74:3.
25. Wolner-Hanssen P, Krieger JN, Stevens CE, et al. Clinical manifestations of vaginal trichomoniasis. JAMA 1989;261:4.
26. Krieger JN, Tam MR, Stevens CE, et al. Diagnosis of trichomoniasis. Comparison of conventional wet-mount examination with cytologic studies, cultures, and monoclonal antibody staining of direct specimens. JAMA 1988;259:8.
27. Bennett JR, Barnes WG, Coffman S, et al. The emergency department diagnosis of *Trichomonas* vaginitis. Ann Emerg Med 1989;18:5.
28. Krieger JN. Treatment of "difficult genitourinary tract infections." Urol Clin North Am 1987;14:2.
29. Campbell WF, Dodson MG. Clindamycin therapy for *Chlamydia trachomatis* in women. Am J Obstet Gynecol 1990;162:2.
30. Stamm WE. Diagnosis of *Chlamydia trachomatis* genitourinary infections. Ann Intern Med 1988; 108:5.
31. U.S. Preventive Services Task Force. Chlamydial infection. Am Fam Physician 1990;42:3.
32. Cates W, Wasserheit JN. Genital chlamydial infections: Epidemiology and reproductive sequelae. Am J Obstet Gynecol 1991;164:6.
33. Lucas LM, Smith DL. Nongonococcal urethritis: Diagnosis and management. J Gen Intern Med 1987;2:199.
34. Zimmerman HL, Potterat JJ, Dukes RL, et al. Epidemiologic differences between Chlamydia and gonorrhea. Am J Pub Health 1990;80: 11.
35. Faro S. *Chlamydia trachomatis:* Female pelvic infection. Am J Obstet Gynecol 1991;164:6.
36. Magder LS, Harrison HR, Ehret JM, et al. Factors related to genital chlamydia trachomatis and its diagnosis by culture in a sexually transmitted disease clinic. Am J Epidemiol 1988;28:298.
37. Martin DH. Chlamydial Infections. Med Clin North Am 1990;74:6.
38. McGregor JA, French JI. *Chlamydia trachomatis* infection during pregnancy. Am J Obstet Gynecol 1991;164:6.
39. Leu RH. Complications of coexisting chlamydial and gonococcal infections. Sex Transm Dis Postgrad Med 1991;89:7.
40. Jones RB. New treatments for *Chlamydia trachomatis.* Am J Obstet Gynecol 1991;164:6.
41. Johnson RB. The role of azalide antibiotics in the treatment of chlamydia. Am J Obstet Gynecol 1991;164:6.
42. Faro S, Martens MG, Maccato M. Effectiveness of ofloxacis in the treatment of *Chlamydia trachomatis* and *Neisseria gonorrhoeae* cervical infection. Am J Obstet Gynecol 1991;164:5.
43. Corrado ML. The clinical experience with ofloxacin in the treatment of sexually transmitted diseases. Am J Obstet Gynecol 1991;164:5.
44. Le Saux N, Ronald AR. Role of ceftriaxone in sexually transmitted diseases. Rev Infect Dis 1989;11:299.
45. Schmid GP. Approach to the patient with genital ulcer disease. Med Clin North Am 1990;74: 1559.
46. Judson FN. Gonorrhea. Med Clin North Am 1990;74:6.
47. U.S. Preventive Services Task Force. Gonorrhea. Am Fam Physician 1990;42:3.
48. Covino JM, Cummings M, Smith B, et al. Comparison of ofloxacin and ceftriaxone in the treatment of uncomplicated gonorrhea caused by penicillinase-producing and non-penicillinase-

producing strains. Antimicrob Agents Chemother 1990;34:1.

49. Schmid GP, Sanders LL, Blount JH, et al. Chancroid in the United States. Reestablishment of an old disease. JAMA 1987;258:22.

50. Jessamine PG, Ronald AR. Chancroid and the role of genital ulcer disease in the spread of human retroviruses. Med Clin North Am 1990; 74:6.

51. Boyd AS. Clinical efficacy of antimicrobial therapy in *Haemophilus ducreyi* infections. Arch Dermatol 1989;125:10.

52. Dangor Y, Ballard RC, Miller SD, et al. Treatment of chancroid. Antimicrob Agents Chemother 1990;34:7.

53. Schmid GP. Treatment of chancroid, 1989. Rev Infect Dis 1990;12:6.

54. Whiteside C, Fitzgerald FT. Syphilis evaluation and therapy: A study of current practices in a university hospital. J Gen Intern Med 1988;3:6.

55. Handsfield HH. Old enemies. Combating Syphilis and gonorrhea in the 1990s. JAMA 1990; 264:11.

56. Hutchinson CM, Hook EW. Syphilis in adults. Med Clin North Am 1990;74:6.

57. Wooldridge WE. Syphilis. A new visit from an old enemy. Syphilis Postgrad Med 1991;89:1.

58. Rolfs RT, Nakashima AK. Epidemiology of primary and secondary syphilis in the United States, 1981 through 1989. JAMA, 1990;264:11.

59. Tang A, Barlow D. Resurgence of heterosexually acquired early syphilis in London. Lancet 1989; July 15:166.

60. Centers for Disease Control. Continuing increase in infectious syphilis—United States. Arch Dermatol 1988;124:4.

61. Centers for Disease Control. Primary, secondary syphilis—U.S., 1981–1990. JAMA 1991;265:22.

62. Ernst AA, Samuels JD, Winsemius DK. Emergency department screening for syphilis in patients with other suspected sexually transmitted diseases. Ann Emerg Med 1991;20:6.

63. Siegel D, Washington AE. Syphilis—updated approach to an old disease. Syphilis Postgrad Med 1987;81:1.

64. U.S. Preventive Services Task Force. Syphilis. Am Fam Physician 1990;42:3.

65. Fleming WL. Changing factors in syphilis and other venereal diseases. Arch Environ Health 1966;12:101.

66. Zenker PN, Rolfs RT. Treatment of syphilis, 1989. Rev Infect Dis 1990;12:6.

67. Hook EW, Roddy RE, Handsfield HH. Ceftriaxone therapy for incubating and early syphilis. J Infect Dis 1988;158:4.

68. Centers for Disease Control. Increases in primary and secondary syphilis—United States. MMWR 1987;36:25.

69. Roddy RE, Godwin SE, Potts DM. Genital ulcers in women. Lancet 1989; Sept. 2:558.

70. Holmes KK, Kreiss J. Heterosexual transmission of human immunodeficiency virus: Overview of a neglected aspect of the AIDS epidemic. Journal of Acquired Immune Deficiency Syndromes 1988;1:6.

71. Moss GB, Kreiss JK. The interrelationship between human immunodeficiency virus infection and other sexually transmitted diseases. Med Clin North Am 1990;74:6.

72. O'Farrell N. HIV, genital ulceration, and granuloma inguinale. BMJ 1988;296.

73. U.S. Preventive Services Task Force. Genital herpes simplex. Am Fam Physician 1990;42:3.

74. Mertz GJ. Genital herpes simplex virus infections. Med Clin North Am 1990;74:6.

75. Kaplowitz LG, Baker D, Gelb L, et al. Prolonged continuous acyclovir treatment of normal adults with frequently recurring genital herpes simplex virus infection. JAMA 1991;265:6.

76. Brown DR, Fife KH. Human papillomavirus infections of the genital tract. Med Clin North Am 1990;74:6.

77. Spitzer M, Krumholz BA, Seltzer VL. The multicentric nature of disease related to human papillomavirus infection of the female lower genital tract. Obstet Gynecol 1989;73:3.

78. Riva JM, Sedlacek TV, Cunnane MF, et al. Extended carbon dioxide laser vaporization in the treatment of subclinical papillomavirus infection of the lower genital tract. Obstet Gynecol 1989;73:1.

79. Billstein SA, Mattaliano VJ. The "nuisance" sexually transmitted diseases: Molluscum contagiosum, scabies, and crab lice. Med Clin North Am 1990;74:6.

80. Roth WI. Scabies resistant to lindane 1% lotion and crotamiton 10% cream. J Am Acad Dermatol 1991;24:3.

81. Taplin D, Porcelain SL, Meinking TL, et al. Community control of scabies: A model based on use of permethrin cream. Lancet 1991;337:1016.

82. Rasmussen JE. Lindane—a prudent approach. Arch Dermatol 1987;123.

Index

Note: Page numbers followed by the letter *f* designate figures; those followed by the letter *t* designate tables.

ISBN 0-397-51154-X

90000

9 780397 511549